ORAL MYOFUNCTIONAL DISORDERS

ORAL MYOFUNCTIONAL DISORDERS

RICHARD H. BARRETT, B.A., M.Ed.
Speech Pathologist, Tucson, Arizona

MARVIN L. HANSON, Ph.D.
Professor, Department of Communications,
Division of Speech Pathology and Audiology,
The University of Utah,
Salt Lake City, Utah

SECOND EDITION
with 169 illustrations

THE C. V. MOSBY COMPANY

Saint Louis   1978

SECOND EDITION

Copyright © 1978 by The C. V. Mosby Company

All rights reserved. No part of this book may be reproduced
in any manner without written permission of the publisher.

Previous edition copyrighted 1974

Printed in the United States of America

The C. V. Mosby Company
11830 Westline Industrial Drive, St. Louis, Missouri 63141

Library of Congress Cataloging in Publication Data

Barrett, Richard H., 1915-
  Oral myofunctional disorders.

  Bibliography: p.
  Includes index.
  1. Tongue thrust. 2. Speech, Disorders of.
3. Orthodontics. I. Hanson, Marvin L.,
1932-   joint author. II. Title. [DNLM:
1. Deglutition disorders. 2. Malocclusion.
3. Tongue habits. WI210 B274o]
RC429.B37 1978   617′.522   78-7029
ISBN 0-8016-0497-4

CB/CB/B 9 8 7 6 5 4 3 2 1

PREFACE
TO SECOND EDITION

The broad acceptance that greeted the first edition of this book has been the source of deep gratification for us. Its distribution surpassed anything that we could have expected, and with very few exceptions reactions have been positive. Since we cannot hope to thank each of the original purchasers, we express our heartfelt appreciation to them and to readers of the present edition collectively.

This edition represents our effort to repay our profession with an ever better volume. We have tried to remain alert to change and innovation and to incorporate these concepts into our work and our writing. Chapter arrangement throughout the book has been extensively reorganized into what we believe to be a more lucid and logical sequence.

The most striking change, however, has resulted from numerous requests for coverage of additional topics. We had feared that the first edition was extending somewhat beyond its limit, but we were evidently conservative in our view. Accordingly, we have added five new chapters, covering anatomy, physiology, an expanded discussion of orthodontic procedures, the treatment of additional oral habits not included in the first edition, plus alternative procedures for tongue thrust correction.

By thus expanding our area of attention, we hope that the present edition will prove more valuable to the reader, more comprehensive as a reference, and more usable as a text, since it may preclude the need for supplemental texts while focusing specifically on orofacial concerns.

The goal to which we had aspired, that of stimulating scientific investigation, voiced in the preface to the first edition and intimated elsewhere, remains largely unfulfilled. Much research remains to be done, especially as oral myology moves into previously little-known areas such as kinesiology, facial pain, and temporomandibular joint dysfunction. It is ironic that despite a laggard approach to research in this area in many dental schools, and in the face of negative literature and position papers, notwithstanding a resurgence in mechanical appliances and lingual surgery as cure-all remedies, the demand for oral myofunctional services has increased greatly in the interval since our previous edition. We remain optimistic that sincere research, conducted by knowledgeable investigators, will follow.

The most common complaint about our first volume arose from the illustrations: the photographs were deemed excellent, while the line drawings were thought unsatisfactory. With this in mind, we have turned again to Mr. Tunney Wong, who earned the plaudits with his camera, talent, and skill in the transmutation of indifferent color slides into usable prints. On the other hand, we belatedly discovered Miss Cindy Cohen, who has largely replaced the previous drawings with more accurate depictions, while working under considerable time pressure to provide the beautiful anatomic illustrations for our new chapters. We feel that these represent a major improvement.

Our gratitude extends also to those who have made requests, who have offered suggestions, and who have critically analyzed our changes and additions. We hope that we have met their expectations.

Richard H. Barrett
Marvin L. Hanson

v

PREFACE
TO FIRST EDITION

Prefaces are supposed to indicate the scope of a book, give some statement of its purpose, and acknowledge the contributions of a variety of outside sources. The preface also provides authors with a chance to chat informally, to confirm the reader's wisdom in having purchased or borrowed the book, and to give an excuse for having written the work in the first place. We believe this volume to be long overdue.

Where does one find a truly complete description of *normal* deglutition, much less abnormal? The welter of opinion concerning the etiology of anomalies, the significance of various manifestations, the requirements for correction of aberrant function, and even the legitimacy of the problem itself—all have proliferated to the point of confusion. They have needed to be pulled together and placed in some kind of perspective so that in the future they may be validly sorted and weighed.

Some fear arises from the fact that this book represents an adventure into an area that is susceptible to scientific research but thus far has not had the benefit of sufficient solid, controlled evaluation. We have tried to construct valid theory from the data now available; nothing can appear more devastating than theory, cast in irrevocable print, after research has established the factual status.

With a mixture of fear and hope, we expect this book to grow old quickly. It is our sincere desire that every aspect of this theory and therapy be ripped apart and subjected to quantitative scrutiny. Perhaps we are not being too optimistic if we also retain the hope that the result will not be mere destruction but that a sounder structure will thus arise—that something positive will re-

sult. The reader should feel free to disassemble, test, and question, but should replace each plank with something better. It requires no great skill to destroy; to build well requires some genius.

The original title of this book was to have been "Tongue Thrust: Theory and Therapy." During the past decade, however, the domain of the therapist who once treated principally tongue thrust has been greatly expanded, and the term "oral myologist" is now coming into wider use. Such a clinician treats many related disorders. We have accordingly enlarged our purview. We have tried to be complete, scientific, and somewhat eclectic in our coverage.

It was necessary to direct the content toward two distinct and quite dissimilar groups: dentists and speech pathologists. Within these separate populations, it was further necessary to provide for such disparate individuals as the student and the experienced professional, the clinician and the researcher. In addition, we have hoped to make provision for those in other professions, such as dental hygienists, whose personal accomplishments and position might qualify them to deal with oral myofunctional disorders.

Since the book is directed toward people with training in such varied professions, we have assumed very limited prior preparation on the part of the reader. We have included chapters on some basics of dentistry for the benefit of speech pathologists and material on speech development for those not conversant in that area. The first part of the book is intended to supply background for the student and to point up areas of needed study for the researcher, whether in speech or dentistry. We have attempted to treat controversial areas without drawing unwarranted conclusions from our own biases. All of the information included should be understood by anyone attempting to work with these disorders.

Part two is simply a treatment manual, setting forth in rather great detail the methods that we have found most effective in correcting orofacial abnormalities. It is designed as a step-by-step guide for the clinician; the researcher may readily find the points of difficulty or doubt. It is somewhat oriented toward the field of speech, since we must speak from our own background; it is hoped, however, that it will not be incomprehensible to those in allied fields who find this subject pertinent to treatment. We believe strongly in the importance of close, interprofessional working relationships among all specialists who treat the patient.

We hope to offend as few dentists as possible as we delineate matters that are primarily dental. In any field it is difficult to accept ideas from someone who is not a member of the club, an interloper from a different profession. Also, there is always some risk, in writing outside one's area of competence, that misinterpretations will be expressed through lack of full knowledge. We have tried to confine our excursions into dentistry to only what seemed essential material and have checked with dental authorities, not once but many times, in our effort to be accurate.

Still, a harvest of true worth is sometimes reaped by planting the basics of two or more fields in a single brain. Separate minds may examine a concept and believe that they are in complete agreement as to its nature, yet retain only partial awareness of the full scope of the concept as it extends beyond their personal scan. The "cross-disciplinary" approach frequently has this result. Combining various individual views within a single head may produce a hybrid strain, an original discipline. Certainly, concepts of oral myofunction have been synthesized from many fields.

We have intended this work to be fit as a textbook for courses offered to dental students, speech pathology majors, and directly for oral myologists. The learning of all the material included herein does not prepare the student to administer therapy. Book reading must be supplemented by extensive supervised work with patients of all ages, representing all the disorders the field encompasses. Nevertheless, we offer the book as a place to begin.

A tremendous debt of gratitude owed to a great many people must be acknowledged. At times we have felt ourselves to be more anthologists than originators. The dentists who gave us early guidance and support, remaining patient with groping blunders, comprise the front rank; they were our original co-authors. Many long-suffering patients, who submitted graciously to a series of ineffectual early techniques and who then reported, with surprising good nature, their experiences, opinions, and suggestions, did much to mold the program. In addition, the many students and clinicians who have studied with us, singly and in groups, provided stimulation as well as valued and often continuing friendships. Many have thereafter focused their attention on myofunctional disorders, sending back frequent notes on their observations, suggestions for overcoming some of the difficulties in therapy, and the joyful discovery of a new procedure. These offerings have become so blended in the program presented here that it would not be possible to single out for deserved credit each contribution. They were individually appreciated, and still are.

Richard H. Barrett
Marvin L. Hanson

CONTENTS

PART ONE

BACKGROUND AND THEORY

A □ FUNDAMENTALS

1 Introduction, 3

Tongue thrust, 3
Normal swallowing, 4
Overview of controversies, 4
Oral myofunctional disorders: an interprofessional problem, 5
Orthodontic treatment, 7
Related oral habits, 7
Potential for change in therapy, 8
Conclusion, 8

2 Fundamentals of speech, 9

Speech development, 9
Disorders of speech, 11
Relationships between dentition and speech, 15
Conclusion, 16

3 Some fundamentals of dentistry, 18

The tooth and its supporting structures, 18
Dental orientation, 19
Dental development, 22
Wasteland of dental "occlusion," 25
Malocclusion, 27
Dental treatment of the young child, 29
Additional important terms, 31
Conclusion, 32

4 Orthodontic concepts and procedures, 37

Personal observation, 37
Appliances, 37
Procedures, 44

5 Anatomy for the oral myologist, 52

Terminology, 52
Divisions of anatomy, 53
Some types of tissue, 53
Osteology, 54
Neurology, 59
Myology, 69

6 Applied physiology, 86

Forces affecting the tooth, 86
Temporomandibular joint, 90
The nasal airway, 96
Effects of playing wind instruments, 98

B □ TONGUE THRUST

7 History, 102

British contributions, 103
American contributions, 106
Recent developments, 111
Conclusion, 111

8 Etiologies, 114

Bottle feeding, 114
Genetic influence, 117
Thumb sucking, 118
Open spaces during mixed dentition, 118
Tonsils and adenoids, 119
Allergies, 119
Mouth breathing, 120
Macroglossia and microglossia, 120
Anesthetic throat, 120
Brain injury, 121
Soft diet, 121
Psychological arrest, 122
Orthodontic treatment, 122
Oral trauma, 123
Sleeping habits, 123

Oral sensory deficiency, 123
A developmental theory, 124
Conclusion, 130

9 Controversies, 133

Does tongue thrust exist? 133
Is it a normal or an abnormal behavior? 135
What should it be called? 137
Is tongue thrust related to dental malocclusion? 137
Does tongue thrust cause malocclusion? 138
Are tongue thrust and malocclusion both related to other physiological behavior patterns? 148
Should tongue thrust be treated? 149
Will tongue thrust correct itself with maturation? 150
How can tongue thrust be treated? 150
Who should treat tongue thrust? 152
When should therapy begin? 152
Is treatment for tongue thrust successful? 154

10 Implications for the dental specialist, 162

General dentistry, 162
Oral surgery, 162
Pedodontics, 164
Periodontics, 165
Prosthodontics, 167
Orthodontics, 168

11 Normal and abnormal deglutition, 169

Normal swallowing, 169
Abnormal swallowing, 172
Classification of abnormalities, 175
Conclusion, 183

PART TWO
TREATMENT
A □ FUNDAMENTALS

12 Diagnosis and prognosis, 187

Diagnostic questions, 187
Diagnostic procedures, 189
Prognosis, 195
Summary, 197

13 A review of treatment approaches, 198

Appliance therapy, 198
Surgery, 201
Hypnosis, 201

Oral myotherapy, 202
Kinesiology, 209
Biofeedback, 209
Summary, 210

14 Other oral habits, 212

General considerations, 212
Etiologies, 212
Influences on speech, 213
Oral habits and malocclusions, 214
Specific oral habits, 215
Summary, 218

15 Philosophy of treatment, 220

A psychophysiological approach, 220
Cooperation of clinician and dentist, 224
Conclusion, 227

B □ PROCEDURES

16 Sucking habits, 228

General orientation, 228
Corrective procedures, 232
Tongue sucking 238

17 Step 1: lip exercises, 239

Preliminary remarks, 239
Parental procedures, 240
Prologue for the patient, 243
Therapy procedures, 245
Testing the need, 248
Strengthening exercises, 250
Repositioning exercises, 253
Conclusion, 256
Assignment, 258

18 Step 2: foundation of deglutition, 259

Evaluation of previous week, 259
Procedures, 260

19 Step 3: potential of anterior tongue, 267

Evaluation of previous step, 267
Tongue-lifting exercise, 269
Positioning of blade of tongue, 270
Molar occlusion, 271
Resting position, 272

20 Step 4: posterior tongue, 277

Evaluation of previous week, 277
Repositioning of posterior tongue, 279

21 Step 5: coordinating the total swallow, 285

Evaluation of previous week, 285
Moment of truth, 286
Assignment, 291
Therapy materials, 294

22 Step 6: the conscious habit, 296

Evaluation of previous week, 296
Rapid drinking, 298
Initiating the habit, 298
Velar control, 303
Rest posture, 304

23 Step 7: the subconscious habit, 305

Evaluation of conscious readiness, 305
Rationale of subconscious procedure, 307
Patient orientation, 309
Waking but subconscious swallows, 313
Assignment, 313

24 Step 8: final concerns, 316

Evaluation of total pattern, 316
Tests for subconscious function, 317
Tying loose ends, 319
Conclusion, 321

25 Recheck period, 322

Early tests of completion, 323
Later tests of retention, 327
Relapses *do* occur, 331

26 Alternative procedures of Hanson, 334

The hierarchy of areas of emphasis, 334
Organismic principles, 335
Behavior modification, 335
Neuromuscular facilitation, 339
Correction of dentalized speech sounds, 339
Lessons, 339
Recheck visits, 356
Conclusion, 357

Appendix 1 □ Forms used in therapy, 358

Case history form, 358
Letter to parents, 358
Report forms, 358
Rest posture chart, 358
Sucking habit calendar, 358

Appendix 2 □ Materials and sources of supply, 366

PART ONE

BACKGROUND AND THEORY

Section A ☐ FUNDAMENTALS
Section B ☐ TONGUE THRUST

Chapter 1

INTRODUCTION

This book is about oral myofunctional disorders, but a great preponderance of attention will be paid to the tongue, particularly its protrusion.

Mankind has suffered from protrusion of the tongue ever since the first physician hit on the idea of using the dorsum as a divining rod for gastrology, ordered, "Stick out your tongue!" and then prescribed castor oil. The ancient ritual of examining the patient's tongue goes back at least to Hippocrates, who identified a number of symptoms and could diagnose hangover from the harsh, parched condition of the tongue after a debauch. Avicenna noted the necessity of scraping the tongue when it was black to prevent its noxious vapors from causing inflammation of the brain.

The tongue has long been considered a prime site for torture and punishment, and mere amputation was rather merciful compared to the carving and mutilation that once was a favorite pastime; dragging a bound victim with his tongue attached to a wild horse was tried on numerous occasions. Judas Maccabaeus was not content with cutting out the tongue of Nicanor, but made a point of feeding it to the birds. From a legal standpoint, paternity cases have been settled by placing a live coal on the mother's tongue, conviction of slander has resulted in partial glossectomy, and a woman who complained of paying her taxes had her tongue nailed to a tree.

In more recent times, a British physician of the eighteenth century, aptly named Testy, examined scrapings from the tongue of a drink-sodden wine porter under a microscope. He reported seeing bodies shaped like pears, plums, eggs, etc., which quickly hatched into minute crocodiles, ostriches, and ravens. He went on

to construct a mirror of character from lingual papillae, finding them multibranched in prattlers, smooth in orators, sharp and bending in liars, and horned in cuckolds.

The tongue possesses a greater variety of skills than any other part of the body. It controls taste, creates air currents that suck in liquids, and supervises dental development. It escorts and directs the voice into articulate speech and is the infant's bridge between the internal and external milieu, the compass by which it explores its new world. It pilots food between the teeth in mastication and steers it into the pharynx in deglutition, although not always in an ideal fashion. It receives, in turn, little consideration. We parch it with smoke and pickle it in alcohol; we freeze it with ice cream, burn it with soup, bite it in frustration, and stick it out to display aggression.

TONGUE THRUST

We push the tongue against our teeth and protrude it between them. The several names for this behavior will be discussed in a later chapter; for now, we will call it "tongue thrust." It is not a simple act, for it involves intrinsic and extrinsic lingual muscles and muscles of expression and mastication. It may occur while the tongue is at rest, during speech, or during swallowing. As in other new areas of knowledge, simple dichotomies give way eventually to complex and subtle shadings. Whereas for many years there were two types of swallows, the tongue thrust and the normal swallow, each with its set of identifiable characteristics, we now recognize that the only difference between a tongue-thrust swallow and a normal one may often be the few millimeters separating the maxillary alveolar ridge from the mandibular in-

3

cisal edges; all other aspects of the swallow may be identical. Even the same child, especially during the mixed dentition stage of development, may swallow normally on one mouthful of food, shift the anterior positioning of the tongue on the next swallow, and swallow with a tongue thrust.

Nevertheless, some of the components of the traditionally described tongue-thrust pattern are found in many children with abnormal swallows, and in our diagnostic procedure we take careful note of them. Their presence, however, is meaningful only if there is an actual anterior or lateral positioning of the tongue against the teeth. Borrowing from several early writers in the field, yet not restricting our description to any one of them, we give the following "classic" description of a tongue-thrust swallow:

The child takes a rather large bite of food. He chews it without making full use of facial muscles to move the food onto the grinding surfaces of the molars and onto the tongue. Instead, the tongue moves the food, first against the teeth, then later, away from the teeth. Chewing is inefficient, and no well-formed bolus results. Scattered portions of food are moved posteriorly, by the creation of an anterior seal, between the tongue tip and blade, anterior teeth, and one or both lips. The molars are not occluded, and the tongue remains wedged between the upper and lower teeth, all around the arch. The circumoral muscles, and especially the mentalis, contract, the muscles of mastication remain flaccid, and suction carries the food back to the pharynx. When the swallow is completed, the tongue has not been effectively cleared of food particles, nor have the teeth. The tongue then often carries out a cleaning procedure by pushing again against the anterior and side teeth.

NORMAL SWALLOWING

In marked contrast to the ineffectual tongue-thrust swallow, the "classic" normal swallowing pattern is offered:

The child takes a moderate-sized bite of food and chews with the lips closed, allowing cheek and lip muscles to move the food toward the tongue as he chews. He chews just long enough to allow the saliva to mix with the food and form a cohesive bolus, right in the middle of the upper surface of the tongue. The tongue tip is positioned against the upper alveolar process, the sides of the tongue are positioned against the gums along the sides of the arch, and no food is allowed to escape laterally or anteriorly during the swallow. The molars are occluded, the lip and cheek muscles are relaxed, and the food is moved posteriorly by a lifting or squeezing action of the tongue. First the blade lifts, and then the posterior portion lifts, while the tip and sides of the tongue retain their contact with the alveolar process. When the swallow is completed, the teeth and tongue are free of food particles.

OVERVIEW OF CONTROVERSIES

Years of experience and research have taught us that neither of the above descriptions accurately portrays the swallowing patterns of specific, individual children. There are as many variations as there are children. It is this variability among children, as well as within the patterns of a given child, that has given rise to so many controversies in the area of tongue thrust. These controversies will be treated in greater depth in Chapter 9 but will be introduced here because they can provide the reader with insight into the present "state of the field."

1. *Does tongue thrust exist?* There is no general agreement that tongue thrust is a real entity or syndrome. Some writers have expressed difficulty in categorizing enough elements of the behavioral pattern in any manner that would result in labeling any behavior as "tongue thrust."

2. *If it exists, is it normal or abnormal?* A number of incidence studies find the behavioral pattern termed tongue thrust to exist in significantly large percentages of the population. The behavior has been identified in over 50% of infants and preschool children. Many investigators question whether a behavior found in a majority of a given population should ever be termed abnormal.

3. *What should it be called?* In addition to tongue thrust, other names for the behavior are deviant swallow, reverse swallow, perverted swallow, deviate deglutition, visceral swallow, infantile swallow, and abnormal swallow.

4. *Is tongue thrust related to dental malocclusion?* Many children who have malocclusions are tongue thrusters. On the other hand, many children who have malocclusions are not tongue thrusters, and many others who swallow by pushing their tongue against their anterior teeth, retain excellent teeth with no malocclusion.

5. *Can tongue thrust cause malocclusion?* There is no doubt about the ability of constant light pressures to move the teeth. This principle is the basis of orthodontic work. There is a question, however, of whether intermittent lingual pressures are capable of moving them.

6. *Can malocclusion cause tongue thrust?* Many orthodontists who believe this is true contend that correction of the malocclusion results

in elimination of the tongue thrust. If so, there would be no need for clinicians to work with habit patterns.

7. *Is there a relationship between tongue thrust, malocclusion, and other physiological behavior patterns?* Often listed as etiological contributors to the development of tongue thrust and malocclusion are thumb sucking, feeding problems in infancy, allergies, and enlarged tonsils. Bottle feeding, particularly, was blamed for several years.

8. *Should tongue thrust be treated?* Since the incidence of tongue thrust appears to decrease with increasing age, should the children be left alone and maturation allowed to do its work?[2] Do we have enough scientific evidence of the efficacy of treatment to warrant its use?

9. *How can it be treated?* As suggested, one approach is to modify the occlusion or the configuration of the dental arches. Another approach is to use mechanical restraints, such as dental cribs, to make it unpleasant for the tongue to rest or move to a forward position. A third approach is myotherapy. Which approach is most effective with most children? When would myotherapy be contraindicated?

10. *Who is best prepared to treat tongue thrust?* Should the treatment be the province of one specific, already existing profession, or should preparation for treating tongue thrust include training in several disciplines and prepare the therapist especially for work with this and related problems? Because this question is germane to the philosophy of this book, we will give our answer to it in the present chapter. Most of the other questions will be discussed at some length in Chapter 9, as well as in the remainder of the book.

ORAL MYOFUNCTIONAL DISORDERS: AN INTERPROFESSIONAL PROBLEM

Among specialists whom we have trained to do an effective job of therapy are orthodontists, dentists in general practice, pedodontists, speech clinicians, dental assistants, dental hygienists, and physical therapists. Each of them brought to training knowledge and experience in at least one important area of the problems to be treated. All needed to have their fields of knowledge broadened considerably before they were able to see the total child with the total problem and deal effectively with it.

DENTISTS. The dentist, with his knowledge of oral anatomy and the developmental aspects of the problem, is in a particularly advantageous position to administer oral myotherapy. However, overhead expenses in his office usually make his personal participation in the therapy impractical. Most of the dentists whom we have trained have also had their assistants or hygienists trained and have merely supervised their work. In other cases, the dentists have worked directly with the patients long enough to feel comfortable with therapy and then trained their own assistants to do the work. The growing emphasis in the profession of preventive dentistry makes attention to this problem very appropriate. Throughout the history of the emergence of oral myology as a profession, the dentists have without a doubt played the key role. It is in the dentistry journals that the vast majority of clinical and research reports are to be found. Since 1839, when Rodrigues attributed malocclusion to improper muscle function,[2] dentistry has carried out many attacks on muscle imbalance. Most of them have been mechanical in nature, because of the orientation of the dentist. As the specialty of orthodontics developed and awareness of the importance of *function,* as well as physical structure, grew, recognition of muscular irregularities became more acute and combative efforts intensified, although awareness that the process of *deglutition* was involved came rather late.

Dentists are in a uniquely favorable position to motivate the children to carry out those instructions which will help to assure their having attractive and healthy teeth. Therapy can readily be administered using a dental chair. It takes very little outlay to supplement the equipment and material normally found in a dentist's office with the special items needed to carry out therapy for tongue thrust. Many dentists, particularly in smaller communities, find themselves with no available resource person adequately trained in oral myotherapy, but with patients whose needs are critical. They have found it worthwhile, and even pleasant, to administer the therapy themselves. The general dentist, pedodontist, orthodontist, and periodontist all have vested interests in abnormal oral habits.

SPEECH PATHOLOGISTS. Over the years, dentists have recognized that the training and experience of speech pathologists place them in a very favorable position for working with oral myofunctional problems. They understand oral anatomy and physiology and are trained to change habits involving oral musculature. The majority of the oral myotherapists we are acquainted with who have been working in the field for ten years or more were originally invited to carry out therapy by an interested dentist, and many began their practice in that dentist's office. The requirement of the American Speech and Hearing Association that certified speech pathologists must hold a master's degree or its equivalent, together with the growth in the number of Ph.D.s in speech pathology, has served to foster an interest in research in that field. As a matter of course, a small but significant percentage of speech pathologists have become interested in the field of oral habit problems, and some significant research has been carried out by their profession. In addition, the national Joint Committee on Dentistry and Speech Pathology-Audiology has brought the two professions together and resulted in very profitable exchanges of ideas and information.

The speech pathologist is usually able to carry out a full or part-time private practice with a relatively small investment. His equipment needs are minimal; therefore, daily operating overhead is small compared to that of the dentist. He can usually carry out the treatment using the same office and furniture that he uses in his work with other disorders. His training as a speech pathologist allows him to treat the speech problems that incidence studies have found to occur in 25% to 40% of children with tongue thrust. Although he requires supplemental training to be prepared to identify dental anomalies, with this training he is able to provide a more complete habilitative program for the patient than any other professional.

DENTAL HYGIENISTS AND ASSISTANTS. Dental hygienists and assistants, we have found, are very adaptable to the training required to become oral myologists. Although their training and experience limits them to knowledge of the dentition, their experience in working with patients has been found to be helpful. It is convenient for the dentist to have these people see his patients because they are already working in his office and he does not need to make a referral outside his office to another specialist. He is able to observe firsthand the progress of therapy and the attitude of the patient. Since most referrals for oral muscle training come from dentists, some patients who might not ordinarily act on the suggestion of the dentist to see a therapist in some other location, might do so if the person who provides the treatment is in the dentist's office.

There are disadvantages to this arrangement, however. There is an air, often a characteristic odor, as well as a certain feeling of apprehension associated in the mind of the patient with a dentist's office. This disadvantage can be compensated for by having the therapist work in a separate room furnished with nondental type of furniture and designed to create an atmosphere of its own. In our experience, motivation is also a little easier when the dentist's office and myotherapy room are in separate locations. We customarily advise our patients in as positive a manner as possible that repeated failure to carry out assignments adequately leads to dismissal from therapy. It is a little more difficult to comply with these conditions when the therapist sees the patient periodically as he visits the dentist in whose office the myotherapy is conducted. Neither of these disadvantages need be serious, however, and we are acquainted with several hygienists and dental assistants who work very effectively in the dentist's office.

PHYSICAL THERAPISTS. Physical therapists are, of course, well trained in the "myotherapy" part of oral myotherapy. Their training needs to be extended considerably to provide them with the necessary background with which to treat disorders involving oral musculature. The physical therapist understands the necessity of consistent, goal-oriented exercise for muscle strengthening, as well as for habituation of motor response patterns. This understanding, along with his experience in motivating and providing therapy for people in a one-to-one relationship, facilitates his preparation in the field of oral myotherapy.

ORAL MYOLOGISTS. Several universities offer training courses in tongue thrust and related disorders, but few of the programs make this training mandatory for completing a degree. At the present time, we estimate that over 90% of the clinicians or therapists working with oral muscular disorders received important specific training in this area after receiving their professional degrees. An oral myologist should be an individual who:

1. Knows the anatomy and physiology of the oral region
2. Understands the vegetative and communicative functions of the teeth and orofacial musculature
3. Has an adequate understanding of developmental processes, including dental, physiological, and speech development
4. Has training and experience in the field of human motivation

5. Understands basic principles effective in changing deep-rooted habits
6. Has had appropriate training and supervised experience in treating oral myofunctional disorders

Unless, at some time in the future, a specialized degree is obtainable to prepare a person to work in this area, we believe that oral myotherapists should hold a degree or certificate in one of the specialties previously discussed. The International Association of Oral Myology, formed in 1972, has a qualifying examination which its applicants must pass in order to become members. The examination is comprehensive, and the applicant must, in order to be certified with that organization, demonstrate his clinical competence to one who already holds certification. The organization promises to be an effective agent in developing and maintaining standards of excellence in the profession.

ORTHODONTIC TREATMENT

Whoever provides the therapy for the patient with an oral myofunctional disorder should do so with the cooperation of the orthodontist. Each specialist can be of immense help to the other. In our experience, a great majority of the referrals come from the orthodontist, who has already told the patient that without therapy for tongue thrust, orthodontic treatment would almost certainly fail. Nearly all the orthodontists who refer to us refuse to begin their treatment with a patient with tongue thrust until they receive a final report from the oral myologist stating that the patient has habituated correct muscle patterns. This requirement motivates the patient to cooperate in the myotherapy. The therapist, in turn, advises the patient that he is eager for him to do well in therapy in order that a satisfactory report can be sent to the orthodontist to avoid any delay in the initiation of dental treatment. The orthodontist is, through the communications he receives from the therapist, provided with a useful index of the degree of cooperativeness of the patient and of the parents. In addition, treatment timing depends on factors that both specialists are required to assess.

RELATED ORAL HABITS

There are numberless things that children do with their mouths that seem to us to be contributory to speech disorders and dental problems. Some contribute also to the development of psychological problems, and many seem to accompany, or be the result of, emotional distur-

bances. Since the specialist who works with tongue thrust needs to be trained to alter behavior that occurs at a subconscious level, involving oral musculature, it seems logical that he should also be ready to treat other deeply rooted habits as well. We have dealt with the following problems with some degree of success. All these problems are amenable to treatment, and the training of an oral myologist should include attention to each one.

DENTALIZATION OF CONSONANTS. The linguoalveolar consonants (/t/, /d/, /n/, /l/, /s/, and /z/) are often produced linguodentally by children with a tongue-thrust problem. Particularly frequently involved are the sibilant sounds. The voiced and whispered forms of the /th/ sounds, normally produced by approximating the tip of the tongue and the posterior biting edge of the upper and lower central incisors, are often produced with an exaggerated tongue protrusion.

THUMB OR FINGER SUCKING. A few children suck their thumbs in a way that does not seem to be detrimental to the occlusion. The majority, though, exert a relatively constant and heavy pressure against the anterior teeth when they do so. Certainly a normal swallow is not possible so long as the finger or thumb is in the mouth.

LIP LICKING. This habit is self-perpetuating. The licking coats the lips with saliva, which dries, becomes sticky, and fosters repeated licking. Children who come to us for treatment very often have chapped and cracked lips that usually become healthy again when the lip licking ceases. On its way to the lips, the tongue pushes against the teeth. When the tongue is repeatedly protruded, we believe it is encouraged to remain in the relatively forward resting position.

LIP OR CHEEK BITING. This habit is often unilateral and results in asymmetry of the dental arch.

EXTERNAL PRESSURE APPLIED TO THE MANDIBLE OR MAXILLA. Some children and adults habitually lean against their hands or fists, with the elbow on the arm of a chair or on a desk. Others push against the outside of the jaw with an object, such as a pencil or a telephone.

TONGUE SUCKING. We are not sure of the effects of tongue sucking on the arch configuration or on the anterior teeth. We know that it often involves the anterior positioning of the tongue against the teeth.

HABITUAL BITING OR RESTING OF OBJECTS BETWEEN THE UPPER AND LOWER FRONT TEETH. Some children hold a pencil, eraser, or other object between the upper and lower front teeth habitually. If the object is made of a hard material, there may be an effect on the cutting edge of the teeth. If the object protrudes into the oral cavity, it may affect the resting posture of the tongue and hence affect the manner of swallowing.

BRUXISM (TEETH GRINDING). When teeth grinding occurs habitually over a long period of time, it has a detrimental effect on the chewing and grinding surfaces of the teeth.

MOUTH BREATHING. Mouth breathing tends to be accompanied by a habitual, forward, low posturing of the tongue, and research has found it to be related to the presence of tongue thrusting.

ABNORMAL LINGUAL AND LABIAL RESTING POSTURES. When the lower lip is habitually positioned lingual to, and pressing against, the upper incisors (as in many cases of extreme overjet), or when the tongue rests against the front teeth day and night, a light, continuous pressure is exerted against the lingual aspect of the anterior teeth that is much akin to the force utilized by the orthodontist. Many believe these resting postures to be more effective movers of teeth than the more powerful, but less frequent, tongue thrust during swallows.

POTENTIAL FOR CHANGE IN THERAPY

Hoffman and Hoffman[1] state that swallowing is almost entirely reflexive in nature, and successful retraining of a reflex is not to be expected. Other writers have agreed with them that efforts in swallowing therapy are futile—that permanent modification of patterns is impossible to accomplish.

Perhaps the existence of the present book is sufficient evidence that we disagree with this opinion. We would not propose that it is *easy* to effect such a change. Swallowing is at least partially reflexive in nature and certainly occurs subconsciously most of the time. The portion of the swallow that we deal with in therapy, however, is the anterior phase, which *is* amenable to

treatment. We will present evidence in later chapters that the transfer from a tongue-thrust pattern to one involving little or no contact between the tongue and the anterior dentition is a normal development in most children and that our therapy merely mirrors a normal developmental change.

CONCLUSION

The field of oral myofunctional disorders remains today a jungle area, inadequately explored, inaccurately mapped, intriguing to most therapists, and imperative to the orthodontist. Some professionals have carved out niches here and there, and every point of view around the entire periphery has attracted supporters. We have had a plethora of opinions; we have a great dearth of facts. Hundreds of studies are needed. For the graduate student seeking a research problem, the following pages present a smorgasbord.

Although it is hoped that this book will stimulate research, its primary goal is clinical. Our intent has been to include philosophy, rationale, and details so that the specialists alluded to in this chapter could, with appropriate supervision, apply the material herein properly. Regardless of the degree of scientific knowledge that we bring to the therapy situation, the application of any program will still contain a large portion of art; the most soundly conceived routine will be only as effective as the clinician's skill in explaining, demonstrating, motivating, and perceiving.

REFERENCES

1. Hoffman, J. A., and Hoffman, R. L.: Tongue thrust and deglutition: some anatomical, physiological, and neurological considerations, J. Speech Hear. Disord. **30:**105, 1965.
2. Salzmann, J. A.: Orthodontics: principles and prevention, Philadelphia, 1957, J. B. Lippincott Co.

Chapter 2

FUNDAMENTALS OF SPEECH

Speech has long been a subject for discussion and concern in the field of dentistry. The conscientious pedodontist must take cognizance of the speech development of his young patients. The orthodontist for many years has been aware of the influences of speech on dentition.[4] The periodontist sees dysfunction and disease caused by faulty speech habits,[8] and after the teeth are destroyed and gone, the prosthodontist still finds that one of the basic considerations in fashioning a denture is its accommodation to speech.[5,9] The general dentist has a share in all these concerns.

SPEECH DEVELOPMENT

In Chapter 3, some dental terminology and procedures will be outlined for the speech pathologist so that he may understand something of the language and work of the dentist. No effort will be made to develop the speech clinician into a dentist, obviously; only a sightseeing tour is planned, with certain places of interest to be pointed out. The intent in the present chapter will be simply to define a number of speech parameters and to point out some guideposts. For the non–speech professional who is seriously interested in learning more about speech correction, the books listed at the conclusion of this chapter are recommended highly.

The dentist should be expected to recognize abnormal speech. If he is to fulfill his obligation to his patient, he should have some awareness of normal speech development and a close acquaintance with those defects which are associated with dental anomalies. He should know specifically what effect dental correction will have on speech patterns and what types of defects require professional attention.

The dentist should realize that very few dental irregularities *impose* defective speech; one has only to look and listen to find many cases with structural deformity and yet with compensatory movement—movement of some element of the anatomy in an uncommon way—that has been acquired and has resulted in perfectly normal speech. Of course, this compensatory movement requires some additional effort by the child, greater motivation, a degree of coordination, and a happy combination of intelligence and chance. It is something that can be taught, but this aspect will be discussed later in the chapter.

Acquisition of speech

Speech is literally "hot air." It is a column of breath supported by the lungs, acted on first by the vocal folds of the larynx, and thereafter molded, reinforced, and resonated by the various tissues, organs, and cavities of the throat, nose, and mouth; it is influenced and often colored by the personality and emotion of the speaker. It is emitted as a series of hums, hisses, and explosions, each produced in a distinctive way or in one of a limited number of distinctive ways. Through common agreement, stereotyped over the years, we accept these noises as meaningful. There is nothing inherently binding in those sounds; our ancestors might have chosen other noises, and in some cases they did, in other languages or in English sounds that have been lost in evolutionary processes. The point is that the sounds we accept as normal are those which are most closely adapted to the structure and function of the normal anatomy, those which can be produced most *easily* by the average adult.

Still, speech is something more than the mechanical ability to produce sounds; learning to talk is learning in a very true sense, and as such it entails all functions of the entire individual as these functions pertain to the use of language.

9

Gestures speak at least as loudly as words; yet it never occurs to us to teach a child gesticulation. The child learns to form certain sounds and later to combine them into a meaningful word. Still later he is taught to transcribe the word with his hand in writing, but at what point did he acquire the ability to stand on the shore and print this word in the sand with his toe? Learning reverberates throughout the nervous system.

As the understanding of speech development becomes more refined, it thus becomes apparent that we are not dealing simply with the acquisition of individual sounds or words but rather with a much more complex skill involving the whole of language use. This more global concept encompasses the buildup of vocabulary, true enough, but in the context of a larger structure, including such considerations as the implications and ramifications of language. Words are not learned as separate noises but as symbols of meaning. The process is thus not confined to the oral cavity; a tactile sensation, a taste, or an odor may trigger a verbal response. This weight of meaning is later transferred in a specific manner to the visual level, if reading skills are to develop normally, and to the manual level of writing. We should not be surprised to discover, therefore, that the child who is handicapped in speech may write illegibly, have a disability in reading, and have other learning deficits, despite normal intellectual capacity.

We are probably going a bit beyond the comfort zone for readers who have no special passion for speech, and we did not intend to make this discussion more complex than necessary. Although some reference to speech concepts is unavoidable, we will not pummel them unduly in the sections below; they should, however, be kept in mind. As we deal with various sounds, it will be safer to think of them as elements in an overall pattern of *language,* not as isolated and sterile vocal emissions. The central nervous system constructs a total configuration of *verbal behavior,* including the many connotations of that behavior as understood by the learner, and including also the nonverbal meaning and expression which this term implies.

It is basic to remember also that speech is not an inherited function. We inherit the apparatus with which to breathe and chew and swallow, and a central nervous system with which to coordinate, direct, and understand. If this original equipment functions and develops normally, as it usually does, we lay on it the added responsibility of producing speech. We have no organ or structure present in our body for the sole purpose of speech, except for an area of the brain that is reserved for later occupancy. The basic function of our "speech" mechanism is vegetative. Speech is a *learned* behavior, and every individual must perform his own learning.

Order of learning

It should be noted first that clinicians do not discuss "letters" of the alphabet, but speech *sounds;* /s/ is "sss" not "*e*ss." English is not a phonetic language; some symbols or letters may represent several sounds or none at all. Thus /c/ may mean either /k/ or /s/, which are unrelated sounds, whereas /x/ is either /ks/ or /gz/, making both /c/ and /x/ superfluous and ambiguous symbols. Certain combinations of symbols are absolutely inexplicable in the English language, and it has been necessary to devise a special system, the International Phonetic Alphabet, in order to carry on the work of speech correction. Conventional symbols will be used below, followed by an identifying word where confusion might arise.

About 75% of our consonants occur in "pairs," voiced and voiceless cognates that are produced in identical fashion, differing only in that one is accompanied by vibration of the vocal folds, whereas the other is "whispered." Thus /s/ and /z/ are distinguished from each other by the fact that although /s/ does not employ laryngeal sound, or voice, /z/ does so but is otherwise the same. Other pairs are /k-g/, /p-b/, /ch-j/, etc.

Very rarely does a speech defect involve vowel production; vowels are usually mastered in the early vocal play of the infant, partially because they necessitate no major interruption of the voice stream, as is required by the consonants. If vowel distortion is a factor, it is usually wise to consult a professional speech therapist.

Growth and development are important concepts for the speech clinician as well as for the orthodontist. Speech sounds are not acquired *in toto* but develop in a fairly predictable fashion. Children tend to learn first those sounds which require the fewest muscles, the largest muscles, and the least degree of coordination between muscles. Based on the ability to execute gross sounds, progress is made in a somewhat physiological manner toward the more sophisticated sounds. Accordingly, the earliest consonants used in speech tend to be the bilabials (/p/, /b/, /m/, /w/), followed by sounds produced by the front of the tongue (/t/, /d/, /n/). Shortly thereafter come the sounds made by the posterior tongue (/k/, /g/ as in "go," /ng/), then a slightly more difficult group consisting of /f/, /v/, /th/ (voiced and voiceless), /sh/, /zh/, and /l/, and finally the highly coordinated /r/, /s/, /z/, /ch/, and /j/. The remainder, such as /h/, /hw/ (*wh*at), and /y/, are acquired at various points along the way.

This process requires from four to six years, beginning with the crying and cooing of the infant and progressing to a meaningful word at 14 or 15 months of age, on the average, with girls being somewhat more precocious than boys. The average child has mastered speech by 5 years of age, and many at still earlier ages; however, certain children may approach 6 years of age and be considered normal in speech, providing their only errors occur on one or two of the most difficult sounds.

Due to the serial order of mastery, note that severely distorted sounds may be considered perfectly normal speech at one age but be classified as a speech defect at a later date. That is, if several of the late-arriving sounds are misarticulated at 4 years of age, it is not thought to constitute a speech defect, whereas the same speech at 6 years of age would be difficult to judge as normal. Again, we do not expect the 2-year-old to be proficient with /k/ and /g/, but the child of 5 years who has not mastered them, and who still says "*d*un" for gun, and "*t*anny" for candy, should receive immediate attention from a speech clinician; every day that passes thereafter makes it less likely that he will "grow out of it."

DISORDERS OF SPEECH

Speech defects cover a broad range of conditions, in most of which there are no dental implications—only a need for recognition.

The lay person often needs only one category with which to classify all speech defects: *tongue-tie*. Diagnosis is quick and easy since it does not require oral examination; the concept is broad enough to encompass brain injury, physical defects, emotional disturbance, and faulty learning. Correction is simple: clip the lingual frenum. Far more cases have been referred to the writers with the lay diagnosis of "tongue-tie" than all other disorders combined. In point of fact, of several thousand such cases, precisely

four have in reality suffered ankyloglossia. Several abnormal frena have been seen accompanied by normal speech, and many speech defects have been seen after frenectomy. Our classification, then, should be a bit more definitive. We will also benefit from a brief glimpse at why such disorders occur.

Causes of speech defects

At least 75% of all speech defects trace their origin to some sort of breakdown in the learning process mentioned above. Given the intact central nervous system of the average child, average hearing acuity, and *normal* structure, faulty learning still occurs. A corollary thought should be noted: A learning procedure implies a teacher; few children have the services of parents who are also speech pathologists, but whether parents are aware of it or not, and whether they teach poorly or well—they teach. The mechanistic approach of simply holding up a round object and repeating the word "ball" may have unexpected results—or none. Normal speech development is fostered when speech is a satisfying activity, when it is associated with pleasurable feelings or rewarded by the gratification of wants and needs. When early speech efforts are met with indifference or impatience, we should expect some delay in future acquisitions. Numerous studies have shown, for example, that an orphanage environment disposes toward delayed and defective speech; some parents, even with admirable intentions, provide scant improvement insofar as speech development is concerned. Overstimulation of the child may prove as detrimental as none. Parental demands may be of the wrong type, or ill-timed, or made with the wrong attitude. It seems truly miraculous that so many youngsters attain normal speech.

A principal tutor is the speech the child hears about him, the pattern set by parents, siblings, etc. If the child is not exposed to normal adult speech, he is robbed of a pattern. If the child simply points and grunts, it being understood that one grunt means "drink of water," whereas two grunts mean "potty," most motivation to learn is destroyed. This also occurs when an older sibling "translates" every speech effort. If the child is either overprotected or rejected, if he is ill at a critical time or for too long a time, if he is exposed to more than one language, if an endocrine imbalance interposes, or if any of several other conditions arise, the learning process, and therefore speech, may be impaired.

Lowered intelligence, brain injury, emotional shocks or conflicts, physical trauma, poor coordination—and dental abnormalities—all serve as possible causes of speech defects. Any of the foregoing circumstances may prove to be operational *concurrently with* malocclusion, a sobering thought that lends caution to the therapist's diagnosis: the malocclusion is so much easier to identify than an obscure brain injury or an unreported domestic situation.

One category of disorders arising from damage to the central nervous system is deserving of specific mention: the various manifestations of *dysarthria*. The resultant incoordination of the speech musculature has perhaps been best described by Van Riper:

Tongues may be clumsy; the lips may flutter tremulously, the jaw may fail to move on time or move sidewise; the larynx may be wrenched out of place; the chest may be expanding as in inhalation at the very time the child is trying to talk. The degree of involvement may be either widespread or almost hidden to all but the expert eye. . . . We also find *apraxias* associated with the dysarthrias in some of our cases, and in others, the apraxia occurs alone. By apraxia we mean the inability to make a movement voluntarily which can otherwise be produced involuntarily. Some children, for example, can curl up the end of their tongues to lick a tantalizing bit of peanut butter from an upper lip but cannot, no matter how they try, do the same thing voluntarily. Such a child might be able to pick up a toothbrush and move it around but could not brush his teeth. It almost seems as though the failure is in the ability to command these muscles.*

Speech is learned by the central nervous system and as noted above is based partly on normal hearing; the deaf child babbles for a time in infancy, and then drops such activity because it is not reinforced. The child who hears normally is stimulated by the sounds in his environment; through auditory feedback, he probably judges his own speech efforts for a time, comparing them with the outer stimuli. If he is able to duplicate a given sound, fine; if duplication proves too difficult, he will substitute the easiest sound which in his opinion is the nearest approximation to the stimulus, whether it be another speech sound or only a noise, or he will simply omit the sound. Whatever his solution, it becomes a *pattern of response*, and after the pattern is established it is turned over to the unconscious system as a unit, the child no longer being aware of a difference between his speech and the original stimulus. He then becomes indignant at any criticism, for he actually "hears" his own speech as normal. "Command" speech therapy, telling the child to stop saying "yitto" and say "little," is whistling in a high gale.

Since normal articulation of speech is based, at least in part, on normal swallowing behavior, it must follow that any gross malfunction of the musculature in basic function, as in deviate deglutition, would be a strong influence toward misuse of these muscles in their secondary role.

Incidence of speech defects

You should expect that approximately one in every ten children whom you see will have some type of speech disorder; about half of this group, or one in twenty, will display a severe defect. Children with speech defects tend to avoid speech and to avoid troublesome words if speech becomes necessary. It is possible to carry on quite a conversation with a stutterer and suddenly realize that he has smiled, gestured, inserted a few animated monosyllables, but has not uttered a single sentence. Only by eliciting a fair sample can speech be evaluated. Many of the "minor" problems go undetected, even though such a problem may be a source of serious concern and definite liability to the patient. Table 2-1 shows an estimated distribution of the more se-

Table 2-1. Estimate of incidence of speech defects*

Type of disorder	Individuals per 1000 population	Percent of total population
Functional articulation	35	3.5
Stuttering	7	0.7
Voice disorders	5	0.5
Delayed speech	5	0.5
Impaired hearing (with speech defects)	5	0.5
Cerebral disorders (brain injury)	2	0.2
Cleft-palate speech	1	0.1
Total	60	6.0

*From Van Riper, C.: Speech correction: principles and methods, ed. 4, Englewood Cliffs, N.J., 1963, Prentice-Hall, Inc., pp. 119-120.

*Based on data from Van Riper, C.: Speech correction: principles and methods, ed. 4, Englewood Cliffs, N.J., 1963, Prentice-Hall, Inc.

vere defects in the total population, not merely in children, and is reportedly the most conservative that can be scientifically defended. Quick arithmetic indicates that some 12 million Americans are handicapped in speech.

Functional articulatory problems are understood to be those for which there is no organic basis, a mere accidental sort of thing resulting from faulty learning, mental or emotional problems, etc. It is suggested that a second look be taken at "functional" disorders: such factors as malocclusion and abnormal swallowing behavior may provide an *organic* basis for some portion of these cases. As has been indicated, functional defects outnumber all other types combined by a wide margin.

Defects of special interest to the dentist

ARTICULATION. Articulation problems constitute about three fourths of the case loads of most speech pathologists.

1. *Lalling* is the distortion of sounds that require vertical lifting of the tongue tip, such as /r/, /l/, /t/, and /d/. The child is frequently described as having a "lazy tongue" and in the private opinion of many speech pathologists is showing one side effect of abnormal swallowing. The child whose tongue rides the floor of his mouth, in deglutition and in mouth breathing, has little inclination to raise his tongue into the stratospheric region required for the normal production of these sounds. The establishment of a normal rest posture, based on normal swallowing behavior in which the tongue functions with some force in the anterior palatal region, would therefore seem to be indicated prior to any efforts made toward correction of the speech sounds.

2. *Lisping* comes in assorted styles and sizes, and should be of particular interest to the dentist. The most common of all speech defects is the *frontal lisp,* which actually consists of substituting the /th/ sounds, voiceless and voiced respectively, for /s/ and /z/. It is not a muscle deformity or tongue stricture, merely the replacement of /s/ and /z/ by /th/, albeit in a few cases the /th/ is made with excessive protrusion of the tongue. In more severe cases the other sibilants, /sh/, /zh/, /ch/, and /j/, are also produced with the tongue in a similar interdental position. The fact remains, *there is no deforming force in producing /th/.* It is a frequently occurring sound, and people use it daily without

jeopardy to their dentition. Aside from English, the /th/ sounds do not occur in any major language except Danish and Greek (to a minor degree in Castilian Spanish), and yet similar malocclusions are found in other countries. The forces exerted during speech are too light in action, and too rapidly executed and released, to have any bearing on the posture of oral structures. In those cases in which teeth are being pushed around, it is probable that the abusive force is embodied in an abnormal pattern of deglutition accompanying the lisp, a rather common occurrence, it now appears.

The *lateral lisp* has a distinctive and very juicy sound. In forming a normal /s/, the apex of the tongue is lifted in proximity to the upper alveolar ridge, with a longitudinal groove or depression down the midline. A tiny jet stream of breath is directed along this groove and delivered with sharp force across the incisal edges of upper and lower teeth, thus setting the air into high-frequency vibration. Children without incisors often produce an excellent sound by directing an airstream against the irregularities of the alveolar ridge itself. A lateral lisp occurs, however, when the apex of the tongue actually contacts the ridge or palate, blocking forward progress and forcing the air laterally over the sides of the tongue and across the bicuspids or first molars, and creating the impression that the vestibular space and the air immediately surrounding it are a maelstrom of saliva particles. An analogous effect is brought about when the apex of the tongue moves obliquely into the cuspid region, throwing the airstream to one side only. You can produce a lateral lisp by whispering a sustained /l/ sound. At the risk of seeming repetitious, the authors have seen few cases of lateral lisping that were not accompanied by a unilateral tongue thrust during deglutition. Whereas many speech pathologists consider lateral lisping to be one of the most difficult to correct of all speech defects, these cases have appeared to yield readily—once normal swallowing habits have been established.

It should be noted in this connection that posterior open bite probably occurs *only* as a result of abnormal tongue pressures during swallowing, as does unilateral open bite in the cuspid region. It might be that anterior open bite, when frontal lisping is also present, has the same uniform etiology. Thus treatment procedure might well follow the order of swallow, speech, occlusion; that is, normal swallowing behavior should be established first; the lisp may then be corrected easily, and should be, for continued malfunction of the musculature in speech can readily subvert the recently acquired pattern of deglutition. Only then should the malocclusion proper be attacked. However, the dentist may need to employ unusual speed in this latter endeavor, in order to stay ahead of nature: most posterior open bites tend to close spontaneously once abnormal tongue pressures are removed. On the other hand, the dental arches exercise a restraint, a boxing in of the tongue in normal activity: an open bite is an open invitation to tongue protrusion. All aspects should be considered. The goal is normal function in a normal environment, for both tongue and teeth.

Some authorities recognize *nasal lisping* and *occluded lisping,* the former being the nasal snort that many cleft cases employ in lieu of /s/ and /z/ and that is rarely seen in other patients, whereas an occluded lisp signifies the substitution of sounds approaching /t/ and /d/ for /s/ and /z/. Nasal lisping might better be considered as part of the generalized condition of the cleft patient; occluded lisping is a common element in the speech of persons with a hearing deficit, specifically of loss in the high-frequency range.

3. *Dentalization of linguoalveolar sounds* is the third articulation problem of particular interest to dentists. The sounds normally produced with the tongue tip against the alveolar ridge are the /t/, /d/, /n/, /l/, and sibilant sounds. Many children with the tongue-thrusting habit tend to produce all these sounds linguodentally. The tongue tip seems to call the anterior teeth "home," and returns there at every opportunity, even including during pauses in conversations. The tongue usually remains positioned anteriorly when not in use and is ready to thrust against the teeth during every swallow of saliva. This habit, in addition to resulting in distorted speech, creates a visually unattractive speech pattern that calls much attention to itself.

DELAYED SPEECH. A previous section dealt with the normal acquisition of speech. When that schedule of development has slowed markedly or halted at an early stage, or when vocabulary is so limited that much communication is achieved by gesture, leaving the child with a few words that are barely intelligible, the condition is called "delayed speech." It has been more specifically defined by Berry and Eisenson:

In all, we may consider that the speech of the child is delayed when (a) it fails to appear or is late in appearance; (b) there are deviations in the sound, syllable, and word patterns so marked as to disturb the intelligibility; or (c) the vocabulary and language patterns are below the norm for one of his chronological age and sex. Delayed speech, then, is a matter of manner, quality, and quantity of performance.*

Unfortunately, many of these children are allowed to reach school, from which they are often rejected, before parents seek professional assistance. The physician pats the child on the head with the customary, "Don't worry, he'll grow out of it." A few persons are seen in their twenties, still waiting to "grow out of it," whatever "it" is. The time to deal with this problem is the earliest possible moment after the child has passed the upper normal limit for any given sound as specified above. The dentist who is able to recognize the symptomatology of delayed speech, and transmit this knowledge to parents, can perform a great and valuable service to his patient. This service may or may not come under the heading of dentistry, but how will we gain the essential information as to whether he is going to have a damaging lisp if we do not teach him to talk?

HYPERNASALITY AND HYPONASALITY. Hypernasality (rhinolalia aperta) may be a concomitant of deviate swallowing; the velopharyngeal mechanism frequently functions abnormally, allowing speech to be directed through the nose excessively. There are many other bases for hypernasality, including, of course, organic anomalies such as cleft palate and palatal paralysis. Hyponasality (rhinolalia clausa), the sound of a constant head cold, is often due to adenoids or a nasal stenosis arising from polyps, a deviated septum, or chronic edema. Referral to a medical specialist is indicated.

HEARING LOSS. Auditory impairment has a direct influence on speech: if the child perceives speech in a distorted manner, his speech will reflect the distortions. Although there are implications for both fields in some cases, neither speech nor dental correction will suffice; the otologist and the clinical audiologist should be consulted. Speech correction may be indicated later.

---

*From Berry, M. F., and Eisenson, J.: Speech disorders: principles and practices of therapy, New York, 1956, Appleton-Century-Crofts, p. 86. By permission of Prentice-Hall, Inc.

RELATIONSHIPS BETWEEN DENTITION AND SPEECH

There are many situations in which the dentist is capable of rendering real assistance to the speech pathologist. Although some patients seem to have the resourcefulness and the ability to overcome dental abnormalities that affect their speech, many others do not. We will discuss in this section some conditions wherein the dentist, by modifying structure, can provide the patient with better equipment with which to produce normal speech.

We shall continue to eliminate cleft lip and palate from discussion, for although these conditions require services from both dentist and therapist, it is believed that a plethora of printed material already exists. Also excluded will be all the rare conditions that are seen once or never in a lifetime by the average dentist; so few children are born with astomia, aglossia, anodontia, a bifid tongue, or a missing jaw.

A considerable amount of material has been written on the subject of dental impairment caused by faulty speech, but very little of a valid and specific nature has been said in print on the potential of dental treatment to improve speech. An excellent treatment of this topic is found in Bloomer's chapter on speech defects associated with dental malocclusions and related abnormalities.[2]

Snow[10] found a positive correlation between the misarticulation of certain consonants and the condition of upper central incisors. Fairbanks and Lintner[3] made a series of dental comparisons between two groups, one with superior speech and one with inferior articulation. They found no significant difference in the height or width of the dental arch and palate, in molar or anterior occlusion, nor in degree of overjet; only open bite conditions were significantly more frequent in the inferior group.

Rathbone[6] called attention to the need for dental recognition of defective speech, devised a test by which the dentist might evaluate speech competency, but advised referral of the patient to a speech correctionist for training.

Rathbone and Snidecor[7] reported a study of ten patients with marked speech defects. Orthodontic treatment was instituted with not only traditional goals in mind but also some thought to effective structures for speech. Although no formal speech therapy was performed, their patients showed a reduction of faulty sounds from a mean of 6.4 to a mean of 1.5. Unfortunately, no ages were given for their subjects, so that no estimate can be formed as to the effect of growth and development, if any, or of other factors that might have influenced the result.

What changes in the patient's speech should the dentist expect to find after correction of dental abnormalities? More to the point, what dental irregularities should be assailed with expectation of improving speech habits? Note first that if there is malocclusion accompanied by speech defect, there is a strong possibility of tongue thrust; if present, the abnormal swallowing behavior may be the basis for both of the other anomalies, or it may be an adaptive pattern. The dentist should make a careful judgment as to the order of importance of each item.

Anterior open bite is perhaps the most rewarding condition; when uncomplicated by defective deglutition, any sibilant sound (/s/, /z/, /sh/, /zh/, /ch/, /j/) *may* be corrected simply by closing the bite. If other sounds are defective, it would be logical to expect their improvement.

Posterior open bite or crossbite would have little effect on speech unless a lateral lisp is in evidence, in which case a lateral tongue thrust is probably responsible for defects of both speech and occlusion. Closed bite and dental spacing have little direct effect on speech, as do high or narrow palates or malposed individual teeth; the latter may interfere with connected discourse but is not associated with a specific speech disorder.

Maxillary protrusion can affect speech in several adverse ways. If incisal labioversion is severe, many patients find it anatomically impossible to occlude the lips for the bilabial plosives /p/, /b/, and /m/; instead these sounds are produced by approximating the lower lip and upper teeth, thus relieving the upper lip of one of its major functions and leading to its further retraction and incompetence. The resultant sound is often acoustically normal but cosmetically unpleasant. Reducing the protrusion and then instituting a program of lip exercises to restore function to the upper lip usually eliminates the speech defect.

If maxillary incisal protrusion is accompanied by gross mandibular retrusion, generalized distortion of many consonants may be noted. In these cases correction of structure should certainly have precedence.

Maxillary protrusion in Class II cases may

also be a major factor in frontal lisping. Reducing the protrusion in this case gives no assurance of speech improvement, but some children find it difficult to perform the necessary tongue positioning to achieve sharp sibilants when the discrepancy between arches is great.

Frequently speech defects that are found in conjunction with Class III cases may be a product of malocclusion. Although some pseudo Class III cases are the product of tongue thrust, the genuine article can cause great speech disturbance. If there is contraction of the maxillary arch, a common circumstance, the apex of the tongue perforce contacts the incisal edges of the maxillary teeth rather than the alveolar and palatal surfaces, thus distorting many sounds. The /f/ and /v/ sounds are often "inverted," that is, produced by touching upper lip to lower teeth rather than by the customary contact of lower lip to upper incisal edges. These sounds in some cases are produced by approximating the lips, which eliminates dental contact and results in obvious distortion of speech. Dental or surgical correction of the structure should be the first step, followed by speech therapy if still necessary.

The above is a fairly complete inventory of the conditions wherein the dentist may expect to render speech correction through modification of structure. Additional sounds may be improved by combining dental treatment with correction of abnormal swallowing; however, the dentist who implies to his patient that treatment will have more far-reaching effects than specified above has stepped beyond the limit of accepted practice.

A final and converse thought in this connection is that even though the denture, prosthesis, or appliance placed in the patient's mouth may not *improve* speech, at least it should be so designed as not to *impede* speech.

People without any teeth at all sometimes speak essentially normally. The flexibility of the tongue, lips, and other articulators permits extensive compensatory action.

Bloomer[2] summarizes relationships between structure and function as follows:

1. Normal structure + normal movements = normal speech.
2. Abnormal structures + maladaptive movements = defective speech.
3. Normal structures + maladaptive movements = defective speech.
4. Abnormal structures + adaptive movements = normal (compensated) speech.*

He concludes:

Considered diagnostically, the relationship between speech and orofacial structures is a complex one. Any decision as to the etiologic significance of orofacial abnormality in an individual instance of defective speech must be interpreted with due regard to the total dynamics of speech and the multiple causes of speech disorders. The diagnostician must evaluate physical growth, the timing of environmental and physioanatomical forces as they inflect the emerging patterns of speech, and the ways in which behavior in turn modifies the directions of physical growth. Thus he must consider not merely the effects of orofacial structure on speech, but also the possible influence of speech habits upon the formation of the dental arches and dental occlusion. He must weigh the effects of personality upon orofacial growth and speech, and the influence which the malfunctions of orofacial structures and speech have upon the personality and upon the life outlook of the individual.†

CONCLUSION

A summary of normal speech development has been presented, along with a brief classification and description of abnormalities, and a discussion of the frequency of their occurrence. It was noted that in most of these conditions formal speech therapy is recommended for proper management.

Also, a résumé was given of those conditions in which speech might be corrected solely through dental treatment, and a few were noted for which dental treatment would not be indicated as a substitute for speech therapy.

There are now some 15,000 speech clinicians scattered about who are certified by the American Speech and Hearing Association, plus several thousand who are active in the field but who do not have their Certificate of Clinical Competence. Most clinicians would be delighted to give advice on the speech problems of your patients. Unfortunately, very few have had formal training in therapy for tongue thrust. This will change as momentum builds and new knowledge is gained.

---

*From Bloomer, H. H.: Speech defects associated with dental abnormalities and malocclusions. In Travis, L. E., editor: Handbook of speech pathology and audiology, New York, 1971, Appleton-Century-Crofts, p. 716.
†Ibid., p. 752.

It may be advisable to stress again what defective speech is *not*. It is not abnormal to see the tongue during connected speech. In particular, it is *normal* for the apex of the tongue to touch or extend beyond the incisal edges in forming /th/ sounds. It is *not* the demonstration of a pernicious lip habit each time a child forms an /f/ or /v/ sound: the lip must contact the upper teeth, even though an effort must be made if malocclusion is severe. The muscular force exerted during normal function on the dentition is far below the level required for deformity.

REFERENCES

1. Berry, M. F., and Eisenson, J.: Speech disorders, New York, 1956, Appleton-Century-Crofts.
2. Bloomer, H. H.: Speech defects associated with dental abnormalities and malocclusions. In Travis, L. E., editor: Handbook of speech pathology and audiology, New York, 1971, Appleton-Century-Crofts.
3. Fairbanks, G., and Lintner, M. V. H.: A study of minor organic deviations in "functional" disorders of articulation. 4. The teeth and the hard palate, J. Speech Hear. Disord. **16**:273, 1951.
4. Palmer, M. F.: Orthodontics and the disorders of speech, Am. J. Orthod. **34**:579, 1948.
5. Pound, E.: Esthetic dentures and their phonetic values, J. Prosthet. Dent. **1**:98, 1951.
6. Rathbone, J. S.: Appraisal of speech defects in dental anomalies, Angle Orthod. **25**:42, 1955.
7. Rathbone, J. S., and Snidecor, J. C.: Appraisal of speech defects in dental anomalies with reference to speech improvement, Angle Orthod. **29**:54, 1959.
8. Ray, H. G., and Santos, H. A.: Considerations of tongue thrusting as a factor in periodontal disease, J. Periodontol. **25**:250, 1954.
9. Slaughter, M. D.: Speech correction in full denture prosthesis, Dent. Dig. **51**:242, 1945.
10. Snow, K.: Articulation proficiency in relation to certain dental abnormalities, J. Speech Hear. Disord. **26**:209, 1961.
11. Van Riper, C.: Speech correction: principles and methods, ed. 4, Englewood Cliffs, N.J., 1963, Prentice-Hall, Inc.

Chapter 3

SOME FUNDAMENTALS OF DENTISTRY

The speech clinician who attempts to modify patterns of deglutition should work in close association with the dentist. The speech pathologist must be capable of understanding and discussing the dental facets of the problem. He should be able to discuss them with the dentist using dental terminology. The speech pathologist, working in the same area of the body as the dentist, may feel that his knowledge of the involved anatomy is excellent—and from a neuromuscular point of view it may be more than adequate—but it is a different knowledge. It is based on different ideas about reaching different goals and couched in different words, extending only superficially into the dental province. The clinician has usually taken courses in psychology. Although not qualified to conduct formal psychotherapy on the basis of mere American Speech and Hearing Association requirements, he gains through his studies insight into normal and abnormal emotional reactions as well as a language with which to understand and join with the psychologist or psychometrician to provide a complete treatment program. Yet, not infrequently, the clinician and the dentist find problems in communication arising from deficits in the clinician's background. This chapter will attempt to bridge those gaps.

THE TOOTH AND ITS SUPPORTING STRUCTURES
Dental anatomy

The tooth is composed of four basic tissues: enamel, dentin, pulp, and cementum (Fig. 3-1).

The *enamel* is the hardest substance in the human body. It is the white, outer surface of the anatomical crown.

The *dentin* forms the body of the tooth, both crown and root. It is yellowish and is composed of a dense, calcified tissue. Much softer than enamel, it is not normally exposed at any point in the natural tooth.

The *pulp* occupies the pulp cavity and the root canals. It is a delicate, fibrous tissue, richly supplied with blood vessels and sensory nerves. It supplies nutritional elements to the main body of the tooth but is primarily concerned with the formation of dentin.

The *cementum* is a layer of modified bone that covers the root of the tooth. Very thin at the cervical line, it thickens toward the apex of the root.

The *apical foramen* is the tiny opening of the root canal at the apex of the root through which pass the blood vessels and nerves supplying the pulp.

Supporting structures

The tooth is supported by four additional tissues, collectively called the *periodontium:* the alveolar process, the periodontal membrane, the mucous membrane and submucosa, and the gingiva (Fig. 3-1).

The *alveolar process* is a band of bone consisting of the portion of both maxilla and mandible that forms and supports the alveoli, or sockets, of the teeth. The alveolar process lies along the occlusal border of the main body of the bone proper and is continuous with it, but it is well to note that whereas the orthodontist is readily able to modify the alveolar process, the bone proper, or *basal bone,* is much less amenable to orthodontic manipulation. Basal bone is the skeletal bone that supports the alveolar bone.

The *periodontal membrane* surrounds the cementum and is composed of bundles of fibers intermixed with connective tissue. The fibers at-

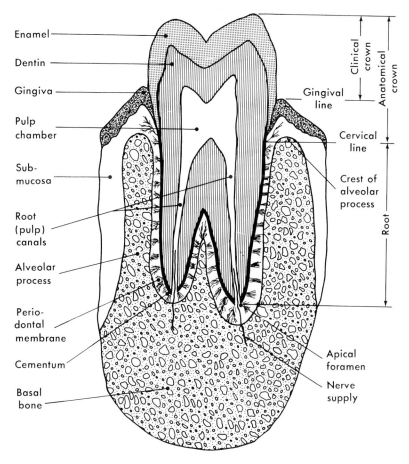

Fig. 3-1. Sagittal section of tooth and alveolus.

tach to the cementum on one side and to the alveolus at the other, thus attaching the tooth to its socket. The connective tissue contains not only blood vessels and lymphatics but also receptor nerves of unusual responsiveness. Differences of only fractions of a millimeter in the thickness of paper can be detected by the proprioceptors located in the periodontal membrane and in the muscles of mastication.[7] The periodontal membrane is also viewed by many dentists today as a ligament, and the tooth-alveolus relationship is seen as a dento-alveolar *joint,* placed in motion by forces of varying pressures acting on the tooth. The basic purpose of the periodontal ligament is, not only to maintain the teeth in their normal position, but also to act as a shock absorber, cushioning occlusal forces as they are transmitted to the bone.[11]

The *oral mucous membrane* consists of two layers: the outer surface epithelium and the *lamina propria.* Between the mucous membrane and the periosteum of the bone lies the *submucosa,* a layer of connective tissue of varying thickness containing blood vessels and nerves.

The *gingiva* (gum) immediately surrounds the tooth and is a keratinized layer of tissue in which no blood vessels are visible, in contrast to the mucous membrane.

DENTAL ORIENTATION
Surfaces of the tooth

Descriptive terminology in dentistry has, of necessity, been altered somewhat from traditional anatomical terms. Because of the curve of the dental arch, a "lateral" surface (the surface farthest from the midsagittal plane) would not indicate corresponding parts of an incisor and a molar; it would describe the surface of an incisor facing a neighboring tooth, whereas it would mean the buccal surface of a molar. Special usage has therefore developed.

The point of orientation is the sagittal midline of the dental arch. The surface of any tooth that lies nearest the median line, following the curve of the dental arch, is called the *mesial* surface, whereas the surface farthest from the median line is called the *distal* surface. Two surfaces of each tooth are thus described.

However, anterior teeth have four surfaces, and posterior teeth have five. The surface lying nearest the lips is known as the *labial* surface in the case of the incisors and cuspids, whereas the corresponding surface of bicuspids and molars is called the *buccal* surface. Opposite this surface, all teeth have a *lingual* surface; it is becoming increasingly popular to simplify this terminology by referring to both the labial and buccal planes as the *facial* surface, while still others prefer the term *vestibular* surface. Thus the anterior teeth have mesial, distal, labial (facial), and lingual surfaces. Bicuspids and molars have additionally an *occlusal* surface: that surface which contacts the corresponding tooth in the opposite dental arch. In the case of anterior teeth this part of the tooth is the *incisal edge* rather than a surface.

The *proximal* surface is an indefinite term simply indicating the surface facing or approximating a neighboring tooth, whether mesial or distal.

Similar terminology is used to locate any line, point, or other feature of a tooth, for example, the *lingual* groove or the *mesial* pit. Where two surfaces approach each other, the area is indicated by dropping off the final letters of the name of one surface, replacing them with "o", and then combining the two names. Thus the *mesiobuccal* ridge, the *distolingual* cusp, etc., differentiate precise features.

The occlusal surfaces of posterior teeth are extremely complex; dentists of an earlier day frequently used the analogy of a "gristmill" in referring to this region. A smooth, flat surface would make trituration of many foods impossible, but simple edges would prove disadvantageous for a number of reasons. Instead the surface is so arranged as to allow the complex

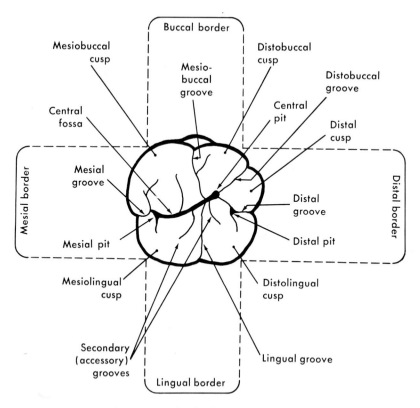

Fig. 3-2. Some landmarks of occlusal surface.

rotary motion of mastication with maximum tooth contact in all ranges of occlusal articulation.

Topographical features

An illustration of the topography of the region is given in Fig. 3-2. The crown of the tooth is characterized by the following principal features: pits, grooves, fossae, cusps, ridges, and inclined planes.

Pits are sharp depressions usually found at the junction of two or more grooves.

Grooves, also called sulci, are long, narrow depressions in the enamel that may extend over the edge of the occlusal surface onto the sides of the tooth. Some are called *primary* or developmental grooves because they are constant and are a developmental part of the particular surface on which they occur. *Secondary,* or accessory, grooves include the other grooves that occur on the occlusal surface; they are less deep and less constant.

Fossae are large depressed areas, some smooth and shallow, others deep and angular. An example of the former occurs on the lingual surface of the maxillary incisors, whereas the latter are found primarily on the occlusal surfaces, where they are formed by pits and grooves, bounded by ridges, and named for the pit they encompass. Thus the *central fossa* surrounds the central pit.

Cusps are the high points, or marked elevations, of enamel, which lead to the names of certain teeth; that is, a cuspid is a tooth with one cusp, and a bicuspid has two cusps. Molars, of course, commonly have four, but some have three or five cusps.

Ridges are long convex elevations of enamel found on all surfaces except the mesial and distal. The incisors have ridges running gingivally from the incisal edge; for other teeth, almost all ridges extend down from the point of a cusp.

Inclined planes are the sloping areas on the occlusal surface that lie between the crests of the ridges and the primary grooves. They are of various shapes and are usually crossed by secondary grooves.

Fig. 3-3 shows the tooth in lateral aspect. It may be noted that the area where two proximal surfaces meet is called the *contact,* or *contact point.* Because of the contour of the teeth, triangular-shaped spaces, called *embrasures,* are created between the crowns; they extend in four directions from the contact area. The occlusal embrasure is noted in Fig. 3-3, as in the gingival embrasure, also known as the *interproximal space.* There are also lingual and buccal embrasures.

Relationship of tooth to arch

It is often necessary to describe the position of a tooth in relation to the dental arch in which it

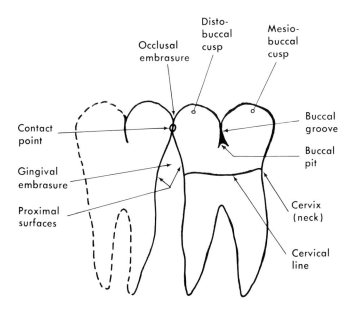

Fig. 3-3. Tooth-to-tooth relationship.

occurs, and thereby to its adjoining teeth. The system most frequently used is Lischer's. He used the proper term to indicate the direction from the normal, added the suffix "-version," and arrived at the following:

Mesioversion—mesial to the normal position.
Distoversion—distal to the normal position.
Linguoversion—toward the tongue.
Labioversion (or buccoversion)—toward the lip (or cheek).
Infraversion—away from (not reaching) the line of occlusion.
Supraversion—extending past the line of occlusion.
Axioversion—wrong axial inclination, tipped.
Torsioversion—rotated on its long axis.
Transversion—wrong order in the arch, transposed.*

The term "supereruption" or "overeruption" is usually acceptable in lieu of supraversion. *Intraversion* and *extraversion* indicate teeth or other maxillary structures that are too near or too far from the median plane. When a tooth is bodily malposed, it is said to be *displaced,* but if only tipped or tilted, it is mesially, distally, lingually, labially, or bucally *inclined.* If the entire incisor segment is inclined labially or lingually, it is usually called *protrusion* or *retrusion,* respectively, and when both upper and lower incisors protrude, the proper term is *bimaxillary protrusion.*

DENTAL DEVELOPMENT
Deciduous and permanent teeth

The subject of oral histology and embryology fills many volumes, at least a few of which should be surveyed by anyone purporting to do serious work with deglutition. Any treatment here would necessarily be so incomplete as to frustrate the research person and bewilder the neophyte. With the firm realization that teeth are not surgically grafted into the mouth, but are subject to the same histological and embryological processes as other tissues, we will outline the more obvious developments.

The enamel organ of the first tooth bud forms at about the fourth or fifth month of intrauterine life. These buds gradually differentiate from their genetic tissues, and calcification of the crown begins. Once the crown is complete, root starts to form, and with root comes eruption.

That is, the newborn is found to have the skeletal bone of the jaws proper, but only rudimentary alveolar bone, which develops only as required to encase the growing teeth. We might pause to note that the fetal tongue protrudes between the gum pads, completely covers the skeletal bone of the lower jaw, and approaches closely, or actually contacts, the lingual surface of the lower lip. This lingual posture is continued by the neonate in nursing, the tongue and lip working in mutual opposition once function begins. The environment into which the tooth is born is thus as stressful as the cruel world into which the baby himself is deposited. Before a tooth has erupted, the developing alveolar bone is subjected to definite shaping forces from the counteracting tongue and lip, so that the teeth must then intrude between two already veteran antagonists, the results of which form the fountainhead of this volume.

The teeth that usually erupt first are the mandibular central incisors, usually at about 7 months of age. Both Moyers[9] and Salzmann[10] state that the time of arrival of the various teeth, providing it is within broad normal limits, is of relatively small importance; the significant factor is the *sequence* in which the teeth erupt. The usual order for the primary dentition is central incisor, lateral incisor, first molar, cuspid, and second molar, with the mandibular tooth erupting one to four months before the antagonist tooth in the maxillary arch. In most cases the

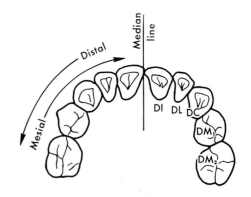

Fig. 3-4. Arrangement of deciduous teeth in dental arch. *DI,* Deciduous central incisor; *DL,* deciduous lateral incisor; *DC,* deciduous cuspid; *DM₁,* first deciduous molar; *DM₂,* second deciduous molar. The term *distal* refers to surface, point, or movement *away* from median line; *mesial* implies surface, point, or movement *toward* median line.

---

*From Lischer, B. E.: Principles and methods of orthodontics, Philadelphia, 1912, Lea & Febiger.

primary dentition is completed between 2½ and 3 years of age.

As indicated in Fig. 3-4, the decidous teeth in each arch total ten, or twenty teeth in the two arches. The mandibular arch is normally the contained arch, that is, the lower teeth fit within the circumference of the maxillary teeth when brought into habitual occlusion.

To simplify the identification of the permanent teeth, it is customary to start with the central incisor at the median line and number the teeth posteriorly around half of the dental arch, as seen in Fig. 3-5. By then adding the prefatory terms of maxillary or mandibular, right or left, all thirty-two teeth are named. This is often shown graphically on dental charts, as in Fig. 3-6.

Numbers are used to show the permanent teeth, and letters indicate deciduous teeth. Note that right and left are oriented as in facing the patient. The heavy vertical line represents the midline, the heavy horizontal line the occlusal plane. Thus the circled number in Fig. 3-6 identifies the mandibular left first permanent molar somewhat more succinctly than words. Carrying this scheme further, it has been found expeditious in the literature to abbreviate the heavy crossed lines of Fig. 3-6 into a mere angle and tuck in the appropriate numeral or letter from the chart, so that 6 would signify the same mandibular left first permanent molar, B would be the maxillary decidous right lateral incisor, etc.

An alternative to the identification procedure shown above is the "universal" numbering system presented in Fig. 3-7. In this case, numbering starts with the upper right third molar, continues around the arch to the upper left third molar, and then drops down to the lower left third molar and comes back around the mandibular arch. Deciduous teeth are handled in similar fashion, again with letters instead of numerals used to indicate the distinction. This plan is believed to be more precise, since every tooth in each arch is provided with its individual designation; there is only one number 28, whereas three other teeth are referred to as "4's" in the traditional system discussed first. The "universal" scheme is used exclusively in military dental services.

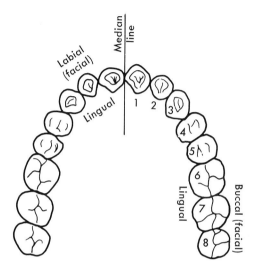

Fig. 3-5. Identification of permanent teeth and their relationship within dental arch. *1*, Central incisor; *2*, lateral incisor; *3*, cuspid (canine); *4*, first bicuspid (premolar); *5*, second bicuspid (premolar); *6*, first molar; *7*, second molar; *8*, third molar (wisdom tooth). The term *labial* indicates surfaces around front of arch extending to distal surface of cuspids, whereas *buccal* describes outside area on each side that lies posterior to cuspids. *Facial* may imply either.

Right	E	D	C	B	A	A	B	C	D	E	Left		
8	7	6	5	4	3	2	1	1	2	3	4	5	6	7	8
8	7	6	5	4	3	2	1	1	2	3	4	5	(6)	7	8
	E	D	C	B	A	A	B	C	D	E			

Fig. 3-6. Dental symbols proposed by Committee on Nomenclature of American Dental Association.

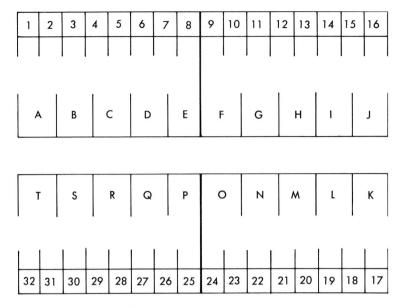

Fig. 3-7. The "universal" numbering system.

Table 3-1. Time of eruption of the teeth

Primary dentition		Permanent dentition	
Central incisors	5- 8 mo.	First molars	5- 7 yr.
Lateral incisors	8-10 mo.	Central incisors	6- 8 yr.
First molars	10-16 mo.	Lateral incisors	7- 9 yr.
Cuspids	16-20 mo.	First bicuspids	8-10 yr.
Second molars	20-30 mo.	Mandibular cuspids	9-11 yr.
		Second bicuspids	10-12 yr.
		Maxillary cuspids	11-13 yr.
		Second molars	12-14 yr.
		Third molars	17 yr. up

Eruption

Many orthodontists feel that the most important phase in the life cycle of a tooth is the process of eruption. Little can be done about this aspect regarding the primary dentition, but elaborate natal plans often precede the permanent tooth, as we shall see in the discussion of "serial extraction." Although the process of eruption continues at a reduced rate throughout the life of the tooth, it is considered primarily as the complex of activities that carry the tooth from its developmental crypt into the mouth and into occlusion with an antagonist tooth. As the roots of a permanent tooth elongate, driving the crown through the gingiva, additional alveolar bone is deposited, and the roots of the deciduous predecessors are resorbed. Although these three processes are usually synchronized, they may be less dependent on one another than has been thought.[9]

As previously noted, the expected time of arrival of the teeth may vary rather widely, and many schedules have been proposed in many books. It is known that eruption is under endocrine control but may be influenced by heredity, pathological conditions in the mouth, or systemic disease. The times shown in Table 3-1 are intended to show some general averages and certainly do not reflect upper and lower normal limits.

The sequence of eruption of the permanent teeth is shown in Table 3-1 and is in part a function of the exfoliation of the deciduous teeth. The normal order, under the ideal conditions

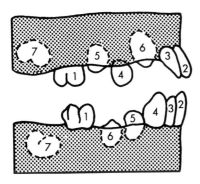

Fig. 3-8. A favorable eruption sequence of permanent teeth.

Table 3-2. Normal sequence of eruption

Mandible	Maxilla
1. First molar	
2. Central incisor	
	3. First molar
4. Lateral incisor	
	5. Central incisor
	6. Lateral incisor
7. Cuspid	
8. First bicuspid	
	9. First bicuspid
	10. Second bicuspid
11. Second bicuspid	
	12. Cuspid
13. Second molar	
	14. Second molar

that customarily prevail, is shown in Table 3-2, and perhaps more graphically in Fig. 3-8. Many studies have shown that any other sequence leads to malocclusion; in some cases the malocclusion can thus be identified prior to its actual development.

Mixed dentition

The mixed dentition stage is the period of time during which both deciduous and permanent teeth are present in the oral cavity. It ordinarily covers some six or seven years, beginning with eruption of the first permanent molar and ending with loss of the second deciduous molars.

During this state of flux, when teeth are coming, going, shifting, turning, and seeking a permanent state of balance, much may appear abnormal to the untrained eye which is in fact mere routine development. Although many malocclusions have their inception at this time, bites that

are open may eventually close, malposed teeth may drift into alignment, and first permanent molars in cusp-to-cusp relationship may, with arrival of the bicuspids, interdigitate normally. It is a time when muscle forces, specifically those of mastication and deglutition, play a major role in developing the dentition. Yet it is a time when the therapist should be in close contact with the dentist, who is able to separate the routine from the incipient abnormality.

WASTELAND OF DENTAL "OCCLUSION"

The path of the tourist gets a bit hazardous in this region. Many authors have described it, seldom are the same words used, and when used they seldom mean the same thing. One small part of the area, "centric" occlusion, has been referred to at various times and by various authorities as: centric position, centric relation, dorsal position, gothic arch central position, habitual rest position, retruded centric relation, retruded rest position, terminal occlusion, terminal occlusal position, true centric relation, unstrained centric relation, true centric position, eccentric jaw relationship, eccentric intercuspation, functional centric relation, functional centric position, normal centric relation, true relaxed centric position, true mandibular centric position, true rest centric position, plus quite a few more. The accompanying description differs to some degree in each case even though all attempt to define the same basic phenomenon. In view of the fact that a list of similar proportion might be offered of synonyms for "speech pathologist," the clinician is advised not to cast stones.

We are safe in assuming that occlusion has to do with the bringing together of the upper and lower teeth. Since the upper teeth are immobile, we may take the next step and view this as a mandibular function. The end product should be the interdigitation of the cusps of the teeth in some manner. However, the concept of occlusion is broad enough to include also the relationship of teeth within each dental arch and the form of the arch itself, as well as the relationship of arch to arch.

The structure of the temporomandibular joint makes possible a wide range of motion other than a simple hingelike closure. Occlusion is thus not a fixed, static position, as is obvious during oral examination when the child, under direction to close the teeth, protrudes the jaw and approximates the incisal edges. Occlusion is best thought of as an act, a motion, a verb; it is what occurs when the mandible moves from the resting position, where there is freeway space (vertical space between the cusps of the two arches) past the point of contact of the multidirectional inclined planes of the cusps—as many as eighteen inclined planes on a lower first molar—through the process of twisting and rotation that is brought to bear on the individual tooth when these inclined planes slide down each other, to a terminal position of interlocking cusps. If one wishes to indicate only the final phase, it is necessary to append the word "position." Occlusion and occlusal position are not synonymous terms.

As speech is a learned function, so, evidently, is occlusion. With eruption of the teeth and the development of their periodontal membranes, sensations of touch and pressure are carried to the brain through the mesencephalic root of the fifth cranial nerve.[9] These sensations in turn monitor and modify the motor impulses transmitted to the muscles that control mandible posture. With experience, the muscles learn to position the mandible in such a way that torque or other stress on the roots of the teeth is minimal while still providing a maximum of dental contact. The teeth are then in "occlusion."

It is well to remember that it is the neuromuscular system that coordinates and integrates mandibular movement. The constant feedback from the periodontal membrane serves as a guide, the musculature seeks a state of balance, and we find an intimate relationship between the interdigitation of the teeth, the status of the controlling musculature, and the integrity of the temporomandibular joint. It is the interaction of all these anatomical features which makes possible an accurate posture and pattern of movement that can be constantly reproduced.[11]

It is true that teeth are in "occlusion" during deglutition, which means that there is cusp-to-fossa contact of opposing teeth reinforced by the temporal, masseter, and other antigravity muscles. It is well to keep in mind, however, a dynamic concept of the occlusal position as being only the terminal phase, momentarily maintained, of the broader synergy of occlusion that also includes masticatory movement and the physiological rest position.

Graber's[6] brief chapter on "normal occlusion" is highly recommended for lucidity and historical material. Ideas are still fluid and often in sharp conflict, particularly as pertains to temporomandibular joint function and dysfunction, and although the orthodontist seeks a stable occlusion, he also seeks a stable *concept* of occlusion. However, a few specific definitions are now possible, based on the foregoing.

centric occlusion (1) The relationship of the teeth to each other when the jaws are closed so that the lingual cusps of the maxillary bicuspids and molars, and the buccal cusps of the mandibular bicuspids and molars, rest in the deepest parts of the sulci of the maxillary bicuspids and molars. (2) The relationship of the upper and lower teeth to one another when the jaws are completely closed at rest.

normal or ideal occlusal position Terms that can then be used to indicate the best possible occlusion of which a given mouth is *potentially* capable. Characteristics include dental arches of concentric curves in which (1) the maxillary arch is slightly larger than the mandibular arch; (2) there is maximal contact of dental surfaces on which the direction of force coincides as nearly as possible with the long axis of the teeth; (3) minimal torque results from the twisting effect of inclined planes sliding in contact; and (4) muscle forces are in equilibrium; and the mesiobuccal cusp of the maxillary permanent first molar articulates in the buccal groove of the mandibular permanent first molar. Such an occlusion is seen in Fig. 3-9.

eccentric occlusion Any occlusal position other than the ideal occlusal position. Since nature constantly deviates from perfection, this term is useful.

habitual or usual occlusal position The occlusal position customarily used by the patient; it may be an ideal occlusion or a completely eccentric one.

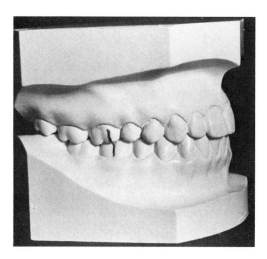

Fig. 3-9. Normal centric occlusion of permanent teeth. All teeth are in contact, with normal molar relationship.

retruded occlusal position A controversial position in which the heads of the condyles are in their most retruded position and the teeth are in occlusion. It has been proposed as a definition of centric occlusion, but it is a strained position and probably has greater value as a research tool than in practical application.

bite When a dentist remarks that "her bite is good," he refers to the fact that the basic features of the patient's habitual occlusion are satisfactory, but he in no way implies that there are not individual teeth, or several of them, which are malpositioned in some way.

One concept that seems to be poorly understood by laymen is the distinction between "overbite" and "overjet." In normal occlusion, the incisal edges of the mandibular teeth occlude against the lingual surface of the maxillary antagonists in such a way that approximately one third of the mandibular crown is concealed, as shown in Fig. 3-10. This overhang is sometimes called "vertical overbite" but more commonly is known simply as *overbite*. It is a strictly vertical dimension. If the incisors are in edge-to-edge relationship during habitual occlusion, there is zero overbite. When a space or vertical distance remains between the incisal or occlusal surfaces during habitual occlusion, the result is called *open bite*. Excessive overbite, where the upper arch so engulfs the lower that little or none of the mandibular incisor is visible, is referred to as *closed bite*.

On the other hand, *overjet* is an anteroposterior dimension and implies the distance on the horizontal plane between the lingual surfaces of the upper incisors and the labial surfaces of the lower incisors.

Crossbite is seen in Fig. 3-11 and refers to one or more teeth that are malposed buccally, lingually, or labially with reference to the opposing tooth or teeth.

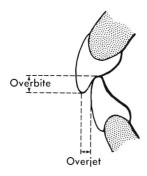

Fig. 3-10. Distinction between overbite (a vertical dimension) and overjet (a horizontal dimension).

MALOCCLUSION
Etiology of malocclusion

The field of orthodontics has made remarkable progress in the past few years toward becoming a more exact science, much as we have been attempting in speech pathology. Both are relatively young specialties, and both are intensively seeking out explanations and remedial procedures for the various phenomena with which they are presented.

It has been evident for some time that more pervasive concepts of multiple causation must supplant older theories of a simple cause-and-effect relationship. There is strong interplay and interdependence of extrinsic and intrinsic factors of prenatal and postnatal influences in the emergence of malocclusion.

If one holds in mind the invisible lines connecting each category with every other, one of the more complete classifications of etiological factors is offered by Graber:

Extrinsic factors (general)
1. Heredity (the inherited pattern)
2. Congenital defects (cleft palate, torticollis, cleidocranial dysostosis, cerebral palsy, syphilis, etc.)
3. Environment
   a. Prenatal (trauma, maternal diet, maternal metabolism, German measles, etc.)

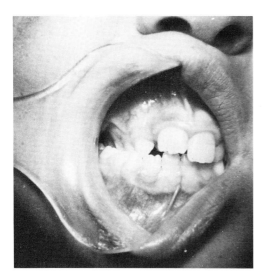

Fig 3-11. Unilateral crossbite. Mandibular molars are not contained within upper arch.

b. Postnatal (birth injury, cerebral palsy, TMJ injury, etc.)
4. Predisposing metabolic climate and disease
  a. Endocrine imbalance
  b. Metabolic disturbances
  c. Infectious diseases (polio, etc.)
5. Dietary problems (nutritional deficiency)
6. Abnormal pressure habits
  a. Abnormal suckling (forward mandibular posture, nonphysiologic nursing, excessive buccal pressures, etc.)
  b. Thumb and finger sucking
  c. Tongue thrust and tongue sucking
  d. Lip and nail biting
  e. Abnormal swallowing habits (improper deglutition)
  f. Speech defects
  g. Respiratory abnormalities (mouth breathing, etc.)
  h. Tonsils and adenoids (compensatory tongue position)
7. Posture
8. Trauma and accidents

Intrinsic factors (local)
1. Anomalies of number
  a. Supernumerary teeth
  b. Missing teeth (congenital absence or loss due to accidents, caries, etc.)
2. Anomalies of tooth size
3. Anomalies of tooth shape
4. Abnormal labial frenum
5. Premature loss
6. Prolonged retention
7. Delayed eruption of permanent teeth
8. Abnormal eruptive path
9. Ankylosis
10. Dental caries
11. Improper dental restorations*

It might be well to read this list one more time, noting that some thirty items are included, one of which is abnormal swallowing (two, if you noticed that "tongue thrust" was listed apart from deglutition). Twenty-eight other possible factors are included. Teaching a child to swallow correctly does not assure beautiful teeth or effortless orthodontic treatment. But it helps.

Classification of malocclusion

The man who brought order out of chaos in the young field of orthodontics was Dr. Edward H. Angle (1855-1930). He inspired zealous adherents and bitter antagonists, but his intense efforts resulted in a systematization of knowl-

*From Graber, T. M.: Orthodontics: principles and practice, ed. 2, Philadelphia, 1972, W. B. Saunders Co., pp. 568, 571.

edge formerly unknown. His name lives on in the name of a professional journal and a professional organization but is probably voiced most often in connection with the Angle system of classification of malocclusions. He did not have the benefit of modern research, and many of his ideas proved erroneous, but the Angle classification is used quite extensively today much as it was presented in 1907, despite seventy years of attacks on its adequacy. Angle was preoccupied with the position of the maxillary first permanent molar as the foundation on which to build, "the key of occlusion," and thus saw occlusion as a static horizontal relation of arch to arch, neglecting considerations on the lateral and vertical planes and the dynamics of dental function. The following is a restatement of the Angle classification (Angle, 1907, pp. 36-59), with Lischer's terms (1912, pp. 89-96) shown in parentheses:

Class I (neutrocclusion). Those malocclusions characterized by normal mesiodistal relationship between the mandible and maxilla. The mesiobuccal cusp of the maxillary first permanent molar articulates in the mesiobuccal groove of the mandibular first permanent molar, as shown in Fig. 3-12. Malocclusion occurs in the anterior segments; one or many teeth may be deflected from their normal course.

Class II (distocclusion). Those malocclusions in which there is retrusion of the mandible, the lower arch being distal from normal in its relation to the upper arch. The mesiobuccal groove of the mandibular first permanent

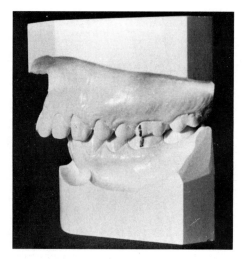

Fig. 3-12. Angle Class I relationship. First permanent molars are in normal posture; malocclusion is confined to anterior teeth.

molar articulates posteriorly to the mesiobuccal cusp of the maxillary first permanent molar.

> *Division 1.* Bilaterally distal, the maxillary incisors being typically in extreme labioversion (Fig. 3-13). Angle noted that these cases were primarily associated with mouth breathing.
>
> *Subdivision.* Unilateral distocclusion, molar relationship normal on one side of the dental arch.
>
> *Division 2.* Bilateral distocclusion in which the maxillary central incisors are near normal or slightly retruded, whereas the maxillary lateral incisors have tipped labially and mesially (Fig. 3-14).

Class III (mesiocclusion). Those malocclusions in which there is protrusion of the mandible, a mesial

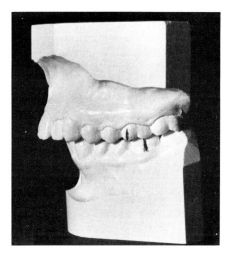

Fig. 3-13. Angle Class II, Division 1, malocclusion. Entire mandibular arch is retruded, with upper incisors in labioversion.

relationship of mandible to maxilla. The mesiobuccal groove of the mandibular first permanent molar articulates anteriorly to the mesiobuccal cusp of the maxillary first molar (Fig. 3-15).

DENTAL TREATMENT OF THE YOUNG CHILD

Despite the fact that many schoolchildren now aspire to the status symbol of full bands, many millions of American children with malocclusion will never see an orthodontist. It has been estimated that over 50% of our population have dental irregularities; obviously, a much smaller percentage receives orthodontic treatment.

The American Dental Association has long urged the forestalling of problems before they occur, and it has laid this responsibility on every dentist to protect the dental interests of the majority of children. Dental service should be viewed in the progression: prevention, interception, correction. Time is the differentiating factor. If handled early, many dental defects can be avoided; if allowed to start, many can still be redirected before permanent damage ensues; if all else fails or if nothing has been attempted, only formal correction of the abnormalities remains.

Preventive orthodontics

Preventive orthodontics should be the concern of the general dentist and pedodontist. Its aim is

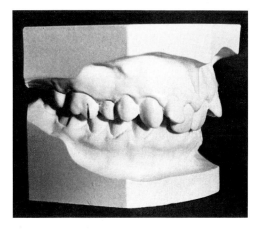

Fig. 3-14. Angle Class II, Division 2, malocclusion. Note characteristic posture of upper incisors.

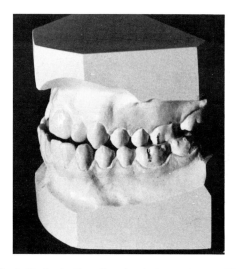

Fig. 3-15. Angle Class III malocclusion. Entire mandibular arch is protruded. In extreme form (prognathism), mandibular arch engulfs the whole of maxillary arch.

to eliminate or minimize the need for orthodontic attention at a later date.

The repair of caries is important; maintaining the primary teeth in good condition and position until they are replaced normally by the permanent teeth is a vital step in preventing malocclusion. The entire critical eruption cycle should be guided as necessary by close observance of the pattern of resorption of the deciduous roots and by the judicious use of space maintainers when early loss is sustained. Attention should also be given to gingivitis or other periodontal disease, tooth injury, ectopic eruption, supernumerary teeth, and other factors that influence the eruption of the permanent dentition.

Serial extraction of teeth, when indicated, is a preventive measure; it will be discussed separately, as will occlusal equilibration, which can be a major factor in both preventive and interceptive services.

The labial frenum may require careful evaluation by the dentist, for proper management can be most essential when diastema is truly the product of the frenum. The upper labial frenum normally attaches to the alveolar crest at birth but usually migrates in a superior direction as teeth and alveolar ridge develop; in some cases this migration is incomplete, and instead a body of tough, fibrous membrane develops between the maxillary central incisors, as seen in Fig. 3-16. Surgical excision of this unyielding mass may allow closure of the diastema, although some dentists believe that it should not be done

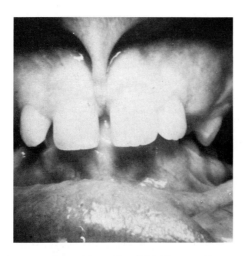

Fig. 3-16. Abnormal maxillary labial frenum. Hypertrophied frenum has failed to migrate upward, thus maintaining diastema between central incisors.

until the permanent canines have completed eruption. Anterior spacing may be a part of normal development, it may be hereditary, or it may be the product of abnormal function of the tongue. In those cases in which tongue pressure is maintaining the space, early frenum excision allows scar tissue to form at the site. The cicatricial mass is as resistant as the original frenum, and the result is therefore disappointing. If the tongue malfunction is corrected prior to the oral surgery, mesial drift or the eruption of the permanent second molars may quickly eliminate the space.

It is in the area of oral habits that we may yet make our greatest advances in preventive orthodontics, and it is here that the oral myologist may make an important contribution. It is possible that far greater numbers of malocclusions result from aberrant orofacial myofunction than is realized even now. We know very little, really, of the etiology of either malocclusion or tongue thrust. We are still at the stage of opinion (Chapter 8). We may state our opinion that once we learn enough to *prevent* abnormal deglutition, we will remove a large segment of malocclusions before they develop; in the interim, we can prevent some malocclusions, and help to correct others, by *treating* abnormal deglutition.

Interceptive orthodontics

Rather than maintaining an occlusion that is still normal, the interceptive program attempts to restore normal occlusion in a mouth already going astray. Many of the procedures mentioned as preventive measures may be extended into use here. Certainly oral habits play a major role; elimination of thumb sucking, lip habits, cheek biting, tongue thrust, etc., is fundamental. Occlusal equilibration, extraction of supernumerary or ankylosed teeth, and education of parent and child concerning the importance of dental health, are all as essential here as in prevention. It has been reliably estimated that over one fourth of all malocclusions can be intercepted, given proper procedures at the proper time.[4]

Interceptive procedures, however, generally imply a wider use of mechanical force. Some of the simple removable appliances described in the following chapter may be employed. A central incisor erupting in a crossbite position may be corrected in two or three weeks by the carefully directed use of a tongue depressor. Abnormal spacing in the anterior maxillary segment may be closed by various means, although indiscriminate measures can lead to serious problems. Lip exercises or the playing of a wind instrument may be prescribed to stimulate a flaccid upper lip, which in turn is allowing incisal protrusion. The propensity of the dentist for mechanical appliances has led to the use of a wide array of wire and plastic devices that exercise muscles, stop finger sucking, correct tongue thrust, and prevent mouth breathing.

Preventive and interceptive measures influence incipient malocclusions or modify developmental factors that induce the problem. Given some of the etiological factors previously listed, malocclusions become inevitable. The following chapter will deal primarily with corrective procedures, the final step in the series.

ADDITIONAL IMPORTANT TERMS
Equilibration

Occlusal equilibration was once the province of the periodontist only, but the general dentist has recently been acquiring new skill in this area. It often also forms a routine part of the final stage of orthodontic treatment.

Occlusal equilibration involves the detailed study of the occlusal contact of each tooth with its antagonist, the elimination of premature or interfacing occlusal contacts, the "wheel balancing" of the entire stomatognathic system, and through these a distribution of the load to all elements in equal proportion during mastication and deglutition. The *stomatognathic system* consists of the bones of the skull, plus the mandible, hyoid, clavicle, and sternum; the muscles and ligaments attached thereto; the dento-alveolar and temporomandibular joints; the vascular, lymphatic, and nerve supply systems; the soft tissues of the head; and the teeth. Note again that the tooth-alveolus articulation is treated as a joint.

The goal of equilibration is to assist nature in making compensatory adjustments throughout the stomatognathic system that will allow the forces dealt to and through the teeth to be distributed within normal limits to all components of the system.[11] This prevents harmful stress on any given structure and provides for equal wear of all occlusal surfaces, thus smoothing the operation of the stomatognathic system and enhancing its integrity.

When this system is viewed as an interrelated whole, it becomes apparent that any influence affecting one element must echo through the entire system. It would seem logical that any aberration of deglutition sufficient to force certain teeth out of occlusion would throw an intolerable load on the teeth remaining in occlusion, would result in abnormal function of other parts, and would destroy the normal integration of the total stomatognathic system.

The actual process of equilibrating the occlusion may be quite intricate. Basically, it consists of making study models of both arches, making a record of the patient's bite on sheets of wax, identifying from these sheets any points where there is premature contact of cusps as the patient closes in occlusion, and then reshaping the teeth by grinding away the unwanted contact or by forming an inclined plane that will direct the bite into a normal position. When properly done, the forces of occlusion, working through the inclined planes of the teeth, can actually move certain teeth into a more functional position and restore harmony to the stomatognathic system.

Serial extraction

The adjectival element in "serial extraction" is the operant word. This concept is not related to routine tooth extraction but rather is a carefully planned and precisely timed program involving removal of selected teeth over a period of four or five years, either in combination with mechanical treatment or, in ideal cases, as the sole procedure in preventing the development of malocclusion.

Ordinary tooth sacrifice during orthodontic treatment is not rare, for the removal of four bicuspids is commonplace. The critical task in any orthodontic program is not moving teeth but finding a place to put them. It seems that nature is generous in proportioning the teeth but does not squander a fraction of a centimeter on alveolar parking lots. Thus when the orthodontist adds up the width of all the teeth in an arch and then measures the total length of the arch itself, he usually finds a shortage of bone. No successful attempt has ever been made to increase permanently the available alveolar distance despite the fact that until 1940 most orthodontic treatment was aimed at "expanding the arch." Since the tooth-to-arch ratio must be balanced, an ear was finally turned to those who, for years, had been practicing and preaching a reduction in the number of teeth in the arch. Dr. Angle had promulgated an almost worshipful regard for each tooth and believed that every one was necessary for a normal dentition.

Now that the principle of essential tooth sacrifice has been accepted, programs first proposed 200 years ago have been perfected for orderly and optimum removal in a physiological sequence. This is serial extraction. Although individual differences may demand a change in continuity, a frequently employed program starts at 5 or 6 years of age with removal of the four deciduous cuspids, thus allowing the eruption and optimal alignment of the permanent lateral incisors. At a later date, or at the same time if the patient has not been seen sufficiently early, the first deciduous molars are extracted in hopes of encouraging the eruption of the first bicuspids ahead of the cuspids. Since nature does not always cooperate, it occasionally becomes necessary to surgically remove the bud of the undeveloped first bicuspid, but this measure is avoided if possible. Most orthodontists prefer to wait until the first bicuspids begin to erupt, and then remove them, allowing the permanent cuspids to drop distally into the space created. In well-handled cases the patient finishes with normal occlusion, short only the expendable first bicuspids and having undergone no mechanical treatment. More often, some banding procedure is also necessary. The presence of an abnormal muscular force, such a tongue thrust, jeopardizes any serial extraction program. However, when myofunctional therapy is provided shortly after eruption of the permanent lateral incisors, it serves as a strong adjunct to the extraction program, and the results can be most gratifying.

Resection

In a few cases of adult malocclusion, mostly Class III, the only recourse is ostectomy (or the sliding of cut sections of the mandible along one another). In occlusion, teeth should be in a relatively perpendicular relationship with basal bone; otherwise, occlusion itself becomes a traumatic force. If placing the teeth in occlusion would require such extensive tipping as to be injurious, resection may be required. In the true prognathic Class III jaw, heredity is presumed to be the guilty factor, and muscle training seemingly has little influence. We have seen very rare cases of adults with such severe Class II, Division 1 malocclusions, aggravated by abnormal swallowing habits, that maxillary resection was performed. It was thought essential to abate the tongue pressure prior to surgery in these cases.

CONCLUSION

This has been a brief, broad, "shotgun" glance at the vast field of dentistry. Included have been only terms and concepts about which the speech pathologist might reasonably be expected to converse intelligently in the process of dealing with problems of deglutition. The references listed after this chapter contain a great storehouse of information and are heartily recommended to those who wish to delve deeper.

The glossary provided immediately hereafter includes most of the essential terms. The clinician should have some recognition of each term. The majority of the items have been used or discussed in this chapter, some will appear in the chapter to follow, while the others seemed to require only definition.

GLOSSARY OF DENTAL TERMS

aberrant Wandering or deviating from the usual or normal course.

abrasion The wearing away of tooth substance by mechanical means.

abutment A tooth used for the support or anchorage of a fixed or removable prosthesis.

alignment The line of adjustment of the teeth.

alveolar process The ridge projecting from the lower surface of the body of the maxilla or the upper surface of the mandible containing the alveoli of the teeth.

alveolar septum The bony wall that separates individual alveoli.

alveolus; pl., alveoli A tooth socket. A cavity in the jawbone that envelops the root of the tooth.

anatomical crown The portion of the tooth that is covered by enamel.

anatomical landmark A readily recognizable anatomical structure used as a point of reference in establishing the location of another structure or in determining certain measurements.

angle A sharp bend formed by two borders or surfaces. A point. The angle of a tooth is the line or point where two or more surfaces meet.

ankyloglossia (tongue-tie) Partial or complete fusion of the tongue with the floor of the mouth or the alveolar crest; caused by lingual frenum being abnormally short or abnormally attached.

ankylosis Abnormal immobility and consolidation of a joint. Stiffened; held by adhesions. An ankylosed tooth is fused to alveolar bone, with obliteration of the periodontal membrane.

anodontia Total congenital lack of teeth, often combined with lack of sweat glands, persistence of fetal hair, lanugo, and defects of the nails. See also **oligodontia**.

antagonist A tooth in one jaw that articulates with a tooth in the other jaw.

anterior tooth Any one of the incisors or cuspids in either jaw.

apex; pl., apices The pointed extremity of any conical part. The terminal end of the root of a tooth.

apical base The basal bone portion of maxilla and mandible; that immediately adjoining portion upon which the teeth and alveolar process rest.

apical foramen The opening of the pulp canal at the apex of the root of a tooth.

aplastic Having imperfect development.

aptyalia Deficiency or absence of saliva.

articulation (of teeth) The contact relationship of maxillary and mandibular teeth as they move against each other.

articulator A mechanical device that represents the temporomandibular joints, to which maxillary and mandibular models may be attached.

attrition The wearing away of the incisal edges and occlusal surfaces of the teeth in the act of mastication or by the opposing teeth of the opposite jaw in the course of normal use.

axial surface Any surface of a tooth that is parallel with its long axis. The labial, buccal, mesial, distal, and lingual surfaces are axial surfaces.

balanced occlusion An ideal relationship of the mandibular and maxillary teeth to one another in centric position and throughout all the movements of the mandible.

balancing occlusion The dynamic relationship of the mandibular and maxillary teeth to one another during the excursion of the mandible from balancing position to centric position.

balancing position The static relationship of the mandibular and maxillary teeth to one another on one side of the dental arch when closure is made with the mandible moved laterally to the opposite side.

basal bone The bone of the maxilla and mandible, excepting the alveolar processes.

bicuspid A tooth having two cusps or points. Man has eight bicuspids, also called premolars. They are situated between the cuspids and the molars, two on each side in both jaws. They are named from the median line distally as maxillary or mandibualr first and second bicuspids.

bifid Separated into two parts.

bifurcation Division into two branches. The division of a root into two parts. The division of a groove into two branches. The anatomic area where roots divide in a two-rooted tooth.

bruxism Grinding of the teeth, especially during sleep. Also called stridor dentium.

buccal Pertaining to the cheek. The buccal surface of a tooth is the surface next to the cheek.

calculus (tartar) A hard, mineralized deposit attached to the teeth.

canine (1) Of, pertaining to, or like that which belongs to a dog. (2) The third tooth from the medial line. See also **cuspid.**

Carabelli cusp The cusp located on the lingual surface of many maxillary first permanent molars. It is also known as the Carabelli tubercle and as the fifth cusp. (Named after Georg C. Carabelli, Vienna dentist, 1787-1842.)

caries A localized progressive disintegration of a tooth.

beginning with the solution of the enamel and followed by bacterial invasion; a "cavity."

cementoenamel junction The line on the surface of a tooth that marks the meeting of the cementum and enamel. The cervical line.

cementum The layer of bonelike tissue covering the root of a tooth. It differs in structure from ordinary bone in containing a greater number of Sharpey's fibers.

central fossa The depressed area in the occlusal surface of the molars that surrounds the central pit.

central incisor The first tooth on either side of the median line in either jaw. Also called the first incisor.

central lobe The middle portion of enamel when the surface or part has three lobes.

centric occlusion (1) The relationship of the teeth to each other when the jaws are closed so that the lingual cusps of the maxillary bicuspids and molars, and the buccal cusps of the mandibular bicuspids and molars, rest in the deepest parts of the sulci of the maxillary bicuspids and molars. (2) The relationship of the upper and lower teeth to one another when the jaws are completely closed and at rest.

cervical border The extreme margin toward the root of any axial surface of the anatomical crown of a tooth. It is located at the cervical line.

cervical ledge The slight elevation of enamel around the periphery of the crown immediately above the cervical line.

cervical line (1) The line of the anatomical neck of the tooth; to be distinguished from the gingival line. (2) The line around the surface of a tooth where the enamel and cementum meet.

cervix The neck or any necklike part. The cervix of a tooth is the portion of the tooth surface adjacent to the junction of the crown and root.

cicatrix A scar left by a healed wound.

cingulum; pl., cingula The lingual lobe of anterior teeth which is located mostly in the cervical third of the lingual surface.

clicking (TMJ articulation) A snapping or cracking noise evident on excursion of the mandibular condyle. See also **crepitus.**

clinical crown (1) The portion of the tooth that projects from the tissues in which the root is fixed. (2) The portion of the tooth that is visible in the mouth.

comminution The act of breaking, or the condition of being broken into small fragments.

condyle The rounded eminence at the articular end of a bone. That portion of the mandible that articulates with the temporal bone of the skull to form the temporomandibular joint.

contact area The portion on the surface of a tooth that touches the adjacent tooth in the same arch.

crepitus (1) A grating sound heard on movement of ends of a broken bone. (2) The cracking sound emitted by a dysfunctioning temporomandibular joint.

crypt A follicle or tubule; a small glandular sac or pit.

curet (curette) An instrument having a sharp, spoon-shaped blade, used for debridement of periodontal pocket, tooth root, and bone.

curettement Scraping or cleaning the walls of a cavity or surface by means of a curet.

cusp A pronounced elevation or point on the crown of a tooth.

cuspid The third tooth from the median line, lying between the lateral incisor and the first bicuspid. The incisal edge of cuspids is raised to form a single point or cusp. There are four cuspids in all. They are named maxillary right and left and mandibular right and left cuspids. Also called canine.

cutting edge Same as incisal edge.

debridement Slitting a constricting band of tissue. the surgical removal of lacerated, devitalized, or contaminated tissue.

deciduous tooth One of the teeth of the first dentition, so called because they are shed to give place to the permanent teeth. Also called *temporary* or *milk* teeth.

dental dysplasia Abnormal development of bone, resulting in insufficient space to accommodate all teeth.

dentin, dentine The hard tissue that forms the main body of the tooth. It surrounds the pulp and is covered by the enamel and cementum.

dentinocemental junction The line of meeting between the dentin and cementum.

dentinoenamel junction The line of meeting of the dentin and enamel.

dentition The kind, number, and arrangement of the teeth.

diastema; pl., diastemata A space between two teeth, commonly between the central incisors. Also called *trema.*

distal Away from the medial line following the curve of the dental arch.

dorsum (1) The back or posterior surface of any organ or part. (2) The upper surface and back of the tongue.

dysphagia Inability or difficulty in swallowing; may result from hysteria, paralysis, muscle spasm, narrowing of pharynx or esophagus, etc.

ectopic eruption In an abnormal position; a tooth erupted out of its normal sequence in the dental arch.

edentulous Absence of teeth due to loss, as contrasted to anodontia, in which teeth never existed. Edentulous space: site of tooth loss either through trauma, extraction, or natural exfoliation of deciduous tooth.

embrasure An opening with sloping sides; the sloping space adjacent to the contact.

    buccal e. The embrasure opening outward toward the cheek in the posterior teeth.

    gingival e. The embrasure opening from the contact toward the alveolar process. The interproximal space.

    incisal e. The embrasure opening from the contact toward the incisal edges of anterior teeth.

    labial e. The embrasure opening from the contact toward the lips in anterior teeth.

    lingual e. The embrasure opening from the contact toward the tongue.

    occlusal e. The embrasure opening occlusally from the contact in posterior teeth.

enamel The hard, mineralized tissue that covers the dentin of the crown of a tooth.

endodontics The specialty of dental science concerned with the diagnosis and treatment of diseases of the dental pulp.

endodontium The dental pulp.

endogenous Growing from within; developing or originating within the organism, or arising from causes within the organism.

epithelium The epidermis of the skin; the surface layer of mucous membranes, consisting of one or more layers of cells varying in form and arrangement.

erosion The loss of tooth substance due to a combination of chemical action and abrasion.

eruption The emergence of a tooth through the soft tissues to appear in the oral cavity.

exogenous Originating or deriving from outside the organism; being produced or growing from without.

extrusion The hypereruption or migration of a tooth out of its normal plane of occlusion.

facet A small abraded spot on a tooth.

facial surface The surface of a tooth that is next to the lip or cheek; the vestibular or outer surface.

fissure A fault in the surface of a tooth caused by imperfect joining of the enamel of the different lobes. Fissures occur along the lines of developmental grooves.

fossa; pl., fossae A round or angular depression in the surface of a tooth. Fossae occur mostly in the lingual surface of incisors and the occlusal surface of posterior teeth.

freeway space The space between maxillary and mandibular antagonist teeth when the mandible is suspended in postural rest position.

frenulum; pl., frenula A small frenum. Sometimes applied to lingual frenum.

frenum; pl., frena A fold of mucous membrane that serves to check the movement of a part or organ.

    lingual f. Fold along midline of inferior surface of tongue extending to floor of mouth.

    labial f. Folds at the midline that attach the upper and lower lip to alveolar tissue.

gingiva The gum; the fibrous tissue covered by mucous membrane that covers the alveolar processes of the jaws and surrounds the necks of the teeth.

gingival line The line of contact of the extreme border of the gingiva to the tooth; to be distinguished from the cervical line.

gingival papilla The part of the gingiva that lies in the gingival embrasure.

gingival sulcus The space that develops in the soft tissues surrounding the tooth, bounded by the tooth surface on one side and the epithelial lining of the gingiva on the other.

gingivally A direction from any part of the tooth toward the gingival line.

gnathic Pertaining to or affecting the jaw or cheek.

gnathology (1) The science of the masticatory system, including physiology, functional disturbances, and treatment. (2) A specialized field of dentistry concerned primarily with positioning the teeth in healthy relationship with the temporomandibular joint; also called orthognathics.

groove A linear depression in the surface of the tooth.

hyperplasia The abnormal multiplication or increase in the number of cells in a tissue; an increase in size of a tissue or organ resulting from proliferation of cells.

hypertrophy The enlargement or overgrowth of an organ or structure due to an increase in size of its constituent cells, but not resulting from an increase in the number of cells.

hypoplasia Defective or incomplete development.

iatrogenic Any adverse condition in a patient occurring as the result of treatment; a detrimental condition induced or caused by a doctor.

idiopathic Of unknown causation.

incisal edge The sharp angle formed by the union of the labial and lingual surfaces of anterior teeth. The cutting edge of the anterior teeth.

incisal papilla An oval or pear-shaped nipplelike prominence of the gingiva immediately behind the upper central incisors. Also called *palatine papilla.*

incisor Any one of the four front teeth of either jaw.

inclined plane A sloping area found on the occlusal surfaces of bicuspids and molars. It is bounded by the primary grooves and the crests of the ridges. Each normal cusp has two inclined planes named for the direction in which they face, that is, the lingual cusps have mesiobuccal and distobuccal inclined planes, and the buccal cusps have mesiolingual and distolingual inclined planes.

intercuspation The cusp-to-fossa relationship of the maxillary and mandibular posterior teeth to each other.

interdigitation The interlocking or fitting of opposing parts, as the cusps of the maxillary and mandibular teeth; intercuspation.

interproximate space The V-shaped space between the proximal surfaces of adjoining teeth; it extends from the contact to the crest of the alveolar process.

keratin A protein that forms the basis of hair, nails, and any horny tissue, including the organic matrix of tooth enamel.

labial surface The surface of an anterior tooth that lies closest to the lips.

lamina dura Alveolar bone proper, or cribriform plate. It lines the inner surface of the alveolus and offers attachment for the fibers of the periodontal membrane.

lamina propria Connective tissue of the oral mucous membrane.

lateral incisor The second tooth from the median line on each side in either jaw. Also called the *second incisor.*

leukoplakia (smoker's tongue) Formation of white, thickened patches on the mucous membrane of the tongue or cheek. These cannot be rubbed off, show a tendency to fissure, and may become malignant.

lingual surface The tooth surface that is next to the tongue.

lobe One of the main morphological divisions of the crown of a tooth.

long axis An imaginary line passing lengthwise through the center of the tooth.

luxation Dislocation of a joint, as the temporomandibular articulation, or displacement of organs.

malar Pertaining to or affecting the cheek.

malocclusion Imperfect or irregular position of the teeth.

mammelon One of the three rounded prominences on the incisal edge of anterior teeth when they first erupt.

mesial Toward the median line following the curve of the dental arch.

molar One of the large grinding teeth of which there are three on either side in both jaws. They are situated distal to the bicuspids and named from before backward as maxillary or mandibular first, second, and third molars. The first molar is also called the *six-year* molar; the second molar, the *twelve-year* molar; and the third molar, the *wisdom tooth.*

occlusal surface The surface of a bicuspid or molar that makes contact with a tooth of the opposite jaw when the mouth is closed.

occlusion The contact of the teeth of both jaws when closed or during these excursive movements of the mandible that are essential to the function of mastication.

oligodontia Congenital absence of one or a few teeth.

operculum (1) Any covering. (2) The hood or flap of mucosa over an unerupted or partially erupted tooth.

orthodontics The profession or science of straightening teeth.

papilla Any small, nipple-shaped elevation.

    incisive p. The elevation of soft tissue covering the foramen of the incisive canal; crosses upper gingiva along midline behind maxillary central incisors.

    interdental p. Gingiva filling the interproximal spaces between adjacent teeth.

    lingual p. Any one of the tiny eminences covering anterior two thirds of tongue, including circumvallate, filiform, fungiform, and conical papillae.

pedodontics Specialized care of children's teeth.

periodontal membrane The fibrous tissue that is attached to the cementum of the tooth and to the surrounding structures.

periodontics Phase of dentistry dealing with treatment of diseases of the tissues around the teeth.

periodontium The investing and supporting tissues surrounding the tooth—the periodontal membrane, the gingiva, and the alveolar bone.

periosteum Tissue that covers the external surface of a bone.

pit A sharp, pointed depression in the enamel.

posterior tooth One of the teeth situated distal to the cuspids. Bicuspids and molars are posterior teeth.

primary groove A sharp V-shaped groove that is a constant and developmental part of the tooth. Marks the union of the lobes.

prosthodontics That branch of dentistry pertaining to the replacement of missing teeth by artificial devices, whether with dentures, or fixed or removable bridges.

proximal surface One of the surfaces of a tooth, either mesial or distal, that lies next to an adjacent tooth.

pulp The soft tissue containing blood vessels and nerve tissue occupying the central cavity of a tooth.

pulp canal The part of the pulp cavity that traverses the root of a tooth.

pulp cavity The entire central cavity in a tooth; it contains the dental pulp.

pulp chamber The enlarged portion of the pulp cavity, which lies mostly in the central portion of the crown.

resorption The gradual loss of the tooth structure or of bone resulting from an altered biochemical state in a localized area.

ridge A long, elevated portion of the tooth surface.

root The portion of a tooth that is covered with cementum.

root canal Same as *pulp canal.*

ruga; pl., rugae Irregular, sometimes branching ridges across the hard palate, radiating from the incisal papilla and the palatine raphe.

secondary groove A groove of lesser importance. Secondary grooves differ from primary grooves in that they are usually rounded, or U-shaped, at the bottom, and they do not mark the boundaries of the lobes.

septum A dividing wall or partition. One of the thin plates of bone separating the alveoli of the jaw.

stomatognathic Pertaining to the unified structure and function of mouth and jaw with all appurtenant tissues and organs as a cohesive system.

subluxation Incomplete or partial dislocation.

succedaneous tooth Permanent tooth that succeeds or takes the place of a corresponding deciduous tooth.

sulcus; pl., sulci A well-defined, long-shaped depression in the surface of a tooth, the inclines of which meet at an angle.

supernumerary Exceeding the regular number. An extra tooth, often peg shaped.

supplemental lobe An additional lobe. A lobe that is not usually associated with the typical form of a tooth.

trismus Inability to open the mouth due to spasms of the muscles of mastication.

trunk The main body of the root of a multiple-rooted tooth. That portion of the root from the cervical line to the division of the root.

tubercle A small, rounded, or pointed elevation of enamel. Tubercles occur frequently on the cingula of anterior teeth and occsionally on various parts of other teeth.

working occlusion The dynamic relationship of the mandibular and maxillary teeth to one another during the excursion of the mandible from working position to centric position.

working position The static relationship of the mandibular and maxillary teeth to one another on one side of the dental arch when the mandible is moved laterally to that side.

REFERENCES

1. Angle, E. H.: Malocclusion of the teeth, ed. 7, Philadelphia, 1907, S. S. White Dental Manufacturing Co.

2. Arey, L. B.: Developmental anatomy, ed. 6, Philadelphia, 1954, W. B. Saunders Co.

3. Best, C. H., and Taylor, N. B.: The physiological basis of medical practice, ed. 7, Baltimore, 1961, The Williams & Wilkins Co.

4. Burlington Orthodontic Research Center: Progress report series no. 6, 1960-1961, Toronto, 1961, University of Toronto.

5. Case, C. S.: Dental orthopedia, Chicago, 1921, C. S. Case Co.

6. Graber, T. M.: Orthodontics: principles and practice, ed. 2, Philadelphia, 1966, W. B. Saunders Co.

7. Langley, L. L., and Cheraskin, E.: The physiological foundation of dental practice, St. Louis, 1956, The C. V. Mosby Co.

8. Lischer, B. E.: Principles and methods of orthodontics, Philadelphia, 1912, Lea & Febiger.

9. Moyers, R. E.: Handbook of orthodontics, Chicago, 1973, Year Book Medical Publishers, Inc.

10. Salzmann, J. A.: Orthodontics: principles and prevention, Philadelphia, 1957, J. B. Lippincott Co.

11. Shore, N. A.: Occlusal equilibration and temporomandibular joint dysfunction, Philadelphia, 1959, J. B. Lippincott Co.

12. Sicher, H., and DuBrul, E. L.: Oral anatomy, ed. 6, St. Louis, 1975, The C. V. Mosby Co.

13. Strang, R. H. W., and Thompson, W. M.: Textbook of orthodontia, ed. 4, Philadelphia, 1958, Lea & Febiger.

14. Zeisz, R. C., and Nuckolls, J.: Dental anatomy, St. Louis, 1949, The C. V. Mosby Co.

Chapter 4

ORTHODONTIC CONCEPTS
AND PROCEDURES

This chapter will continue on the same level as the preceding one; that is, it is strictly intended for consumption by nondental personnel, and any other use would be most unfortunate. It is offered for the reader who is without dental background, especially of an orthodontic nature, in an effort to supply some rudimentary acquaintance with this setting.

This chapter is a blend of many rationales and dogmas, and so it may fit poorly the routine of a given working orthodontist; in the process of synthesizing we lose individual thought and opinion, levelling the best and worst into a general average. Since we are not undertaking to instruct dentists or to describe a specific orthodontic philosophy, perhaps we may be forgiven this glimpse through the eyes of a lay observer into the world of the orthodontist.

PERSONAL OBSERVATION

The speech pathologist is strongly urged to pay a series of visits to one or more orthodontists, watch them work, become familiar with some of their procedures—what makes a headgear work, how bands are applied, and how force is transmitted to the teeth—and learn the nomenclature of some of the materials and appliances.

Avoid the term "orthodontia," for it may strike a nerve; after many harsh years of differing opinions, general agreement has been reached that both the profession and the treatment will be known as *orthodontics*. Do not speak of "braces," for this term refers either to prostheses for arms and legs or to antediluvian dentistry, when prefabricated monolithic devices were locked onto the teeth; use instead such terms as "bands" or "appliance," or other specific apellation.

Get acquainted with plaster *study models* (you have seen many in the illustrations of the preceding chapter) and realize that they are not quick impressions of teeth but are carefully produced re-creations of the dental arches exactingly oriented to reflect either the Frankfurt or occlusal plane. When stood upright on their posterior surface, with incisors uppermost and the two halves approximated, they form a precise duplicate of the patient's occlusion as of the date taken. Models, infrequently known as "casts," are precious to the orthodontist, representing time, effort, and money, and cannot be replaced at a later time when the patient's occlusion is no longer identical. They chip and break easily. The quality of interpersonal relations may hinge on careful handling of models.

APPLIANCES

As in speech therapy, the atitude and skill of the operator is often of far greater importance than the method used. Nevertheless, there are several schools of thought in orthodontics, all aimed at the same result but using different techniques and appliances. It is advisable to learn the philosophy of the dentists with whom you associate.

Most appliances were first invented by individual dentists, many of whom then patented the device. Thus many appliances and systems came to be known simply by the name of their creator. Appliances fall into two general categories, removable and fixed.

Removable appliances

Originally, all appliances were removable and in effect were dentures with built-in springs, prongs, hooks, pressure screws, etc. They have been traditionally the method of choice in Europe, where they were developed to a high degree. In the United States, where attention has been focused on fixed appliances, removable devices are used primarily in mild, uncomplicated conditions, or in interceptive or preventive orthodontics, or as retaining devices following full correction with a fixed appliance. The general practitioner, the pedodontist, and other nonspecialists in orthodontic treatment often feel more comfortable with removable appliances; they are usually more simple to construct and can be fabricated at less expense to the patient. Some of them utilize the palatal vault or the bone inferior to the lower teeth for anchorage and can thus be used at an early age. They often involve an acrylic body to the lingual, with wire or elastic bands on the labial surface; others apply force from the lingual surface and are entirely metal.

Acrylic is the "bailing wire" of the dentist: he can fix anything with it. Acrylic resin reaches the dentist in two containers, one holding a powder, the other liquid. By mixing small amounts of the two and molding the mixture quickly, he has an instant plastic which, depending on the product, may be clear, white, or pink. It forms the plastic portion of dentures, for example.

There are two broad categories of removable appliances: (1) those that attempt to stimulate muscle activity which can be harnessed by the appliance and directed into the service of moving teeth; and (2) those that rely on the appliance itself or some attachment thereto as the means to generate the force required in tooth movement. This sorting arrangement is not entirely satisfactory, since it provides no pigeon-hole for the appliances intended to maintain static position and prevent tooth movement. For ease of discussion, therefore, we will divide them instead into two different classes, *loose* and *attached*. By and large, loose appliances include those in type 1 above, while attached removables take in those of type 2 plus the holding devices. There is minor overlapping.

LOOSE REMOVABLE APPLIANCES. Loose removable appliances include, among others, the oral shield, the Andresen appliance, the Bimler appliance, the Frankel appliance, and the positioner.

An *oral shield* is simply a thin sheet of acrylic that is placed between the anterior teeth and the lips (the oral vestibule) and that extends distally to the maxillary second molars. It is accurately fitted to the individual mouth and is used to correct mild labioversion of maxillary incisors, close spaces in this region, stimulate lip action, and correct tongue thrust.

The *Andresen appliance* (Fig. 4-1) is also known as an "activator," the "Norwegian system," or commonly as a "monobloc." Again it is acrylic, and in one continuous body lingual to the dental arches it lines the mouth, conforming to the contours of the lingual surfaces. It frequently has a shelf that fits between the upper and lower teeth, with a replica of the occlusal surface of each tooth molded into the acrylic; however, these depressions are placed in a more

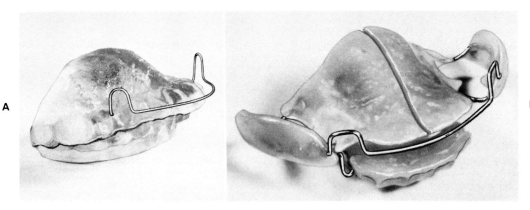

Fig. 4-1. Andresen appliances. **A,** Conventional monobloc, designed to contain tongue. **B,** Activator with modifying attachments. (Courtesy Rocky Mountain/Orthodontics.)

advantageous position than in the existing bite. The appliance is quite loose fitting and falls if not held in position by the tongue or by closing the teeth. The aim is to stimulate muscle action, setting up new reflexes that will, in turn, be beneficial in maintaining normal occlusion, such as closing the teeth and lifting the tongue during deglutition, while the mandible is guided forward.

The *Bimler appliance,* as seen in Fig. 4-2, is composed basically of wrought wire with acrylic wings flaring up lingual to the buccal teeth and connected by a U-shaped wire called a Coffin

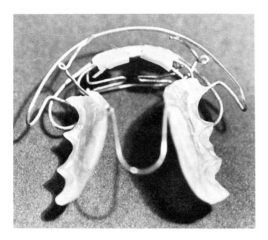

Fig. 4-2. Bimler appliance, with acrylic palatal wings connected by Coffin spring.

spring. The molded continuous wire is adapted to the labial surface of the upper arch and may have additional springs attached in a given case. The anchorage obtained in the buccal segments permits movement of the anterior teeth, both upper and lower.

The Bimler combines some of the principles of the labiolingual (fixed) arch technique with features of the Andresen (removable) activator, to produce an appliance that is designed for use in the early mixed dentition stage. It attempts to recruit both the growth and the orofacial muscle forces of the patient to the service of repositioning teeth, guiding growth into favorable patterns, and improving oral behavior.

The *Frankel appliance* may take one of many strange forms. It is also constructed mainly of an elaborate wire framework, but is primarily tissue-borne rather than tooth-borne; in fact, it often does not actually touch the teeth. In the molar region it is equipped with acrylic pads that hold the buccal wall away from the dental arch and support the distal ends of the wire framework; the acrylic may extend between the upper and lower buccal teeth, as in the monobloc, or be augmented by another acrylic "lip plumper" behind the lower lip to reduce mentalis muscle activity. As with the Bimler and several other removables, the concept behind the Frankel "function regulator" is to change existing muscle pressures in such a way that desirable tooth movement and growth responses will result.

A *positioner* is made of rubber or flexible plas-

A
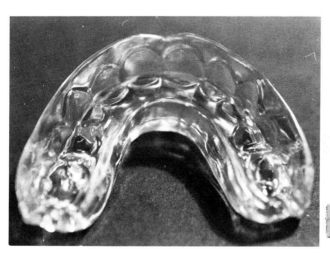

B
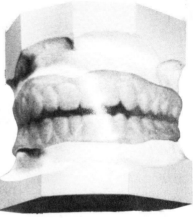

Fig. 4-3. Positioner made of flexible plastic. **A,** View of positioner showing imprint of every tooth. **B,** Positioner in place. (Courtesy Rocky Mountain/Orthodontics.)

tic, and as one unit it surrounds the crowns of all teeth in both arches. Such an appliance is seen in Fig. 4-3. It is used as the final step of treatment by some orthodontists. When the fixed appliance is removed, impressions are taken, the teeth are cut off these models and reset into an ideal relationship, and the positioner then duplicates this ideal. It is worn principally at night, and the teeth are gently guided into their ultimate positions.

ATTACHED REMOVABLE APPLIANCES. Some of the more common types of attached removable appliances are the bite plane (or bite plate), the space maintainer, the stabilizing plate, the retainer (with variations), extraoral appliances, and the entire system of orthodontic treatment based on the Crozat appliance.

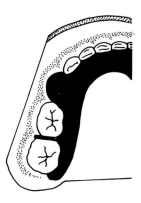

Fig. 4-4. Acrylic space maintainer. Wire clasp between first and second molars holds plate in place.

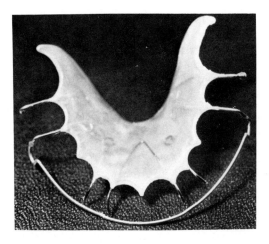

Fig. 4-5. Hawley type of retainer. Acrylic palate supplies anchorage for labial wire.

A *bite plane* is a palatal structure made almost entirely of acrylic and dependent on the mucosa and the teeth themselves for anchorage. It may have springs attached to stabilize it in the molar area, or hooks by which a very light elastic may be held around the upper incisors, or in some cases it may overlay the entire dental arch. Its main feature is a smooth sloping shelf against which selected teeth occlude, tipping them into a more desirable position. If the shelf is made level, such an appliance becomes known as a bite *plate* and may be used to open the bite; for example, if only mandibular incisors meet the plate, molars are held out of occlusion and thus encouraged to erupt further.

A *space maintainer* (Fig. 4-4), as the name implies, is used to maintain the space where a deciduous tooth or teeth have been lost, pending the arrival of permanent teeth. The acrylic covers the lingual surface of both the teeth and the mucosa, and extends into the edentulous space or spaces. It also prevents overeruption of teeth in antagonist position to the space by providing a surface on which they can occlude.

A *stabilizing plate* is an acrylic plate somewhat similar to the body of a space maintainer, except that it is molded precisely to the contour of the lingual surface of the arch (often mandibular) and has metal shafts that fit into tubes welded to molar bands. Its purpose is the positive maintenance of the molars in a desired position. It is little used, and then only in the more difficult cases.

The *Hawley retainer* is used to maintain the new positions of teeth at the conclusion of active treatment with a fixed appliance. It consists of an acrylic body accurately fitted to the lingual surfaces of the teeth, the maxillary version often being a replica of the entire palatal arch, rather than the partial arch shown in Fig. 4-5. A variety of wires are incorporated, depending on the program that has been carried out or the problem to be solved, the wire fitting around the labial surface. Variations of the Hawley, which therefore should not be referred to as Hawleys, have been endless. Dentists have found the principle invaluable in a number of early or relatively minor problems. The labial wire can be activated to produce stress against certain malposed teeth, a light elastic can replace the wire to close anterior spacing or reduce minor protrusion, space maintainers may be incorporated, etc.

Extraoral appliances were once described as "skullcap therapy," from their origin in the last century when some fairly weird harness contraptions were placed over the head and attached to the teeth. Today such appliances bear the more respectable title of "headgear" and are in widespread use. The type shown in Fig. 4-6, *A*, is designed for use with a full-banded appliance on the upper arch. The metal hooks of the headgear fit into special brackets that are welded to the bands. The cloth or plastic straps may go around the head in any of several arrangements and supply external anchorage. Although tooth movement can thus be actuated at an early age, the basic idea is to take advantage of growth and development, restricting and retarding the downward and forward growth of the alveolodental portion of the maxilla, while the mandibular bone continues its physiological growth pattern and "catches up" with the maxilla. The reverse is also possible in Class III cases, by using a "chin cup" on the outer surface of the chin rather than an intraoral attachment.

A *cervical strap* is pictured in Fig. 4-6, *B*. More commonly called a "neck band" and more commonly used than a headgear, it replaces the head straps with a single band, usually elasticized, which goes around the neck. A "face-bow" of steel wire is welded to the front of a heavy labial arch wire in one of various positions; the face-bow extends from between the lips around the outside of the cheeks, ending in a loop that attaches to the cervical strap. A pair of maxillary molars are fitted with bands bearing tubes on the buccal side to receive the ends of the arch wire. By modifying the arch wire, the face-bow, or their union, the dentist can produce a range of forces. This appliance is less cumbersome and more comfortable, but it provides less control of forces when teeth are being moved.

The *Crozat appliance* has won many fiercely loyal and vocal adherents, and the dentist so dedicated is often known as a "Crozat man." He is most frequently a pedodontist or general dentist, and usually belongs to a study club composed of other Crozat proponents for the purpose of sharing ideas and experiences, for this deceptively simple appliance can be most fickle in the unskilled hands of one who has not delved deeply into its vagaries. Few orthodontists use the Crozat, for their training is otherwise; few dental schools offer instruction in this procedure. Nevertheless, some dramatic successes can be shown by the true expert to result from the use of the very light forces of this nearly invisible appliance.

As with most appliances, individual dentists invent personal variations, so that no two appear quite the same—partly due also to the unique needs of the patient. A few varieties are depicted in Fig. 4-7; all have features in common. The most distinctive characteristic is the close-fitting but uncemented molar bands that hold the appliance in place. The wire body, usually of precious alloy, is generally fitted to the lingual of the mandibular arch, while a high labial arch wire typifies the upper appliance. From this maxillary arch wire, separate prongs often extend down to the labial surface of each tooth, the placement on the tooth and the tension of the individual fingers regulating tooth movement. Beyond these basic details, the manifestations of the appliance be-

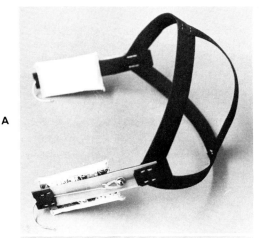

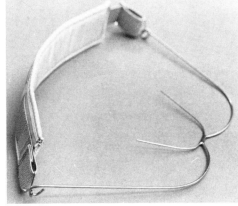

Fig. 4-6. Two types of headgear. **A,** Anchorage is supplied by cranial straps fitted over patient's head. **B,** The "neck band," in which anchorage is achieved by cervical strap worn around patient's neck.

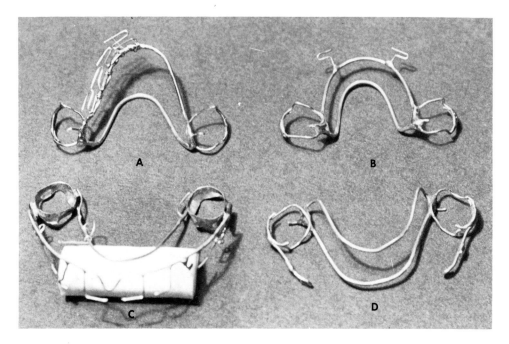

Fig. 4-7. Some types of Crozat appliances. **A,** Correcting unilateral imbalance. **B,** Labial hooks to receive elastics. **C,** Propped on cotton roll to display finger springs, which may take various designs. **D,** Basic construction.

come too complicated to describe in a brief space.

Fixed appliances

The basic element of all fixed appliances is the orthodontic *band.* This is the metal band that is cemented around the crown of the tooth and to which are welded various types of *brackets* (Fig. 4-8). The bracket is the attachment by which the *arch wire* is affixed to the band. The bracket is precisely formed in many styles to fit the particular arch wire chosen for use.

The arch wire is the muscle of the appliance; it is a high-tension stainless alloy (occasionally precious metal) which, when expert hands connect it in various ways to the bracket, produces the pushing, pulling, rotating forces required in treatment while maintaining exact control over every individual tooth to which it is attached. The arch wire is affixed to the bracket in one of several ways: some brackets have lock pins, and others have locking caps that slide over the wire, but probably the most commonly used method is the ligature (usually referred to as "tie wire"). This is a fine steel wire that is hooked into slots in the bracket, embraces the arch wire, and is

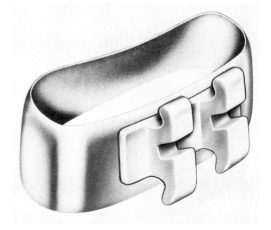

Fig. 4-8. Incisor band with bracket welded in place. That pictured here is called "Siamese" bracket. (Courtesy Rocky Mountain/Orthodontics.)

then twisted into a "pigtail" that is partially snipped off and the remainder tucked between arch wire and bracket. Assorted hooks may be welded to the bands to receive elastic bands. By using elastics of different sizes to interconnect the upper and lower arches, or different teeth

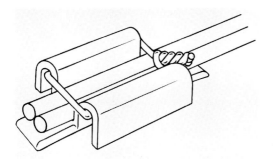

Fig. 4-9. Twin wire technique. Note style of bracket, ligature wire, and "pigtail." (Courtesy Rocky Mountain/ Orthodontics.)

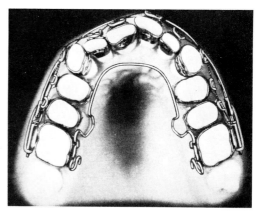

Fig. 4-11. Labiolingual appliance showing many adaptations in single arch. Additional teeth are banded and other modifications incorporated. (Courtesy Rocky Mountain/Orthodontics.)

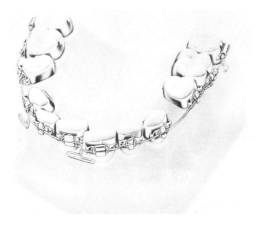

Fig. 4-10. Upper arch banded with edgewise appliance. This is extraction case: first bicuspids have been removed. Note tube welded to bands on second molars; these receive labial arch of headgear. (Courtesy Rocky Mountain/Orthodontics.)

within the same arch, a still wider range of movements is possible. These are the elastics that the patient forgets or refuses to wear and that pop out in your face when the patient laughs or sings.

It is primarily in the refinement of fixed appliances that the controversies previously referred to have arisen. The six major systems or methods now in use are (1) the round wire, (2) the twin wire, (3) the edgewise wire, (4) the universal appliance, (5) the labiolingual arch wire, and (6) the light wire.

ROUND WIRE. The original concept of a multiband procedure was to connect the bands with a single round archwire that would supply the de-

sired forces. It moves teeth, but the crowns easier than roots.

TWIN WIRE. This involves the use of two light wires lying parallel in the same bracket rather than one heavier wire and achieves greater physiological tooth movement (Fig. 4-9).

EDGEWISE WIRE (Fig. 4-10). One of Angle's early contributions was a "ribbon," or flattened wire, rectangular in cross section, that could be adjusted to achieve greater control of the apices of the teeth. He later discovered that by turning the ribbon "edgewise," using brackets machined so that the rectangular wire was inserted with its long dimension horizontal, he achieved better control over individual teeth.

UNIVERSAL APPLIANCE. The universal appliance combines the use of one flat wire and one round wire in different channels of the same bracket.

LABIOLINGUAL ARCH WIRE (Fig. 4-11). Only molars are banded, two in each arch, with tubes instead of brackets welded to the bands. A single, heavy, round arch wire is fitted on the labial surface near the gingiva and attached by inserting the ends into the tubes. A similar arch wire is usually placed on the lingual surface. Movement is accomplished by means of vertical spurs and finger springs welded to the arch wire. Inevitably, there are many innovations and variations.

LIGHT WIRE. The light wire method is usually referred to as the "Begg light wire technique," or "differential force technique." It was developed in Australia by Dr. P. R. Begg in a neighborhood somewhat less than opulent and where high-tension wire, common in the United States, was difficult to find. He devised a method of using wire of small gauge, which he bent into a series of coils, box loops, round loops, etc., and bracketed lightly to the bands in a manner that allowed the convolutions of the wire to press in various desired directions. It requires true expertise in evolving its meanderings and has a surrealistic appearance, but with the development of improved wire it has been adopted by a large number of orthodontists.

PROCEDURES

A surprising number of people phone an orthodontist, brush their teeth well, and keep their appointment with the expectation that they will walk out with a full-banded appliance in their mouth. Actually, it will be a few weeks to a few years before the bands make their appearance. It might be helpful to "walk through" a hypothetical case and examine what transpires between that first phone call and the removal of the last appliance some years later.

The first appointment in many cases is merely a matter of getting acquainted, during which the orthodontist makes a gross evaluation of the problem, compiles some case history data, observes the general oral status and function of the patient, and, if myofunctional anomalies are found, may refer the patient forthwith for correction of deglutition, a sucking habit, incompetent lips, or other obstacle in the orthodontic path. The dentist may then wish to delay further action for a few months, waiting for molars to complete eruption, for noxious habits to be eliminated, or for other reasons. In areas where there is an overabundance of orthodontists, the tendency is to band the patient first and ask questions later.

Records and cephalometrics

The orthodontist usually does not want specific measurements of the patient until treatment is imminent. Accordingly, a later appointment is made for this purpose, generally called a record session or "taking records." At this time the dentist acquires the raw material for a detailed evaluation of the patient. Profile and full-face photographs are taken, impressions are made of both dental arches for construction of study models (record casts), and intraoral radiographs are taken of each segment of the arches.

Often a second set of models is made, called working models; the teeth from this set can be cut off and remounted in a malleable plastic, making it possible for the dentist to manipulate them as he simulates the effect of the treatment he is planning. An oriented roentgenographic lateral headplate is made, and such other information as the dentist may desire is obtained.

The oriented x-ray film of the full head provides the dentist with invaluable information, but it is knowledge that must be teased out. The film is traced onto paper, and certain fixed points, or landmarks, are located and noted. By analyzing these points, by connecting some of them with others and measuring the angles of the lines thus formed, by noting relationships of teeth, jaws, and cranium, and by combining dimensional and angular criteria, the dentist is able to identify abnormalities of both form and function, project growth and development, and thus diagnose and plan treatment. Later x-ray films can be superimposed to check progress.

Depending on the amount of research which the myotherapist intends to do, some awareness should be gained in the area of cephalometrics. Cephalometric analysis is a tedious, painstaking process and will not be even abstracted here. The inquisitive reader should take a formal course on the subject or ask a friendly orthodontist to supply long-term tutelage. If nothing else, one should appreciate the laborious hours an orthodontist usually devotes to studying a case before he begins or even discusses actual treatment.

COMPUTER ANALYSIS. A diagnosis can be made only by a qualified clinician evaluating a live patient. Nevertheless, some of the tedium can be removed from the process described above. Some orthodontists are now utilizing a "Fundamental Computerized Cephalometric Analysis" offered by Rocky Mountain Data Systems. The dentist submits a data sheet accompanied by both lateral and frontal x-rays; these data are examined, the films are analyzed by technicians, and over 50 points of measurement are located and translated into "computer talk." All of this material is fed into the computer, where it is compared to stored data from over 20,000 previous patients. The resulting print-out contains complete details of both diagnosis and treatment planning, including projected growth and development expectations both with and without treatment. Another set of x-rays is analyzed at the end of treatment to evaluate results. A number of other services are available in this program; the most important for the oral myologist is the consideration that all of this system is made available for research under proper conditions.

Temporomandibular joint analysis

As the orthodontist analyzes his records and begins to plan his treatment and establish goals for a particular patient, he finds almost invariably that certain compromises must be made. Some physical characteristics do not square with others; correcting one problem may preclude the repair of another—it may be absolutely essential to gain 4 millimeters of space whereas the only tooth that can safely be extracted is 7 millimeters in width, etc.

While making these decisions, he must have in mind the ultimate facial appearance of his patient, some ideal which he will approach as nearly as conditions permit. Angle chose Apollo Belvedere as the epitome of facial symmetry, and attempted to build this profile into each patient. In the early days, esthetics was almost the only goal of orthodontic treatment, along with the effort to place the occlusal surface of each tooth in static contact with its natural antagonist. Given the fixed nature of the maxillary arch, this often resulted in a mandibular placement far from harmonious with other cranial structures, rendering serious insult to the temporomandibular joint (TMJ).

It is difficult to forsake established principles. Only in very recent years have orthodontists begun to study the effects of their treatment on the requirements of the TMJ. It is now apparent that quite serious health problems, of a seemingly unrelated nature, may readily supervene when even moderate stress proves intolerable to the temporomandibular joint over a period of years. The conscientious orthodontist takes this into account as he studies and plans. We will look at this problem in Chapter 6.

A new breed is beginning to emerge, the gnathologist, a specialist within a specialty, whose primary interest is protection of the TMJ.

Conference appointment

Some time after records are taken, often two or three weeks, the orthodontist has made a full analysis and is ready to discuss his plan of treatment with the patient or the patient's parents. A discussion period is arranged, during which the dentist explains what he will do, how he plans to accomplish it, makes an estimate as

to how long it will take, what it will cost, and how he expects payment; usually a contract is signed containing many of these provisions. The dentist will request that any cavities be repaired before treatment can begin, and outline the cooperation that he will expect of patient and parents. This may be the last chance that parents have to ask questions directly of the dentist, but unfortunately they seldom know which questions to ask; future information will be exchanged via the child, who often forgets or gets it wrong.

Extractions

During the above conference, the dentist will also reveal his decision as to extractions. He will have measured the total length of the bone in each arch, and added up the combined width of the teeth within each arch. When the arch perimeter is inadequate in which to place each tooth in a healthy position, when permanent teeth are ankylosed, or when one or two other conditions prevail, he may refer the patient to an oral surgeon for extractions, and will send an "extraction letter" specifying exactly which teeth are to be lost, usually the first or second bicuspids.

It is not sound orthodontics to extract only one or two teeth as a means of gaining space; if one bicuspid goes, four should go, one from each quadrant, since the symmetry of the arch must be maintained and the teeth in the two arches must be capable of intercuspation in a reasonably normal manner at the conclusion of treatment. Nonextraction treatment is invariably to be preferred, when it is possible; the sacrifice of permanent teeth is not a step taken lightly, although a few dentists treat almost every patient as an extraction case, robbing the tongue of essential space and sometimes creating a "dish face," in which the midportion of the face has a concave appearance.

In any event, extraction sites must heal before an appliance is installed. With careful timing, it is often possible to initiate myofunctional therapy at this juncture, as long as it can be completed before the appliance is scheduled.

Expansion devices

Some patients, particularly those displaying certain types of oral muscle dysfunction, exhibit what has been called a "collapsed upper arch," a palatal vault where the lateral segments of the basal bone itself have developed so little lateral

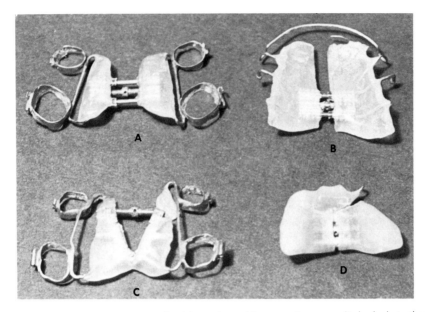

Fig. 4-12. Palatal expansion devices. Each of those pictured incorporates an acrylic body, but others are made entirely of metal. **A,** Expansion screw has been turned to its fullest extent. **B,** Labial wire rather than bands. **C,** Hinged at posterior extremity, this expands anterior palate. **D,** Cut from its original bands, this has second expansion screw designed to move anterior segment forward, while expanding buccal segments laterally.

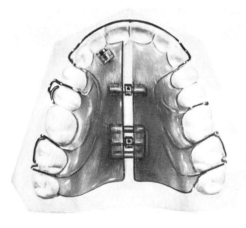

Fig. 4-13. Expansion device in place. (Courtesy Rocky Mountain/Orthodontics.)

dimension as to be incapable of containing the tongue or of supporting the teeth in any sort of normal alignment. In these cases, some orthodontists turn to a procedure called "splitting the palate," or R.P.E. (rapid palatal expansion). Devices for expanding the arch vary somewhat,

from a pair of turnbuckles embedded between two blocks of acrylic, to the somewhat lighter wire arrangement shown in Figs. 4-12 and 4-13. The patient is supplied with a key with which to rotate the expansion screw a prescribed number of turns each day, breaking open the midline suture of the palate and thus creating a greater horizontal dimension. This can usually be achieved in only two to three weeks, after which a retaining appliance is installed, or the expansion device simply left in place, until the suture area has recalcified as it is filled in by the deposition of new bone.

Again, this is not a procedure that can be used indiscriminately, for there are at least two conditions in which it is contraindicated. One occurs when the upper molars still occlude in a normal lateral relationship with the lowers. Unless the molars are in bilateral crossbite, expansion may set the maxillary teeth so far buccally as to make any normal relationship with mandibular molars impossible; it would be necessary to tip the lower teeth at a most unphysiological angle to accomplish any kind of interdigitation.

The other inadvisable condition results from the abnormal muscle function itself that so frequently accompanies these cases. We will stress in later chapters the fact that any untreated malocclusion is in a state of dynamic muscular balance. When maxillary teeth are suddenly thrust against the musculature of the buccal wall, with no provision for compensatory alteration of the environmental forces, there is risk of relapse or even greater damage to the teeth.

Should the patient be scheduled for R.P.E., the oral myologist might safely carry out some preliminary lip and cheek procedures, but should never attempt to complete therapy for abnormal deglutition until the expansion device is removed. When therapy is extended prematurely, the realization comes rather quickly that the appliance itself forces the tongue into an abnormally low posture. This prevents any semblance of normal function in swallowing, and thus assures a return to tongue thrusting, even in the relatively brief time that the appliance is in situ.

It has seemed more logical to wait until the expansion device is replaced by a retainer or full bands. The retainer can be removed for practice sessions, interferes little with routine function, and once the tongue begins to exert palatal pressure it makes an excellent substitute for the retainer. The tongue is nature's expansion device.

Separation of teeth

The patient might reasonably expect, after submitting to all of the foregoing preliminaries, that he is finally ready to acquire bands, but it is not to be. He has yet to make the acquaintance of one of the less pleasant aspects of treatment, the separator wire.

Even in severe malocclusion, most of the teeth are pressed tightly together at the contact point. Still, the orthodontist must have the thickness of two bands and two layers of cement, one over each contact point, between each tooth and its neighbor on either side in order to place the bands. The answer lies in separation of the teeth.

There are several methods by which to accomplish this. Probably the most common is to place small loops of brass or stainless steel wire around each contact point, then twist the ends together, drawing the loop tightly around the contact, and tucking the ''pigtail'' into the gingival embrasure. Another common procedure is to use a commercially available product, a tiny molded, bone-shaped piece of elastic material; when grasped at each end and stretched, it can be drawn between the contacts and released, wedging them apart as it returns to original

thickness. Other dentists employ elastic thread or very small elastic bands for this purpose. The teeth are usually separated within two or three days, and the separator devices begin to fall out, frequently to be ingested. They stop hurting after the first day.

Banding the teeth

The separator session is frequently combined with a fitting session, during which bands are selected for each tooth and grossly fitted; they are adapted precisely at this, the banding appointment, after which the brackets are welded in place and the band cemented to the tooth.

Great variation occurs at this point. Some dentists prefer to band all teeth in one marathon session, others band one arch and wait a week or more for the other, while some install one segment at a time over several weeks or months: upper molars, lower molars, upper anteriors, lower anteriors, etc. Some place and activate the arch wire as soon as bands are in place, others attach it only loosely at this time, still others wait a week or so before installing the arch wire.

A few factors in addition to personal preference enter in, but most orthodontists follow a customary routine that the oral myoclinician does well to learn: when active therapy has been completed before banding, it is advisable to recheck the status within two weeks after the sudden dramatic change in the orofacial environment occasioned by a full-banded appliance.

There is an inclination to live life without dental occlusion for a few days after banding, in the fear that biting will increase the discomfort. In fact, those who choose hamburgers over soup for their first postappliance meal seem to fare much better; the sooner the jaws are closed with some force, the quicker the bands are forgotten. Danger lies in the proclivity of some patients to place the tongue interdentally as a cushion, a precaution against unexpected closure; newly acquired swallowing and resting patterns can deteriorate rather quickly under this influence.

Once banded, the patient begins the routine of returning every two to four weeks for adjustment of the arch wire as the teeth are slowly moved into alignment. (The mechanics of how this is accomplished is afforded a special section below.) For now, we may note that by bending the arch wire into various configurations, and combining its force with elastics, headgear, or other supplemental pressures, the desired changes are effected.

Recent innovations

One promising development has been the appearance of the "arch wire with a memory." This is an alloy called Nitinol made of nickel and titanium; it is drawn into a fine wire, .019 inch in diameter, which is quite flexible and easy to manipulate. It is formed into the desired curve, heated briefly to 800° C., then quenched in cold water.

It can thereafter be bent to conform to the present shape of the patient's arch and ligatured in place. Body heat is sufficient to trigger the efforts of the wire to return to the shape built into its memory, exerting desirable force not found in conventional alloys or stainless steel arch wire.

Claims for Nitinol include the ability to reduce treatment time by 50% for the patient while increasing comfort, since it is not necessary to tighten it so much or to replace it every month or two. The orthodontist saves valuable chair time otherwise spent in arch wire changes.

Nitinol was developed by researchers in the space program, where it has several applications. It was brought into orthodontics by Dr. George F. Andreasen, chairman of the Department of Orthodontics at the University of Iowa. Considering the long history of the Andresen appliance, Andreasen may prove a trip-word for the unwary.

The cosmetic affliction that some patients feel as a result of wearing bands, and the revulsion that comes with time when they are repetitiously labelled "metal mouth," "railroad track," "brace face," or "tin grin," has spurred some orthodontists to develop less unsightly appliances (Fig. 4-14, *A*). One or two will be described in case the clinician is suddenly faced with something unfamiliar.

Direct bonding is a concept that reappears at intervals and is now in a resurgent phase because of improved techniques and materials. This involves etching the tooth by washing the surface with an acid solution, thereby clearing the microscopic crevices in the enamel of all foreign matter, then bonding the bracket directly to the tooth without benefit of any type of band (Fig. 4-14, *B*). This results in some loss of control in moving roots, but can be effective when both patient and dentist are careful. The brackets pop off when the patient chews hard or coarse food, and sometimes when he does not.

The effect can be made more "invisible" by using clear plastic brackets bonded to the tooth with a clear adhesive that leaves only the arch wire a metal feature. This demands some additional compromise, since the arch wire can distort and cut the bracket, and excessive force can fracture brackets. Nevertheless, there are a number of advantages to direct bonding, whether with metal or plastic brackets; tooth separation is unnecessary, as is closing spaces after band removal, the uncomfortable force-fitting of tight bands, etc.

Indirect bonding has been tried using several methods. The effort grew out of some dissatisfaction with direct bonding, in which human

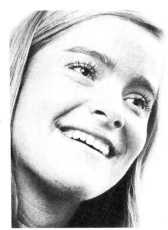
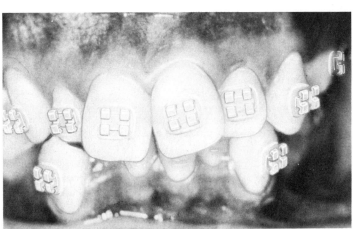

A

B

Fig. 4-14. Direct bonding. **A,** Patient wearing "almost invisible" appliance. **B,** Plastic brackets bonded directly to teeth. (Courtesy Rocky Mountain/Orthodontics.)

limitations often influence the method. That is, when the bracket is placed against the tooth in direct bonding, it may be turned or moved just slightly from its optimal position; this throws awry the action of the arch wire. Accordingly, dentists have experimented with placing the brackets in ideal alignment on the working models but only lightly attached so that errors of placement can be corrected. The brackets can then be embedded superficially in a matrix of some sort and transferred in toto to the real teeth of the patient. Given an orthodontist who is part magician, it works.

Straight wire appliances are beginning to appear in some quarters. Using conventional methods, the orthodontist spends an appreciable amount of his time in bending arch wire in and out, up and down, in order to achieve the desired movement of the teeth. The straight-wire concept is that most of this bending can be eliminated by using a system of brackets which has the necessary angulation "built in." That is, these brackets are made in varying thicknesses to stand out from the band to whatever degree required by the individual tooth, and are precisely tipped to accomplish torquing, angulation, and other details of tooth positioning. Most of the shaping and forming of the arch wire is then unnecessary, a relatively straight wire can be ligatured in place, and the treatment is built into the bracket. These brackets are also being produced for use with direct bonding techniques.

Tooth movement

TYPES OF MOVEMENT. There are five general types of tooth movement used in treatment: tipping movement, bodily movement, rotation, extrusion, and intrusion. It should be borne in mind that the orthodontist is not merely uprighting teeth into a previously prepared slot, as if moving a gearshift lever. He is literally moving the entire tooth, complete with alveolus, through bone. This maneuver is accomplished through the physiological processes of *resorption* and *deposition,* shown in Fig. 4-15. Bone is vital, living tissue undergoing constant revision and is more responsive to force than is often appreciated. Pressure against the bone causes resorption of existing bone until the pressure is eased; tension or pulling on the surface results in the deposition of new bone until a balance of forces is restored.

Orthodontists usually refer to this process as "physiological tooth movement." A different

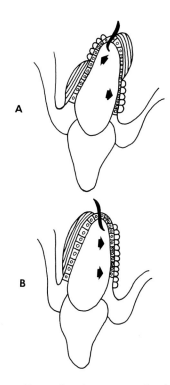

Fig. 4-15. Types of tooth movement. Results of pressure applied lingually to crown of central incisor (periodontal membrane greatly enlarged). **A,** Tipping movement: periodontal membrane is crushed at alveolar crest lingually and at apex labially; fibers are stretched at opposite diagonal. Scalloped lines show bone resorption, and concentric lines indicate bone deposition. **B,** Bodily movement: entire membrane is compressed lingually and stretched on labial side.

appreciation of their work may be gained through the realization that to benefit the patient, the orthodontist is actually injuring the tissue, inflicting a deliberate but controlled pathology. The periodontal membrane governs the consequences. Pressure against the crown of the tooth is transmitted through the root, reducing circulation in the periodontal membrane in areas where the membrane is compressed while straining its attachments in other places. The reaction of tissue to such insult effects tooth movement.

Tipping movements are relatively fast even with moderate pressures, for the periodontal membrane recovers quickly; bodily movement, compressing a much greater portion of the membrane, requires a longer recovery time. It is thus common for the patient wearing an appliance effecting bodily movement to see the orthodontist only at three-week intervals for adjustment.

Total time during which the appliance is worn may vary from a few months up to two years or slightly longer, but long treatment periods of three to eight years often indicate an untreated tongue thrust or some other etiological agent.

MESIAL DRIFT. Mesial drift is nature's orthodontic procedure, not the dentist's, but it is a condition that the dentist must control at times. It is the tendency of the teeth to shift toward the midline of the dental arch until contact is established with another tooth. The forces at work in the normal mouth militate to this end, so that if a tooth is extracted, the teeth distal to the resulting space "drift" mesially through the bone by the natural occurrence of resorption and deposition, as described above. As neighboring teeth rub together in function, the proximal surfaces wear away and flatten; mesial drift keeps them in contact, nevertheless. When a deciduous tooth is lost prematurely, we have noted that a "space maintainer" is frequently employed to combat mesial drift and to hold a place in line for the future arrival of the permanent tooth destined for that space. Mesial drift can be a beneficial force when permanent teeth must be extracted. Abnormal tongue pressures can prevent mesial drift in extraction cases, causing an undesirable spacing of the teeth.

FORCE. The optimum force that should be applied in order to move teeth has not yet been established; it will be a difficult formula to devise, for many unknown factors remain. One proposal has been 20 to 26 grams (less than 1 ounce) per square centimeter of root surface, the capillary pulse pressure of the body through which teeth erupt and drift naturally. In actual practice a greater force is often used, but it must be kept under rigid control to avoid such unpleasant sequelae as root resorption, sheared alveolar crests, and poor gingival health.

AGE. The age factor is of vital concern to the dentist, for he must utilize growth processes to achieve some of the necessary changes. The growth spurt that usually occurs when a child enters puberty is often prime time to the orthodontist. The apices are fully formed and closed, so that major tooth movements are possible without danger of root impairment. Prior periods of rapid body growth are also precious, but the puberty cycle is the "last chance" timing for some aspects of Class II and Class III treatment.

That is, this cycle essentially completes the growth of the basal bone forming the jaws. Thereafter, the orthodontist is not able to take advantage of growth by restraining development in one arch while the bone of the opposing arch "catches up" as it continues normal growth and development. Such restraint or encouragement of growth is the purpose behind some uses of the headgear appliances discussed earlier.

By no means does this indicate that there is no help for the adult patient; remarkable changes have been effected in patients over 40 years of age when orthodontic treatment followed correction of the swallowing pattern. Individual teeth have been moved for 70-year-old patients in order to place a prosthesis.

ANCHORAGE. "For every action, there is an equal and opposite reaction." This law of physics will concern the therapist more directly in matters of deglutition, but it is basic to the dentist in tooth movement. To apply force to a tooth, there must be a point of resistance to that force, a "skyhook" by which to lift. In the past, it was usual to wait until the permanent molars were present in the mouth and to use their more securely affixed root structure to effect movement of anterior teeth. However, some seven or eight types of anchorage have now been devised, including the extraoral resistance inherent in the headgear in which the neck or occiput supplies anchorage.

Retention period

Joy is unrestrained on the day bands are scheduled to be stripped from the teeth. Lips that have been drawn together, concealing the appliance, are now rehearsing broad smiles, to exhibit beautiful unencumbered teeth. Still, one important phase remains to be completed: the retention period.

Once the bands are stripped off, the teeth are usually buffed and polished, and some occlusal equilibration is often done to encourage healthful intercuspation and make other fine adjustments. Typically, at this same appointment, "finish models" are taken, sometimes for later comparison with the original study models but also as a guide for constructing retention appliances. The patient will return two or more days later to receive retainers, as it requires a few hours to fabricate them.

Extensive changes have been wrought in the tissues of the mouth as a result of orthodontic pressures. We referred earlier to orthodontic treatment as "controlled pathology." Just as the orthopedic surgeon must splint and brace his handiwork until bones have knit and tissues healed, so too the orthodontist must immobilize the reorganized mouth until it is able to withstand environmental forces unassisted. Additionally, spaces between the teeth required for the bands must now be closed.

We have pointed out the great diversity of orthodontic approaches and appliances. The dentist understands quite well the physiology of tooth straightening, and so is able to arrive at the desired result along many different routes. However, the actual body of scientifically proven data concerning retention is discouragingly small, with the result that there is remarkable uniformity in retention procedures: a cuspid-to-cuspid fixed bar behind lower incisors and a Hawley-type removable on the upper arch. It has been done this way for many years, and few dentists challenge the system.

The lower appliance is made by rebanding the long-rooted lower cuspids and connecting the two bands with a light bar of stainless steel adapted closely to the lingual surface, thus preventing any sort of distal movement of the lower incisors. If an anterior crossbite has been corrected, the upper teeth themselves act as the retainer.

The upper retainer varies somewhat in design, depending upon whether or not there have been extractions. With acrylic fitted precisely to the lingual surfaces and a static wire around the labial surface, the upper teeth are effectively locked in place.

Occasionally an orthodontist will remove the bands earlier than he would otherwise do, and use a positioner as both a "finisher" and a retainer. The teeth from the finish models are cut off and mounted in wax as described earlier, so that the impression of each tooth within the positioner reflects ideal position; the patient bites into this guidance system four or five or more hours per day while awake and continues through the night. Positioners are frequently less acceptable to the patient, and in most cases must still be followed by the conventional retainers described above.

The length of time during which retainers are worn depends on two factors in addition to the preference of the dentist. One consideration is the type of tooth movement that has been carried out; teeth that have been rotated require much more time than those that have been shifted or tipped. The second factor is the age of the patient. When treatment has been concluded during body growth, much of the necessary reorganization of tissue has occurred spontaneously as a part of the growth process, reducing the time required for retention. Adult patients must be retained over a longer period in order to be secure.

The duration of the retention period may thus vary from a few months to several years. Patients have been seen who have been in retention for 20 years or more; we might add that the authors have not seen such a case who displayed a healthy mouth or even reasonably normal occlusion. Long retention is demanded only when teeth are placed in a posture which is inharmonious with their environment. The antagonistic stress generated even by normal surrounding tissues can result in thickening of the periodontal membrane and other ills leading to dental breakdown.

Whatever the continuance of retainers, when the last appliance is removed the patient's musculature resumes command of tooth posture. Given normal function, a beautiful, healthy, permanent result emerges; it has been the conviction of some orthodontists that retention devices should not even be required in the thoroughly treated mouth.

In contrast, an untreated tongue thrust makes its presence known rather quickly at this juncture. No amount of retention is adequate when the dentition is subjected to abnormal environmental forces. Some dentists maintain quite a vocabulary of euphemisms for use in these cases: "settling," "post-treatment adjustment," "God's will," and "preeminence of the morphologic pattern"—any of these sounds less offensive than the term *orthodontic relapse*.

We should make one final point concerning retainers. These appliances are designed to resist force only on a horizontal plane, but exert no vertical pressure and are thus incapable of counteracting the effect of a tongue placed interdentally. Open bite cases may begin to reopen with dramatic suddenness even with retainers in place, once relieved of the interarch elastics used to close the bite.

Chapter 5

ANATOMY FOR THE ORAL MYOLOGIST

Anatomy is an area of absorbing interest to the nonanatomist only in the context of gender. It is a subject like basic mathematics (and unlike spelling) in which it is hard to be original or creative—basic anatomy changes little. We strain our mind almost to the breaking point in attempting to understand the workings of the human mind. Mostly, anatomy is memorization.

There is no scarcity of textbooks on either anatomy or physiology, some of which run to over 1200 pages and many of which are specialized in nature and thus able to eliminate extraneous material and focus on a certain portion or system of the body with some depth. For those who have not established friendly relationships with one or more of these books, especially those exploring the head, neck, and torso, we heartily recommend making their acquaintance. Yet we know of none that relates specifically to the act of deglutition or the vagaries and associated concerns thereof. Hence we will devote a handful of pages to this pursuit.

As with several of the preceding chapters, each of which is intended for only those readers whose needs include the specific category of information given, this will be a sharply circumscribed presentation of anatomy; physiology will be discussed in the next chapter. We will look backward through the large end of the telescope at only those nerves, muscles, and structures that have pertinence for the oral myologist. However, we will try to explain in the course of the two chapters *why* and *how* these elements relate to oral function.

There is a threat of gross misunderstanding when we delimit so drastically the extent of our inspection. It is essential that there be an ever-present awareness of the *oneness* of the miraculous human body, every fiber affecting and being affected by every other cell as well as the sum of the parts. The function of an oral muscle may be influenced by tension in a remote or seemingly unrelated muscle, by body posture or temperature, by emotion or state of mind, by diet, and by many other factors. Such considerations will be laid aside for the moment, along with the skin and flesh that we must strip away, in order to view the tissues we seek and to offer a brief and partial explanation of their purpose.

TERMINOLOGY

As a general rule, the language of anatomy is specific, requiring some agreement among discussants for full understanding. Variations do occur; Latin names are often Anglicized (as will be the case here in most instances) but we will define a few of the terms essential to an orderly perusal of this material. In addition, we will conclude this chapter with a brief glossary of anatomic terminology. In order to avoid duplication, we will eliminate terms recorded in the dental glossary at the end of Chapter 3. Should we unintentionally use a term not shown in either glossary, desperation may drive the reader to one of the formal texts listed in the references.

Viewing the erect body face-to-face, we should establish our directions, for some minor reorientation is necessary for readers with a dental background. The dentist's ''mesial'' becomes the anatomist's ''medial'' and no longer accommodates the concept of traversing a curved dental arch, but instead implies a direction squarely toward the vertical midline. Its opposite becomes ''lateral,'' denoting direction away from the vertical midline. Two other terms that alter in meaning as they commute between dentistry and anatomy are ''proximal'' and ''distal.'' Proximal, as used in this chapter, indicates direction toward a point of attachment, while distal denotes the opposite, or away from the point of attachment; these words are used primarily in describing features of the limbs, to indicate relative distance from the attached end.

Four other words should be clearly understood; the meaning of these is the same in both fields:

ventral (anterior) Toward the front
dorsal (posterior) Toward the back
cephalad (superior) Toward the head
caudad (inferior) Toward the tail or lower end

In order to examine the interior of the body and some of its organs, it is helpful to divide the structure into sections, removing one section for easy viewing. The direction of these cuts, or *anatomic planes*, must be clear:

sagittal plane A division vertical to the ground and front-to-back, yielding right and left parts or sections. When the division is made to coincide with the vertical midline, it is called the *median* or *midsagittal* plane.
frontal or **coronal plane** A lateral or side-to-side division, vertical to the ground, separating the front section from the back.
horizontal or **transverse plane** Division across the structure, parallel to the ground, forming upper and lower sections.

DIVISIONS OF ANATOMY

The study of the structure and function of the human body is made more meaningful, efficient, and economical in terms of time and effort by dividing the total into cohesive units of special interest. Were we concerned solely with muscle function, we might confine our attention to *myology*, that segment of anatomy devoted to the study of muscles. Such an exclusive perusal would have little meaning, however, without some knowledge of *osteology*, the study of bones; most muscles derive their name from points of attachment to the skeleton or other body structures, and their function can be understood only in relation to their effect on the tissues thus connected. It is further necessary to have some concept of *neurology*, the study of nerves within the nervous system that control the muscles, and on occasion it would be helpful to know something of *angiology*, the study of the vascular system supplying blood to the muscles.

Among the many other divisions into which anatomy is segmented are: (1) *cytology*, the study of cells; (2) *histology*, the study of cell groups as they form the component parts of the body; (3) *embryology*, the study of the growth of cells from the fertilized ovum to full differentiation; and (4) *syndesmology*, study of joints or articulations. Other specialized areas are concerned with the *visceral system*, the *respiratory system*, the *digestive system*, the *urogenital system*, etc.

SOME TYPES OF TISSUE

Groups of cells joined for a common purpose and functioning in harmony form a tissue. There is a great variety of tissues, of many types, sizes, and composition. In fact, we may view the human body as a fantastically intricate mass of differentiated tissues, such as cartilage, bone, blood, and connective tissue (all of the preceding are sometimes referred to as connective tissue) held in place and set in motion by muscular tissue, which in turn is activated under the governance of neural tissue.

While confining our attention to the area of the head and neck, we will examine these tissues in order. We do so with the understanding that body tissue may be classified in several other ways and into many other categories. And we will save the inspection of muscle tissue until last, since a fuller comprehension and a broader view of their structure and function will then be possible.

It seems expedient to eliminate herein any extensive discussion of *blood* and the *vascular system*, since these are of less specific importance to the oral myotherapist. Some mention will be required later as they relate to the reposturing of certain labial tissue.

Nor will we go into any great detail at this point concerning *connective tissue*. Those tissues that have an application to this field will be pointed out in the context of muscle function. For now, we may note that the connective tissue that we encounter will consist primarily of four types: loose, dense, regular, and special. All are collagenous, with abundant interlacing processes, and may pervade, support, and bind together other tissues and organs and form ligaments, tendons, and aponeuroses. *Loose* connective tissue is strong, inelastic, and white. *Dense* connective tissue is thicker, more compact, and more elastic. *Regular* connective tissue is composed of parallel bundles of fibers that have great resistance to stretching, and accordingly is the type found in tendons and ligaments. Connective tissue with *special properties* varies rather widely, its composition depending in part on its location and function; examples are mucous membranes, adipose (fat) tissue, the connective tissue of the periodontal membrane, etc., each differing in some respect from the others.

Cartilage

Cartilage is a dense mass with a very uncomplicated structure. It contains no blood vessels or nerves, receiving its nutritive elements from surrounding tissue. It is the precursor of bone in the embryo; the fetal skeleton consists primarily of "temporary" cartilage. Ossification occurs on a varying timetable, depending on the location and precise consistency of the cartilage. Much is complete at birth although the fontanels or "soft spots" of the neonate skull will require some further time; the transition to bone happens in "permanent" cartilage only with advanced age, or never.

Cartilage may be classified according to its internal structure into three types: hyaline, elastic (also called yellow fibrocartilage), and white fibrous.

HYALINE. Encompassing several subtypes, hyaline cartilage is the most abundant type. It has a shiny bluish-white appearance and has considerable elasticity despite being quite firm in texture. Hyaline cartilage encrusts the ends of bones that are encased in joints, its smooth surface providing ease of movement. Bars of hyaline cartilage connect the anterior ends of the ribs to the sternum or to each other, lending enhanced elasticity to the walls of the thorax. It also combines elasticity with stability in vital airway passages in the nose and trachea.

ELASTIC. For our purposes, we need only note that elastic cartilage, more elastic and flexible than hyaline cartilage and with a faint yellow tinge, makes up the epiglottis, much of the larynx, the eustachian tube, and the external auditory canal.

FIBROUS. The color of fibrous cartilage is white, since the cartilaginous tissue is mixed with varying amounts of white fibrous tissue. The latter ingredient adds toughness to the elasticity of cartilage, making its appearance appropriate in joints subject to frequent or extended movement, and to cushion joints that are exposed to sudden or violent shock. Therefore, it is hardly surprising to find this type of cartilage in the temporomandibular joint, the most frequently and stressfully used of all joints; even this tough, resilient tissue, in this location called the *articular meniscus,* is not always equal to the strain and abuse to which it may be exposed.

Fibrous cartilage is also found in wrist and knee joints, forms discs between the bodies of the vertebrae (where they also rupture on occasion), and forms a thin coating over the surface of the grooves through which the tendons of certain muscles glide.

SYNOVIAL MEMBRANE. We cannot conclude this section without some general description of the structure of joints and the critical synovial membrane. When joints are immovable, as those between bones of the skull, the margins of the bones are separated only by a thin membrane, called the *sutural ligament.* When slight movement is involved, as in the joints between the vertebral bodies, we have noted above that the osseous surfaces are joined by fibrous cartilage. However, freely movable joints present quite a different structure. In order to achieve a full range of motion, the surfaces of the bones are completely separated, this division sometimes being further increased by a rim of fibrous cartilage surrounding and thus deepening the articular cavities. That portion of the bone forming the joint is covered by cartilage, as previously described, the joint is strengthened by ligaments which attach to the articulating bones, and the joint enveloped by a capsule of fibrous tissue. The interior of the fibrous capsule is lined with the *synovial membrane,* which secretes a lubricating fluid, facilitating the action of the joint.

OSTEOLOGY

The adult skeleton consists of over 200 named bones; we must be concerned with only about one-eighth of these, but it is essential that we lift our eyes from an over-fascination with mere maxillary and mandibular bone.

Bones may be classified according to their shape into four groups: *long,* found in the arms and legs; *short,* located mostly in wrists and ankles; and the two with which we will deal, *flat* and *irregular.* Flat bones exist where there is need for extensive protection, as in the upper skull. Irregular bones have peculiar and often individual shapes, as in the sphenoid bone of the skull.

Bone is distinguished from cartilage by having a very dense intercellular matrix containing mineral salts, mainly calcium compounds. Depending on its composition, bone is classed as either dense (compact) or spongy (cancellous).

The outer portion of each bone is composed of a layer of dense bone, which has the appearance of a continuous hard mass, with a central portion in most cases containing a space called the medullary or marrow cavity. Spongy bone makes up all of a few bones and a portion of most bones, and consists of intercrossing and connecting osseous bars of various thicknesses and shapes; while appearing quite porous and flimsy, the arrangement of these bars provides the bones with maximum rigidity and resistance to stress or changes in shape, adding strength without adding weight. Regardless of its composition or structure, all bone is plastic and responsive to pressure.

The outer surface of each bone, except for articular surfaces, is covered by a closely attached layer of dense fibrous tissue called the *periosteum;* the periosteum is richly supplied with blood vessels and nerves, and plays an important role in providing blood and sensory innervation to bone.

A number of the bones with which we are concerned are characterized by irregularities, projections and depressions that have specific descriptive terms, some of which are defined in the box at the right in order to clarify our discussion.

We will confine our attention to the bones of the skull plus the hyoid bone, with a fleeting glance at an upper vertebra or two. Even some in this limited purview will be merely listed, despite their importance in other contexts.

The skull is composed of 21 bones joined closely together and one, the mandible, that is freely movable. This does not include the three tiny bones of the ossicular chain in each middle ear cavity.

It would be helpful at this point if we could supply each reader with an actual skull, for many features are easily determined by examining the skull as a whole; some are seen in Fig. 5-1, which also identifies the cranial bones. The two large sockets housing the eyeballs are the orbits. Between and slightly below the orbits is the pear-shaped nasal opening, divided vertically by the nasal septum. The nasal bone itself appears quite short, without its fleshly extension of cartilage; but within the nasal opening on each side can be found three scroll-like bony processes, the nasal conchae or turbinates. The zygomatic arch, or cheek bone, flairs from the side of the skull and circles around beneath the orbit. Behind the orbit and above the zygomatic arch, the external surface of the sphenoid bone swoops in to form

the temple, or temporal fossa, with only minor participation of the temporal bone itself. The mastoid process is the bulky projection behind and below the external auditory canal. Viewed from below, the foramen magnum is the large opening through which the spinal cord emerges. The hard palate forms the floor of the nose, while the floor of the brain case can be seen from above to consist of three large uneven depressions called the anterior, middle, and posterior cranial fossae.

TERMS PERTAINING TO BONE

process An arm or projection; any marked bony prominence
tubercle A small rounded process
tuberosity A large rounded process
condyle A rounded, knuckle-like process
spine A sharp, slender process
crest A narrow ridge of bone
ala A wing; a wing-like structure or appendage
head A part supported on a constricted portion, or neck
fossa A depression in or upon a bone
sulcus or **groove** A furrow
fissure A narrow slit
foramen A hole or orifice through which blood vessels, nerves, and ligaments pass
meatus or **canal** A long tube-like passageway
antrum or **sinus** A nearly closed cavity or chamber in a bone, or one having a relatively narrow opening

---

Cranial bones

Eight bones are incorporated into the cranium: two parietal, two temporal, and one each frontal, occipital, sphenoid, and ethmoid. These blend into the fourteen bones of the facial skeleton, with little to mark the distinction. Since our interest in bone is primarily in its function of providing attachment for muscle, we will not discuss certain of the cranial bones.

FRONTAL BONE. An exception to the preceding statement is the frontal bone, the saucer-shaped bone forming the forehead and the upper part of the orbit; it also forms part of the septum between the brain case and the nasal cavity. While it does serve as attachment for a few muscles, it also houses the frontal sinuses and nasal cavity. With our demanded concern for nasal breathing patterns, it behooves us to note that the frontal sinuses play an important part by expanding the

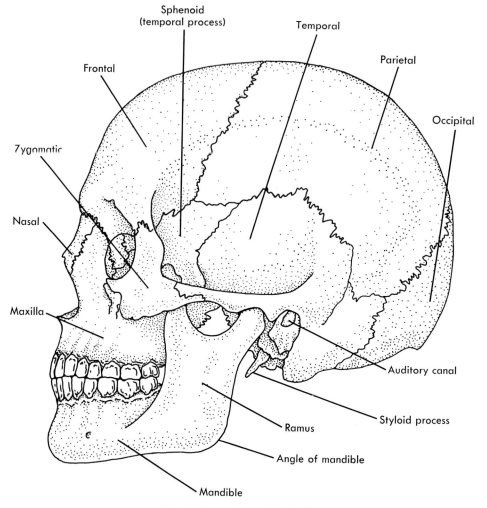

Fig. 5-1. Some bones of the skull.

area available to the nose in warming, humidifying, and filtering the inhaled breath.

The frontal sinuses are two large members of the group connecting directly with the nasal passage, a group known collectively as the paranasal air sinuses. The frontal sinuses are located superior to the orbits, vary greatly in size and shape, and empty into the middle meatus of the nose. Their contribution will be detailed in Chapter 6, after we encounter some of the other sinuses.

TEMPORAL BONES. On either side of the cranium are the two temporal bones forming part of the lateral wall of the base of the skull. The temporal bone is usually divided for study into five parts; the *squamous, petrous, mastoid, tympanic,* and *styloid* portions.

The squamous is the large, fan-shaped portion which forms a part of the temporal fossa, and from which arises the temporalis muscle. Projecting from the lower part of the squamous region is the long arch of the *zygomatic process,* the inferior border of which provides origin for the masseter muscle. The zygomatic process articulates with the temporal process of the zygomatic bone.

The petrous portion is shaped like a pyramid and is wedged in at the base of the skull between the sphenoid and occipital bones. The middle and inner ear are contained in this portion, along with other features of the auditory system. On its inferior surface is the origin of the levator veli palatine muscle, part of the bony portion of the cartilaginous eustachian tube, as well as the root of the styloid process. Just anterior to the styloid, where the petrous and squamous portions join, is the round, smooth *mandibular fossa* for the lodgment of the head of the mandibular condyle.

The mastoid portion lies inferior to the squamous, and is the most posterior part. It forms the bulky prominence that can be felt behind the ear. Beneath this portion is the *mastoid process,* a large cone-shaped projection which provides attachment for the digastric and sternocleidomastoid muscles, among others.

The tympanic portion forms most of the bony portion of the external auditory meatus (canal) and provides attachment for the cartilaginous segment of the canal. It also contains the tympanic sulcus, a groove which receives the tympanic membrane (eardrum).

The *styloid process* is a long, slender, bony spike projecting downward and forward from the temporal bone. This is the point of attachment of the stylopharyngeus and styloglossal muscles, and the stylohyoid and stylomandibular ligaments.

ETHMOID BONE. The ethmoid bone is found immediately below and behind the frontal bone, is spongy in composition, and is very irregular in shape. Basically, it consists of a cribriform (horizontal) plate, a median perpendicular plate, like the stem of a T, and two lateral masses, or *labyrinths,* suspended from the ends of the cribriform plate. The cribriform plate helps to complete the floor of the anterior cranial fossa. The perpendicular plate forms part of the nasal septum. On either side the labyrinths form part of the orbit and the lateral wall of the nasal cavity. In addition, the inner face of the lateral mass bears a thin curving sheet forming the middle and superior nasal turbinates. Between these two lies the superior meatus; the middle meatus lies beneath the middle turbinate. The labyrinths also contain the ethmoid air cells, or ethmoid sinuses, which communicate with the nasal cavity.

SPHENOID BONE. The sphenoid bone is often likened in appearance to a bat or butterfly with outspread wings; it also has many characteristics of a figure from an inkblot test, and requires almost as many words to interpret. It is situated at the anterior part of the base of the skull, just posterior to the ethmoid and immediately in front of the temporal, and binds the other cranial bones together. The relatively large body is shaped somewhat like a cube, with a great and a small wing projecting from each side, the small wings lying superior to the great wings. At the base of the great wings, the two pterygoid processes project downward, flanking the posterior opening of the nose; the lower end of each process is divided into two flat sheets of bone, the medial and lateral pterygoid plates or laminae. The lower end of the medial plate, the longer and narrower of the two, ends in a hook-like projection, the hamulus of the pterygoid.

The body of the sphenoid bone is hollowed into two separate spaces, the sphenoid sinuses. On the upper surface superior to the sinuses is a small fossa or pit, the sella turcica, which cradles the hypophysis (pituitary gland).

The lateral pterygoid plate is broad, thin, and flaring; its lateral surface gives attachment to the external pterygoid muscle, while its medial surface provides attachment for the internal pterygoid. The medial pterygoid plate, along the full length of its posterior edge, serves as attachment for the pharyngeal aponeurosis; the superior constrictor muscle takes origin from its lower third.

At the divergence of the lateral and medial plates a V-shaped space is created, the pterygoid fossa. Above this fossa is a small oval depression, the scaphoid fossa, which gives origin to the tensor veli palatine muscle; the tendon of the tensor veli palatine glides around the hamulus.

The facial skeleton

Fourteen bones surround the nose and mouth and comprise the facial skeleton—six paired and two unpaired. Some will be discussed briefly here.

The *nasal bones* are two small oblong bones placed side by side, forming by their junction the bridge of the nose. The *zygomatic (malar) bones* form the midportion of the zygomatic arch and an upward projection forms part of the floor and lateral wall of the orbit. The *inferior nasal concha* (inferior turbinate) is a shell-like scroll of spongy bone that projects medially into the nasal cavity, separating the inferior from the middle meatus. It articulates principally with the maxilla. By mentioning that the *lacrimal bones* form part of the medial wall of the orbit, we have disposed of eight of the facial bones.

VOMER BONE. The vomer (plowshare) is one of the unpaired bones. It is a midline structure whose long, sloping, anterior border forms the lower and posterior part of the nasal septum. It is frequently deflected to one side at its anterior end, resulting in a deviated septum and consequent interference with nasal breathing. Its upper border thickens and then divides into two alae for articulation with the inferior surface of the sphenoid. Its posterior border is free and forms the wall between the posterior nares.

PALATINE BONES. The palatine bones are located at the posterior end of the nasal cavity, behind the maxilla and in front of the medial pterygoid plate of the sphenoid.

The palatine bones are L shaped, with one reversed so that they join at the tips of the lower (horizontal) arms, their union forming the nasal crest on the superior edge and the posterior nasal spine on the posterior border. The posterior nasal spine gives attachment to the muscle of the uvula. The superior surface of the horizontal part forms the back part of the floor of the nasal cavity, while the inferior surface forms, with the corresponding surface of its mate, the posterior fourth of the hard palate. The posterior border is free, and serves for the attachment of the soft palate.

The vertical portion forms part of the lateral walls of the nose, and on this surface bears three shallow depressions corresponding to the three nasal meatuses.

MAXILLARY BONES. Some problem in conceptualization arises here, since many of us were originally taught to say "maxilla" rather than "maxillae." We have referred to this bone in previous chapters as singular, and will continue to do so as soon as the exigencies of the present chapter are behind us. For the sake of accuracy we must report, however, that the maxillae are really two, twin bones so deftly joined, in most cases, as to present a deceptively unitary appearance. The exception, of course, is found in cases of cleft palate, a failure of the two bones to fuse normally during embryonic development. The combined maxillae are exceeded in size only by the mandible among the bones of the face. The mandible also represents the fusion of two halves (the symphysis menti) but remains in unwed solitude among the pages of descriptive atlases.

Each maxilla (right and left) consists of a body and four processes: the *frontal, zygomatic, alveolar,* and *palatine* processes. The body has a pyramidal shape, and contains the large maxillary sinus which follows the same form. The sinus cavity extends laterally over the maxillary molars; at times only a thin layer of bones lies between the floor of the sinus and the apices of the molar roots. In rare cases no bone at all separates the apices and the sinus, only the soft tissue of the periodontal membrane on the tooth and the mucous membrane lining the sinus.

The frontal process forms the lateral wall of the lower part of the nasal cavity. The zygomatic process is the lateral projection that articulates with the zygomatic bone and forms the anterior end of the zygomatic arch. The alveolar process, thick and spongy, is the dental arch. The palatine process is the horizontal shelf of bone within the dental arch which forms the greater portion of the floor of the nose and about three-fourths of the hard palate. As we have seen, the horizontal plate of the palatine bone supplies the other fourth.

THE MANDIBLE. The mandible consists of a horseshoe-shaped body and a strong ramus extending upward and slightly posteriorly from each free end of the horseshoe. The fusion of the two halves of the mandible is at the *symphysis menti,* which is elevated to form the mental protuberance at the point of the chin. The surface of the mandible is marked by two lines: externally, the *oblique line* is a slight ridge running downward and forward from the anterior border of the ramus, while internally the *mylohyoid line* is a marked horizontal ridge below the alveolar process.

In the upper portion of the ramus is the *mandibular foramen,* through which pass the nerves and arteries for the lower teeth. Overhanging the foramen on the inner surface is a spine of bone called the *lingula.* The *mylohyoid groove* extends downward and forward from the foramen, and is distinct from the mylohyoid line described above.

Each ramus ends in two prominent extensions, the *coronoid* and the *condyloid processes.* The coronoid is the anterior process to which attach the temporalis and masseter muscles. The condyloid process consists of a condyle, or head itself, and a neck from which the head arises. The head articulates with the mandibular fossa of the temporal bone, forming the only freely moving joint in the skull, the temporomandibular joint. Between the two processes is a broad, deep depression called the *sigmoid notch,* while inferiorly the rami join the main body at a location known posteriorly as the *angle* of the mandible.

Adjacent bones

Three other bones must be considered that are not part of the skull—the hyoid bone, because of its great importance to the muscles with which we deal, and the first two vertebrae because they provide helpful landmarks.

HYOID BONE. The hyoid bone has been called "the skeleton of the tongue" because of its many attachments of muscles supporting the tongue. It is the only bone in the human skeleton not articulating or connecting more intimately with any other bone.

The hyoid is another horseshoe-shaped bone, lies below the mandible and roughly parallels the body of the mandible in its orientation. It is suspended in its position at the upper border of the larynx by two thin fibrous cords attached to the styloid processes of the temporal bone, the stylohyoid ligament.

The hyoid consists of a body and two pairs of processes, the greater and lesser cornua (horns). The body is quadrilateral, with a faceted anterior surface that is somewhat convex. The posterior surface is smooth and sharply concave. The epiglottis stands within the arch of this bone, and is separated from the body of the hyoid by the hyothyroid membrane and by loose connective tissue.

From each end of the body, the greater cornua curve laterally and posteriorly, tapering somewhat before swelling to a tubercle at the tip. The lesser horns are small, cone-shaped, and project upward and backward from the superior surface of the body at or near the attachment of the greater cornua. The apex of the lesser cornua provide the inferior attachment of the stylohyoid ligament, the tether of the hyoid. In addition to ligaments, a dozen or so muscles have attachment to some portion of the hyoid bone.

CERVICAL VERTEBRAE 1 AND 2. The first cervical vertebra is called the *atlas*, because it supports the globe of the head; the second vertebra is named the *axis*, because it provides the pivot on which the atlas turns.

The atlas is a ring of bone with no body and no spinous process, but with a rounded prominence rising from its anterior surface, the *tubercle of the atlas*, identifiable on most lateral head films. There is also a posterior tubercle with which we are less concerned. Nodding movements occur between the atlas and the skull.

The axis is characterized by the *dens*, a tooth-like process that projects upward from the anterior region of the body. The dens articulates within the atlas; rotating movements of the head occur around the dens.

NEUROLOGY

The unimaginable complexity of the human nervous system renders any superficial description almost nonsense. While full comprehension of some of the finer details is still frustratingly absent from our knowledge, the deliberate omission of known particulars is quite difficult on a selective basis. Where do we draw the line? Do we restate a few obvious facts and insult the sophisticated reader, or chance the wrath of the student by including yet more words to memorize? The danger of aiming between the extremes is that we hit nothing, but that is our target.

We will start at the top and work down, but may find ourselves going in both directions at once in some instances. Should vertigo ensue, refer to the outline below: it sets the limits of our excursion, lists the order in which each item will be addressed, and shows to some degree the relative position of component parts in the overall scheme.

THE NERVOUS MECHANISM

I. Central nervous system (CNS)
  A. Brain
    1. Cerebrum
      a. Hemispheres
        (1) Fissures
          (a) Major
          (b) Sulci
        (2) Convolutions (gyri)
        (3) Lobes
      b. Cerebral Cortex
        (1) Motor areas
        (2) Sensory areas
        (3) Association areas
      c. Basal ganglia
        (1) Corpus striatum
        (2) Thalamus
        (3) Hypothalamus
    2. Cerebellum
    3. Brain stem
      a. Midbrain
      b. Pons
      c. Medulla oblongata
  B. Spinal cord
II. Peripheral nervous system
  A. Somatic (cerebrospinal)
    1. Spinal nerves
    2. Cranial nerves
  B. Visceral (autonomic)
    1. Sympathetic
    2. Parasympathetic

Despite the fantastic intricacy of human flesh in all its many forms, it would be but a collection of aimless baubles without the nervous system. Through the nervous system, the body lives. The bone, cartilage, and other connective tissues of the basic skeleton depend on muscle contraction for movement, and on glandular secretions to integrate and chemically regulate that motion. In most cases, muscles contract and glands secrete only upon orders from the nervous system. By means of the neural network we are able to perceive and interpret sensation, from both inner and outer environments, and to translate these stimuli into action, use them to appreciate our existence, store them for future reference, or employ them in homeostasis (to maintain the integrity of the body and its parts).

The nervous system in general is organized into two divisions, the *central* and the *peripheral* portions.

The central nervous system

Two elements make up the central nervous system (CNS), the *brain* and the *spinal cord.* These are enclosed throughout within three membranes, or *meninges.* Named from without inward these are the *dura mater, arachnoid mater,* and *pia mater.* They consist of fibrous connective tissue containing a great many blood vessels, and invest the entire surface of the system, even dipping down between the convolutions of the cerebral cortex.

BRAIN. The brain consists of the *cerebrum,* the *cerebellum,* and the *brain stem.*

Cerebrum. The brain is the largest and most complex mass of nervous tissue in the body, and the cerebrum constitutes the major portion of the brain, filling the entire upper part of the cranium. It is divided front to back by the *longitudinal fissure* into right and left *hemispheres,* which are heavily interconnected below by the *corpus cal-*

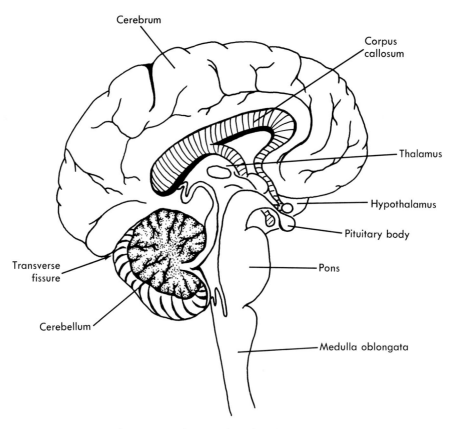

Fig. 5-2. Sagittal section through midline of brain.

losum (see Fig. 5-2). Each hemisphere is further divided by four additional fissures, the *transverse,* the *central* or *fissure of Rolando,* the *lateral cerebral* or *fissure of Sylvius,* and the less well-defined *parieto-occipital* fissure. The location of the transverse fissure is shown in Fig. 5-2; the others appear in Fig. 5-3.

The transverse fissure separates the cerebrum from the cerebellum. The other three help to divide each hemisphere into four lobes, as seen in Fig. 5-4, the *frontal, parietal, temporal,* and *occipital* lobes. The lobes receive their names from the bones about them. In a general sense, each lobe is thought to subserve specific functions; however, localization of brain function can be misleading if carried too far. In no case is the control of a function limited to a single center; all parts of the cerebrum interconnect, making any activity the result of changes in excitability throughout the system. With those reservations,

we may state that the frontal lobe is hypothetically the center for memory and personality, allowing man to ponder on sensory data, to conceive and will the motor acts of his body. The temporal lobe is concerned primarily with audition. The parietal lobe is essentially a general-body sensory lobe, while the occipital lobe is related to vision.

The surface of the cerebrum is extensively wrinkled; only one-third is actually exposed, two-thirds lying within the folds, called *sulci.* A sulcus is more shallow than a fissure. Rising from the sulci are *convolutions,* or ridges. Portions of convolutions are called *gyri;* for example, the *anterior central gyrus* forms part of the precentral convolution lying anterior to the fissure of Rolando, in the frontal lobe, and appears to be the center for most voluntary motor actions. The terms "convolution" and "gyrus" are often used synonymously.

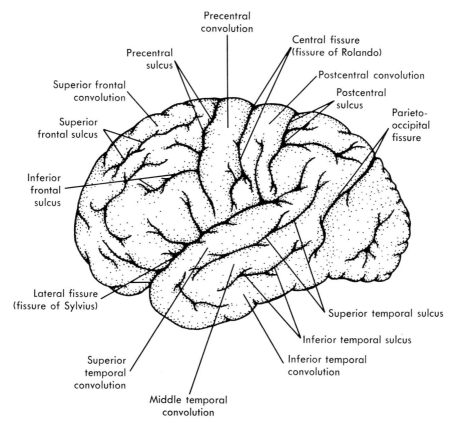

Fig. 5-3. Lateral surface of left cerebral hemisphere, showing fissures, sulci, and convolutions of cerebrum.

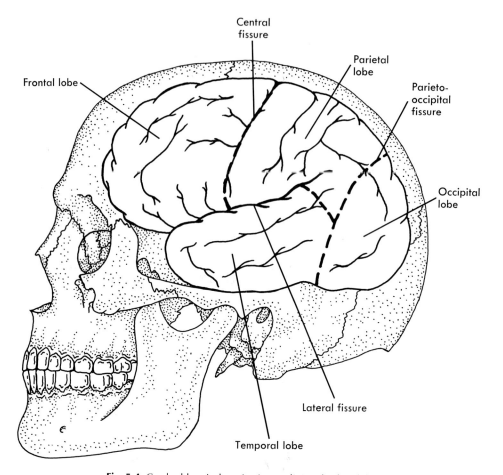

Central fissure

Parietal lobe

Parieto-occipital fissure

Frontal lobe

Occipital lobe

Lateral fissure

Temporal lobe

Fig. 5-4. Cerebral hemisphere in situ, outlining the four lobes.

This creased and corrugated surface of the cerebrum is composed of *gray matter*. It derives its color by being composed primarily of the gray nuclei, or cell bodies proper, of nerve cells. *White matter,* on the other hand, is formed to a larger extent by the *axons* (arms or processes) of nerve cells. Axons run from the cell body to their terminal branches and may be up to 3 feet long.

Most nerves are mixed nerves containing both sensory (afferent) and motor (efferent) fibers. Students have despaired for generations in the attempt to find a reliable mnemonic device by which to remember the contrast between *afferent* and *efferent,* just as many people are troubled by the distinction between *affect* and *effect.* Affect means to influence, to sway, to touch; effect means to accomplish, bring about, or execute. The fact that "execute" and "efferent" both begin with an *e* might be an aid.

Cerebral cortex. The layer of gray matter forming the surface, or rind, of the hemispheres is called the *cerebral cortex.* It is here that "brain mapping" has been carried to its furthest extent, most often during the course of surgical procedures or following various injuries or lesions of cortical regions. As a result of such exploration and observation, areas numbered from 1 to 52 have been identified and their boundaries and functions defined. These areas are then assigned to one of three manifestations of cerebral function: the *motor cortex,* the *sensory cortex,* or the *association cortex.*

For example, the anterior central gyrus referred to above is designated as area 4, and is part of the motor cortex. If the upper or dorsal part of area 4 is explored with a stimulating electrode, movement in the lower extremities of the body results.[12,13] Stimulation of the middle portion of area 4 brings movement of the upper extremities, while excitation of the lower or ventral part results in movement of muscles of the face, tongue, and jaw, and occasional vocalization. It is thus apparent that the motor cortex contains cells whose large axons connect with those motor neurons of cranial and spinal nerves that innervate skeletal muscle. Stimulation of other areas of the motor cortex, of course, leads to contraction of different muscles.

For the oral myologist, one salient fact should be stressed at just this point. While mastication and salivation appear to be somewhat secondary to the entire portion of area 4 concerned specifically with motor control of lips, jaw, tongue, and deglutition, the ventral tip of this region is a segment reserved entirely for swallowing.[7,13] That is, a center exists in the cerebral cortex for voluntary, conscious control of deglutition. By definition, a reflex consists of activity initiated at a subcortical level. Remember that, the next time you hear the total swallowing act described as a reflex. The reflex aspects of deglutition are itemized in Chapters 9 and 11.

The sensory cortex is concerned with the interpretation of sensory stimuli. It is located mainly in the postcentral convolution, lying posterior to the fissure of Rolando and thus in the parietal lobe. However, as noted above, the receptive areas for vision are in the occipital lobe, and those for hearing are in the temporal lobe.

The association cortex comprises the greater part of the lateral surfaces of the occipital, parietal, and temporal lobes, and of the frontal lobe anterior to the motor areas. In effect, the motor and sensory areas form small islands, surrounded on all sides by tissue designated as association areas. No definite functions have been localized in much of this region, but it is known that it is made up of association fibers connecting motor and sensory areas, and some of its specialized abilities are understood. For instance, area 22, located in the parietal lobe, is quite complex. It is, in part, the auditory psychic area where spoken speech is understood. Another part of area 22 is a musical memory area, and if stimulated the subject hears tunes or songs, often forgotten ones.[7] Still another part is concerned with speech in a different way, and injury here results in aphasia, the diminution or loss of language; thoughts and feelings remain, but the subject cannot express them since he cannot associate them with words.

The regions of the cerebral cortex comprising the four lobes are the best known, because they are the most important and the most accessible. Areas below the surface, being less accessible, are less understood. With decortication, the removal of the cerebral cortex, man is reduced to a simple reflex animal. Actions become involuntary and all responses that depend upon memory of acquired experience are lost.

Basal ganglia. Within the interior of the cerebral hemispheres are well-defined areas of gray matter known as the basal ganglia. These include the *corpus striatum,* the *thalamus,* and the *hypothalamus.* The corpus striatum serves to exert a steadying and smoothing effect on voluntary movement. The thalamus acts as a relay station for sensory pathways, for through and alongside the thalamus pass most of the impulses transmitting sensation. It has been called "the seat of emotion," the center for primitive, uncritical sensation. The hypothalamus appears to serve many purposes, decreasing heartbeat, increasing temperature, and perhaps having an influence on sleep. It also influences the pituitary gland which regulates hormonal secretion, and is the main subcortical control center for regulation of sympathetic and parasympathetic activities.

In summary, the cerebrum not only constitutes a larger proportion of the central nervous system in man than in other forms of animal life, it has developed its greatest complexity. Here are found the areas that govern all our mental activities—reason, intelligence, will, and memory. It is the instigator and coordinator of voluntary acts, functions that other animals must leave to involuntary control. It is unique in man in that it provides the means for codification of experience into a symbolic process—language—enabling man not only to communicate in the present, but also to learn from preceding generations and to pass knowledge on to his heirs. It exerts strong control, both facilitatory and inhibitory, over many performances often considered to be reflex acts: micturition, defecation, laughing, weeping—even swallowing, as we noted. A wondrous instrument!

Cerebellum. The cerebellum appears to be a miniature of the cerebral hemispheres attached to the brain stem by massive bundles of nerve tissue. It occupies the lower and posterior part of the skull. Like the cerebrum, it has a cortex of gray matter and an interior of both gray and white matter, and is divisible into two lateral hemispheres. The cerebellum helps to maintain posture and equilibrium and acts as a reflex center, through which coordination and refinement of muscular movement is achieved.

Brain stem. Immediately anterior to the cerebellum lies a massive bundle of nerve tissue called the brain stem. This issues from the base of the cerebral hemispheres and continues downward to connect directly to the spinal cord. It is composed of three areas: the *midbrain* (mesencephalon), a short, constricted portion that connects directly with both the cerebellum and the base of the brain and that leads to a large rounded structure known as the *pons,* which in turn narrows down to the *medulla oblongata.* The latter is continuous with the spinal cord at the foramen magnum, and is sometimes categorized as the superior aspect of the spinal cord rather than the inferior area of the brain.

The midbrain houses important correlation centers as well as nuclei concerned with motor coordination. The pons (bridge) is so named because it is not only the union between the two halves of the cerebellum, but is also the bridge between the midbrain and the medulla. It is a point from which major trunk lines depart to other important centers, and itself contains centers from which emerge three of the cranial nerves that serve head and neck muscles.

The medulla oblongata serves as an organ of conduction for the passage of impulses between the brain and the spinal cord. It also houses the nuclei from which radiate four other cranial nerves (to be discussed below), two of which innervate the muscles of the tongue and palate. Additionally, vasoconstrictor and respiratory centers are found here, along with centers for defecation, salivation, coughing, sneezing, sucking, vomiting—and swallowing.

Note that the brain stem as a whole might be considered a general housekeeping center, concerned with vital processes and visceral and somatic functions, all of which may be modified by impulses entering from the cerebellum and the cerebral cortex. Nerve fibers ascending and descending between the cortex and the lower centers form innumerable interconnections, directly or indirectly, with every center and organ in the entire nervous system. Sensory impulses are interpreted, evaluated, acted upon, or stored. Excitatory impulses are shaped or even extinguished by the inhibitory influences of other centers. Each area exerts some authority in its specialized field over every other center and over the functioning of the total system, thereby helping to maintain the integrity of the body as a

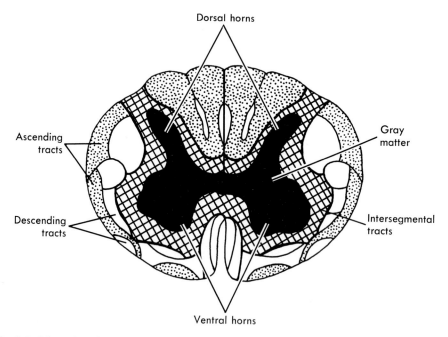

Fig. 5-5. Schematic cross section of spinal cord, showing gray matter and numerous ascending, descending, and mixed tracts. Intersegmental (mixed) tracts completely surround gray matter.

whole. This allows many routine chores to be carried out quite efficiently at a subcortical level, even deglutition in many circumstances.

THE SPINAL CORD. The spinal cord lies protected within the canal of the vertebral column. It is continuous with the brain stem at the foramen magnum, and extends downward to the upper border of the second lumbar vertebra. It is much shorter than the vertebral canal in which it rests, and does not fit as snugly as does the brain in the cranial cavity. Rather, it is suspended within the canal, protected by the meninges, the three membranes that enfold the entire nervous system.

Also unlike the brain, the gray matter of the spinal cord is located internally, arranged in the form of the letter H, and is surrounded by white matter, as indicated schematically in Fig. 5-5. The white matter is composed of parallel bundles of nerve fibers which are grouped together into functional units called *tracts*. Tracts may be either *ascending* (sensory), *descending* (motor), or *mixed* (intersegmental), the latter containing both ascending and descending fibers and surrounding entirely the gray matter of the spinal cord.

The descending tracts carry impulses downward from the cortex to the motor cells in the ventral horns of the gray matter (the lower arms of the H). This is the voluntary motor pathway by means of which we exercise conscious control over body movements. Axons of the cell bodies in the ventral horns emerge through openings in the meninges and attach to striated muscles, bringing about contraction on demand.

Ascending tracts carry sensory impulses upward to higher levels of the spinal cord and to the brain. The cell bodies of these fibers are contained in the dorsal horns. The gray matter also contains a great number of connecting (internuncial) neurons; these allow for the passage of impulses from the dorsal to the ventral roots of the spinal nerves, or from one side of the cord to the other, or from one segment of the cord to another. Some sensory neurons are thus able to make connections with other neurons within the cord itself, thereby making many spinal reflexes possible.

Peripheral nervous system

The peripheral nervous system consists of those nerves that connect the brain and spinal cord (CNS) with all other parts of the body. Generally speaking, the peripheral system controls rapid activities, such as smooth and skeletal muscle contraction, so that response to the environment is immediate. The peripheral system of nerves is a combination of two parts, the *somatic* (pertaining to the body wall) or *cerebrospinal system,* and the *visceral* or *autonomic system.*

SOMATIC SYSTEM. The somatic system includes those parts of the brain, spinal cord, and the nerve fibers, both sensory and motor, that control skeletal (striated) muscles, as well as the end organs, both receptors and effectors, of the body wall.

While much reflex activity is available, this cerebrospinal system is also characterized by consciousness, awareness of sensation and mental activity, and purposeful, planned response to environmental needs. Habitual responses develop, making consciousness of the act unnecessary, but this differs from true reflex.

The primary motor system originates from large cells of the cerebral cortex that are shaped like pyramids; hence the name, *pyramidal pathway.* As they descend, the axons of pyramidal cells make myriad interconnections with fibers from every other center below the cortex, each making its contribution to the nature of the ultimate response. Many of the connecting fibers are organized themselves into the *extrapyramidal system;* this self-controlled system originates deep in the cerebrum, around the basal ganglia, and serves to integrate motor function. It is often referred to as the ''old pathway,'' since phylogenetically it probably preceded the pyramidal pathway which has now usurped much of its original function.

As the pyramidal neurons pass downward through the various subcortical regions, a large number terminate in the pons and medulla, where they serve the cranial nerves. These are called *corticobular* fibers, while those that continue on caudad are termed *corticospinal.*

When the corticospinal fibers arrive at the lower boundary of the medulla, the great majority cross to the other side of the brain stem. This crossing produces a bulge, called the *pyramidal decussation.* A small percentage, about one-fifth, remain ipsilateral until they cross just before they terminate at some level in the spinal cord. It is because of this decussation that the right hemisphere of the cortex controls the left side of the body and vice versa.

All pyramidal fibers of the corticospinal system terminate around the large motor cells in the ventral column of gray matter in the cord. Their impulses are there transmitted to spinal nerve fibers, which in turn bring about volitional movements.

Note once again the constant stream of impulses fed into the pyramidal fibers at every level by multitudinous centers, from the cortex down to the feedback of the sensory system, before a "summation" of all influences results in the "final common pathway." These supplemental impulses may call for compensatory movement, or reinforce, change, or actually inhibit the primary impulse. We can only protrude our tongue with cooperation from the muscles that retract the tongue, or close our lips with inhibition of the perioral muscles that open them. The efficiency of the individual in controlling his muscle activity is determined by the balance between excitatory and inhibitory impulses; to the degree that an imbalance exists, there is clumsiness, inefficiency, or even complete disruption of the system.

We should also point out that any disruption or damage to the motor nerve fiber reduces innervation of the muscle it serves, and paralysis ensues; the paralysis may be partial or total, depending upon the number of nerve fibers impaired. With total disruption of nerve supply, the muscle atrophies. Of more importance to the clinician, however, is the concept of tonicity, which is the result of a constant flow of low-level innervation to a muscle, causing a state of mild but continuous contraction with little or no evidence of fatigue. Tonus can be voluntarily established, then turned over to lower centers in the brain and spinal cord for maintenance.

Spinal nerves. We will spend little time on spinal nerves. This is a complex subject, but has a lesser urgency for the oral myologist. We may note that there are 31 pairs of spinal nerves; listed from the neck downward, these consist of 8 cervical pairs, 12 thoracic, 5 lumbar, 5 sacral, and 1 coccygeal. Each pair emerges into the body by way of the intervertebral foramena, openings at the juncture of the vertebrae in the spinal column. Each nerve is compounded of both sensory and motor roots and, as seen above, the sensory root exits through the dorsal horn of the vertebra while the motor root leaves by way of the ventral horn.

After leaving the cord, each spinal nerve gives off four branches: (1) a *dorsal* branch (posterior primary branch), running to the muscles and skin of the back (motor root to the muscles, sensory root to the skin); (2) a *ventral* branch (anterior primary branch), which supplies the muscles and skin of the sides, front, and extremities of the body; (3) a small *meningeal* branch, going back to the meninges of the cord; and (4) an *autonomic* branch, which connects with ganglia located along but outside the vertebral column. More about this last branch when we discuss the autonomic system.

Cranial nerves. For the oral myoclinician, we can now examine the ignition system, the spark that strikes motion into the muscles entrusted to our care. The cranial nerves supply all areas superior to the throat, with superficial assistance from two of the cervical pairs of spinal nerves.

Twelve pairs of cranial nerves emerge from the undersurface of the brain and pass through openings in the base of the cranium. They are designated by Roman numerals I through XII, according to the order in which they arise from the brain, and also by names which describe their nature, function, or location. Thus, cranial I, the olfactory nerve, is the highest and most anterior, and is so named because it is concerned solely with the sense of smell, while XII, the hypoglossal nerve, arises from the lower portion of the medulla just superior to the spinal cord, is the lowest of the twelve, and is named for its function of serving lingual muscles.

Three of the cranial nerves are entirely sensory in function, five are purely motor, while four are mixed, having both sensory and motor roles.

Some of these nerves have little importance in the present context, whereas others should be conceptualized, their functions understood, their interweaving realized. The most efficient manner in which to present this material is to exhibit it in chart form, as seen in Table 5-1. In order to better visualize the function of these nerves, Fig. 5-6 lists the specific muscles served by four nerves having major importance for us. Only superficial information is provided for nerves in which we have less interest, but their existence is noted in Table 5-1.

Note that in cranial V, VII, IX, and X, the four with mixed function, fibers of the sensory and motor branches within each nerve have interconnections at subcortical levels, making possible reflexive action. The nuclei of origin of motor nerves and the nuclei of termination of sensory nerves are connected with the cerebral cortex.

VISCERAL SYSTEM. The visceral system is not

Table 5-1. Cranial nerves

Num-ber	Name	Type*	CNS Connections	Function
I	Olfactory	S	Mammillary bodies, thalamus, other cranial nerves for salivation, reflexive swallowing	Smell: from receptors in nasal mucosa to olfactory cortex
II	Optic	S		Vision
III	Oculomotor	M		Movement of eyeball, lid, etc.
IV	Trochlear	M		
V	Trigeminal—3 branches:		To thalamus, then postcentral gyrus of cortex	
	1. Ophthalmic	S	Arises from lateral surface of the pons	Pain, touch, and temperature from top of head, conjunctiva and upper lid, skin and mucosa of nose
	2. Maxillary	S		Pain, touch, and temperature from cheek, upper lip, hard palate, upper jaw and teeth, maxillary sinuses
	3. Mandibular	S		Pain, touch, and temperature from lower lip, lower jaw and teeth, mouth, anterior tongue, external ear
		M	With nerves VII and IX for reflex movements; from cortex for voluntary muscle movements	Contraction of muscles of mastication
VI	Abducens	M		Lateral eye movement
VII	Facial	S	From nucleus in lower pons to thalamus and postcentral gyrus	Taste from anterior two-thirds of tongue
		M	Reflex connections with extrapyramidal and spinal tracts, and with nuclei of V	Contraction of muscles of expression, scalp, stapedius, and posterior belly of digastric Secretion of salivary glands, mucous membrane of nose and mouth
VIII	Acoustic—2 divisions:	S		
	1. Cochlear			Hearing
	2. Vestibular			Equilibrium
IX	Glossopharyngeal	S	From nucleus in medulla to thalamus and postcentral gyrus of the cortex	General sensation from pharynx, velum, posterior tongue, eardrum
			Reflex connections with cardiac center of medulla, with sympathetic system for regulation of respiration and blood pressure	Taste from posterior third of tongue
		M	Reflex connections with nuclei of X; with extrapyramidal and spinal tracts for gag reflex and reflexive swallowing	Pharyngeal movement during swallowing
X	Vagus	S	From sensory nucleus in medulla to thalamus and postcentral gyrus of cortex	Pain, touch, temperature from auditory canal, meninges; general sensation from pharynx, larynx, trachea, esophagus; sensation of nausea, etc.

*Sensory, S; motor, M.

Continued.

Table 5-1. Cranial nerves—cont'd

Num-ber	Name	Type*	CNS Connections	Function
		M	Reflex connections with extra-pyramidal and spinal tracts; with thalamus; with nuclei of V, VII, IX	Swallowing: contraction of muscles of velum, pharynx Speech: contraction of intrinsic muscles of larynx Secretion: glands of stomach and intestines Innervates all visceral organs in thorax and abdomen
XI	Accessory (or spinal accessory)	M	Connections with spinal tract for postural reflexes	Speech: contraction of some muscles of larynx, pharynx, velum, uvula Head and shoulder movement: contraction of trapezius and sternocleidomastoid
XII	Hypoglossal	M	Reflex connection with extra-pyramidal and spinal tracts, and with sensory nuclei of V, IX, X	Contraction of tongue muscles in speech, mastication, swallowing

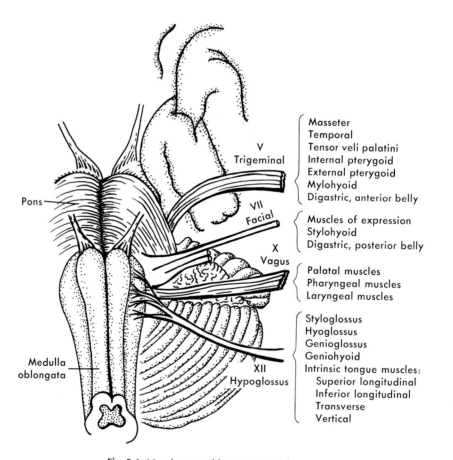

Fig. 5-6. Muscles served by some cranial nerves.

normally under voluntary control, from which fact it derives its title of *autonomic* system. It consists of all parts of the nervous system that serve the smooth muscles of the blood vessels and the viscera, including the heart, digestive tract, genitourinary system, and glands.

Basic to an understanding of the autonomic system is a definition of *ganglia;* a ganglion is a cluster of neural cell bodies (gray matter) located outside the brain or spinal cord. Certain nerve fibers of the CNS provide connections to the ganglia, as we saw while describing the spinal nerves; these are called preganglionic fibers. Other fibers, the postganglionic fibers, extend peripherally to the muscle or gland they serve. Since much of the function of this system involves reflex activity, the ganglia are able to retain considerable control over their own neurons. Accordingly, the visceral system possesses a certain independence of the cerebrospinal system. There is no specific consciousness of these activities; the heart muscle contracts automatically; we do not will the glands to secrete. Nevertheless, the two systems are so closely integrated, and have so many overlapping neural attachments, that either is able to elicit responses from the other.

Anatomically, the visceral system is divided into *sympathetic* and *parasympathetic* divisions. Each division has its own responsibilities, but in many ways they have an antagonistic function. For example, the sympathetic dilates the eye, stimulates the heart, and inhibits the bladder, while the parasympathetic constricts the iris, inhibits the heart, and stimulates the bladder.

In general, but not without exception, we can say that the sympathetic system *mobilizes* and *spends* the resources of the body whereas the parasympathetic system *conserves* and *stores* bodily resources. Of course, as with every other element of the nervous mechanism, these two systems never act independently of each other but are brought into correlated activity according to the demands made on the body by the external world. Through their antagonistic yet coordinated action, a comparatively stable equilibrium of the internal environment is maintained under many different conditions of work and rest.

Sympathetic. The preganglionic fibers of the sympathetic system emerge from the vertebrae comprising the great central section of the spinal column, the thoracic (chest) and lumbar (trunk) portions. Just outside the spinal cord, however, these axons leave the main root nerve and enter a ganglion, where they end upon the cell bodies of other neurons. A chain of ganglia, called the *ganglionic cord,* lies along each side of the spinal cord throughout its length, and these house the cell bodies of the autonomic nerves, from which rather lengthy axons extend to the tissue or organ each subserves.

This system has been known historically as the "fight or flight" mechanism, since its functions include so many preparations for emergency situations. Stimulation of these fibers produces vasoconstriction and accelerated heartbeat, with a resulting rise in blood pressure, erection of hair, gooseflesh, depression of gastrointestinal activity, secretion of adrenalin into the bloodstream, plus several other preliminaries that ready the body to flee or to stand and give battle.

Parasympathetic. The parasympathetic or craniosacral system joins two unlikely components from opposite ends of the CNS, the brain stem and the sacrum, the lower portion of the spinal cord. From the second, third, and fourth sacral nerves come fibers serving the colon, rectum, bladder, and genital organs. All other organs and tissues of the visceral system receive innervation from the cranial component; this is composed of fibers emanating from cranial nerves III, VII, IX, and X, but in a fashion quite different from the thoracicolumbar pattern.

We noted that the ganglionic chain of the latter system lies just outside the spinal cord, with long postganglionic fibers running to visceral structures. To the contrary, the ganglia of the parasympathetic system are always located in or very close to the organ innervated; this requires long preganglionic fibers but postganglionic fibers that are quite short. This arrangement also precludes any organized ganglionic chain by which nervous effects can be interrelated. From such a structural difference we might surmise a resultant functional contrast: the sympathetic division tends to act more diffusely and as a whole, whereas the parasympathetic system is more highly differentiated, capable of independent and specific activity in each of its parts.

MYOLOGY

Based on the information in the preceding pages, we are prepared at last to examine the muscles from which we derive our professional title.

General considerations

Before looking at individual muscles a number of general factors applying to all muscle tissue should be understood. A muscle consists of a bundle of elongated cells that are called *fibers,* unified by an intercellular substance and supported by a framework of connective tissues. All motion in the body is a product of the contractility of muscle fibers.

Muscles are distinct from ligaments, tendons, and aponeuroses. The latter three are composed of strong, fibrous connective tissue, are inelastic, and do not contract, but serve as the attachment of muscles to bones or other parts. Ligaments also bind together the articular ends of bones, support certain visceral organs, and are usually sheet-like in form. A tendon is a narrow ribbon-like band; an aponeurosis is a broad, flat tendon.

MUSCLE CLASSIFICATION. Muscles are classified according to their structure and function into three categories: *smooth (visceral), striated (skeletal),* and *cardiac.* Smooth muscles are those of the stomach, intestines, and blood vessels, and since they are under the control of the autonomic nervous system they are not subject to conscious voluntary action. They are called smooth muscles because their cytoplasm has no transverse striations. They are composed of spindle-shaped cells held together by fibrils.

Cardiac muscle is striated, but not distinctly so. Its cells are elongated, branching, and multinucleated, and are grouped in bundles. Its contraction ejects blood from the heart and, of course, is not under voluntary control.

The striated muscles, those with which we deal, are so called because the cytoplasm of the cells has fine transverse bands that are visible microscopically. The fibers are arranged in compact bundles separated by fine connective tissue sheaths; these sheaths extend into the muscle from an outer connective tissue framework that carries blood vessels and nerves. These are the voluntary muscles.

ATTACHMENT. In describing muscle attachments two terms are used, *origin* and *insertion.* Actually, muscles do not originate at one point and insert into another, but convention decrees that we identify the attachment nearer the center of the body, or the one more fixed, as the origin, and the more peripheral attachment, or the one more movable, as the insertion. The supposition would be that contraction of the muscle would create movement from the insertion toward the point of origin; in function, this is not always the case.

In general, muscles are attached to bones; however, some muscles are affixed to cartilage while others encircle blood vessels (vasoconstrictors) or attach to visceral organs, etc. Occasionally a muscle is anchored directly to the periosteum of bone, but more commonly the attachment is made by means of a tendon or aponeurosis.

NERVE SUPPLY. Each muscle is supplied with at least one nerve that transmits impulses from the CNS, causing the muscle to contract. While each motor nerve fiber is capable of innervating up to fifty muscle fibers, those muscles that perform delicate tasks have a larger proportion of nerve fibers, ranging down to only six muscle fibers for each nerve fiber. A motor nerve fiber with the muscle fibers it serves is called a *motor unit.* Sensory nerves feed back information regarding the degree and strength of contraction to the central nervous system.

The many interconnections and interrelationships of the nervous system find some reflection in muscular tissue. No movement is the result of action by a single muscle. Many other muscles function simultaneously to a greater or lesser degree, supplementing, stabilizing, smoothing, or simply relaxing antagonistic tension, in order to execute the desired action.

TYPES OF CONTRACTION. Striated muscle is capable of two types of contraction, both of which should be understood by the clinician. When a muscle bundle contracts, lifting a weight, the muscle becomes shorter and thicker, but its tonus remains the same. Since the tone of the fibers is not changed, this contraction is called *isotonic.* On the other hand, if the muscle is forced to contract against a weight that it cannot lift, the tension in the fibers increases, but the muscle length is not altered. Since the length of the fibers is unchanged, this contraction is called *isometric.* Most muscle contraction is of the isotonic type, but complex muscular activity requires the coordinated development of both types.

Musculature

Of more than 600 muscles in the body, we will study approximately 40. While it will be necessary to discuss some of these individually, we will again present much of the information in chart form.

MUSCLES OF EXPRESSION. The array of muscles

customarily grouped under the heading of "muscles of facial expression" includes a number situated about the eyes, nose, and scalp. We will eliminate those as being nonessential to our specific purposes. Nevertheless, we are left with ten muscles in which we have a rather intense interest, those listed in Table 5-2. The location of each can be seen in Fig. 5-7. All are innervated by cranial VII, the facial nerve.

Orbicularis oris. We may logically consider first the orbicularis oris, the most complex of the facial muscles, the only one not demonstrably paired in the two sides of the face, and the one creating most anguish for the clinician in many cases. The orbicularis oris encircles the lips and is the sphincter of the mouth, its tonicity alone usually adequate to achieve bilabial contact in the resting face. A slight increase in tension suffices to maintain closed lips during mastication, while extreme contraction puckers the lips.

The complexity of the orbicularis oris arises partly from the fact that its fibers appear to be borrowed from other perioral muscles; technically it has no origin or insertion, and might be considered in a sense to be a composite of many muscles, a hub where representatives from surrounding muscles meet to form a unified network. As a result, this muscle is not simply a circular band. As the fibers pass along the borders of the lips, there are intimate interconnections between the decussating fibers of the upper and lower lip, but many fibers then pass on at various oblique angles into the neighboring muscles. It has now been shown that contraction of orbicularis oris does not necessarily result in equal force of the upper and lower lip; one or the other lip may be weaker, a condition that would not exist if the muscle were a continuous band.

Two minor muscles that we will not pursue hereafter serve to stabilize the orbicularis oris by providing bony attachment. The upper one consists of two bands, lateral and medial, on either side of the midline; the lateral band connects the orbicularis with the alveolar border of the maxilla near the lateral incisor tooth, while the medial band connects to the septum of the nose. The interval between the two medial bands is recognized on the surface of the lip as the *philtrum*, the vertical depression beneath the nasal septum terminating at the vermillion line. The lower lip is attached to the mandible, lateral to the mentalis, by the second of these two muscle slips.

We will now move clockwise around the or-

Table 5-2. Muscles of facial expression*

Muscle	Origin	Insertion	Function
Orbicularis oris	None. Derives fibers from other muscles in the area. Encircles mouth.		Closes mouth: compresses or puckers lips
Quadratus labii superior	Frontal process of maxilla; lower border of orbit; zygomatic bone	Upper lip, laterally from midline	Elevates upper lip
Caninus	Canine fossa of maxilla	Upper lip, at angle of mouth	Elevates outer end of upper lip
Zygomatic	Zygomatic bone	Upper lip, at angle of mouth	Pulls corner of mouth up and back
Buccinator	Alveolar processes of maxilla and mandible; pterygomandibular raphe	Fibers of other labial muscles	Compresses cheek; unifies action of interconnecting muscles
Risorius	Fascia over masseter	Skin at angle of mouth	Retracts angle of mouth
Triangularis	Oblique line of mandible	Lower lip at angle of mouth	Depresses angle of mouth
Quadratus labii inferior	Oblique line of mandible	Integument of lower lip	Draws lower lip down and back
Mentalis	Incisive fossa of mandible	Integument of chin	Raises and protrudes lower lip
Platysma	Fascia covering thoracic muscles	Skin and tissue of lower face; mandible below oblique line	Depresses mandible; wrinkles skin of neck and chin; depresses outer end of lower lip

*All innervated by cranial nerve VII.

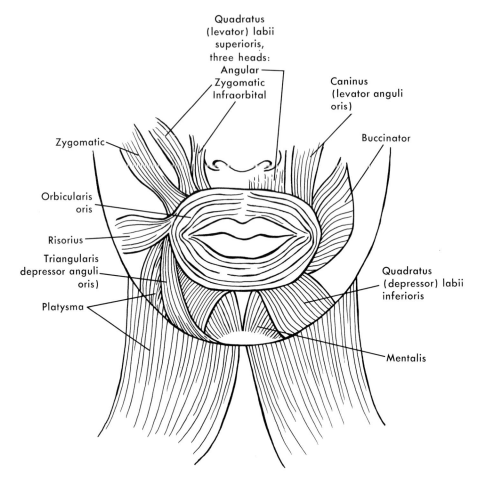

Fig. 5-7. Muscles of expression in lower face.

bicularis oris, although the overlapping of muscles will prevent this from being precise.

Quadratus labii superior. The quadratus labii superior (levator labii superioris) lies nearest the midline of the muscles above the mouth, some of its fibers even inserting into the alar cartilage of the nose. It has three heads: the *angular,* whose origin is the frontal process of the maxilla near the nose, the *infraorbital,* with origin at the lower border of the orbit, and the *zygomatic,* arising from the zygomatic bone. All three run inferiorly and insert into the upper lip from the midline laterally.

Caninus. The caninus has origin in the canine fossa below the infraorbital foramen of the maxilla, and thus lies quite near the superior quadratus. Its fibers descend vertically to the angle of the mouth, its insertion in the upper lip

mingling with fibers from the orbicularis, triangularis, and zygomatic muscles.

Zygomatic. The origin of the zygomatic muscle is from the zygomatic bone, placing it lateral to the caninus. Its fibers descend obliquely with a medial inclination and insert into the corner of the mouth, blending with fibers of the nearby muscles.

Buccinator. The buccinator covers the entire lateral wall of the mouth, constitutes the essential muscular coat of the cheek, and will be discussed in more detail in Chapter 6. It arises in the molar region from the outer surfaces of the alveolar processes of the maxilla and mandible, and posteriorly from the anterior border of the pterygomandibular raphe, a dense band of deep fascia in the pharynx.

Buccinator fibers converge as they approach

Table 5-3. Muscles of mastication*

Muscle	Origin	Insertion	Function
Masseter	Superficial: lower border of zygomatic arch Deep: medial surface of zygomatic arch	Superficial: outer surface of lower ramus and angle of mandible Deep: outer surface of upper ramus and coronoid process	Lifts mandible vertically
Temporalis	Temporal fossa of skull	Coronoid process and anterior margin of upper ramus	Elevates and retracts mandible
Internal pterygoid	Lateral pterygoid plate; palatine and maxillary bones	Lower margin of inner surface of ramus	Elevates and protrudes mandible
External pterygoid	Upper head: greater wing of sphenoid Lower head: outer surface of lateral pterygoid plate	Neck of condyle and articular disc of TMJ	Draws mandible forward; depresses mandible; moves mandible to side

*All innervated by the mandibular branch of cranial nerve V.

the angle of the mouth. The central fibers intersect and pass on, those from the upper portion dipping down to become continuous with the fibers of the orbicularis oris in the lower lip, lower central fibers rising to continue around the upper lip. Fibers from the upper and lower regions of the buccinator continue forward into the corresponding lip without decussation.

In basic function, contraction of the buccinator compresses the cheek, keeping it firmly in contact with the teeth, and thus aids in chewing by preventing food from escaping into the buccal vestibule.

Risorius. The risorius is a narrow bundle of fibers originating in the fascia overlying the masseter. It runs horizontally forward, tapering somewhat before it inserts into the skin at the angle of the mouth.

Triangularis. We now dip below the horizontal midline to the triangularis muscle. This muscle has origin in the oblique line of the mandible, where it is continuous with the fibers of the platysma muscle. From this broad origin the fibers converge into a narrow bundle and insert into the angle of the mouth.

Quadratus labii inferior. The quadratus labii inferior (depressor labii inferioris) is a small square muscle also arising from the oblique line of the mandible, but anterior to the triangularis. Its fibers run upward and medialward to insert into the integument (skin) of the lower lip where it also blends with the orbicularis oris.

Mentalis. In our clockwise journey we have now arrived at 6 o'clock, the lower vertical midline, where we find the mentalis muscle, the only facial muscle with fibers running *away* from the lips. Its origin is the incisive fossa of the mandible, from where it descends alongside the frenum of the lower lip to insert into the skin covering the chin. It is often described in anatomy texts without conscious irony as a "small" muscle; the oral myologist battles to reduce the seemingly mountainous bundle that results from excessive use. Even when not overdeveloped, it varies in size more than any of the other facial muscles.

Platysma. The last of this group is the platysma muscle, whose fibers forms a broad sheet, sometimes scattered, just below the skin of the neck. It originates in the superficial fascia covering the muscles of the thorax. Its fibers rise upward and medially over the side of the neck, cross the mandible, and insert at various places, some into the mandible below the oblique line, others into the skin and tissue of the lower face. Contraction of the platysma wrinkles the skin of the neck and chin, draws the outer part of the lower lip down and back, and assists the external pterygoid in lowering the mandible.

MUSCLES OF MASTICATION. The four muscles itemized in Table 5-3 are termed the "muscles of mastication," although a number of other muscles have accessory functions in varying degrees during actual mastication. A detailed description of the masticatory process is found in Chapter 11.

Of the four muscles under discussion here, three (the masseter, temporal, and internal pterygoid) serve to elevate the jaw, and are often grouped as the "antigravity muscles." The fourth, the external pterygoid, lowers the mandible. All are supplied from the motor part of the mandibular branch of cranial V, the trigeminal nerve. This branch is sometimes referred to as the "masticator nerve."

The masseter is a thick, powerful muscle consisting of two parts, a superficial and a deep portion, as shown in Fig. 5-8, A. The superficial portion arises as a thick aponeurosis from the zygomatic process of the maxilla and the lower border of the zygomatic arch. These fibers run downward and backward, and insert into the angle of the mandible and into the lower half of the outer surface of the ramus. The deep portion, smaller but more muscular, arises from the medial surface of the zygomatic arch; its fibers pass downward and forward, where they insert into the upper half of the ramus and the outer surface of the coronoid process. Contraction of the masseter lifts the mandible vertically against the maxilla.

Temporalis. The temporalis, also seen in Fig. 5-8, A, is a fan-shaped muscle whose origin covers the entire temporal fossa. As the fibers descend, they converge to end in a tendon which passes beneath the zygomatic arch and inserts into the coronoid process and the anterior border of the ramus of the mandible. From this attachment the temporalis is enabled to retract the mandible as it elevates.

Internal (medial) pterygoid. The internal pterygoid (Fig. 5-8, B) is another thick, quadrangular muscle. It arises from the lateral pterygoid plate and from the nearby surfaces of the palatine and maxillary bones. Its fibers angle downward, backward, and outward to find insertion by a strong sheet of tendon into the inner surface of the ramus along its lower margin. In this posture it acts to pull the mandible forward.

External (lateral) pterygoid. The external pter-

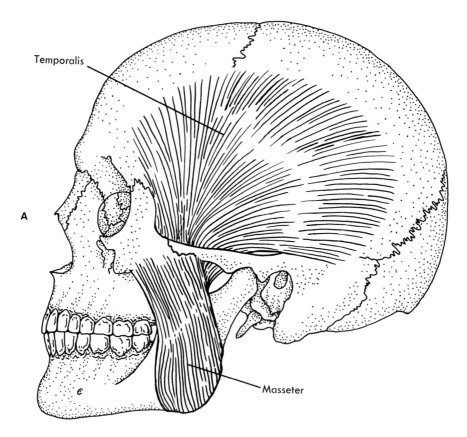

Fig. 5-8. Muscles of mastication. **A,** Masseter and temporalis. **B,** Internal and external pterygoids.

ygoid is a short, thick muscle that tapers backward from twin origins almost horizontally to the condyle of the mandible. It too is shown in Fig. 5-8, *B*. One of its heads arises from the outer surface of the greater wing of the sphenoid bone, the other from the outer surface of the lateral pterygoid plate of the sphenoid bone. Its fibers incline slightly outward as they pass back to their insertion on the front of the neck of the condyle. Some fibers also insert into the front margin of the articular disc of the temporomandibular joint. The action of the external pterygoid is in part to tip the mandible down, opening the jaw, but its primary function is to draw the mandible forward. This protrusion of the mandible results when the external pterygoid of both sides contract in unison. When both the external and internal pterygoids of one side work alternately with those of the other side, they produce lateral movement of the mandible.

MUSCLES OF THE TONGUE. The tongue, the target of much of the oral myologist's efforts, is composed almost entirely of muscles. It must then be obviously essential that the clinician know and understand the eight constituent muscles of the tongue. Four of these are contained entirely within the tongue, the *intrinsic* muscles, and are responsible for changes in the shape of the tongue; four others originate from nearby skeletal structures, thus are *extrinsic* muscles, and are accountable for most movements of the tongue.

The tongue is divided into lateral halves by a median fibrous septum that extends the entire length of the tongue. This division is outlined on the surface, beneath by the lingual frenum, the vertical fold of mucous membrane along the midline that attaches the tongue to the soft tissue below, and above by the midline groove running front to back on the dorsum of most tongues. All lingual muscles are thus paired, each half of the tongue boasting a full set of eight.

Intrinsic muscles. The intrinsic muscles of the tongue are displayed in Table 5-4. They are

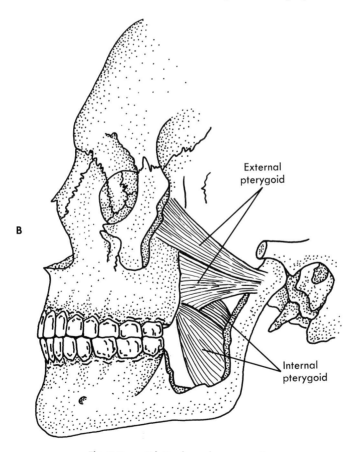

Fig. 5-8, cont'd. For legend see opposite page.

Table 5-4. Intrinsic muscles of the tongue*

Muscle	Origin	Insertion	Function
Superior longitudinal	Submucosa near epiglottis; median septum of tongue	Edges of tongue	Shortens, widens tongue; turns tip and sides up, forming concave dorsum
Inferior longitudinal	Lower portion of root of tongue	Apex (tip) of tongue	Shortens, widens tongue; depresses tip, forming convex dorsum
Transverse	Median septum of tongue	Mucosa at side of tongue	Narrows, elongates tongue
Vertical	Upper surface of tongue	Lower surface of tongue	Flattens, widens tongue tip

*All innervated by cranial nerve XII.

Table 5-5. Extrinsic muscles of the tongue

Muscle	Cranial nerve	Origin	Insertion	Function
Genioglossus	XII	Inner surface of mandible near symphysis	Median septum of tongue; body of hyoid bone	Various fibers protrude and retract tongue; depress midline of tongue; elevate hyoid bone
Hyoglossus	XII	Body and greater cornu of hyoid bone	Side of the tongue, posterior half	Depresses and retracts tongue; depresses side of tongue
Styloglossus	XII	Styloid process of temporal bone	Lateral margin, full length of tongue	Draws tongue upward and backward; elevates side of tongue
Palatoglossus	X	Anterior surface of velum	Side of posterior tongue	Constricts faucial isthmus, elevates posterior tongue

named for their planes of direction within the tongue and, although there is considerable interweaving of fibers, they remain to a great degree separate bundles or layers. Fibers from the extrinsic muscles also blend in, providing the tongue with the potential for an infinite versatility while maintaining firm coordination between the position and the shape of the tongue.

We need add little here to the information in Table 5-4. The *superior longitudinal* is a thin layer lying immediately beneath the mucous membrane on the dorsum of the tongue. The *inferior longitudinal* is a narrow band on the under surface of the tongue, between the genioglossus and hyoglossus. The fibers of the *transverse* pass laterally from the midline to the lingual edges. The *vertical* is found only at the borders of the forepart of the tongue. All are innervated by cranial XII, the hypoglossal nerve.

Extrinsic muscles. The four extrinsic muscles of the tongue are shown in Table 5-5 and pictured in Fig. 5-9. The palatoglossus muscle is included, since it is a lingual muscle; however, it is also

associated with the soft palate and its function may be best understood in that context. Accordingly, it will be described in the following section.

Genioglossus. The genioglossus muscle derives its name from the Latin *genion* (chin) and the Greek word for tongue *(glossa);* the Latin term for tongue is *lingua.* This muscle not only constitutes a large physical proportion of the tongue, it does most of the work. It also poses one of the major challenges for the clinician, since lack of a normal balance of tonus among the three segments of the genioglossal fibers allows the tongue to drift forward and downward to a familiar but undesirable interdental resting posture.

The genioglossus is a flat, triangular muscle, somewhat resembling a fan held perpendicularly, the handle representing its point of origin. This origin is a short tendon from the lingual surface of the mandible at the symphysis, from where the fibers fan out in three directions. The lower fibers extend back and down where they

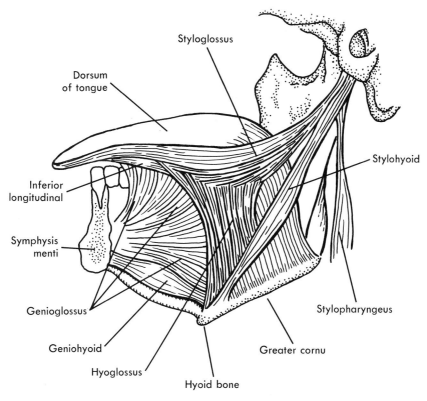

Fig. 5-9. Extrinsic muscles of tongue.

attach to the upper part of the body of the hyoid bone. The middle fibers pass back and upward, while the superior ones curve up and forward; combined, they enter the entire length of the tongue from root to tip to insert along the median fibrous septum.

The anterior fibers withdraw and depress the tip of the tongue. They also work in concert with the middle fibers to draw the entire dorsum of the tongue downward into a concave channel, as in sucking action. The middle portion alone draws the base of the tongue forward and thereby protrudes it. The inferior fibers pull the hyoid bone upward and forward, a part of the synergy of actions involved as the entire larynx moves up and forward during deglutition.

Hyoglossus. The hyoglossus is a thin, rectangular sheet of muscle that arises from the side of the body of the hyoid bone and from the entire length of its greater cornu. It runs vertically upward to enter the side of the tongue, then pass medially to insert into the medial septum of the tongue. Its fibers interlace with intrinsic muscle

fibers. Its contraction pulls the tongue down and back; when the hyoid bone is fixed, it depresses the sides of the tongue.

Styloglossus. The styloglossus originates from the styloid process of the temporal bone. As it passes downward and forward to the side of the tongue, it divides into two segments, the longitudinal and oblique portions. The longitudinal portion enters the side of the tongue near its dorsal surface, and blending with the fibers of the inferior longitudinal muscle, runs to the tip of the tongue. The oblique portion overlaps and penetrates the hyoglossus muscle as it runs transversely to the midline of the tongue. The styloglossus retracts the tongue and draws its sides upward.

MUSCLES OF THE SOFT PALATE. Looking over the tongue toward the back of the mouth, as in Fig. 5-10, several features are to be noted. The soft palate (velum) extends from its junction with the hard palate without perceptible demarcation, the continuous mucous membrane concealing the line of the union. The attachment of the velum to

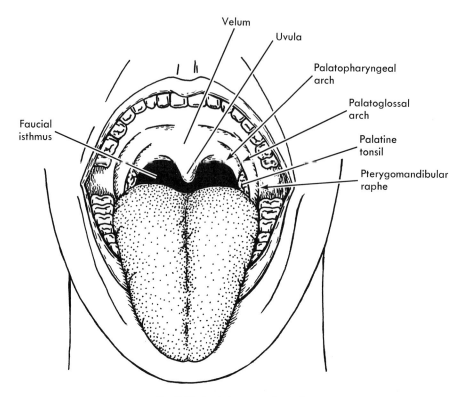

Velum

Uvula

Palatopharyngeal
arch

Palatoglossal
arch

Palatine
tonsil

Pterygomandibular
raphe

Faucial
isthmus

Fig. 5-10. Posterior area of mouth.

the hard palate is achieved by the *palatine apo-neurosis*, a thin, firm, fibrous plate emerging from the posterior border of the hard palate. When lifted, the velum reveals the uvula suspended from its lower midpoint, as well as the posterior pharyngeal wall behind. Laterally the soft palate blends into the two *pillars of the fauces* (throat), one behind the other, which connect the velum with the lateral pharyngeal wall and the base of the tongue, respectively. The posterior pillar is called the *palatopharyngeal arch* and the anterior is termed the *palatoglossal arch;* each is formed by a muscle described below. Between the two arches on either side lie the tonsils, technically the *palatine tonsils*. The lateral space between the anterior faucial pillars, the opening into the pharynx, is called the *faucial isthmus*.

We may then examine the velum more closely. This mobile structure, like the tongue, is largely composed of muscles. Because these muscles enter the palate from various outside locations, some above, some below, and some behind the velum, it is given the ability to move in many

directions as it combines or separates the oral and nasal cavities, the nasal cavity and the pharynx, etc. The six muscles thus employed are itemized in Table 5-6, and some are depicted more graphically in Fig. 5-11.

Note that we enter here into a gray area where voluntary contraction of muscles begins to give way to reflex contraction; posterior to the velum, direct voluntary control over muscle is lost, contraction occurring only as a secondary reaction to some volitional action in the mouth. That is, we cannot deliberately set in motion the chain of constrictor muscles lining the pharyngeal wall; we can only perform a voluntary act that will trigger their reflexive contraction.

The importance of the foregoing lies in the fact that, among the patients we see, many display inactivity, or inappropriate activity, of the palatal muscles. While voluntary control of these muscles may not be exercised, it is accessible, and needs to be established in most cases.

The muscle of the *uvula* is not one to cause concern. The entire uvula is vestigial, serving no known purpose. It is listed because it exists.

Table 5-6. Muscles of the soft palate

Muscle	Cranial nerve	Origin	Insertion	Function
Uvula	X	Posterior nasal spine; palatal aponeurosis	Body of uvula	Elevates uvula
Tensor veli palatini	V (mandibular branch)	Scaphoid fossa; spine of medial pterygoid plate; posterior border of hard palate	Palatal aponeurosis; cartilage of eustachian tube	Tenses velum: opens eustachian tube during deglutition
Levator veli palatini	X	Lower surface, petrous portion of temporal bone; side of eustachian tube	Throughout velum to midline	Elevates velum toward posterior pharyngeal wall; dilates orifice of eustachian tube
Palato-pharyngius	X	Lower: mucous membrane along posterior border of velum Upper: midline of velum	Posterior thyroid cartilage; aponeurosis of pharynx	Depresses velum; constricts faucial isthmus; elevates pharynx
Palatoglossus (see also: "Extrinsic muscle of tongue")	X	Anterior surface of velum	Side of posterior tongue	Constricts faucial isthmus; elevates tongue
Velopharyngeal sphincter	X	Midline of velum	Posterior median raphe of pharynx	Aids in moving velum posteriorly; creates ridge on posterior pharyngeal wall

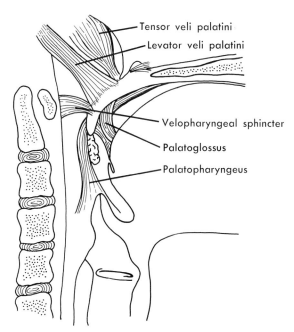

Fig. 5-11. Muscles of soft palate.

The *tensor veli palatini* and the *levator veli palatini* need little discussion beyond that shown in Table 5-6. Both are named for their function.

The *palatopharyngeus*, as indicated above, forms the posterior faucial pillar. Its upper and lower fasciculi unite into a compact bundle to curve out and down behind the tonsil.

The *palatoglossus* forms the other (anterior) pillar of the fauces, arching down in front of the tonsil. Since both ends attach to mobile structures, its contraction may either draw the sides of the tongue up and back, or draw down the sides of the velum, depending upon which end of the muscle is more firmly fixed at the moment.

The *velopharyngeal sphincter* has fibers that pass horizontally around the sides of the pharynx, from the midline of the velum to the midline of the posterior pharyngeal wall. This muscle also has dual, but in this case simultaneous, functions. It draws the soft palate posteriorly, and is thought to pull forward a horizontal fold of the posterior pharyngeal wall known as Passavant's pad. This action occurs during one phase of swallowing.

MUSCLES OF THE NECK. Moving dorsad, we have now reached the outer boundary of our province; as previously noted, the sequential layer of muscle lining the wall of the pharynx is beyond our supervision. We have described three muscles that enter this region, the palatoglossal, palatopharyngeal, and velopharyngeal muscles. Five other muscles reside in the area, the *superior, middle,* and *inferior constrictor,* aided from below by the *stylopharyngeal* and *salpingo-*

pharyngeal muscles. These function in series to change the shape of the tube in deglutition, constricting the diameter of the pharynx, as the bolus is progressively squeezed into the esophagus.

Inferior to the tongue there are four additional muscles in which the clinician should have an

Table 5-7. Suprahyoid muscles

Muscle	Cranial nerve	Origin	Insertion	Function
Digastric				
Anterior belly	V	Interior mandible near midline	Body and greater cornu of hyoid bone, via intermediate tendon	Depresses mandible or elevates hyoid bone
Posterior belly	VII	Inner surfaces of mastoid process		
Mylohyoid	V	Mylohyoid ridge of mandible	Body of hyoid bone and midline raphe	Lifts hyoid bond and base of tongue up and forward
Geniohyoid	XII (aided by first cervical)	Inferior mental spine at symphysis of mandible	Body of hyoid bone, anterior surface	Draws hyoid bone and base of tongue forward
Stylohyoid	XII	Styloid process of temporal bone	Body of hyoid near greater cornu	Lifts hyoid bone up and backward

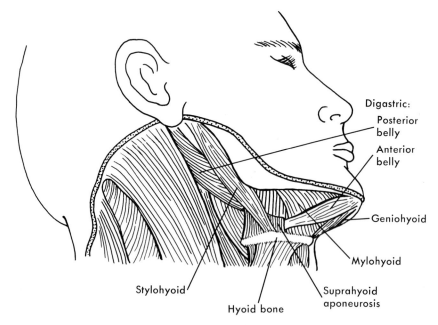

Fig. 5-12. Suprahyoid muscles.

interest, those treated in Table 5-7 and seen in Fig. 5-12. These all lie above the hyoid bone, to which each one is attached, and accordingly they are known as the suprahyoids. Four other muscles, the infrahyoids, attach to the hyoid bone from below; as with the constrictors, the infrahyoids are beyond our grasp on a direct basis. The infrahyoids consist of the *sternohyoid, sternothyroid, thyrohyoid* and *omohyoid* muscles, and serve at the conclusion of the swallowing act to return the hyoid bone and the larynx to a neutral position.

The *digastric* muscle is a fleshy, sling-like muscle consisting of two bellies arising from opposite points but joining near the middle. The anterior belly originates on the inner and lower border of the mandible close to the symphysis and loops downward and backward. The posterior belly arises from the mastoid notch of the temporal bone and swings downward and forward. The two bellies meet at a round intermediate tendon which in turn gives rise to the *suprahyoid aponeurosis,* a broad fibrous layer that attaches to the body and greater cornu of the hyoid bone. It is somewhat unusual in that the two bellies are not served by the same nerve, the anterior being innervated by the trigeminal, cranial V, while the posterior belly receives fibers of the facial nerve, cranial VII.

The *mylohyoid* has added interest because it forms a muscular sheet that is the floor of the mouth. It arises from the entire length of the mylohyoid line of the mandible, from the symphysis menti to the third molar region. The posterior fibers run medially and slightly down to insert into the body of the hyoid bone. The middle and anterior fibers meet their fellows from the opposite side at a midline raphe which runs from the symphysis to the hyoid bone.

The *geniohyoid* and the *stylohyoid* muscles work from opposite anteroposterior origins to move the hyoid bone forward and backward.

A GLOSSARY OF ANATOMIC TERMS

abduction To draw away from the midline.

adduction To draw toward the midline.

adipose Pertaining to various tissues which store fat cells.

afferent That which conducts toward the center, usually related to sensory nerves.

ala; pl., alae A structure or appendage which has wing-like characteristics.

amorphous Shapeless; without distinct form or structure.

ansa Any loop-like structure of bone or nerve.

antrum Any nearly closed hollow or cavity, usually applied to those cavities or sinuses located in the various bones.

apex The topmost part of a structure which is conical or pyramidal in shape; tip of the tongue.

aponeurosis A broad, flat sheet of connective tissue serving for the attachment of muscular fibers.

areolar Related to the fleecy, mesh-like organization of connective tissue which occupies the interspaces of the body.

articular Pertaining to surfaces or structures which meet to form a joint.

astrocytes Nerve cells or bone corpuscles which are star-shaped.

atlas The first cervical vertebra.

atrium Chamber, sinus, or cavity in the heart, lung, ear, and larynx.

atrophy A wasting of any part due to lack of nutrition; caused by disuse, injury, disease, or interference with blood or nerve supply.

auricular Related to the auricles of the heart, or of the ear, or to the external ear in general.

autonomic A self-controlling structure or system; usually related to a portion of the nervous system uncontrolled by the brain or spinal cord.

axis The second cervical vertebra; also the pivot-point, the center, or line running through the center.

axon The portion of the neuron that carries stimuli away from the cell body, usually the longest portion of the neuron.

bolus A rounded or pill-shaped mass; a mass of food ready to be swallowed.

bronchiole Name applied to each of the divisions resulting from the forking of the trachea.

buccinator The trumpeter; a flat muscle located in the cheek, which helps to compress the cheeks.

cancellous Having a latticework structure, as the tissue of spongy bone.

capitulum A small, rounded protuberance on a bone surface.

capsule An enveloping membrane acting as a container.

cardiac Pertaining to the heart, or esophageal orifice of the stomach.

carotid The artery which runs to the brain, or to the head in general; the principal artery of the neck.

cartilage A dense, nonvascular body tissue capable of withstanding considerable pressure or tension; it furnishes strength, shape and flexibility.

caudad Toward the tail or lower end.

caudate Possessing a tail.

cephalad Toward the head or upper end.

cerebellum The small portion of the brain located behind and below the cerebrum. Its major responsibility is coordination of bodily actions.

cerebrum The largest portion of the brain. It is incompletely divided into two major hemispheres and contains many convolutions and fissures.

cervical Related to the region of the cervix or neck.

choana Posterior opening into the nasopharynx of the nasal cavity.

cilia Hair-like process projecting from epithelial cells. They line the respiratory tract, waft only in one direction, and wave mucus, pus, and dust particles upward from the bronchi and backward from the nasal passage.

coccygeal Pertaining to the last four bones of the spine.

collagen An insoluble fibrous protein, the chief constitutent of the fibrils of connective tissue. It is characterized by swelling in water solutions, by conversion to gelatin and glue on prolonged heating in water, and by conversion to leather on tanning.

collagenous Containing or composed of collagen.

concha Shell-shaped; the concavity of the external ear; any of the nasal turbinates.

condyle A rounded protuberance at the end of a bone forming an articulation, as on the mandible.

contralateral Situated on, pertaining to, or affecting the opposite side, as opposed to ipsilateral.

cornu (plural, **cornua**) A structure shaped like a horn.

coronal Any structure resembling a crown; the anatomical plane which divides the body into front and back sections.

corpus Any mass or body.

corpuscle A small body; specialized bodies located in nerves, epithelium, bone, blood, etc.

cortex Any outer layer of substance; usually applied to the outer layer of the brain (cerebral cortex) or of bone.

cranial Related to the head or upper end.

cribriform Perforated like a sieve.

cricoid Signet-shaped; the cricoid cartilage in the larynx which acts to support the thyroid and arytenoid cartilages.

cuneiform A wedge-shaped structure; cartilages located near the arytenoid cartilages of the larynx.

cutaneous Pertaining to the skin.

cytology The study of cellular structures.

cytoplasm Protoplasm; cell plasm lying external to the nucleus.

decussate A crossing action which results in an X formation; usually applied to nerve groups of the central nervous system.

deferens That which carries away from the center; usually applied to nerves or ducts.

deglutition The act of swallowing.

dendrite The portion of the neuron which carries stimuli toward the cell body, usually a short portion.

diaphysis The portion of a growing bone called the shaft.

diarthrosis A freely moving joint such as the elbow, wrist, temporomandibular, etc. (also, **diarthrodial**).

digastric Double-bellied muscle of mastication located near the floor of the mouth.

distal Away from the point of attachment, away from the midline.

dorsal Pertaining to the back or rear side.

ectoplasm The outer layer of the protoplasm which forms a cell membrane.

edema An abnormal swelling owing to an accumulation of serum in a tissue or part.

efferent That which conveys away from the center; usually applied to motor nerves.

embryology The study of cell growth and the development of an organism.

end-organ (1) The special structure in which nerve fibers terminate at the periphery; (2) one of the larger, encapsulated endings of the sensory nerves.

endo- Prefix meaning within, or inner.

enervate To make weak; to lessen the nerve, vitality, or strength of.

epi- Prefix meaning upon, above, or upper.

epiphysis The ends of a growing bone which form the boundaries for the diaphysis or shaft.

epithelium The cellular, outer substance of skin and mucous membrane which is without blood supply.

esophagus Part of the digestive system; the tube connecting the pharynx and the stomach.

eustachian tube The tube which leads from the middle ear to the pharynx; also known as *auditory tube*.

extrinsic Derived from or situated without; external.

falciform Sickle-shaped.

fascia A tough band or sheet of fibrous connective tissue that encloses, supports, and separates muscles and some organs.

fasciculus A bundle or cluster of nerve or muscle fibers which gather to make up whole nerves or muscles.

fauces The space leading from the mouth into the pharynx.

fenestra Window or opening; the opening in the middle ear that leads to the inner ear.

fibril A small fiber; a very small filament, often the component of a cell or fiber.

fissure A groove or sulcus; usually applied to those clefts found in tissues.

fixate The act of making static, fixed, or relatively immovable.

flaccid Soft, flabby; usually applied to muscles which have lost their quality or tonus.

follicle A small sac or gland capable of excretion.

foramen An opening or passage that is a regular part of a structure.

fossa A furrow, cavity, or depression that is a regular part of a structure.

fusiform Having a spindle shape.

ganglion (plural, **ganglia**) A concentration of nerve-cell bodies lying outside the brain or spinal cord and serving as a nerve center.

glossal Pertaining to the tongue.

glossodynia Neuralgic pain in the tongue.

glottis The opening between the vocal folds which disappears when the folds approximate.

gyrus (plural, **gyri**) A rise, fold, or promontory located in membranous tissue; usually applied to the con-volutions of the cerebral hemispheres of the brain.

hamulus Any hook-shaped structure; usually applied to the pterygoid process of the sphenoid bone.

hiatus A space, gap, foramen, or opening in any struc-ture.

histology The study of tissues.

homeostasis The state of equilibrium of the internal environment in the living body with respect to var-ious functions.

hormone A chemical secretion of the ductless glands which is carried in the bloodstream and which acts to stimulate the activity of organs.

hyaline Type of white, pearly cartilage commonly found throughout the body.

hyoid The U-shaped bone located below the tongue and above the thyroid cartilage.

hyper- Prefix meaning in excess of some normal state.

hypo- Prefix meaning less than some normal state.

inferior Below; toward the caudal end of the body.

infundibulum A funnel, canal, or extended cavity; usually applied to a passage connecting the nasal cavity with ethmoid bone or with the area at the upper end of the cochlear canal.

innervate To stimulate a part, as the nerve supply of an organ.

insertion Point of attachment for muscles; usually ap-plied to the most movable point of attachment.

integument A covering; the outermost surface of the body, or skin.

interstitial Located in the spaces between cells, or be-tween essential parts of an organ.

intrinsic Anything wholly contained within another structure; usually applies to muscles which are ex-clusively attached to one organ or structure, as in-trinsic muscles of the tongue.

ipsilateral Situated on the same side.

jugular Pertaining to the neck; usually applied to the large vein of the neck.

lacrimal Pertaining to the tears and the ducts from which they arise.

lacuna A small, hollow space; usually applied to bone cavities.

lamina A plate or flat layer of bone.

larynx The structure responsible for voice; the en-larged upper end of the trachea; the voicebox.

lateral Away from the midline, toward the periphery.

ligament Tough, fibrous connective bands which sup-port or bind bones and various organs.

lobe A globular part of an organ usually delineated by fissures or cleavages.

lumbar Pertaining to the portion of the back located between the thorax and the pelvis, commonly re-ferred to as the loins.

lumen The cross-sectional space within a tubular struc-ture.

lymph A clear, watery fluid secreted by the lymph glands in order to expedite the removal of waste from tissue cells.

malar Pertaining to the cheekbones.

mandible The bone of the lower jaw; the inferior max-illa.

mastoid Nipple-shaped; a process of the temporal bone.

maxilla A jawbone, especially the upper one; the supe-rior maxilla.

meatus Any passage or opening, usually canal-like.

median Situated in the midline.

medial Toward the midline or median plane.

medulla The marrow; the inner portion of an organ, in contrast to the outer portion or cortex.

medulla oblongata The most inferior portion of the brain; the uppermost portion of the spinal cord after it enters the foramen magnum.

membrane A thin sheet of tissue which sheathes or divides organs and surfaces.

meninges Specialized membranes which encase the brain and spinal cord.

meniscus Concavoconvex lens; an interarticular car-tilage of crescent shape found in certain joints, as the temporomandibular.

metabolism The regular chemical modifications of sub-stances which occur in the growth and development of the body.

morphology The study of forms and structures.

mucus The sticky secretion which covers the mem-branes of many cavities and passages that are ex-posed to the external environment.

muscle Specialized tissues composed of contractile cells or fibers which furnish the body with motive power.

mylohyoid A muscle connected to the mandible, the hyoid bone, and median raphe.

myo- A Greek combining form signifying relation to muscle; meaningful only when used as an attached prefix.

nares The anterior openings of the nasal cavities which communicate with the external environment, i.e., the nostrils.

nasopharynx The part of the pharynx located above the velum or soft palate.

neuron The basic structural unit of the nervous system; composed of a cell body, axon, and dendrites.

nucleus A small round body within every cell which acts as the functional control center; refers also to a mass of cell bodies in the brain or spinal cord.

occiput The back part of the skull.

orbicular Circular; muscle about an opening, as the orbicularis oris muscle encircling the mouth.

orifice An entrance or opening into a body cavity.

origin The relatively fixed muscular attachment.

oropharynx The part of the pharynx located between the velum, or soft palate, and the hyoid bone.

ossicle A small bone; often applied to the bones of the ear.

ossify The act of becoming bone.

osteoblast A cell concerned with the formation of bone.

osteology The study of structure and function of bone.

ostium A small entrance or opening.

pedicle Stalk-like process or stem.

peduncle A supporting part of another structure; a band running between sections of the brain.

perioral About or surrounding the mouth.

periosteum The fibrous sheath which covers all bones except at their articular surfaces.

peristalsis A wave of contraction passing along a tube.

petrous Resembling stone; relating to the petrous portion of the temporal bone.

pharyngeal Pertaining to the pharynx or throat.

plasma The fluid portion of the blood during circulation.

platysma A plate; usually applied to the neck muscle connected to the mandible and the clavicle.

plexus A collection, concentration, or network of parts of the nervous or vascular systems.

pons A bridge; that portion of brain stem which is between the medulla oblongata and the midbrain.

posterior Toward the back or rear side.

protoplasm The basic material of every living cell.

proximal Toward the point of attachment; toward the midline.

pterygoid Wing-shaped, alate; usually applied to two large processes of the sphenoid bone or to the muscles that arise from these.

pulmonary Pertaining to the lungs.

ramus A branch; usually applied to parts of nerves, vessels, or bone.

raphe A line or seam formed by the union of two parts.

reticular Like a network; often applied to the network of fibers passing between the pons and the medulla oblongata.

risorius A muscle connected to facial fascia and the angle of the mouth.

rostral Toward the head end.

sacrum The triangular bone composed of five united vertebrae and forming the base of the vertebral column.

sagittal Arrow-like; usually applied to the plane which divides the body into right and left portions.

sarcolemma A membranous sheath encasing each striated muscle fiber.

scaphoid A bone or process shaped like a small boat.

segmentation Division into similar parts or segments.

sensory Nerves, organs, or structures related to the process of sensation and carrying stimuli from the exterior toward the cerebrospinal system.

septum A partition or dividing wall, such as the nasal septum.

sinus Any cavity having a relatively narrow opening, as those located in the facial bone.

somatic Pertaining to the body, or to structures of the body wall.

sphenoid Wedge-shaped; a complex bone of the interior skull.

sphincter Any muscle or combination of muscles which provides a closure for a natural body opening.

squamous Scale-like; the upper anterior portion of the temporal bone.

sternum The breastbone.

striated Streaked; usually applied to a special type of muscular fiber which effects voluntary movement.

styloid Resembling a stylus; a process of the temporal bone which furnishes attachment for muscles and ligaments.

sulcus A fissure or groove in bone or tissues, especially of the brain.

superficial Confined to the surface; lying on or near, or affecting only the surface or surface layers.

superior Above; toward the head or cephalic end.

suture A stitch or seam; the line of union in an immovable articulation, as those between skull bones.

symphysis A line of fusion between two bones which are separate in early development, as the symphysis of the mandible.

synapse The junction between the axon of one nerve cell and the dendrite of another.

synarthrosis A type of joint in which the skeletal elements are united, resulting in restricted or complete lack of movement in the joint.

syndesmosis Restricted movement of a joint because of connective tissue attachments.

synergy A coordination or cooperation between two or more agents or organs which results in smooth, economical activity.

synostosis Restricted or lack of movement of a joint due to a bony connection.

synovia A lubricating fluid secreted in joints, bursae, and tendon sheaths.

synovial Pertaining to synovia.

systemic Affecting the body as a whole.

tendon A cord-like fibrous connective tissue serving for the attachment of muscles with points of origin and insertion.

thorax That part of the body which is located between the clavicle and the diaphragm.

thyroid The shield-like cartilage of the larynx which rests on the cricoid cartilage and furnishes an attachment for the vocal folds; also a gland.

tonus A state of partial contraction of a muscle which produces a healthy, resilient quality in the muscle.

trachea The cartilaginous and membranous tube extending from the larynx to the bronchial tubes; commonly referred to as the windpipe.

transverse Usually applied to a plane which extends horizontally from one side of a structure to the other; a cross section.

tuberosity Protuberance, eminence, or round process of a bone.

turbinate Any structure shaped like a top and filled with pits, hollows or swirls; usually applied to bones of the nasal passage.

vagus Wandering; the pneumogastric or tenth cranial nerve.

vein A vessel which conveys blood toward the heart.

velum The soft palate; the posterior and muscular portion of the roof of the mouth.

ventral Toward the front or abdomen.

ventricle A small cavity.

vertex The topmost part; the top of the head.

vestibule An antechamber; a small space or cavity at the beginning of a canal.

viscera Generic term for the organs of any large body cavity; most frequently applied to the organs in the abdomen.

zygoma The long arch that joins the zygomatic processes of the temporal and malar bones.

REFERENCES

1. Carlson, A. J., Johnson, V., and Cavert, H. M.: The machinery of the body, ed. 5, Chicago, 1962, University of Chicago Press.

2. Eckstein, G.: The body has a head, New York, 1970, Harper & Row, Publishers.

3. Francis, C. C., and Martin, A. H.: Introduction to human anatomy, ed. 7, St. Louis, 1975, The C. V. Mosby Co.

4. Fried, L. A.: Anatomy of the head, neck, face, and jaws, Philadelphia, 1976, Lea & Febiger.

5. Goss, C. M., editor: Gray's anatomy, ed. 27, Philadelphia, 1959, Lea & Febiger.

6. Grant, J. C. B.: An atlas of anatomy, ed. 6, Baltimore, 1972, The Williams & Wilkins Co.

7. Grollman, S.: The human body: its structure and physiology, ed. 2, New York, 1969, Macmillan, Inc.

8. Langley, L. L.: Physiology of man, ed. 4, New York, 1971, Von Nostrand Reinhold Company.

9. Miller, M. A., and Leavell, L. C.: Kimber-Gray-Stackpole's anatomy and physiology, ed. 16, New York, 1972, Macmillan, Inc.

10. Palmer, J. M., and La Russo, D. A.: Anatomy for speech and hearing, New York, 1965, Harper & Row, Publisher.

11. Quiring, D. P.: The head, neck, and trunk, Philadelphia, 1947, Lea & Febiger.

12. Rasmussen, R., and Penfield, W.: The cerebral cortex of man, New York, 1950, Macmillan, Inc.

13. Roberts, L., and Penfield, W.: Speech and brain mechanisms, Princeton, N.J., 1959, Princeton University Press.

14. Shearer, W. M.: Illustrated speech anatomy, Springfield, Ill., 1963, Charles C Thomas, Publisher.

15. Taber, C. W.: Taber's cyclopedic medical dictionary, ed. 9, Philadelphia, 1963, F. A. Davis Co.

16. Woodburne, R. T.: Essentials of human anatomy, ed. 5, New York, 1973, Oxford University Press.

Chapter 6

APPLIED PHYSIOLOGY

An entire volume might now ensue, detailing the implications of the preceding chapters. Many facets must necessarily yield to limitations of space; several will be reserved for later, where their application to myofunctional concerns can be shown more directly; a few areas demand elucidation herewith. In particular, we would like to explore normal and abnormal function as applied to three structures of the body: the tooth, the temporomandibular joint, and the nasal airway. We also have some thoughts concerning the influences of muscial instruments in this context.

FORCES AFFECTING THE TOOTH

It is our position that myofunctional disorders interfere with normal dental development and thereafter interfere with the orderly correction of dental anomalies. Some abnormal forces are so pervasive that they have repercussions throughout dentistry and myotherapy. These general saboteurs, individually or in coalition, may also provide the basis for many of the delimited intruders that plague us in only one special area. The sources of their power will be examined.

Tongue thrust is at root a problem of *pressure*. Nevertheless, it is not some independent agency capable of generating its own power, or a force that is foreign to the human mouth. Instead, it is a perversion of natural forces, a rearrangement of normal pressures into a harmful distortion. It might be enlightening, therefore, to examine some of the *normal* forces of the orofacial complex, noting as we go the consequences of disrupting or modifying each component of force.

A look at Fig. 6-1 will give some idea of the stressful environment of the tooth. The illustration does not, however, reveal all the pressures to which the tooth is subjected, for this would require a third and even a fourth dimension,

since time is also a factor. Thus, although the complete dynamics involved will demand some mental imagery, we may nonetheless use this figure as a point of reference.

Forces of occlusion

The forces of occlusion have been described in earlier chapters. They are powerful, occur only during normal mastication and deglutition, and are greatly reduced in abnormal function. The extent of the pressure parallel to the long axis of the tooth has been variously reported as from 100 to far more than 200 pounds per square inch in forceful occlusion. This force is essential and healthful, maintaining vitality in the mouth, strengthening the antigravity musculature, encouraging upright teeth in a symmetrical arch, and stimulating the deposition of firm alveolar bone of a dense texture.

Tongue thrust abates this critical force as the tongue is interposed between the dental arches. Antigravity muscles sag, fostering an undesirable orofacial rest posture. Molars are allowed to tip or wander. Once the tooth is malposed, any instance of occlusion then becomes an additional microtrauma, a force for evil rather than a beneficial influence.

Some degeneration of alveolar bone must also result. The so-called "law of transformation of bone" was formulated over a hundred years ago but has been confirmed in more recent studies.[11] Osteoporosis indicates a reduction in the density of bone and may stem from lack of function or pressure. This process becomes more evident in extraction, when a tooth is left without an antagonist in the opposing arch. Alveolar bone surrounding such a tooth is easily penetrated by x rays and becomes a fading image on radiographs. It has been found, however, that restoration of pressure by the artificial replacement of an an-

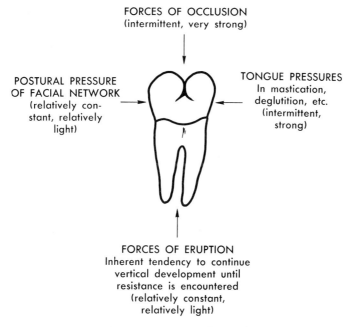

FORCES OF OCCLUSION
(intermittent, very strong)

POSTURAL PRESSURE
OF FACIAL NETWORK
(relatively con-
stant, relatively
light)

TONGUE PRESSURES
In mastication,
deglutition, etc.
(intermittent,
strong)

FORCES OF ERUPTION
Inherent tendency to continue
vertical development until
resistance is encountered
(relatively constant,
relatively light)

Fig. 6-1. Forces exerted on teeth.

tagonist will cause rejuvenation of the alveolar process.

Forces of the tongue

The forces of the tongue are at work primarily during mastication and deglutition and may be reduced or absent during normal rest, speech, and other auxiliary functions. The combined strength of the eight muscles comprising the tongue represents a potential of some magnitude.

In normal function these forces are primarily directed against the palate, which is arched and otherwise so constructed as to withstand such pressures with ease; in fact, it depends on these pressures for its normal development. Any residual tongue pressure exerted in the horizontal plane during swallowing is readily absorbed by the teeth in normal occlusion: if the cusps are properly interlocked, the inclined planes provide reciprocal bracing and thus a stable, rigid wall that is self-sufficient; pressure is transmitted by this wall to the alveolar process, where it has a beneficial expanding effect.

So much attention has been accorded the tongue as an instrument of villainy—the creator of a variety of malocclusions in abnormal movement—that little comment has been made concerning the influence of the tongue in forming *normal* structures during dental development.

Thus it might be advantageous to inspect this function for a moment. The tongue probably has little effect on the growth or shape of the basal bone; rather, the jaws develop toward a potential shape largely determined by heredity. This growth potential may be modified by poor nutrition or illness during a critical period or impeded by endocrine imbalance, ankylosis of the temporomandibular joint, trauma, etc. Nevertheless, basal bone is little influenced by the teeth it bears or the forces of its environment.

However, the normal structure of the alveolar processes, and the arrangement of the crowns of the teeth into the dental arch, are subject not only to the genes but also to other natural forces operating in the area. Strictly speaking, these structures—the teeth and the alveolar processes that support them—are *not skeletal features:* they grow *from* the skeleton but are nevertheless separate from it. They are parts of what is called the "exoskeleton" and are thus not subject to the same laws of growth and development that govern basal features. The shape of the initial arch is set by basal bone, but as the crowns of the teeth erupt away from skeletal bone into the oral environment, muscular forces supercede the diminishing influence of basal bone in the development and maintenance of the individual arch form.

The alveolar process is usually seen as a bone

of convenience, or a bone of adaptation, the function of which is to support the teeth in whatever position they may assume. As such, the alveolar process does not possess the property of expansive growth and thus cannot widen the arch or effect tooth movement.[29]

The tongue supplies the *only* sturdy, vigorous force on the dental arch from within outward and must play a major role in growth. Acting independently of the dental arch, this muscular organ is situated inside the denture and is ideally constructed to expand and maintain arch form. With glossectomy comes collapse of the dental arch.

The tongue is thus a vital element in normal development; it is from the essential nature of this required influence that the tongue derives much of its potential for evil. When its forces are displaced from palatal and alveolar locales directly onto the teeth or when mechanical advantage is lost in the molar region due to the separation of teeth by the tongue during deglutition, powerful abnormal forces are released with which the tooth is not prepared to cope.

Forces of eruption

It has long been a basic tenet of dentistry that teeth seek occlusal antagonists: they tend to continue eruption until met by resistance. However, the process does not stop even then; having made contact with an antagonist, the "prefunctional" phase of eruption comes to an end, but even so the process continues throughout the life of the tooth.[25]

In normal function this moderate but constant force compensates for abrasion and other loss from the occlusal surfaces, maintaining the relative position of the teeth in the occlusal plane and thus their ability to meet in forceful relation. Removal of an antagonist, and failure to provide a replacement, usually results in renewed eruption as the remaining tooth elongates in its search for resistance.

In many types of tongue thrust the interdental presence of the tongue unsettles the forces of occlusion and may result in the infraeruption of some teeth while allowing hypereruption of others. The teeth at the site of the thrust meet untimely resistance and stop erupting prematurely, leaving the familiar open bite. In the case of incisal thrusts, the maxillary alveolar process itself may appear to be displaced superiorly. With retraction of the tongue in myotherapy, eruption resumes and the bite tends to close.

Quite a different effect is occasionally seen in teeth situated in a different part of the arch, away from the site of the thrust—that is, teeth that are held out of occlusion by tongue thrust but that do not contact the tongue. In some anterior thrusts, the molars may actually supererupt, thus opening the bite still more and requiring intrusion of the molars as part of orthodontic correction. In extreme cases, supereruption may even lead to mandibular resection.

Nevertheless, the force of eruption is a *normal* force, one that is routinely utilized to open the closed bite, as when a bite plate is inserted to hold molars out of occlusion until they erupt sufficiently to meet before incisors overclose. In a few cases we have found that some spontaneous intrusion of elongated molars has followed the establishment of firm molar occlusion in myotherapy.

Forces of the facial network

The muscles of the lips and cheeks are so interlaced and interconnected that action by one finds an echo in all; such reverberation is ordinarily mild. However, some of these muscles are so closely adapted to each other in their influence on dental structures as to function almost as a unit. One such unit has frequently been referred to as "the buccinator mechanism" (Fig. 6-2); it has also been called the "strap effect," since it can be seen that there is a continuous band of muscle fiber encircling the dental arches and anchored at the base of the occiput. Starting with the decussating fibers of the orbicularis oris, joining right and left fibers in the lips, upper and lower strands intermingle and run laterally and posteriorly around the corner of the mouth, connecting with fibers of the buccinator, which in turn insert into the pterygomandibular raphe just behind the dental arch. The fibers of the buccinator mechanism here interweave with fibers of the superior constrictor and continue posteriorly and medially to anchor at the pharyngeal tubercle of the first cervical vertebra, the atlas.

In normal function, reciprocity among components is found, with adjustments in muscle activity available as compensations are required. It has been noted that even in the newborn the perioral musculature displays a smoothness in function quite in contrast to the jerky, uncoordinated movement of more distal or caudal muscles.

One function of this elastic band is to maintain the integrity of the dental arch by exerting a relatively constant enclosing force on the teeth.

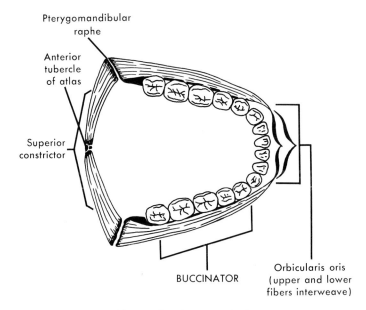

Pterygomandibular
raphe

Anterior
tubercle
of atlas

Superior
constrictor

BUCCINATOR

Orbicularis oris
(upper and lower
fibers interweave)

Fig. 6-2. Buccinator mechanism.

It serves as the antagonist mechanism for the tongue. Even in postural rest there is the restraining influence of the buccinator mechanism. Although these forces have been found to be much less than the pressure of the tongue during deglutition, they are operative over a much longer period of time.

In abnormal swallowing, the compensatory movements noted above may work to restrain the malocclusion but may also serve to *increase* the discrepancy in some cases. An open-mouth rest posture, for example, removes the entire influence of the muscle band, allowing all anterior teeth to develop in labioversion, whereas an over-developed mentalis muscle may be accompanied by such constant and extreme force against the mandibular dentition that the lower incisors develop in linguoversion, or the contiguous skeletal jaw may be retarded in development. In the latter instance, even basal bone is influenced by soft tissue.

Forces of torque

Although not a factor if each tooth is in proper occlusion, there are also rotating pressures—the twisting forces that are supplied by firm intercuspation of the teeth and to a lesser degree by the surrounding muscles. It is not uncommon for teeth to erupt at a slight tangent or in some posture less than optimal in relationship to adjacent or antagonist teeth. The normal forces of torque tend to correct such errors, uprighting and turning the teeth, and guiding them into a position of easy function as the inclined planes of posterior teeth slide down each other in forceful occlusion.

This force is supplied in adequate measure *only* during normal deglutition, since there is no other constantly recurring situation in which the cusps are brought into contact with force—not during mastication as we shall see later. These forces are thus largely unavailable to the teeth in abnormal swallowing, so that the cusps strike in an unhealthy manner during any remaining instances of tooth-to-tooth contact.

Forces of mesial drift

The forces of mesial drift fill in the last gap on the peripheral surfaces of the tooth and consist of distomesial pressure supplied by adjacent teeth at the contact points of the crown. This pressure was recognized by Angle, who referred to it as the "anterior component of force." It is the product of several factors, such as the cumulative effect of all orofacial muscle pressures and the axial inclination of the root structure, which is such that, when the teeth are brought firmly together, the crowns are propelled toward the front of the mouth, etc. It has the effect of closing gaps, which unifies and stabilizes the dental arch, and it compensates for wear at the contacting surfaces of adjacent teeth. It depends in part on continuity of the dental arch.

We noted earlier that mesial drift must be a concern for the pedodontist when early tooth loss requires a space maintainer to assure living space for a succedaneous tooth. To the contrary, this movement can be of assistance to the orthodontist when extractions are necessary during treatment, helping to restore and maintain contact of proximal teeth.

Some types of abnormal deglutition tend to disrupt the beneficial forces of mesial drift, as when mandibular or bimaxillary thrusts create diastemata in the lower arch. Almost any type of thrust poses a threat to the orthodontist in extraction cases, and even in some nonextraction instances: mesial drift may not be able to compensate for abnormal muscle pressures, thus destroying the integrity of the dental arch and resulting in unsightly spacing between the teeth after retention. Such unpleasant outcomes, discouraging for both dentist and patient, are precluded when myofunctional therapy is planned into treatment.

Atmospheric force

Several authorities have assigned some value to atmospheric pressure, particularly during deglutition. It is postulated that, with a partial vacuum created in the oral cavity, atmospheric pressure in the nasal cavity would have the effect of forcing the bony palate to descend, especially during periods of rapid body growth and in the early years when the palatal bones are thin, are lightly calcified, and react readily to pressure. Descent of the palate helps to expand the upper arch, a highly coveted situation. Whether the force thus generated is genuine and sufficient has not been established. The vacuum itself would seem to provide a greater influence than the air driving downward from above the palate. In any event, such force as might be present would be totally lacking in deviate swallowing, with its reversal of intraoral air pressure.

Summary

With the possible exception of atmospheric force, it can be seen that the forces exerted on the tooth are so varied and of such magnitude that the tooth would surely be crushed and destroyed before long if nature had not had the foresight to endow the tooth with its hardy enamel armor and resilient periodontal ligament.

Yet all these forces are *natural* forces, and *each force is essential* to the total health of the tooth. It is only when pressures are removed, disrupted, or displaced that trouble arises.

This may also hold true in the disordered mouth: a malocclusion represents nature's best attempt to maintain a balance among all the elements of the stomatognathic system. The clinician should be aware of a concept of which orthodontists frequently remind each other: an untreated malocclusion *is in dynamic balance at any particular time.* Disturbing this balance cannot be done with impunity; the dentition may be harmed by careless handling. If we keep in mind the relatively slight pressures employed in orthodontics to effect major physiologic response in the alveolar bone, we gain a proper respect for the state of equilibrium that may be only precariously maintained in a given mouth. Anyone proposing to tamper with this balance should have a very clear understanding of the dynamics involved and be prepared to compensate for every change, so that the end product is a revised equilibrium, not a still more harmful imbalance.

TEMPOROMANDIBULAR JOINT

As in the preceding section, we must examine the *normal* physiology of the temporomandibular joint before we can appreciate its dysfunction or abuse.

The TMJ may be palpated by placing a finger immediately forward of the ear, then opening and closing the mouth. A clearer concept may be gained by placing a fingertip inside the ear, then opening and also moving the mandible from side to side.

Construction of the joint

Shown in Fig.6-3 are the three elements composing this joint: (1) the mandibular condyle; (2) the articular fossa (the glenoid fossa) of the temporal bone; and (3) the articular meniscus, often referred to simply as the *disc.*

The knuckle-like head of the condyloid process has a thicker lateral dimension than is apparent in head films or lateral drawings. It swells up in all directions from the neck, providing a relatively broad expanse of slick, cartilaginous, articulatory surface.

The articular fossa may also be somewhat deceiving in structure, since it is partially concealed behind the zygomatic process of the temporal bone in lateral view. The bone sur-

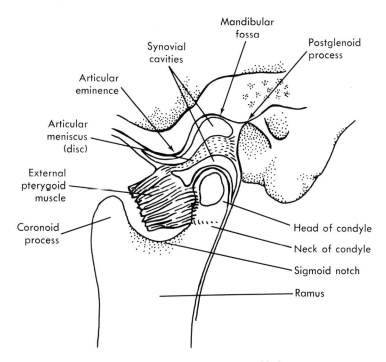

Fig. 6-3. Sagittal section of temporomandibular joint.

rounding the rim of the fossa is fairly thick, but as it domes up to the roof of the fossa it becomes quite thin centrally, where it separates the disc and the condylar head from the middle cranial fossa, the lodgment of the temporal lobe of the brain. The front portion of the fossal rim is known as the *anterior articular eminence,* or *articular tubercle,* or *eminentia.* Posteriorly, the fossa is bounded by a bony ridge, the *postglenoid process.*

The disc, or articular meniscus, is a body of dense fibrous cartilage lying between the head of the condyle and the articular fossa, extending somewhat forward under the anterior eminence. This oval plate is thinner at the center than around the edges, with an undersurface concave in shape, conforming to the head of the condyle. However, anteroposteriorly its upper exterior has a double curve; the posterior portion is convex front-to-back, adapting to the fossa, while the anterior portion is concave, dipping under the articular eminence.

The joint is encased in a fibrous *capsule,* a sheath or sac of tissue that is attached superiorly around the circumference of the glenoid fossa; below, it attaches around the neck of the condyle. The capsule is composed of two layers, an exterior of fibrous tissue reinforced by accessory ligaments, and an inner layer, the synovial membrane, that secretes the lubricating fluid, *synovia,* into chambers above and below the disc.

The meniscus is attached medially and laterally to the neck of the condyle, so that the disc is carried with the condyle in some movements. Posteriorly it attaches to a thick layer of loose, vascular connective tissue which fuses with the capsule but which allows anterior movement of the disc without stress. Anteriorly, the disc is fused to the capsule; fibers of the external pterygoid muscle penetrate the capsule and insert into the disc at its capsular attachment, enabling the muscle to pull both meniscus and condyle forward in unison.

The surface of the thin dome forming the top of the glenoid fossa is devoid of cartilaginous armor, which suggests that the head of the condyle was not designed to press upward into the depths of the fossa during any aspect of function. To the contrary, the surface of the posterior slope of the eminence, like the articular surface of the condylar head, is covered by fibrous cartilage, indicating that these parts of the joint are able to provide resistance to force.

The entire complex of the TMJ is suspended from the skull by a system of three ligaments, guy wires which steady and brace while still allowing for freedom of movement within a prescribed range. The *temporomandibular* ligament connects above to the zygomatic arch, and below to the outer and posterior surface of the neck of the condyle. Medially, the mandible is anchored by the *sphenomandibular* ligament; this is attached above to the spine of the sphenoid bone, and below to the inner surface of the mandible at the lower border of the mandibular foramen. The *stylomandibular* ligament is the posterior support; it extends from the styloid process of the temporal bone to the posterior border and angle of the mandible.

Movement of the joint

The musculature of the temporomandibular joint was discussed in the previous chapter. It is of interest that the structure of the joint, and the alignment of the muscles, provide a versatility of movement unique to the human species. A significant amount of controversy persists concerning the various positions and movements of the mandible and the implications arising from these; much of the strife regarding "centric" occlusion has its origin here. As was the case in Chapter 3, some care is required in traversing this area.

There is not even harmony with respect to the resting position from which movement starts. Some insist that normal posture should find the head of the condyle seated well within the depths of the fossa; others point out that the head of the condyle is angled slightly forward, and should hold the disc against the posterior slope of the articular eminence at rest.

There is agreement that we are not dealing with a simple hinge-like movement such as found in even the highest order of apes. The division of the joint by the meniscus into upper and lower compartments results in a compound joint. The statement of some that it is really two joints is hotly disputed by others, who feel that all movement is a product of combined action by both compartments.

Starting from a resting posture somewhat as seen in Fig. 6-4, *A,* minor opening and closing movements probably occur between the cartilaginous disc and the head of the condyle, as in Fig. 6-4, *B.* Opening the mouth widely, or protruding the jaw, creates movement between the disc and the fossa, the disc in this case moving with the condylar head, represented by Fig. 6-4, *C.* Grinding movements elicit both types of action in the joint, the disc gliding forward and backward over the articular eminence while some rotation occurs between the disc and the head of the condyle. Fig. 6-4, *D,* illustrates the result of extreme opening of the mandible.

A recapitulation of muscle action might now be helpful. The mandible is *lowered* through contraction of the external (lateral) pterygoid, the anterior belly of the digastric, and the platysma muscles (minor influence may be supplied by the mylohyoid and geniohyoid). The mandible is *raised* by contraction of the masseter, temporalis, and internal (medial) pterygoid muscles. It is *protruded* by the simultaneous contraction of the external pterygoid on both sides. It is *retracted* by the contraction of the posterior fibers of the temporalis. *Lateral* movement is accomplished by contraction of the external pterygoid on one side only, and *grinding* movements represent a complex synergy involving many muscles, but characterized by the external pterygoids contracting in alternate fashion.

Note that the activities of this group of muscles in maintaining the position of the mandible are directly influenced by postural reflexes deriving from head and body position. Being subject to such modification, they are also easily stimulated by factors such as oral habits (mouth breathing, digit sucking, tongue thrusting, tooth clenching), emotional tension, respiratory movement, and afferent impulses from oral structures.[24]

We might also pause to note once again the complexity of the nerve supply to this area. It is served primarily by the many branches and fasciculi of four major nerves, the trigeminal (cranial V), the facial (cranial VII), the vagus (cranial X), and the great auricular, which is composed of cervical nerves 2 and 3. Fibers from these nerves anastomose (unite) with each other, with other branches of the same nerve, and with nuclei of the glossopharyngeal (cranial IX). The end product is a network of such intricacy that the brain is not always able to recognize the source of some neural excitations. This accounts for the phenomenon of "referred pain," when pain in a lower molar may be experienced as emanating from an upper tooth. In the same way, pain in the lower molar region often radiates to the TMJ, pain in the joint may be interpreted as an earache or vice versa, and the content of the preceding paragraph is explicated.

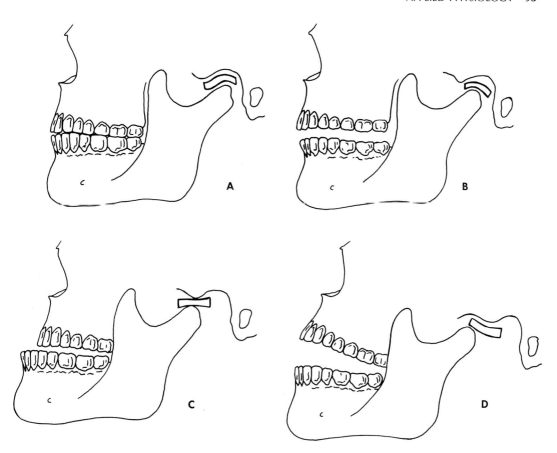

Fig. 6-4. Function of temporomandibular joint. **A,** Normal resting relationship. **B,** Mouth slightly open, movement occurs between head of condyle and meniscus. **C,** Protrusion; meniscus moves with condyle. **D,** Dislocation; premature contraction of elevator muscles has locked head of condyle anterior to articular eminence, stretching all attachments of disc.

Disorders of the joint

The temporomandibular joint is subject to a wide variety of clinical problems. There are many reasons for its susceptibility. Among the more basic factors are the structure of the joint itself, the extremes of use and force to which it is subjected, its vulnerability to influences arising from tooth position, malocclusion, and other agents listed above. In addition, the neural innervation just described involves numerous small nerve centers located around the exterior of the skull, particularly in the region just superior to the TMJ.

Infection in the joint is rare. Tumors occasionally develop in various components of the joint, creating painful excessive pressure on surrounding nerves. Certain types of blows can snap the neck of the condyle, requiring splinting of the mandible until the fracture is reduced. None of these concern the oral myologist. However, almost all of the remaining disorders incorporate aspects of muscle dysfunction, either as a causative factor or as a resultant anomaly.

DISLOCATION. When the mandible is lowered excessively, opening the mouth to an extreme degree, the head of the condyle may slip out of the fossa entirely and come to rest in front of the articular eminence, resulting in dislocation. Because of its looseness, the capsule does not tear in this situation, but is stretched to a harmful extent, as are the muscles and ligaments of the TMJ.

In normal closure, the precise sequence of muscle contraction begins with the posterior belly of the temporalis, which retracts the condyle, bringing the head into position behind the peak of the eminentia. The elevators then replace the head into the fossa. If this sequence is disturbed, and the elevators contract before the mandible is retracted, the jaw will move superiorly while still beneath or slightly anterior to the articular eminence, and the mandible is dislocated (see Fig. 6-4, *D*).

The resultant pain is usually severe, causing muscles to go into spasm; continued spasm of the elevator muscles maintains the punishing malposition, and outside assistance is required in most cases to reduce the dislocation. When such help is needed, or when the dislocation is complete as described, it is called *luxation*. When the dislocation is partial, or when the patient is able to retract the jaw himself, the term is *subluxation*.

Some patients have stretched the capsule and the supporting ligaments to such an extent that they experience constant subluxation. This has several causes, but the effects are invariably harmful. Mechanical influences such as malocclusion should be eliminated first, after which the oral myologist may be helpful in toning the antigravity muscles and in disrupting the habitual thrusting of the jaw which may continue after mechanical correction. A mandibular tongue thrust will frequently be found in these cases.

Two terms, *clicking* and *crepitus*, should be mentioned in this context. They are often used interchangably, but have slightly different connotations.

Clicking. During some excursions of the mandible, many patients hear or feel a click or snap, a sharp popping sensation. This is the sound resulting from the meniscus snapping back and forth over the articular eminence in excessive fashion. This condition has several causes, such as reduced thickness of the disc; or the fibrous attachments of the disc to the condyle may become stretched, causing hypermobility of the meniscus; or constant overstretching of the capsule may result in loss of resiliency, a "sloppy" joint that is quite conducive to clicking.

Crepitus. As a general rule, a condition somewhat more severe is indicated by crepitation. Crepitus is usually defined as the sound emitted when the broken ends of a bone are rubbed together. It has also been likened to the sound of walking in loose gravel. It is often the result of a perforated disc; in this case it is the sound of bone-to-bone contact between the head of the condyle and the fossa or eminentia.

ARTHRITIS. The temporomandibular joint may be the site of arthritis, occasionally even in younger patients. Arthritis is defined as inflammation of a joint. There are two general types of arthritis, that of infectious origin and that of noninfectious origin. We have noted that the TMJ is rarely subject to infection, although in a few cases it is invaded as an extension of generalized arthritis in all joints. More commonly it is prey to the noninfectious type, specifically *osteoarthritis*. Osteoarthritis is characterized by destruction of the articular fibrocartilage, overgrowth of bone, especially around the rim of the fossa, spur formation on the condylar head, and thus impaired function. Osteoarthritis is usually the result of malfunction of the masticatory mechanism, growing out of malocclusion or other harmful jaw relationship, or of improper function of the muscles primarily involving hypercontraction. Any circumstance that brings undue stress or pressure to bear on the protective disc can reduce the cushioning effect of that cartilage and lead to inflammation.

Intolerable stress is avoided by some patients through the use of an unconscious procedure of which the oral myologist should be aware. This is the "myoprotected occlusion" delineated by Picard.[21] After outlining a "mutually-protected occlusion" in which all elements of the stomatognathic system work in harmony to prevent trauma in any one segment, he provides a contrast. He itemizes the steps leading from an occlusal discrepancy, through self-equilibration (bruxing) with the resultant additional stress damaging the investing tissues, to pulpitis, periodontal breakdown, TMJ dysfunction, occlusal disease, and pain. When the system exceeds its limit of tolerance, the tongue may be placed as an interocclusal mass during swallowing, since it is then that the teeth occlude with force. Closing on the padded cushion of the tongue relieves all previous ills, and a myoprotected occlusion is instituted. He warns that attempts to alter deglutition before the original causative factors are corrected would deprive the system of its last protection.

OTHER DEGENERATIVE CONDITIONS. In contrast to the arthritic tendency toward formation of extraneous bone are those conditions leading to degeneration and loss of osseous tissue. It is not uncommon to find patients with the severe protrusion accompanying some class II, division 1 malocclusions who habitually carry the mandible forward. This positions the head of the condyle against the descending slope of the eminence with some force; considerable tension in the external pterygoids is required to maintain such a posture. The result may be bone resorption in both the head and the eminence at the focal point of the abnormal pressure.[26] This may also be true of many functional class III patients; in this case, the tongue thrust jams the mandible forward, creating the injurious condyle-fossa relationship.

Something similar is found in patients with an open bite, but for a different reason. In normal function, protrusion of the mandible causes the lower incisal edges to slide down the lingual surface of upper incisors, instantly disarticulating the molars. This prevents the bumping and scraping of cusps between upper and lower molars. Such incisal guidance is lost to the open bite patient, who must then rely on an abnormal function of the joint itself to separate the posterior teeth, a process that may prove traumatic to the TMJ with constant repetition over a period of years. Failure to disengage the molars before protrusion occurs is equally harmful, with repercussions throughout the stomatognathic system; it has the same effect on the neuromuscular system as a "premature contact" or other occlusal interference. Premature contacts may trigger muscle spasm, and the vicious circle of consequences is thereby reinforced.

According to several authorities, a majority of TMJ problems arise from insufficient vertical dimension. In younger patients this may result from delayed eruption of molars, while in adults it commonly follows the extraction of molars without providing replacements. In these cases, the head of the condyle is forced upward and somewhat forward; laminographic x-rays frequently reveal some erosion of the fossa and a decidedly "moth-eaten" anterior surface of the head of the condyle.

MYOFASCIAL PAIN-DYSFUNCTION SYNDROME. A list of symptoms, known for some years as the "Costen syndrome," was first presented by J. B. Costen[5] in 1934. After a period of little attention, recent years have seen an outpouring of literature dealing with this subject, now referred to under five or six titles; temporomandibular joint myofascial pain-dysfunction syndrome, though lengthy, is one of the more common labels. Calling it a "TMJ syndrome" is less precise, but saves time.

The incidence of this condition in the general population has not been established, but it appears to be very widespread; estimates exceeding 20% have been made. The symptoms, all stemming from dysfunction of the TMJ, include pain of the head, face, ear, neck, and shoulder, in various combinations; intermittent vertigo; tinnitus (subjective ringing ear noise); burning sensations in the sides of the tongue; spontaneous subluxation; clicking and crepitation of the joint; occasionally, trismus or restricted jaw movement; difficulty in swallowing; fatigue; forgetfulness[9]; and muscle spasms throughout the body.

The pain-dysfunction syndrome may lead to arthritis of the TMJ as a secondary effect, but is a distinct condition resulting primarily from dysfunction of the masticatory muscles. A majority of patients suffering from this condition never receive proper treatment. They tend to consult physicians who lack dental expertise. They are placed on migraine programs and medications, which prove futile. Their vertigo is ascribed to untreatable inner ear conditions. They are classified as neurotic and referred for psychotherapy. It is true that they may require the combined services of physician, dentist, psychologist and oral myologist before they are restored to full health; nevertheless, a knowledgeable dentist can remove most of their overt symptoms with surprising speed, usually within one or two months.

A point to be stressed is that the oral myologist can perform a great service by being aware of the pain-dysfunction syndrome, particularly during initial examinations. Gelb,[9] as well as Stack and Funt,[26] stress the concept that the precursors of this syndrome are identifiable long before the patient begins to experience clinical symptoms.

A simple procedure is suggested by Hutchison,[15] who routinely includes solicitude for the TMJ in her peripheral examination. She employs an eight-point section in her diagnostic form: (1) pain upon palpation of masseter and temporalis muscles; (2) clicking; (3) limited opening; (4) deviation of the mandible upon opening; (5) fullness or pressure in the ears, or earache without infection; (6) tinnitus; (7) frequent headaches; and (8) evidence of bruxing. Inquiry into these areas usually reveals the presence and extent of any current problem, and may even unmask a potential hazard. Treatment may then be instituted as indicated, or referrals of an appropriate nature can be made.

SUMMARY. The treatment of problems arising from the temporomandibular joint, as with other oral myofunctional disorders, remains the scene of confusion and controversy. It is helpful to realize that almost every affliction of the TMJ is basically a result of abnormal muscle function, and almost always stemming from tension and overcontraction of the muscles. In normal function, the teeth are in firm occlusion only during the act of deglutition, and regardless of the estimate of swallowing frequency, the musculature should be in strong contraction a cumulative total of only a few minutes per day.

However, we live in a stressful society. A universal reaction to stress is sustained TMJ muscle contraction (clenching) and continual overworking of these muscles (grinding) with a resulting combined force far in excess of the limits for which this system was designed. When perpetuated over a period of years, some breakdown must be anticipated.

The well-grounded oral myologist should understand the composition and function of the temporomandibular joint, should be cognizant of some of the symptoms of its dysfunction, and should be prepared to treat the ensuing or causative muscle defects.

THE NASAL AIRWAY

The individual osseous parts of the nasal airway were laid out in the preceding chapter, but somewhat on the order of the scattered pieces of a puzzle. We may now assemble them into a working whole, drape them with membrane, and examine their function.

The nasal cavity

We deal here not with a mere bony skeleton, but with a nose completed by a lower framework of five major cartilages: two lateral, two alar, and the septal cartilage. Several other small pieces fill in odd-shaped crannies near the face. All are connected to each other and to the bones by tough fibrous connective tissue.

The entrance to the nasal cavity is through the *nares,* or nostrils, and the exit into the nasopharynx is through the two *choanae.* Immediately within the nostril is a dilation, the *vestibule,* that is lined with skin which in turn gives rise to stiff, coarse hairs, the *vibrissae.* The skin of the vestibule blends into the mucous membrane, which thereafter lines the passageway throughout.

The medial wall of the passage, the septum, is smooth and flat, the roof very narrow except posteriorly, the floor gently curved from side to side and almost horizontal anteroposteriorly.

The lateral wall is more interesting. This small area is composed of bits of six different bones: the lacrimal, ethmoid, sphenoid, palatine, and maxilla, in addition to the inferior nasal concha, which is a separate bone. The lateral wall is made irregular by the projection of three *conchae,* or *turbinates.* They are called conchae because of their shell-like shape, and turbinates because of their function. They curve gently upward front-to-back, and extend horizontally into the nasal cavity, almost reaching the septum. In effect, they thus subdivide each nasal cavity into three groove-like passageways, the *nasal meatuses.* Each meatus is named for the turbinate above it; the inferior meatus lies below the inferior concha, and the middle and superior meatuses are below the middle and superior conchae, respectively. The *nasolacrimal canal* opens into the inferior meatus; it drains tears from the eyes into the nose and accounts for a "runny nose" when crying.

The paranasal sinuses

Grouped about the nasal passage is a system of cavities, the paranasal sinuses, all of which are pneumatic areas and all of which connect with the nasal passage. While the sinuses serve a variety of purposes, to count them off as mere resonating chambers for the voice, or as a means of lightening the weight of the skull, as is frequently done, is to underestimate their value; for the oral myologist, they have a much greater importance. In the well-ordered nasal passage they perform a wholesome and gratuitous service by expandng and facilitating the labyrinthine channel; in the unused nose they lurk as a morbid and hostile menace as they constrict and impede the airway.

These sinuses are located in four bones: the frontal, ethmoid, sphenoid, and maxilla. They are rudimentary in early life, only the maxillary sinus being definitely present at birth. Through the process of *pneumatization,* bone around invading mucosal sacs is resorbed and the cavities enlarge. The frontal and sphenoid sinuses are radiologically visible at six or seven years of age, while the ethmoid cells, small but numerous, do not develop adult proportions until puberty.[33]

The frontal sinuses communicate with the nasal passage through a short canal, the *frontonasal duct,* which opens into the middle meatus. The sphenoid sinuses and the posterior ethmoid cells open into an aperture above the superior concha, the *sphino-ethmoidal recess;* other ethmoidal cells open into the middle meatus. The maxillary sinuses, the largest of these cavities, occupy the body of the maxilla and communicate with the middle meatus by way of an opening in the upper medial wall of the sinus; since the sinuses lie just external to the lateral nasal wall, drainage is poor in the erect posture, requiring the laying of the head on one side.

The mucous membrane

Mucous membrane lines the entire nasal cavity except the vestibule. It is continuous throughout all of the chambers with which the nasal passage communicates, the nasopharynx behind and the paranasal sinuses above and laterally.

The epithelium forming the surface of the mucous membrane is ciliated; that is, the free ends of the epithelial cells give rise to cilia, microscopic hair-like processes. Eight cilia project from each cell, and beat in a wave-like motion at an incredible rate toward the pharynx; that is in distinction to the bronchi, where the cilia beat *upward,* waving mucus, pus, and dust particles out of the lungs but also toward the pharynx.

The mucous membrane is thick and richly endowed with blood vessels, especially over the conchae; it is thinner in the meatuses and in the sinuses. It contains a layer of glands throughout, in which both mucous and serous alveoli are present; it thus emits both a thick mucoid secretion and a thinner, serous fluid which contains both an acid and the bacteria-destroying substance, *lysozyme,* which is also present in tears. The combined secretions form a sheet which overlies the cilia rather than the epithelial cells proper.

Function of the nasal airway

We are now prepared to put the nasal airway into operation. It might be considered a processing plant for breath, warming, cleansing, humidifying, even sterilizing the air. As breath is inspired, the vibrissae guard the twin openings of the nares, removing gross particles of foreign matter. Since the nasal passage is really quite narrow, air is drawn over the nasal mucosa in a thin stream. The turbinates set the air in whirling motion, speeding its rate, forcing it into sinuses, and circulating it within the nasal fossae. The air is thus brought into intimate contact with the sticky mucous membrane, which traps and holds such microscopic matter as pollen, dust, and bacteria.

Body heat, radiating from venous cavities under the mucosa of the turbinates, effectively warms the inspired air. At the same time, secretions in the nose and in the paranasal sinuses combine in the humidifying process; it is estimated that approximately one quart of fluid is secreted each day in order to properly humidify the breath.

Through the combined actions of the cilia and respiration itself, the clogged and bacteria-laden mucoid blanket is removed and quickly renewed as it is moved posteriorly to be swallowed, blown away, or expectorated.

MOUTH BREATHING. In juxtaposition to the above, we should examine the process of mouth breathing. The antigravity muscles of the mandible and tongue are provided adequate development only during normal deglutition. When robbed of tonicity by tongue thrust, the sheer weight of the mandible, tongue, and their associated structures proves too great for many patients, and in a resting state the mouth falls open. Even though the nasal airway is available, and is used occasionally, the more common result is oral breathing.

All of the beneficial contributions of the nasal airway are now surrendered. Raw, dry, dirty, cold air is drawn into a respiratory system not prepared for such onslaught. Large quantities of moisture are evaporated from the oral and pharyngeal mucosa, much of it lost to the body during exhalation. The lower lip becomes parched and chapped as the air fans back and forth over its surface. The pharyngeal wall becomes less sensitive. The alveoli of the lungs are impaired, along with the ability of the pulmonary alveolar epithelium to perform its essential function in exchanging dissolved gases between the breath and the blood. The mucoid sheet in the nasal passage and sinus cavities stops moving and stagnates; it thickens, which not only reduces the diameter of the passageway, but may also irritate the tissues beneath, causing edema and still further reduction of the airway. Eventually, the nose may become blocked, and the patient has an excuse for mouth breathing.

The nasopharynx may also pose a threat in this situation, particularly during sleep, when swallowing incidence drops dramatically. With saliva being evaporated by the breath stream, the need to swallow is reduced still further. Stagnating secretions in the nasopharynx may then follow an alternative route into the bronchial tree, given a supine position from which droplet infection into the lungs is most likely to occur.

At least some mild sinusitis is commonly observed in mouth-breathing patients. Even this subverts the mucous linings of the sinuses from their normal function in respiration.

RESPIRATORY ALLERGY. A number of patients present themselves for therapy who suffer from true respiratory allergies. When severe and constant, such allergies are felt to be a contraindication for therapy, and we tend to postpone such efforts until the condition is improved. Little achievement of lasting worth can be maintained against the deleterious effects of mouth breathing, and when the result of mouth closure is anoxia, progress in therapy is not a realistic aspiration.

Nevertheless, it has seemed that the milder allergies have proved no insurmountable barrier. In fact, our routine procedures have often seemed to be a boon to the patient who makes a sincere attempt. As he is provided with the muscular ability for effortless mouth closure, and gradually encouraged in nasal breathing, the airway has appeared to improve and the allergic reaction lessen.

This clinical impression was reinforced by a study done by Toronto,[30] a survey that will be discussed further in Chapter 9. Toronto examined a group of former patients of one of the writers (R.H.B.) not only with a view to determining the number who had relapsed, but if possible *why* they had failed. The one consistent finding in the relapse group was continued mouth breathing. However, this group did not include most of those who had originally reported respiratory allergy; instead, they were primarily those whose record revealed poor performance during therapy, who failed to return for follow-up procedures, and who had exerted themselves as little as possible. This led Toronto to the conclusion that while mouth breathing is a major cause of relapse to tongue thrusting, excessive allergies are not.

Summary

Oxygen is the most imperative requirement of the human body; food, liquid, and other needs can be postponed for some time, but life is brief without oxygen. It is therefore not difficult to understand the resistance of some patients to any suggestion that might imperil their source of supply for this precious commodity. Yet a few oral myotherapists reveal some exasperation when their assignments are not met with enthusiasm. Some patience is required. Without a reasonably healthy nasal airway, functioning in a reasonably normal manner, all is lost.

EFFECTS OF PLAYING WIND INSTRUMENTS

Five significant articles in national dental journals deal with this topic. They were written by Strayer,[28] Pang,[19] Parker,[20] Herman,[14] and Wiesner and co-workers.[32] Two of them (Pang and Parker) report on research done by writers, while the other three authors write from clinical experience or report the work of others.

Pang's research design was a double-blind approach, wherein dental occlusions of 76 seventh-grade students were examined. It is difficult to determine the numbers of subjects in the con-

Table 6-1. Wind instruments and occlusion*

Type of instrument	Strayer (theory)	Herman (theory)	Pang (research)
A. Trumpet, trombone, tuba, French horn	Good for overjet; bad for maxillary retrusion	Good for Class II, Division I (overjet)	Good for overjet
B. Clarinet, saxophone	Good for maxillary retrusion; bad for overjet	Good for Class I, Class III; bad for Class II (overjet) and for irregular, sharp teeth	Little effect on overjet; may cause open bite
C. Oboe, bassoon, English horn	Good for hypotonic or short lips; bad for "complicated Class I's"	Good for open bite; good for Class II (overjet)	Good for overjet; may cause open bite
D. Flute, piccolo	Good for Class I and Class III, short upper lips, mentalis habit; bad for overjet	Good for Class II (overjet)	Bad for overjet

*A comparison of the conclusions of three writers regarding the effects of playing wind instruments on dental occlusion: Strayer,[28] Herman,[14] and Pang.[19]

trol, experimental, and subgroups in this research, but a reasonably close calculation would be 46 in the experimental group and 30 control subjects. It is also not clearly stated whether all the experimentals had malocclusions, but members of the control group did all have malocclusions. There were roughly equal numbers of boys and girls. There were 19 Class A instrument players (trumpet, bugle, French horn, trombone, tuba); 21 Class B players (clarinet, saxophone); two Class C players (oboe, bassoon, English horn); and four Class D players (flute, piccolo).

Pang's subjects were examined orthodontically before and after six months of playing in school bands. Control subjects played no musical instruments. A summary of the results of his research is included in Table 6-1.

Parker's study was a roentgenographic analysis of the physiology involved in playing wind instruments. Subjects were 84 school pupils of all ages and both sexes. Excellent data were gathered showing how students position the instruments in the mouth, but several unwarranted conclusions, regarding the effects of playing instruments, were drawn from this research. Subjects were photographed only once, and no before-and-after data were taken. The control group consisted of 30 youngsters with Class II, Division I malocclusions who did not play a musical instrument. The average angle of the central incisors of this latter group was found to be 116.2 degrees, compared to a very consistent 107.6 to 109.0 degree means in the four subgroups of experimental subjects. Parker erroneously concluded that this demonstrated an absence of deleterious effects upon dentition from playing wind instruments. He wrote, "The study indicates that, if the patient is under the proper supervision and is using the correct embouchure, the orthodontist need not concern himself about a clarinet, flute, or saxophone player who may have a Class II, Division I malocclusion."

The articles by Strayer, Wiesner, and Herman were based either on their own experiences with wind instrument players or reports in the literature. The Wiesner paper includes a chapter on the use of protective appliances recommended for musicians, to prevent injury to soft tissues from orthodontic appliances and sharp, irregular teeth.

Table 6-1 summarized claims and findings of Strayer, Herman, and Pang. There is general agreement among the three writers on the beneficial and harmful effects of playing certain instruments. The trumpet and related instruments can reportedly affect overjets favorably. Subjects with overjet should avoid playing the clarinet, saxophone, flute, or piccolo. The oboe, bassoon, and English horn may affect an overjet favorably.

Since only one of the five writers mentioned in the first paragraph of this section actually studied cause and effect, perhaps the opinions of the others should be regarded with less credence. Nevertheless, conclusions reached from clinical experience need not be rejected as invalid, especially when they are in essential agreement with research findings.

As in the treatment of any aspect of human behavior, it is wise to consider the generalizations others have made as you examine the individual patient. Before concluding that the playing of a given instrument will help or harm the teeth or lips of a child, however, several variables should be considered.

1. Relationships between the dental arches—In order for a child with an extreme Class II or Class III occlusion to play any brass instrument he will be required to exert strong effort to align the upper and lower lips. Pang's warning about the possibility that playing a clarinet, saxophone, oboe, bassoon, or English horn may cause open bite should be taken seriously, especially when the patient has a tendency toward such a malocclusion.

2. Intra-arch conditions, such as sharp, irregular maxillary incisors, may result in injury to the lips.

3. Improper positioning of the instrument may produce a lever-like action against the upper incisors.

4. The mouthpiece may be forced against the upper alveolus, lingual to the incisors, and periodontal damage may result.

5. Hypotonia and shortness of the lips may be aided considerably by playing a brass instrument.

6. It is possible that a child with an anterior overjet can be aided by playing a trumpet, but only if the tongue is properly held away from the lingual surfaces of the upper incisors.

7. The eventual necessity for a retainer should be considered. Some forms of retainers reduce the vertical dimension of the maxillary arch to such a degree that it becomes very difficult to play certain wind instruments.

8. Instructors who are unfamiliar with relationships between the dentition and instrument-

playing may teach an embouchure that is either difficult for, or harmful to, the patient. Others who are knowledgeable may have 50 or 60 students in the school band, and hence not become aware of the dental problems of individual players.

Recommendations

Our practice is to consider each patient individually. Interarch and intraarch dental factors, as well as soft tissue conditions are examined carefully. If the child is in the process of selecting an instrument to play, there are several which definitely will not harm the teeth. If he is already playing one that is potentially harmful, he is asked to bring the instrument to therapy and demonstrate its positioning as he plays it. If there is any possibility of damage to the dentition or soft tissues, the clinician contacts the music teacher to explain the situation and ask whether another type of embouchure might be taught. If that is not feasible, it is recommended that he discontinue playing the instrument.

We are conservative in our estimates of improvement to be expected in the dentition or soft tissue from proper playing of an instrument. A child who practices regularly, for long periods of time, may improve the tonicity of the lips, however, and the playing of the instrument may be a helpful adjunct to therapy.

In this area of study, as in all others related to oral myofunctional problems, longitudinal research is needed to determine *long-term* effects on the players with and without malocclusions or adverse orofacial conditions.

REFERENCES

1. Ballard, C. F., and Bond, E. K.: Clinical observations on the correlation between variations of the jaw form and variations of orofacial behavior, Speech Path. Ther. pp. 55-63, Oct., 1960.
2. Blitzer, M. H.: Diagnosing the TMJ pain dysfunction syndrome, Prosthodontics **8**:37-38, May, 1977.
3. Bohl, C. F., and Knap, F. J.: Evaluating occlusal relationship, mandibular dysfunction, and temporomandibular joint pain by palpation, J. Prosthet. Dent. **32**:80-85, July, 1974.
4. Carlsson, S. H., Gale, E. N., and Ohman, A.: Treatment of temporomandibular joint syndrome with biofeedback training, J. Am. Dent. Assoc. Sept., 1975.
5. Costen, J. B.: Syndrome of ear and sinus symptoms dependent upon disturbed function of the temporomandibular joint, Ann. Otol. **43**:1, March, 1934.
6. Emslie, R. D., Massler, M., and Zwemer, J. D.: Mouth breathing: I. Etiology and effects (a review), J. Am. Dent. Assoc. **44**:506-521, 1952.
7. Francis, C. C., and Martin, A. H.: Introduction to human anatomy, ed. 7, St. Louis, 1975, The C. V. Mosby Co.
8. Fried, L. A.: Anatomy of the head, neck, face, and jaws, Philadelphia, 1976, Lea & Febiger.
9. Gelb, H., and Tarte, J.: A two-year clinical dental evaluation of 200 cases of chronic headache: the craniocervical-mandibular syndrome, J. Am. Dent. Assoc. **91**:1230-1236, Dec., 1975.
10. Goss, C. M.: Gray's anatomy of the human body, ed. 29, Philadelphia, 1973, Lea & Febiger.
11. Graber, T. M.: Orthodontics: principles and practice, ed. 2, Philadelphia, 1966, W. B. Saunders Co.
12. Grant, J. C. B.: An atlas of anatomy, ed. 6, Baltimore, 1972, The Williams & Wilkins Co.
13. Greene, C. S., and Laskin, D. M.: Long-term evaluation of conservative treatment for myofascial pain-dysfunction syndrome, J. Am. Dent. Assoc. **89**:1365-1368, Dec., 1974.
14. Herman, E.: Dental consideration in the playing of musical instruments, J. Am. Dent. Assoc. **89**:611-619, Sept., 1974.
15. Hutchison, V.: Personal communication.
16. Leech, H. L.: A clinical analysis of orofacial morphology and behavior of 500 patients attending an upper respiratory research clinic, Dent. Pract. **9**:57, 1958.
17. Overstake, C. P.: Investigation of the efficacy of a treatment program for deviant swallowing and allied problems, Part I, Int. J. Oral Myol. **1**:87-104, July, 1975.
18. Overstake, C. P.: Investigation of the efficacy of a treatment program for deviant swallowing and allied problems, Part II, Int. J. Oral Myol. **2**:1-6, Jan., 1976.
19. Pang, A.: Relation of musical wind instruments to malocclusion, J. Am. Dent. Assoc. **92**:565-570, March, 1976.
20. Parker, J. H.: The Alameda instrumentalist study, Am. J. Orthod. **63**:399-415, June, 1957.
21. Picard, P. J.: Gnathology and the myoprotected occlusion, a hypothesis, Int. J. Oral Myol. **1**:78-82, Jan., 1975.
22. Pomp, A. M.: Psychotherapy for the myofascial pain-dysfunction syndrome: a study of factors coinciding with symptom remission, J. Am. Dent. Assoc. **89**:629-632, Sept., 1974.
23. Schwartz, L., and Chayes, C. M., editors: Facial pain and mandibular dysfunction, Philadelphia, 1968, W. B. Saunders Co.
24. Shore, N. A.: Occlusal equilibration and temporomandibular joint dysfunction, Philadelphia, 1959, J. B. Lippincott Co.
25. Sicher, H., and DuBrul, E. L.: Oral anatomy, ed. 6, St. Louis, 1975, The C. V. Mosby Co.
26. Stack, B. C., and Funt, L. A.: TMJ dysfunction

from a myofunctional perspective, Int. J. Oral Myol. **3:**11-26, Jan., 1977.

27. Stone, S., Dunn, M. J., and Robinov, K. R.: The general practitioner and the temporomandibular joint pain-dysfunction syndrome, J. Mass. Dent. Soc. **20:**262-268, Fall, 1971.

28. Strayer, E. R.: Musical instruments as an aid to the treatment of muscle defects and perversions, Angle Orthod. **9:**18, April, 1939.

29. Swinehart, D. R.: The importance of the tongue in the development of normal occlusion, Am. J. Orthod. **36:**813-830, 1950.

30. Toronto, A.: Permanent changes in swallowing habit as a result of tongue-thrust therapy prescribed by R. H. Barrett, Thesis, University of Utah, 1970.

31. Weinberg, L. A.: Temporomandibular dysfunction profile: a patient-oriented approach, J. Prosthet. Dent. **32:**312-325, Sept., 1974.

32. Wiesner, G. R., Balback, D. R., Wilson, M. A.: Orthodontics and wind instrument performance, Music Educators National Conference, Washington, D. C., 1973.

33. Woodburne, R. T.: Essentials of human anatomy, ed. 5, New York, 1973, Oxford University Press.

Chapter 7

HISTORY

History-making events continue to occur regularly in efforts to modify oral muscle dysfunction. Some, like molten silver pouring into a mold, will have enduring worth. Others resemble the Fourth of July sparkler, emitting an engaging light that turns to dross. Both can burn the fingers of one who handles them too soon.

Events of the last decade will be left to cool for awhile. A brief roster may be in order, but those that triumph over time, as they shape and smooth our profession, will emerge more clearly, and their influence be more accurately weighed, at some distance from the original flash.

Nevertheless, to fully appreciate what we are dealing with and to avoid the errors of the past, at least a summary is required of the evolution of therapuetic concern for these conditions. In reviewing the past we will find that abnormal swallowing has many meanings. Sometimes, writers have used different but synonymous terms for the same phenomenon; sometimes, without being aware of it, they are not discussing the same condition. Efforts have been made to contort the various manifestations into a single affliction; a "syndrome" approach developed, a device that can easily be used inappropriately while still imparting a learned air.

There is considerable concordance between British and American literature on atypical deglutition, but in some areas two viewpoints are expressed that resist homogenization. The British orientation has historically been toward research and theoretical formulation. H. G. Wells noted in his countrymen the proclivity to allow a comfortable time lag of 50 or 100 years between the realization that something ought to be done and the attempt to do it. American dentists, meanwhile, have shown a propensity toward clinical experimentation, of jumping rather willingly on the nearest convenient bandwagon.

The literature has been sparse, something less than scholarly in many instances, and much of it merely expressions of opinions. Research standards have often been low. Orientation has been toward treatment. American dental patients receive the finest care in the world, for all efforts have been focused toward this end. Deglutition has received the same intensive attention. Interest in retraining patients who have abnormal patterns has, however, been clinical rather than academic and pragmatic rather than analytical. The investigator remains frustrated by the unwarranted generalizations found in the books and journals in the field.

Some notice should be taken of the important Scandinavian contributions. Orthodontists there occupy a professional position between what is found in the United States and England, keep abreast of current developments on both sides, and are responsive to new ideas. Much of their literature is available in English translation and contains many articles on tongue thrust.

Elsewhere in Europe, available literature is less plentiful. Historically, the focus of the European orthodontist has been on removable rather than fixed appliances. In the more recent past, many have adopted American techniques, whereas others, particularly in Switzerland, have shifted their attention to surgical orthodontics, doing partial glossectomies for tongue thrust and mouth breathing while performing radical surgery of various types to align teeth.

In the present review, British and American literature will be scanned separately and somewhat chronologically. Rather than trace every reference, we will include only some representative viewpoints. It should be noted that until

1960 all writing on the subject of abnormal deglutition was done by dentists, the sole exceptions being the speech pathologist T. R. Francis and an astute ear, nose, and throat specialist, Gwynne-Evans, both in England.

BRITISH CONTRIBUTIONS

The early spokesmen for the English primarily were Rix, Ballard, Gwynne-Evans, and Tulley. These four made the major contributions, and we will have an adequate understanding of British thought by confining our attention to them. Leech,[24] who reported a single research project that continually crops up in American literature, plus Ardran, Kemp, and Lind,[2-4] who did a series of cinefluorographic studies, will be added for statistical seasoning. The original quartet in this group were all in London, and all became concerned with deglutition during approximately the same time period. Basing their conclusions on their work, a number of British speech clinicians related deglutition to lisping (interdental sigmatism in England), among them Francis[13,14] and Ballard and Bond,[10] but none proposed corrective measures for swallowing.

Rix

Rix published the first of a series of papers on this subject in 1946. He described a characteristic dental impairment consisting of proclinate upper incisors and a high, narrow palatal arch resulting from what he termed the "teeth apart" swallow. He described in some detail two contrasting types of *normal* swallowing, one consisting of the customary closure of lips, with the teeth brought into occlusal contact and the whole dorsum of the tongue coming to lie in contact with the palate. He continued:

I want to emphasize that the spread tongue, thrust with some force from below by the contracted mylohyoids, is operating in a rigid chamber formed at the sides and in front by the occluding teeth and their supporting bone. The chamber is roofed over by the bony vault of the palate, and posteriorly by the tense, sloping soft palate. The tongue operates best in a rigid cavity, and it might be mentioned here that, with the occluded teeth providing the front and side walls, the lips and cheeks on the outside of the walls are not particularly active. There is no need for them to be.*

Rix noted that, with juicy or soft prepared food, quite a different pattern is evoked. The teeth are not occluded and the periphery of the tongue comes in contact with lips and cheeks, the muscles of which are contracted to create a rigid cavity in which the tongue acts. He then observed that certain children utilize something similar to this latter procedure at all times, regardless of the food being swallowed, and could swallow, if teeth were closed, only with some difficulty. He reported 51 who habitually separated their teeth in swallowing in a run of 86 children applying for orthodontic treatment. He later added:

Since the more [the tongue] bulges between the teeth the less efficiently will it carry the food back into the pharynx, the lips and cheeks are put in tension to limit to some extent its excursion between the teeth. . . . There is another point to make. When a mandible is not strapped to the maxilla by the masseter and temporal muscles during the first stage of deglutition, a subtle change takes place in the effort of muscles attaching to both the mandible and the hyoid bone, for they are now deprived of a rigid fixation, direct or indirect, with the skull itself. There must be a fundamental re-arrangement of antagonistic muscle action to poise the mandible and hyoid bone.*

He rejected the idea prevalent until then, that the dental damage resulted solely from mouth breathing, in turn caused by enlarged adenoids. Instead he proposed the concept of residual behavior, feeling that the orofacial pattern was the product of a delay in muscular maturation. He offered the possibility that upper respiratory infections or sore and swollen tonsils made normal swallowing uncomfortable, thus interrupting the maturational process.

He noted certain similarities between some types of atypical swallowing and the suckling of infants; others he felt were "gulping" swallowers. He stated that lisps, without exception, were accompanied by abnormal swallowing.

Gwynne-Evans

A number of major contributions to British thought on deglutition were presented by Gwynne-Evans. He was the first, for example, to suggest that something might be done to *correct* abnormal behavior. Gwynne-Evans[15,16] proposed the Andresen or monobloc appliance, which was discussed in Chapter 4.

---

*From Rix, R. E.: Deglutition and the teeth, Dent. Rec. **66:**103, 1946.

*From Rix, R. E.: Deglutition, Eur. Orthod. Soc. Trans., p. 193, 1948.

Rix had considered atypical swallowing as abnormal behavior. Gwynne-Evans differentiated between "abnormal behavior" and the persistence of infantile characteristics, believing that atypical swallowing was normal behavior but consistent with an earlier stage of development. He believed that muscle behavior is predetermined, patterned, and dominated by the central nervous system; that is, there is an innate plan by which groups of muscles are progressively selected, coordinated, and controlled for the service of the child's future activities. There are frequent delays in normal adjustment toward these higher levels of adjustment. Atypical swallowing represents such a delay, and some stimulus should be supplied to allow the central nervous system to resume a natural sequence of development. Since orthodontic treatment cannot influence the form of the basic bony structures, we should make every effort to assist maturation of muscle behavior and inhibit infantile characteristics, thus allowing normal growth and development to proceed.

After many years of failure to achieve the desired stimulus with a monobloc appliance, Gwynne-Evans[17] became quite pessimistic in regard to the possibility of effecting any change in swallowing behavior. He advanced the idea of "visceral" as opposed to "somatic" swallowing, a concept not readily grasped by the average person. There is an anatomic distinction between somatic muscles, those attached to the body wall, and visceral muscles, or those attached to the intestines and other visceral structures. While somatic muscles are subject to voluntary control, visceral muscles are governed by the autonomic nervous system. Gwynne-Evans believed that the orofacial musculature occupies a functional position between these two systems, being under cortical control in somatic activities, such as speech and normal swallowing, but falling under control of lower centers of the nervous system in abnormal swallowing, during which they display the peristaltic movements typical of visceral muscles. He decided that these visceral tendencies could not be inhibited, that an atypical gradient of development was projected into adult years, and sought to incriminate such factors as innate patterns of emotional and expressive behavior, and the modern proclivity toward soft, mealy food as opposed to the vigorous chewing of a coarser diet.

One of the favorite pursuits of Gwynne-Evans[17,18] was the evaluation of the so-called adenoid facies, which he maintains is unrelated to adenoidal status. Recall that Gwynne-Evans is a physician, a rhinologist, not an orthodontist. He points out that the adenoid facies is not typical of all children who have bilaterally obstructive adenoids but that, to the contrary, all cases of adenoid facies display visceral swallowing behavior and may not even have a proneness to upper respiratory infections. Again, he believes that this is an inherited type and that the dull mental look, narrow nose, and high, contracted palatal arch are genetically controlled.

Gwynne-Evans also made a great point of contrasting sucking and suckling, a discussion that has had some influence and been reflected in some American thinking. Suckling, the nursing activity of the infant, is another inborn reflex, whereas sucking is acquired through a learning process at a later age. He described suckling as being characterized by lips everted to enclose the nipple, lip and cheek muscles contracted to contain the food and to resist the forward and lateral spread of the tongue, a rhythmical pumping action of the jaw, and peristaltic squirting movement of the tongue during swallowing, which is accomplished with an upright epiglottis and no interruption of nasal breathing. At rest, the infant may breathe with the mouth open but is not really breathing *through* the mouth; coaptation of the soft palate and the posterior dorsum of the tongue prevents oral passage of the air.

Sucking, on the other hand, requires the creation of an intraoral negative pressure. Opposing teeth in occlusion, rather than lips and cheeks, supply restraint of the tongue. Developmental descent of the posterior tongue makes nasal breathing dependent on lip closure, and breathing must be suspended during somatic swallowing. Retention of the suckling pattern typifies visceral swallowing.

Ballard

Ballard wrote a dozen or more articles[5-9] relating to orofacial musculature. He believed that everything which occurs in a human mouth or face happens reflexively, but his use of the term "reflex" is clearly not in the usual sense. One of his preferred terms was "endogenous" to account for the posture of lips, mandible, and tongue. It is apparent that he felt adamantly that all muscle behavior is of the central nervous system and is impervious to environmental factors. Thus he rejects any possibility for *educating* a change in posture but asserts that many people *adopt* a change in habitual posture; this they do as a result of inherent physiological necessity.

He stated that all muscle forces, normal and abnormal, are inherited. At one point he said that children under 14 years of age, being incapable of prolonged conscious effort, might be treated subconsciously by means of the monobloc appliance. He, too, despaired of this approach and stated later that reeducation has no useful purpose in orthodontic therapy. If new patterns are required to maintain the orthodontic result, they must come about quite reflexively as a result of orthodontic treatment. Orthodontic correction itself should not be made available to some cases displaying abnormal tongue posture, since the incorrect habits often result in a narrow upper arch and a bilateral lingual crossbite. Treatment in such cases results in relapse.

Tulley

Research, primarily with electromyography and cinefluorography, occupied a large measure of Tulley's attention. Although he agreed with much of the British thinking and contributed to it, he was by far the most optimistic, concerning therapy, of those we have mentioned.

Tulley[43,44] agreed that the orofacial muscles are visceral muscles forming the upper end of the alimentary canal. He regards speech and other mature uses as learned behavior and asserts that during the learning process faulty habits may be acquired. He concurred with Ballard that certain types of abnormal function are endogenous but believed that they are very few and may be due to neuromuscular impairment. He listed two other categories: adaptive and habit. The former is an adjustment of orofacial musculature to abnormal dental and skeletal demands, whereas the latter is a learned reflex response. His position at one time was that swallowing behavior could be retrained by exercises only if it would have changed anyway, and that all other patients swallowed correctly, after therapy, only in the presence of the therapist. Later he became more hopeful, believing that orthodontic correction of the occlusion would spontaneously correct the adaptive and habit types, and even suggesting that patients whose abnormality is endogenous might be helped to fulfill their growth potential.

Following Rix, he distinguished between an atypical swallow with nondispersing tongue behavior, in which the anterior teeth remain upright or retroclined, and the swallow in which the actions of the tongue and lower lip are responsible for dispersal of the incisor relationship. With Gwynne-Evans,[18] he worked out a rudimentary classification in which he described eight basic types of abnormal behavior. Included were patterns with and without circumoral contraction, with teeth open and closed, etc. Tulley reported that his myographic studies disclosed that many adults swallow with teeth apart but that this abnormality is generally associated with malocclusion; he asserted that normal swallowing should be accompanied by firm molar contact.

Ardran and Kemp

Ardran and Kemp were two medical researchers who did a series of radiographic studies relating to deglutition. In their initial efforts they were concerned solely with normal adult deglutition. Their 1955 paper reported observation of 250 adults under 30 years of age without gross facial or dental abnormalities, and with no known defect of speech or swallowing. They described behavior with small and large liquid boluses, and with a small paste or solid lump, and they asked subjects to drink through a straw, drink normally from a glass, and pour liquid rapidly into the mouth, chug-a-lug fashion. Their presentation was of an average pattern for each situation, without inclusion of numerous individual idiosyncrasies.

In their studies with Lind,[3,4] Ardran and Kemp observed infant deglutition in both breast and bottle feeding and found no evidence that a difference existed in the mode of swallowing between the two situations. In both cases the nipple extended to the vicinity of the junction of the hard and soft palates, the tongue protruded over the mandibular gum pad, and a pumping action of tongue and mandible was apparent.

Leech

In 1958 Leech,[24] an orthodontist, reported his study of 500 children, ages 2 to 13 years, in Edinburgh, Scotland. All were patients in an upper respiratory clinic. Leech inquired into many aspects of the problem and sought many interrelationships. Using the twin criteria of facial contraction and tongue thrust between upper and lower incisors, he found that 43% had some form of atypical swallow, 10% had both circumoral contraction and tongue thrust, 25% had tongue thrust alone, and 8% showed only circumoral contraction.

Leech found incompetent lips in 20% of the total group. Nineteen percent had a history of a sucking habit, 4% had anterior open bite (all of whom swallowed improperly), and 93% had hypertrophied tonsils or adenoids or both. He found no relationship between atypical swallowing and lack of breast feeding, did not consider finger sucking an important cause of malocclusion, but found that when incisors were affected in the presence of a sucking habit there was nearly always a tongue thrust present as well.

AMERICAN CONTRIBUTIONS
Angle

Although orthodontics had existed as a profession for some time, the first great systematizer of the field was Edward H. Angle (1855-1930). Most of his writing was done before the turn of the century, and the final revision of his textbook was the 1907 edition.[1] Angle was almost more artist than dentist; he was enraptured with facial symmetry, and his language usage was delightful in portraying his passionate regard for human dentition. He describes the "mischievous" tooth that nudges another out of alignment, "the majesty of pattern" of a lateral incisor, "the beautiful difference" between a cuspid and an incisor, the sacrilege when "these beautiful lines are impaired by grinding any of the marginal surfaces," which is "never anything but a travesty on Nature's beautiful normal patterns."

Angle had no conception that deglutition was a factor in malposed teeth, or indeed that the tongue was in any way responsible except as an obstruction in its resting state. He did recognize the influence of facial muscles, which he likened to hoops upon the staves of a cask.[1] He made frequent use of the term "pernicious" in discussing lip and finger habits, a phraseology that became embedded in orthodontics. He believed that mouth breathing was the chief etiological factor, and in defining his Class II, Division 1 malocclusion, Angle[1] stated that this form of malocclusion is always accompanied and, at least in its early stages, aggravated, if not caused, by mouth breathing due to some form of nasal obstruction.

Angle showed models of severe malocclusions and followed with a remarkably accurate description of tongue thrust. He states:

We are just beginning to realize how common and varied are vicious habits of the lips and tongue, how powerful and persistent they are in causing and maintaining malocclusion, how difficult they are to overcome, and how hopeless is success in treatment unless they are overcome.*

He was personally quite pessimistic in regard to orthodontic treatment for mouth breathing cases and showed a series of relapses due to mouth breathing. He wrote:

The difficulty of breaking the habit is even greater than that of overcoming the pernicious lip habits, resting, as it does, almost wholly with the patient and very few having sufficient character and persistence to overcome it.†

Lischer

One of Angle's contemporaries, as well as antagonist in many orthodontic discussions, was B. E. Lischer. Possibly because Angle had referred to mouth breathing as a habit, Lischer[25] pointedly notes that it is rather the symptom of pathological conditions of the respiratory tract.

He could attribute nothing to the tongue except "perversion" of the teeth in cases of macroglossia and microglossia, agreed that mouth breathing was a deforming influence, and laid stress on thumb sucking and lip biting as etiological factors. It is interesting to note that sixty years ago dentists were decrying bottle feeding of infants as the cause of arrested development of the maxilla and the then current methods of cooking food, which resulted in disuse of the dental organs. We may also observe that dentists were even then pleading for research, Lischer feeling that the lifetime of a single observer was probably too brief to make use of human subjects and that experiments with the lower animals were therefore indicated. Lischer[25] was cognizant of the anthropological work on malocclusion and wrote:

Some authors contend that civilization is a cause, that our modes of life in contrast with primitive man make for retrogression and degeneration. But there is little in the way of direct evidence regarding this, and it is probably only one of those delightful suggestions which are thoughtlessly advanced. Knowing, as we do, that "thousands" of Chinese skulls have been examined, and only one trivial case of irregularity has been observed, and knowing also that the Chinese belong to the most ancient civilization extant, and, further, hav-

---

*From Angle, E. H.: Malocclusion of the teeth, ed. 7, Philadelphia, 1907, S. S. White Manufacturing Co., p. 612.
†Ibid., p. 111.

ing been taught that irregularities are frequent among Hawaiians, we must be careful about laying too much credence on the idea that civilization is anything more than a frequent concomitant of irregularities.*

At the time Lischer published his textbook he had no specific suggestions for dealing with abnormal muscle forces; attention was then focused solely on static position of teeth, and any functional movement of facial structures was almost entirely ignored. Later, as we will see below, he came to have a different regard for musculature.

Rogers

Probably the first writer to propose modification of orofacial muscles was Alfred P. Rogers. He was convinced that general body posture, and particularly an imbalance of numerous groups of facial muscles, resulted in malocclusion. A personal friend, Salzmann,[36] credits Rogers with suggesting corrective exercises to develop tonicity and proper muscle function in 1906; however, his first published paper on the subject was in 1918. He made an early convert of Lischer, who later dubbed the program "myofunctional therapy," by which name it has endured.

For over thirty years Rogers[31-35] carried on his crusade through frequent publications and "restatements." He sought to transform orthodontists from "tooth straighteners" into custodians of the total child. He was concerned with the general physical self-improvement of the patient, including nutritional factors, endocrine function, mental maladjustment, and social habits. He warned against expecting great results from little effort, demanding that exercises be practiced several times daily for months, sometimes years.

Lingual habits did not occupy a major position in his thought. He never became aware of deglutition as a possible deforming influence, and suggested no program related specifically to the swallowing act. He did find many cases of open bite which he thought were the result of tongue sucking. He describes a case in which the temperament and young age of the patient made usual procedures impossible.[33] For this patient he designed an appliance containing four sharp prongs. The appliance was cemented in place and discouraged the patient from tongue sucking.

*From Lischer, B. E: Principles and methods of orthodontics, Philadelphia, 1912, Lea & Febiger, p. 78.

Rogers is perhaps best known for his concept of muscles as "living orthodontic appliances." Although he sanctioned and practiced mechanical treatment, he strongly urged that only the lingual wire appliance be used and condemned the cumbersome expansion appliances, together with their underlying philosophy. He cited cases in which myofunctional therapy alone was responsible for correction of malocclusion and stated that retention devices should be unnecessary.

He developed a series of specific exercises for each facial muscle, to accomplish which he devised a number of ingenious bite plates, rubber exercise straps, a metal orbicularis oris exerciser, etc., some of which the modern speech therapist might view with envy. Rogers' program was widely disseminated, Ballard reporting that it was part of his early training in England.

The Truesdells

The first to interject the idea that deformity arose primarily due to forces exerted during the act of swallowing were Truesdell and Truesdell. In a paper read at a meeting of the Angle Society of Orthodontics in 1924, they proposed that some persons with severe malocclusions appeared to have great difficulty in swallowing, and likened the swallow to a gulp.

In their only published article,[42] Truesdell and Truesdell devoted a majority of the pages to a detailed description of normal swallowing; they followed Magendie's three stages, concentrating primarily on the second stage. They did note, however, that the first stage was critical for dentition, that this phase was a voluntary act and modifications could be made as desired. Unfortunately, they believed that they could render complete change in the lifelong pattern in a matter of minutes. The Truesdells[42] described three classes of abnormalities: (1) abnormalities immediately preceding deglutition, (2) abnormal function of the lips and jaws, and (3) abnormalities in which the tongue is involved as well as the lips and jaws.

The first consisted of "drawing the saliva," using the tongue to suck saliva from the vestibule or to scoop it up from the floor of the mouth. This resulted in a deforming pull on the muscles of expression, although the swallow itself may have been normal. This was the most common abnormality they found and was corrected merely by telling the patient to stop doing it.

The second class of abnormality, and the next

most frequent, occurred when teeth were slightly parted during deglutition, throwing excess strain on the lip and cheek muscles to create the suction for swallowing. Correction was to be achieved by having the patient tense the masticatory muscles rather than facial muscles.

The third and rarest type involved a "rigid tongue," the tip of which was behind the upper incisors, the dorsum held away from the palate but in contact further back and at the sides. The chief problem in correction was to get the patient to close the teeth. Since commands proved of no avail, they devoted 5 to 15 minutes to a frontal assault. The patient was to lean forward, elbow on table and resting his chin on his closed hand, thus keeping teeth in occlusion; he was then to swallow as naturally as possible, with no effort made on his part to force the tongue to press anywhere, to think about something else and let nature take over. The Truesdells reported that as the resulting relaxation of the lips spread throughout the body, the patient began to feel drowsy. The further from normal the swallowing has been, the more complete will be the relaxation after correction.

They reported two possible etiological situations: (1) that tonsils may become infected, sore, or tender, requiring forward placement of the tongue, which would be made easier if the teeth were left open, and (2) the theory they favored, that during shedding of deciduous teeth soreness was engendered in the gum tissue by pressure of the sharp edges of the crowns after the roots were resorbed, inducing teeth to remain apart during swallowing.

Incubation period

Except for Rogers, who contributed a new paper periodically, little was published in the United States that would be of interest to us during a period of some twenty years, possibly because of the approach and occurrence of World War II and the recovery period thereafter. The British theories discussed earlier began appearing toward the middle of this period but had little impact in America. One lone item of terminology, "tongue thrust," seemed to waft across like a water-borne spore and proliferate here, but the basic concepts, the plant itself, sank somewhere in mid-ocean. Thus this term, tongue thrust, was the only name in use and was employed to indicate the entire condition, a condition which obviously was not thoroughly understood. Perhaps they did not accept Rogers'

theories, or perhaps they did not feel prepared to deal with the global problem, possibly because of a strong orientation toward "pernicious habits" of lips and fingers, but in any event, only the salient fact of tongue thrust remained as a disembodied malevolent adversary. While many orthodontists proceeded as though the problem did not exist, others set about devising the multitudinous mechanical devices to combat tongue thrust. Perhaps also it is significant that after Rogers, no article appears describing these contraptions, many of which were barbaric, painful, inhuman, and ineffectual; the rationale seemed to be that the dentist was not punishing the child, only fighting some malicious entity that dwelt within the child's mouth.

For the most part, the whole idea was put aside. It was there in the background, like next year's income tax, not brought to consciousness and examined unnecessarily. Influence was certainly felt from the drastic changes in orthodontic philosophy that were thrust on an unwilling profession during this time. It has been mentioned that the original concept of orthodontic treatment was based on static position of the teeth. A bit later, "function" became the watchword, and all efforts were directed toward expanding the dental arches to achieve a functional climate in which growth of the mandible was stimulated, changes were wrought in the size and relation of the condyle, etc. Failures were attributed to uncooperative patients, particularly in wearing retention devices for several years after treatment. Roentgenographic cephalometry appeared in the 1930s, and studies conducted by this means revealed the shocking discovery that the orthodontist was *not* effecting the changes he had previously claimed; any osseous changes that occurred were found to be the result of natural growth processes and were unrelated to orthodontic pressures. Despair was general. According to Brodie,[12] environmental factors and oral habits were disregarded. Heredity was blamed for malocclusions; correction of the defects was not possible.

Out of the consternation and confusion came new insight, longitudinal studies of growth, and the development of the present philosophy of taking advantage of growth and development.

Strang[37] published the opinion that every malocclusion represents a denture under the influence of, and stabilized by, balanced muscular forces that are inherent in the individual and cannot be changed by any known means of treatment. Huckaba[20] reviewed the thinking of the preceding fifteen years on the reasons for orthodontic relapse, and although he skirted the area, he never once mentioned tongue thrust or deglutition as a possible basis. Instead, he voiced the somewhat fatalistic view that after the orthodontist moves the teeth into new relationships, nature eventually repositions them where they can best serve the patient.

While recognizing the problem, some authors toward the end of this period, even as now, probably did more to hinder than to help. Brodie[11,12] was concerned with the effect of buccinator influence, but although he maintained that growth and orthodontic treatment would solve all problems, he managed to put in a plug for spurs on the lingual surface of incisor bands and a rubber band held between the palate and the dorsum of the tongue. We may also note Whitman,[45] who presented a somewhat oversimplified process of curing all ills by having children hold a Life-Saver on an otherwise unidentified portion of the posterior tongue. He blithely states that the bite will close, and if the patient had a lisp before, it will disappear also. How many orthodontists must have kept the vigil in vain! Whitman was heard from again in 1964, but the intervening years were without noticeable effect. He presented the same basic approach, which he reports finding in a French dental textbook of 1840 vintage, surely the earliest recorded effort to correct deviate swallowing. Whitman states that except for the substitution of candy mints for French-prescribed buttons, the exercises are practically identical. In his later presentation, Whitman detailed an effective but time-consuming procedure for thumb sucking, and a sadly inadequate method for curing a lisp, in addition to his tongue-thrust suggestions.

Klein

A refreshing change appeared when Klein[23] presented a well-prepared and provocative paper, first read before the Rocky Mountain Society of Orthodontists in 1951, which is still worth reading. He ranged through abnormal pressures from Chinese bound feet to the bowed legs of cowboys, discussed swallowing specifically, and in a long list of conclusions included the following:

2. Living bone is extremely susceptible to the guidance and influence of pressure and stimulus.
3. The extent to which living bone can be changed

with pressure or stimulus is controversial. However, even the most conservative group will agree that alveolar bone can be changed and the teeth in that bone regulated with orthodontic treatment (planned, intentional pressure).
4. Abnormal pressure habits (unintentional pressures) also change alveolar bone and regulate teeth in that bone because the bone-building cells on the receiving end of pressure or stimulus cannot differentiate whether that pressure or stimulus is intentional or unintentional.
5. Since changes take place in living bone whether the stimulating factor is intentional or unintentional, one cannot deny abnormal pressure habits as an etiological factor in malocclusion without denying the accepted principle of planned orthodontic treatment. . . .
7. It is during the transition from the deciduous to the permanent arch that much damage takes place, and it is during this transition stage that the avoidance of all abnormal pressure habits is of the utmost importance. . . .
12. The orthodontist and the patient can suffer no possible detrimental effects by eliminating abnormal pressure habits. It is logical to eliminate everything that aggravates malocclusion, everything that nullifies the plan of orthodontic treatment, and everything that is a potential factor in causing treated orthodontic cases to relapse.
13. Prevention of malocclusion is a responsibility that must be accepted by the family dentist as well as by the orthodontist.*

The year 1960 may be considered as the formal opening of the present stage of thinking. Exploration was being made, activity was picking up, and thoughts were falling into place during the five years preceding this; specific pressures exerted by the musculature were being measured; radiography provided an intriguing new vista; a number of people, including Straub, Moyers, Harrington, and Barrett, were experimenting with corrective measures. The Janns visited England and returned with a full cargo of British concepts, which they successfully transplanted. The literature resulting from all of this activity began to pour forth about 1960.

Straub

The man who must remain unchallenged as the Paul Revere of deglutition was Walter J. Straub. He raced about the countryside alerting orthodontists to the impending devastation threatened by malfunction of the tongue, commanded their

---

*From Klein, E. T.: Pressure habits, etiological factors in malocclusion, Am. J. Orthod. **38:**586-587, 1952.

attention, and forced consideration of the problem.

He first presented his theory of bottle feeding as the sole etiological factor, and a description of "perverted" swallowing in 1951.[38] However, the time was not ripe. He suggested that existing methods be used for correction rather than offering his fellow orthodontists anything new, and his paper was largely overlooked at the time. Straub, however, was not to be denied. He employed an anonymous speech therapist, later to become a series of therapists, to work behind the scenes at his office and train his patients to swallow correctly. He compiled a great number of photographs and records for some 500 patients, made a movie on deglutition, compiled a syllabus outlining therapy procedures, and went on the lecture circuit. Starting in 1958, he appeared at dental meetings throughout the United States and even carried his message abroad. He would lecture on his theories, show his movie, together with the film of a postsurgical facial carcinoma case, and distribute copies of his syllabus to all present so that they might immediately begin to correct perverted habits. He enrolled interested dentists, speech therapists, nurses, etc., for short courses at his office near San Francisco, wherein the same materials were expounded and expanded. Part I of his trilogy on "Malfunction of the Tongue" appeared in 1960.[39]

Straub's influence has been tremendous. He stirred a large segment of his profession from a monolithic lethargy regarding management of oral habits. It is possible that the presently intense national concern about matters deglutitory might still be a submerged fumbling without his enthusiastic presentation. Despite the growling arousal of those who would feel more comfortable were the matter still slumbering, knowledge and service can be eventually improved only as a result of such increased attention.

Unfortunately, Straub sent many dentists scurrying out in search of *anyone* in whose hands they could place his syllabus and expect a trouble-free future. Things did not always work out that way: his program was not that satisfactory. Many patients were improperly referred at the wrong time or for the wrong reason to people who were unprepared to deal with them, and many orthodontists were quickly disillusioned. His syllabus experienced many changes and complete metamorphoses, and doubtless inspired some excellent work on the part of knowledgeable therapists, but it remained somewhat impractical and ineffectual in and of itself.

Straub made many original contributions to the practical literature, some valid, some misleading, some erroneous, but all with definite assurance. He was the first in modern times to incriminate conventional bottle feeding of infants.

Straub[40] grouped abnormal patterns into a classification of types. He devised a much-copied therapy program, to be described in depth in Chapter 13.

Moyers

Perhaps best known for his electromyographic research, Robert E. Moyers, professor of orthodontics at the University of Michigan, has long been interested in problems of deglutition. A fairly complete statement of his views on the subject is contained in a lucid, well-organized publication.[27]

While acknowledging that it is difficult to treat well that of which so little is known, Moyers proceeds to outline normal development of orofacial musculature (following Tulley) as well as diagnostic and therapeutic procedures, and prognosis for his three classifications of the problem: simple tongue thrust, complex tongue thrust, and retained infantile swallow.

He treats normal posture of tongue and lips as separate entities. He sees lips as (1) morphologically inadequate, (2) functionally inadequate, and (3) functionally abnormal. He suggests that morphological inadequacy may be more apparent than real, that once the incisors are repositioned, the short upper lip may prove quite adequate. Functionally inadequate lips should receive attention in therapy after orthodontic and tongue therapy. Functionally abnormal lips are those seen in abnormal swallowing in which there is hypertension of the mentalis and even blanching of the skin over the belly of the muscle.

As for the tongue posture, Moyers believes that it should normally rest with the tip on the lingual surface of the mandibular incisors or the mucosa just below. Whereas edentulous adults may tend to retract the tongue from this position, some children tend to protrude the tongue between the incisors or hold it on top of the mandibular teeth. The latter may be an endogenous pattern for which there is no known assistance, or it may be an acquired posture resulting from nasorespiratory disturbance that may be corrected through treatment by an otolaryngologist or later, if necessary, by placing an incisor band roughened on the lingual surface.

Ricketts

Some mention should be made of the contribution of Robert M. Ricketts, clinical orthodontist in Pacific Palisades, California, and now visiting professor at several dental schools in southern California. His primary interest has led him into associated areas of cleft palate, deglutition, etc. He has been in the forefront of the growth and development movement.

Like Straub, Ricketts has employed a speech therapist to handle problems of deglutition, but his movie-colony clientele was probably a great asset when he produced a very smoothly professional and well-organized film on deglutition. The movie, *Tongue Thrust: an Orthodontic and Speech Syndrome,* is available from the University of California at Los Angeles on a rental basis. It contains some excellent background material, but some of the classifications employed are uniquely Rickett's and might require some further amplification.

Harrington

Up to this point every author cited in the American group has been an orthodontist. The first speech clinician to be reckoned with is Robert Harrington. If this discussion were strictly a review of the *literature,* we would probably omit Harrington, since he published only one article, and presented few papers. However, he was actively at work on deglutition in the Los Angeles area during the late 1950s. Since we are in private practice, we feel some empathy for his failure to find time to write. Perhaps many other speech pathologists were also engaged in similar work at the same time. Certainly the Counts[26] were starting, but Harrington was sufficiently precocious to occupy a place on the first panel that presented the "orofacial muscle pressure imbalance pattern" to the national convention of the American Speech and Hearing Association in 1960. Among several who appeared with him were Jann and Jann, from Rochester, New York.

Harrington staked out early the domain of deglutition as the private province of the speech pathologist, seeking dental assistance only in diagnosis and prognosis, not in therapy. He read the British literature and made much of the suckling-sucking distinction. He rejected the term "habit" when applied to abnormalities. Harrington and Breinholt[19] believed that whether abnormal oral habits were the cause of structural problems or the result of them, the habits represented the most efficient method of the organism for accomplishing the acts of chewing, swallowing, and talking.

They specified three etiological factors: (1) chronic nasal congestion, with its accompanying disruption of velopharyngeal function; (2) thumb and finger sucking, encouraging improper use of facial musculature; and (3) faulty eating habits, involving insufficient mastication of a too soft diet or flushing of coarse foods into the gullet with gulps of liquid.

RECENT DEVELOPMENTS

As stated at the outset of this chapter, we will not be impatient to evaluate the events of the past few years. Much has occurred, which may in itself be indicative of a growing awareness. Many people have sought to place their views in print; editors have seemed to show a preference for negative over positive statements, but this may reflect a reticence on the part of some potential authors, pending the resolution of all controversy. Anachronistic lingual spurs are periodically reinvented or reintroduced. There is an obvious increase in the ranks of competent oral myologists, and dental specialists outside the traditional orthodontic fraternity are beginning to seek their services. Of valid research there has been a discouraging poverty.

One of the more stimulating advances has been the continued growth of the International Association of Oral Myology and the publication by this organization of the quarterly *International Journal of Oral Myology,* whose pages have contained some articles of merit. Although quite young, this journal is gaining respect.

CONCLUSION

This has been the evolution of thought concerning deviations in deglutition. Viewed from today it seems a confused, slow-moving, hard-fought, and often contradictory struggle. Few conflicts have been resolved. The controversies to be discussed in Chapter 9 attest to this. We have at least found direction, and a momentum is building that may carry us some distance. We have discovered some areas that need to be explored; the research and experience acquired and shared in the next few years may well prove decisive. Our greatest need is for controlled research conducted by *informed* minds, eclectics who have surveyed the entire field and gained some personal knowledge.

Most authors who have made a study of deglutition itself, as opposed to studying the literature concerning deglutition, are usually tentative in their conclusions, temper their position with a willingness to modify certain observations, and reflect a feeling that the book is not yet closed, that all of the data are not now known and reported.

We are indebted to these people, as well as to those pioneers whose imaginations often exceeded their scientific acumen, happily for those of us who have followed behind.

REFERENCES

1. Angle, E. H.: Malocclusion of the teeth, ed. 7, Philadelphia, 1907, S. S. White Manufacturing Co.
2. Ardran, G. M., and Kemp, F. H.: A radiographic study of movements of the tongue in swallowing, Dent. Pract. **5:**252, 1955.
3. Ardran, G. M., Kemp, F. H., and Lind, J.: A cineradiographic study of bottle feeding, Br. J. Radiol. **31:**11, 1958.
4. Ardran, G. M., Kemp, F. H., and Lind, J.: A cineradiographic study of breast feeding, Br. J. Radiol. **31:**156, 1958.
5. Ballard, C. F.: The upper respiratory musculature and orthodontics, Dent. Rec. **68:**1, 1948.
6. Ballard, C. F.: Some bases for aetiology and diagnosis in orthodontics, Br. Soc. Study Orthod. Trans., p. 27, 1948.
7. Ballard, C. F.: The facial musculature and anomalies of the dentoalveolar structure, Eur Orthod. Soc. Trans., p. 137, 1951.
8. Ballard, C. F.: Ugly teeth, Speech Path. Ther. **2:**1, 1959.
9. Ballard, C. F.: Conclusions résumées actuelles de l'auteur relatives au comportement musculaire (paper), Société Française d'Orthopedic Dento-Faciale, 1960.
10. Ballard, C. F., and Bond, E. K.: Clinical observations on the correlation between variations of jaw form and variations of orofacial behavior, including those for articulation, Speech Path. Ther. **3:**55, 1960.
11. Brodie, A. G.: Appraisal of present concepts in orthodontia, Angle Orthod, **20:**24, 1950.
12. Brodie, A. G.: General considerations of the diagnostic problem, Angle Orthod. **23:**19, 1953.
13. Francis, T. R.: A preliminary note on tongue thrusting and associated speech defects, Speech Path. Ther. **1:**2, 1958.
14. Francis, T. R.: The articulation of English speech sounds in anterior open bite accompanied by tongue thrusting, Speech Path. Ther. **3:**1, 1960.
15. Gwynne-Evans, E.: The upper respiratory musculature and orthodontics, Br. Soc. Study Orthod. Trans., p. 165, 1947.
16. Gwynne-Evans, E.: Organization of the orofacial muscles in relation to breathing and feeding, Br. Dent. J. **91:**135, 1951.
17. Gwynne-Evans, E.: The orofacial muscles: their function and behavior in relation to the teeth, Eur. Orthod. Soc. Trans., p. 20, 1954.
18. Gwynne-Evans, E., and Tulley, W. J.: Clinical types, Dent. Pract. **6:**222, 1956.
19. Harrington, R., and Breinholt, V.: The relation of oral mechanism malfunction to dental and speech development, Am. J. Orthod. **49:**84, 1963.
20. Huckaba, G. W.: The physiologic basis of relapse, Am. J. Orthod. **38:**335, 1952.
21. Jann, H. W.: Tongue-thrusting as a frequent unrecognized cause of malocclusion and speech defects, N. Y. Dent. J. **26:**72, 1960.
22. Jann, G. R., Ward, M. M., and Jann, H. W.: A longitudinal study of articulation, deglutition, and malocclusion, J. Speech Hear. Disord. **29:**424, 1964.
23. Klein, E. T.: Pressure habits, etiological factors in malocclusion, Am. J. Orthod. **38:**569, 1952.
24. Leech, H. L.: A clinical analysis of orofacial morphology and behavior of 500 patients attending an upper respiratory research clinic, Dent. Pract. **9:**57, 1958.
25. Lischer, B. E.: Principles and methods of orthodontics, Philadelphia, 1912, Lea & Febiger.
26. Lore, J. I., Counts, A. B., and Counts, C. R.: A speech pathologist's introduction to the tongue-thrust syndrome, J. Speech Hear. Assoc. Va. **6:**18, 1964.
27. Moyers, R. E.: Tongue problems and malocclusion, Dent. Clin. North Am., p. 529, July, 1964.
28. Rix, R. E.: Deglutition and the teeth, Dent. Rec. **66:**103, 1946.
29. Rix, R. E.: Deglutition, Eur. Orthod. Soc. Trans., p. 191, 1948.
30. Rix, R. E.: Some observations upon the environment of the incisors, Dent. Rec. **73:**427, 1953.
31. Rogers, A. P.: Exercises for the development of the muscles of the face, with a view to increasing their functional activity, Dent. Cosmos **60:**857, 1918.
32. Rogers, A. P.: Muscle training and its relation to orthodontia, Int. J. Orthod. **4:**555, 1918.
33. Rogers, A. P.: Open bite cases involving tongue habits, Int. J. Orthod. **13:**837, 1927.
34. Rogers, A. P.: Place of myofunctional treatment in the correction of malocclusion, J. Am. Dent. Assoc. **23:**66, 1936.
35. Rogers, A. P.: A restatement of the myofunctional concept in orthodontics, Am. J. Orthod. **36:**845, 1950.
36. Salzmann, J. A.: Orthodontics: principles and prevention, Philadelphia, 1957, J. B. Lippincott Co.
37. Strang, R. H. W.: The fallacy of denture expansion as a treatment procedure, Angle Orthod. **19:**12, 1949.
38. Straub, W. J.: The etiology of the perverted swallowing habit, Am. J. Orthod. **37:**603, 1951.
39. Straub, W. J.: Malfunction of the tongue. Part I. The abnormal swallowing habit: its cause, effects,

and results in relation to orthodontic treatment and speech therapy, Am. J. Orthod. **46**:404, 1960.

40. Straub, W. J.: Malfunction of the tongue. Part II, Am. J. Orthod. **47**:596, 1961.

41. Straub, W. J.: Malfunction of the tongue. Part III, Am. J. Orthod. **48**:486, 1962.

42. Truesdell, B., and Truesdell, F. B.: Deglutition: with special reference to normal function and the diagnosis, analysis and correction of abnormalities, Angle Orthod. **7**:90, 1937.

43. Tulley, W. J.: Prognosis and treatment planning in orthodontics, Br. Dent. J. **97**:135, 1954.

44. Tulley, W. J.: Adverse muscle forces—their diagnostic significance, Am. J. Orthod. **42**:801, 1956.

45. Whitman, C. L.: Habits can mean trouble, Am. J. Orthod. **37**:647, 1951.

46. Whitman, C. L.: Correction of oral habits, Dent. Clin. North Am., p. 541, July, 1964.

Chapter 8

ETIOLOGIES

As early as 1927, Rogers[36] blamed tongue thrust on spaces between the teeth found during mixed dentition when the deciduous teeth that had been lost had not yet been replaced by the permanent teeth. Now, more than fifty years later, we still are not certain about the cause of tongue thrust. We can prove that we have not been neglectful in searching out the cause, however, by reviewing fifteen of the twenty or more theories that have been proposed over the years. Many of them were reviewed in an excellent article by Fletcher.[17] Fletcher's list will serve as the basis for our review of etiologies, although we will deviate from it from time to time.

BOTTLE FEEDING

Until recently, much credence was given to the theory that improper feeding of infants resulted in tongue thrust. Straub[39] had reported that of 478 tongue thrusters he had personally seen, only two had been breast-fed, and that the mothers of these two infants had a tremendous supply of milk that flowed freely. He attributed the abnormal swallow to a too rapid flow of milk that caused the infant to thrust the tongue forward in order to prevent being choked. The nipple used on most baby bottles was so long that it almost reached the back of the throat, making it extremely difficult for the infant to place the tongue against the roof of the mouth. The problem was aggravated by the practice of mothers who placed extra holes in the end of the nipple or enlarged the ones that were already there, to make sure that the milk would flow rapidly. The resulting thrusting action of the tongue supposedly also occurred in infants whose mothers had rich supplies of milk.

The best statement of this theory was presented by Picard,[33] who went to Europe, where the concept had originated, and brought back specific research reports. The Germans particularly have censored the use of "drinking nipples" rather than "nursing" nipples, and one of their men, Professor W. Balters, designed the Nuk-Sauger Nursing Program.

According to this statement, in natural feeding the orbicularis oris acts as a seal against the breast; however, mere negative pressure does not suffice to deliver milk into the infant's mouth. A pumping action of the mandible, allowing direct lingual pressure against the nipple to alternate with suction, is required to extract the milk. This milking act thus requires a protrusion of the mandible out of its infantile distal position and the expenditure of considerable effort. It has been found that the digastric muscle is approximately twice as strong in the newborn as it is in the adult.

Picard[33] cites the work of Usadel at the University of Heidelberg, who measured the work output of a 3-week-old infant in various feeding situations. Usadel found that in breast feeding, the infant, consuming 70 grams in a 13-minute span, made 569 milking motions, with 53 rest periods along the way. Similar figures involving the use of the Nuk-Sauger were: 70 grams in 14 minutes, and 605 milking motions, with 50 rest periods. In conventional bottle feeding, less than half this number of milking motions occur, as a rule, despite the fact that twice as much liquid may be ingested. The risorius, triangularis, and other facial muscles that serve as antagonists for the orbicularis oris are brought into use, resulting in everted lips, habitually apart, a "bottle mouth" said to be typical. Picard states:

During conventional artificial feeding the bottle is held in such fashion and the hole in the nipple kept at such diameter that easy flow of milk through light sucking alone is insured.

The infant receives milk in such quantities that he must learn to cope with a surplus rather than to work his jaws for his daily meals. Instead of receiving nutrition as a reward for hard work, he receives it without effort on his part, which starts him out just right for our push-button civilization.

In order to stop the abundant flow of nutrition during swallowing, the infant is forced to hold the tongue forward against the hole in the nipple, or drown. The perverted swallowing-tongue thrust habit is thusly initiated. Because the milk is injected by a long nipple almost directly into the throat, it has little chance to mix with the enzyme ptyalin, which is necessary for the breakdown of higher carbohydrates. Lack of this enzyme and an over-full stomach often leads to the expulsion of the just enjoyed meal.*

During the last decade, considerable evidence has been found that questions the relationship of breast feeding to tongue thrust. Subtelny[40] cited several studies of breast feeding which indicate that differences between swallowing habits in breast-fed babies and those in bottle-fed babies are minor. Weinberg's[43] review of research revealed no significant relationships between manner of feeding and existence of tongue thrust in children. He lists the following research findings:

1. The tongue tip protrudes well beyond the mandibular ridge in newborns during breast feeding and bottle feeding. Patterns of movement in the two types of feeding are not significantly different.[3]

2. No significant difference was found between duration of breast feeding in infancy and distal occlusion of the mandibular teeth. Subjects: 1085 preschool children.[7]

3. No significant relationship obtained between manner of feeding and maxillary protrusion in 1000 children 6 to 12 years of age.[7]

4. There is no greater prevalence of tongue thrust in bottle-fed children.[26]

Najera,[31] in a remarkably detailed study, investigated relationships between early feeding procedures and orofacial morphology and physiology and other related factors. His subjects included an experimental group, consisting of 431 children from a single elementary school and 43 breast-fed patients from various sections of the St. Louis area. Of the 431 children, 31 had been breast-fed exclusively as infants; he combined these with the 43 to form his experimental

group. The remaining 400 children were divided into the bottle-fed and mixed-feeding groups.

Parents of the children completed a comprehensive questionnaire covering the child's medical, dental, feeding, and developmental history. Each child was then clinically evaluated with respect to thirty-seven items, which constituted a fairly complete orthodontic examination.

The 31 breast-fed only children constituted 7.2% of the school group. Two hundred eighty-five (66.1%) were bottle-fed only, and 115 (26.7%) were mixed-fed. He found more breast-fed children in higher-income families than in the lower socioeconomic families. An interesting finding was that the physician's attitude toward manner of feeding greatly influenced the choice of breast or bottle feeding by the mother.

Najera reports results only in terms of percentages. Since no description of statistical tests applied is offered, the reader concludes that when the author speaks of significant differences in data between the breast-fed children and children in the other two groups, he is not using the term "significant" in a statistical sense. This is, of course, a real weakness in the study. For example, he writes:

The breast-fed children exhibited a lower incidence of fingernail biting, thumb sucking, clenching or grinding teeth, and lip chewing.

Of the children who had no habits, the highest percentage was found in the breast-fed group with 56.8%; the mixed-fed 34.8%, and the bottle-fed with 40.4%.*

Some of the percentages reported are found in Table 8-1.

Because of the differences between group sizes (74, 285, and 115), many of these reported differences will not be significant statistically. Other findings are as follows:

1. The breast-fed thumb suckers did not continue the habit past the seventh year.

2. The bottle-fed thumb suckers had the highest percentage of those continuing the habit past the sixth year.

3. The majority of the nail biters in practically all age groups were found in the bottle-fed group.

---

*From Picard, P. J.: Bottle feeding as preventive orthodontics, J. Calif. Dent. Assoc. **35**:90, 1959.

*From Najera, A.: A critical evaluation of early feeding procedures, their implications on oral, facial morphology, and related factors, Thesis, St. Louis University, 1963, p. 103.

Table 8-1. Percentages of various oral habits related to three types of infant feeding*

Oral habit	Percent breast-fed	Percent bottle-fed	Percent mixed-fed
Thumb sucking	13.5	16.2	22.6
Fingernail biting	17.6	36.8	33.0
Grinding teeth	2.7	11.2	8.7
Lip chewing	2.7	4.6	3.5
Finger sucking	6.8	2.1	6.1

*From Najera, A.: A critical evaluation of early feeding procedures, their implications on oral, facial morphology, and related factors, Thesis, St. Louis University, 1963.

Table 8-2. Results of clinical examinations*

Criteria	Percent breast-fed	Percent bottle-fed	Percent mixed-fed
Normal swallowing	75.7	58.2	61.7
Frontal thrust	20.3	38.6	33.0
Orofacial muscle activity	74.3	48.8	58.3
No crowding, upper teeth	86.5	64.6	63.5
Open bite	1.4	6.0	2.6
Normal overjet	40.5	16.5	23.5
Dental protrusion (upper teeth)	39.2	67.0	57.4
Need for orthodontic treatment	29.7	53.7	47.8

*From Najera, A.: A critical evaluation of early feeding procedures, their implications on oral, facial morphology, and related factors, Thesis, St. Louis University, 1963.

In Table 8-2 are selected data on clinical examinations, wherein are listed numbers and percentages for the criteria studied.

We have included in Table 8-1 only those criteria which have relevance to proposed etiologies of tongue thrust and which appear to show differences that may be significant. Data items that seem to fail to differ significantly among the three groups are normalcy of speech, manner of breathing, occlusion according to Angle classification, upper anterior diastemata, crossbite, deep overbite, tapering upper arch, high or low palatal vault, heavy or thin alveolar process, and facial profile analysis.

We would very much like to see these data analyzed statistically. There does seem to be evidence here relating bottle feeding to tongue thrust. A major weakness of the research, however, is the procedure used in selecting subjects. The 43 breast-fed only children were located through the efforts of a mothers' study club and other interested parents. These carefully selected children were combined with the 31 breast-fed children from the randomly selected school group to form an experimental group. Although the author states that the children were similar in the two parts of this group, no statistical evidence of this claim is offered.

Andersen's[1] case histories on 312 first-, sixth-, and twelfth-grade children found most of the tongue thrusters had been bottle-fed, but so had most of the normal swallowers. Tables 8-3 and 8-4 show the high percentage of students among both the tongue thrusters and the non-tongue thrusters who were bottle-fed. Of the 48 students with the tongue thrust, 44, or 91.7%, were bottle-fed, and only 4, or 8.3%, were breast-fed. Among the 264 students without tongue thrust, 218, or 82.6%, were bottle-fed, and 46, or 17.4%, were breast-fed. Although the percentages were higher among the tongue thrusters, the difference between the two is rather low, and on the basis of this study, bottle feeding does not appear to be a highly significant etiological factor in the production of the tongue-thrust syndrome.

Hanson and Cohen[21] studied 214 children, 4½ to 5 years old, and found approximately 50% of the children to be tongue thrusters. There was no significant difference between the number of tongue thrusters who had been breast-fed and the normal swallowers who were breast-fed. This same group of children was seen for four subsequent years by these investigators. At the end of the four years, there was no significant relationship found between bottle and breast feeding and the retention or development of the tongue-thrust swallow.

Hanna[19] studied the relationship between breast feeding and oral habits (excluding tongue thrust) in 589 patients. Only 10% had been completely breast-fed; 27% were breast fed initially and transferred to a bottle later; 63% were bottle fed only. The percentage having thumb- or finger-sucking habits did not vary significantly among the three groups of patients.

Nevertheless, this theory of the etiology of tongue thrust is still accepted by many dentists and therapists.

Table 8-3. Relationship of various factors listed among 48 students at three age levels with tongue-thrust syndrome*

Age	Bottle-fed		Breast-fed		Thumb or finger sucking		Frequent sore throat and colds		Tonsils removed		Total
	Number	Percent	Number	Percent	Number	Percent	Number	Percent	Number	Percent	
6	22	95.7	1	4.3	15	65.0	7	30.4	11	47.8	23
11	14	100	0	0	6	42.9	4	28.6	6	42.9	14
17	8	72.7	3	27.2	5	45.5	5	45.5	7	63.6	11
Total	44	91.7	4	8.3	26	54.2	16	33.3	24	50.0	48

*From Andersen, W. S.: The relationship of the tongue-thrust syndrome to maturation and other factors, Am. J. Orthod. **49:**264, 1963.

Table 8-4. Relationship of various factors listed among 264 students at three age levels without tongue-thrust syndrome*

Age	Bottle-fed		Breast-fed		Thumb or finger sucking		Frequent sore throat and colds		Tonsils removed		Total
	Number	Percent	Number	Percent	Number	Percent	Number	Percent	Number	Percent	
6	71	91.0	7	9.0	18	23.1	34	43.6	26	33.3	78
11	66	88.0	9	12.0	24	32.0	25	33.3	34	45.3	75
17	81	73.0	30	27.0	24	21.6	38	34.2	58	52.3	111
Total	218	82.6	46	17.4	66	25.0	97	36.7	118	44.7	264

*From Andersen, W. S.: The relationship of the tongue-thrust syndrome to maturation and other factors, Am. J. Orthod. **49:**264, 1963.

GENETIC INFLUENCE

We who insist that the parent accompany the child not only on the first visit to our office but also during subsequent training sessions have not been able to avoid the formulation in our minds of certain biases regarding possible genetic etiologies of tongue thrust. So many times the face of the child, together with his lingual habit patterns, mirror those of his mother or father. This is a very fruitful area for research and one that has remained relatively untouched over the years. Our patients have often reported to us that their orthodontists have said, for example, "Your child has inherited his mother's lower jaw and his father's upper jaw." Of course, it is not that simple. We do not inherit one parent's entire set of mandibular characteristics and another parent's complete maxilla. There is a complexity of factors, numberless combinations of which might predispose a child toward a tongue-thrust pattern. Among them are

(1) a tendency toward allergies and upper respiratory congestion; (2) an extremely high or narrow palatal arch; (3) an unusually large tongue; (4) a restricted nasal passageway due to small nares or a deviated septum; (5) hypertonus of the orofacial musculature; and (6) an imbalance between the number or size of teeth and the size of the oral cavity.

One of us (R. H. B.) has on numerous occasions worked with twins who were reportedly monozygotic. In rare instances one of the pair has swallowed correctly. It has been even more rare to find twins with identical types of deviation. In several cases twins who were otherwise identical could easily be distinguished by their dental structures, and the clinician has been known to call a child "Diastema" rather than "Priscilla." The study of twins should prove a fertile area for controlled research.

The same discrepancy has also been noted in a number of cases in which the child had a parent who swallowed abnormally; whereas the parent displayed one type of abnormal swallowing pattern, the child manifested another.

The individual stomatognathic system is basically determined by heredity. The relative size and shape of the various portions of the mandible and maxilla, the anatomy of the teeth, the neuromuscular system by which they function, and the pattern of growth that the individual elements will follow are all determined by genetic constitution. Forces that undertake to establish and maintain a physiological occlusion must act within the limits established by heredity; the action of the lips and cheeks as they seek to balance the expanding force of the tongue, the muscles of mastication designed to bring the inclined planes of the occlusal surfaces into forceful contact, and the pattern of masticatory movement itself are thus initially governed by innate tendency.

Certainly the equipment with which to swallow is inherited. The newborn brings this ability into the outside world and has often swallowed amnionic fluid before birth. There are doubtless strong impulses reverberating through his neuromuscular system that impel him toward a certain mode of function—perhaps toward normal deglutition. We might well inherit a tendency toward abnormal swallowing, much as we inherit a predisposition to stuttering or to tuberculosis. The presence of any genetic factor in the development of the tongue-thrust pattern itself is, at the present time, merely speculative and unsubstantiated by carefully controlled research.

THUMB SUCKING

Most of the standard orthodontic texts list thumb sucking as a major influence in bringing about tongue thrust. Moyers,[29] for example, writes that the tongue-thrust habit often accompanies or is a residuum of thumb sucking.

Since the thumb depresses the tongue and keeps the teeth apart, and since it would seem logically to open the bite, it is not unreasonable to suspect that it also induces malfunction of the tongue in deglutition. There is, however, considerable evidence to the contrary. Jann and associates,[25] who studied a group of 358 children from the first through the third grades, found no relationship between abnormal swallowing and digit sucking in this group of children. Andersen[1] studied a group of 405 first-, sixth-, and twelfth-grade students. Some of the information he received was in the form of questionnaires, 312 of which were returned. Among 48 students

he diagnosed as having tongue thrust, 54.2% had a history of thumb or finger sucking, whereas among the 264 students with normal swallow patterns, only 25% had sucked their thumb or fingers.

We believe that thumb sucking can be regarded as a possible, but relatively infrequent contributor to the development of tongue thrust. In Hanson and Cohen's[21] research, it was found to be significantly associated with the retention or development of tongue thrust in children. Clinically, a small percentage of the tongue thrusters we see have a history of thumb or finger sucking. We regard it, however, as a foe to effective treatment of deviate swallowing. It is not possible to swallow in the normal fashion with the thumb in the mouth. Since many children who have a digit-sucking habit engage in the activity during the night, it is not possible to completely habituate proper swallowing procedures in these children until the digit sucking has been eliminated.

OPEN SPACES DURING MIXED DENTITION

Clinically we have observed that when a child loses a deciduous tooth, especially a canine or an incisor, the tongue frequently protrudes into the space at rest and during speech and swallowing activities. This phenomenon was reported as early as 1927 by Rogers.[36] In Hanson and Cohen s[21] research the total diastema and edentulous space was measured in each child during each of five approximately annual visits during the mixed dentition period. No significant difference in total space was found between children who retained a tongue-thrust pattern or developed it during the years of the research, and those who retained a normal swallowing pattern or developed such a pattern by the age of 8 years. The limitation of this research, however, was that the children were seen only once annually. Ideally, the length of time the edentulous space remained would have been a factor in the computations. Of 75 children who were swallowing normally at the age of 4 years 9 months, however, 25 did develop a tongue-thrusting pattern by the age of 8 years 2 months. We would not want to rule out the possibility of the open spaces contributing to the development of the tongue-thrust.

Gap-filling tendency

An extension of the foregoing is the theory of "adaptive" tongue thrust. The origin of this theory could not be found, possibly because it has been indigenous to dentistry from early times. The theory holds, in essence, that any space around the dental arches not occupied by teeth will tend to be filled by the tongue, due partly to exploratory excursions of the tongue and partly to preventing the escape of food during deglutition. The first of these reasons is understandable, but the second may be poorly founded. If the patient has routinely trapped a bolus on the dorsum of his tongue, locking it in place with a peripheral seal, he would have small cause for alarm about its subsequent escape.

The malocclusion is considered to be preexistent and actually causes deviant swallowing as the tongue adapts to its environment and fills the seductive intermaxillary space. There is some evidence that this is the case. Hanson and Cohen[21] found an increase in incidence of tongue thrust in their longitudinal study when their 178 subjects were 6 years old and missing some central and lateral incisors. In a follow-up study of these same subjects, Hanson and Hanson[20] found a similar increase in incidence when the children were 12 years of age and a number of them were missing, or had partially erupted, cuspids. Ninety-two children were seen at this age, 31 of whom had been tongue thrusting at 8 years of age. Of the 31, 22 were still tongue thrusting, but an additional 23 who had swallowed normally at the age of 8 were now tongue thrusting. A total of 45 of the 92 subjects were now tongue thrusting. This incidence of 48.9% represented an increase of 15.2% over the incidence in the same group of children at the age of 8.

Of the 23 subjects who had not been tongue thrusting at 8 years of age, but were now doing so, 21 manifested incomplete eruption or absence of one or both maxillary canines. Ten of the 21 had otherwise normal occlusions. We would expect nearly all these subjects to resume a normal swallowing pattern after the cuspids had erupted completely.

We believe ''gap-filling'' accounts for a considerable amount of transitional tongue thrusting, and may be related to a relatively small percentage of tongue thrust habits which remain after the temporarily missing teeth have been replaced.

• • •

We list next a triad of interrelated problems: tonsils and adenoids, allergies, and mouth breathing.

TONSILS AND ADENOIDS

Two textbooks in orthodontics published in 1958 (Moyers[29] and Strang and Thompson[38]) attribute the presence of tongue thrust to an abnormal size of the tonsils and adenoids or to the infection of these tissues. The enlarged or inflamed tonsils theoretically contribute by fostering a low, forward posturing of the tongue, and the adenoids by interfering with free nasal breathing. When both are enlarged or diseased, mouth breathing is encouraged, which further contributes to a forward, habitual rest position of the tongue. Hanson and Cohen's[21] research found a significant relationship between enlarged tonsils and the retention or the development of tongue thrust in children, and between mouth breathing and tongue thrust. They also found that children with restrictions in any dimension of the palatal arch (width, height, depth) were tongue thrusting to a significantly greater degree than children with normal palatal configurations. We know of no research, however, that relates inflamed tonsils or adenoids causally to tongue thrust. Indeed, it has not been established that tongue pressures during swallowing are painful. The throat may well be sore, and constrictor movement during any type of swallow may be uncomfortable. Children have been observed to deliberately retract the tongue as though they enjoyed ''scratching'' their infected tonsils with the lingual papillae. It is our belief that grossly enlarged tonsils sometimes occupy space ordinarily filled with posterior tongue, and greatly interfere with the effectiveness of therapy; in such cases we postpone therapy until the condition can be remedied surgically, or until the tonsils atrophy.

ALLERGIES

Allergies affecting the upper respiratory system are similar in their effects to tonsil and adenoid problems and are also cited by Moyers[29] as contributors to tongue thrust.

Carr[13] studied 500 children ages 6 to 14 years. There were five groups of 100 each, labeled ''hospital,'' ''whites,'' ''Indians,'' ''Negroes,'' ''allergy.'' In the first four groups, a mean of 5% had ''V-shaped'' arches and ''overlapping front teeth.'' In the allergy group, 24% were found with these conditions.

Hanson and Cohen's[21] research found inconsistent relationships between allergies, palatal shape, and tongue thrust. In those children in whom the allergies are so persistent or so severe as to contribute to frequent nasal congestion, certainly mouth breathing is encouraged, and a number of studies have found relationships between persistent mouth breathing and tongue thrusting.

MOUTH BREATHING

Holik[23] studied the relationship between mouth breathing and the development of lingual musculature. Among the children who were habitual mouth breathers, 85% were judged as having underdeveloped oral musculature. Holik concluded that there is a definite relationship between habitual mouth breathing and an inferior neuromuscular development in the oral cavity, which he postulated may be a causative factor in distocclusion.

Leech[26] studied 500 upper respiratory clinic patients and found 95 to be mouth breathers. There was a fairly normal distribution of skeletal classes represented in the group of children, with 16 in Class I, 25 in Class II, and 10 in Class III.

Watson and associates[42] describe research by Lyn Aaronson and Backstron, which found that children with long, narrow faces or high, narrow palates have a mean greater nasal resistance to breathing than those with short, wide faces or low, broad palates. Watson and colleagues, in their own research, found no significant relationship between the magnitude of nasal resistance to airflow and skeletal classification, and also found that the breathing pattern of the subject and the skeletal classification were independent of each other. Of course, many of the patients we see for tongue-thrust therapy have a Class I occlusion.

Hanson and Cohen[21] did find a significant relationship between the presence of mouth breathing and the retention or development of tongue thrust in their subjects. It is always difficult, and especially difficult in this case, where there are multiple factors involved, to determine, first, whether a cause-and-effect relationship exists among the factors and, second, whether the relationship is unidirectional or reciprocal.

MACROGLOSSIA AND MICROGLOSSIA

The oral cavity enlarges as the infant develops and more readily accommodates the tongue, which increases in size relatively less. A few patients we have seen appear to have an unusually large tongue. The point at which the tongue is so large as to earn the label "macro" remains a question mark in the minds of most clinicians. In the first year of Hanson's longi-

tudinal research, he attempted to develop a valid and reliable procedure for determining tongue mass. Unable to do so, he eventually did find an effective manner of determining tongue length. Finding no difference between the young children with a tongue-thrust pattern and those with a normal swallow with respect to tongue length, and being somewhat less than satisfied with the significance of this measure without the other important tongue dimensions, he abandoned the measuring of tongue for the remainder of the research. We believe that true macroglossia is a relatively rare condition, although many deviant swallowers give the impression of having an oversized tongue. With the tongue functioning in an abnormally forward position in the mouth, and a resting posture similarly forward, it is easy to understand an interpretation of macroglossia. In fact, this error is so inviting that only a few years ago such competent observers as Ray and Santos[34] reported that all 32 adult patients with tongue thrust selected from their clinic displayed macroglossia. They felt this condition was developmental rather than congenital. This high incidence is not borne out in therapy, however. Once muscles have been retrained, particularly those in the posterior tongue and the velar region, the tongue suddenly assumes a much more normal appearance and in most cases proves to be just the right size in relation to its environment. It would be logical to assume that in true macroglossia there would be deviation in the pattern of deglutition. Many palatal vaults have been seen that have never known dorsal pressure and are far too narrow to accommodate a tongue of any size. No case can be recalled in which macroglossia appeared to be the basic cause of abnormal deglutition. To the contrary, macroglossia has been found in subjects who swallowed normally (see p. 163).

In contrast, cases have been reported in which the tongue was too small. Ballard and Bond[4] describe situations in which the tongue is inadequate to fill the oral space, resulting in a forward-thrusting tongue. Patients with borderline microglossia have been seen and are usually very difficult; they have not, however, proved hopeless. It is believed that although such cases are rare, they probably occur more frequently than macroglossia.

ANESTHETIC THROAT

Whereas the concept of anesthetic throat is gradually losing adherence, there are still some who maintain that a congenital physiological discrepancy, manifested in hyposensitivity of the velum, brings about abnormal handling of the bolus of food and thus tongue thrust. A few have laid the blame for lowered sensitivity on tonsillectomy, believing that the sensory nerves in the faucial region have been injured.

Precisely why this reduced sensitivity, often thought to be confined solely to the uvula, should have far-reaching results has not been adequately explained. It is perhaps the antithesis of the sore tonsil theory proposed by some writers; rather than pain causing retraction of the posterior tongue from the pharynx, it is held that *lack* of sensation in some way produces the reaction of posterior tongue thrust upward against the teeth, to force the bolus into the pharynx.

There has been considerable disagreement as to whether or not an anesthetic throat is actually present in deviant swallowing, some declaring that this is a misconception. One side effect of mouth breathing, especially when combined with the undesirable oropharyngeal muscle patterns found in abnormal deglutition, does appear to be a decreased tendency to exhibit the normal gag reflex with mechanical stimulation of the palatal and pharyngeal areas. This is further discussed under diagnostic procedures (Chapter 10). No basis can be found, however, for attributing etiological significance to this phenomenon even when it is present.

BRAIN INJURY

Another theory has pointed the finger at birth trauma, maldevelopment of the brain, or other dysfunction of the central nervous system. Considering the relatively large area of cerebral cortex reserved for motor control of the tongue, and the five pairs of cranial nerves that serve it, such a theory has some superficial attractiveness. Efforts have been made to approach this problem as a subclinical type of cerebral palsy. Several factors militate against such a concept. In the first place there is the sheer frequency of its occurrence in cases of completely negative prenatal and birth histories. There are also the many cases demonstrating impairment of the neuromuscular system in no other function except in the specific act of deglutition; if brain injury were the cause, all secondary functions—for example, speech—should reflect even greater aberration. Finally, it seems strange, if deviant swallowing were the result of damage to the central nervous system, or genetically determined and established before birth, or impervious to environmental influences, or in any way removed from

the realm of volitional control, that only those aspects which are conscious and voluntary display radical variation. In the presence of proved impairment of the central nervous system, as in cerebral palsy, and athetosis in particular, there may actually be disruption of the *pharyngeal* stage of swallowing. Such has not been demonstrated in deviant swallowing; training the oral stage suffices.

SOFT DIET

A few investigators have objected to the serving of a soft diet containing foods of prechewed consistency. Oral laxity is encouraged, with resulting underdevelopment of orofacial muscles. The mouth hangs open in repose and the tongue lies flat from disuse, although the tongue spreads between the teeth in deglutition because it is not restrained in the dental arch by energic contraction of the muscles of mastication.

Less emphasized in this theory, although perhaps deserving of greater attention, is the influence of mastication on the structure of the palatal vault. It has seemed logical to us that normal function of the stomatognathic system from the time of tooth eruption should encourage the development of a broad, rounded arch as

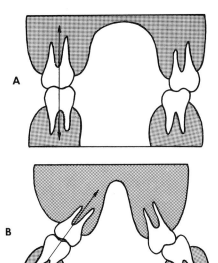

Fig. 8-1. Role of occlusion in formation of palatal vault. A, Firm, frequent occlusion, with normal alveolar development and broad palate. Lower arch contained within upper. B, Lack of molar occlusion, resulting in changed direction of force and abnormal palate. Bilateral crossbite.

shown in Fig. 8-1, *A.* The greater forces that have been measured in firm molar occlusion, the pattern of bone deposition, the influence of the inclined planes of the occlusal surface on the posture of the entire tooth—all these factors should be beneficial but might be lacking if there were a reduction of the frequency of the force of occlusion. The resulting mouth might then resemble Fig. 8-1, *B,* a common sight in deviant swallow. However, something of the same effect might be achieved even with a coarse diet, given the teeth-apart pattern of deglutition; the forces exerted on the occlusal surfaces during mastication are relatively small compared to those of normal deglutition.

This theory seems to us inadequate to be of primary importance, although it may well be a contributing factor in certain cases.

PSYCHOLOGICAL ARREST

The implication of this theory is that deviate swallowers are psychically disturbed or impaired and that their swallowing behavior is simply a manifestation of their psychological rather than physiological arrest. There is the further admonition that therapeutic attention to the overt act of deglutition is additionally traumatic and must therefore be preceded, if not replaced, by long-term psychotherapy. This concept springs directly from the Freudian school at its narrowest, in which all aspects of human adjustment are accounted for by perseveration, or at least by momentary pause at one or another of the arbitrarily identified levels of development. There are ramifications throughout the system, but since the specific activity here involved occurs toward the superior aspect of the digestive tract, we may assume that it represents fixation of the oral rather than the anal stage of development.

It does not seem to us that deviant swallowing is a particularly gratifying form of activity. It is not initiated or practiced in a manner that attracts attention or secures any secondary gain. It has never been shown to produce a pleasurable or comforting sensation. It does not effectively release nervous tension, as does bedwetting, thumb sucking, or beating baby brother. Were the theory valid, we would perforce find overt sequelae in direct therapy; although a number of parents have evidenced some frustration, despair, and other ego weakness, we have yet to observe an instance of evil consequence in the child. To the contrary, it has been frequently noted that success in therapy, the conquest of one small aspect of self, has led to an improved attitude and adjustment in other matters; this should remain, however, an incidental aspect.

It is believed that we may largely ignore this concept from any consideration as an etiological basis. Seven or eight psychiatrists in the Tucson area have thus far had occasion to submit their own children to the rigors of therapy in Barrett's office. They have constituted expert and interested observers; yet no detrimental effects of treatment have been found in their children.

Nevertheless, a side issue that perhaps might be related should be noted in this connection: Deviant swallowers, when viewed as a group, may prove to be a bit more sensitive than their smoothly swallowing fellows. It has been found prudent over the past several years to inquire as to the emotional status of the child before undertaking therapy; perhaps it is an artifact of maternal attitude, but the first sentence in reply to this question almost always contains the word "sensitive" or a synonym. The implications of this phenomenon, if true, are only conjecture; it does occur with remarkable frequency.

ORTHODONTIC TREATMENT

There is a fairly common assumption that some instances of malfunction develop during the course of orthodontic treatment and as a direct result of such treatment. We are inclined to disagree with this theory as a general rule. A full-banded appliance, in most cases, appears to discourage tongue pressure against the teeth, not invite it. The aberrant pattern of deglutition has probably been present from the start. In many cases of deep overbite, the teeth obscure the tongue from the view of the examining dentist. When the bite is opened and the teeth are aligned, the same pattern of movement brings the tongue into contact with the teeth in a new way and against different surfaces, so that removal of the appliance brings forth incisal protrusion or an open bite in the mouth where this type of malposition never previously existed. Since the posttreatment malocclusion is dissimilar to the original, the dentist feels that he must in some way produce tongue thrust. We believe that the problem has, in most cases, been the result of inadequate diagnosis prior to the initiation of orthodontic treatment.

This is not to say that such instances never occur. In some cases in which it is necessary to reposition the mandible, an occlusion may be enforced over an extended span of time in which interdigitation of the cusps becomes impossible. The resultant cusp-to-cusp relationship of the arches may then make any effort at closure a painful procedure, experienced not only in the mouth but also extending up to the temporomandibular joint. An automatic muscle reaction would then be to cushion the shock of occlusion, protecting the cusps by interposing the tongue. Given adequate repetition, the result would be an induced tongue thrust. Should there be a residual strain on the temporomandibular joint after the dentist has moved the teeth into position, the thrust might not be merely transient.

ORAL TRAUMA

If there have been cases of deviant swallowing as the result of orthodontics, they might be grouped with the rare examples under this heading. A number of patients have been seen, mostly adults, in whom a traumatic condition persisted for a sufficient time to effect changes in deglutition. Most have involved faulty prostheses. One patient had a molar segment denture that was so painful that any tongue pressure on that side was intolerable. Although he was assured that the pain was unreal or would go away, it continued. After some months an unusual deviation in swallowing became apparent: all the teeth distal to the midline on the side opposite the fixed denture began to separate and move buccally and labially. A change in dentists served to eliminate the painful prosthesis, but retraining in deglutition proved necessary before orthodontic treatment succeeded in realigning the native teeth. Somewhat similar have been the cases where a heavy bar was placed laterally across the palate to brace the prosthesis; if overly thick, such a bar can effectively block the bolus in its distal passage, causing some unusual distortions in deglutition, with resulting malocclusion. Still others have been found to resemble the documented cases presented by Palmer,[32] in which the tongue is placed between the dental arches to cushion the sensitive area resulting from impacted wisdom teeth.

The total number of these cases has been small; yet they serve to demonstrate that tongue thrusting may be instigated in the adult mouth where there has been no history of prior malocclusion.

SLEEPING HABITS

Some of our patients have reported that when they sleep on their back on a low pillow, an open-mouth position results; the tongue rests in the mandibular arch and moves forward against the teeth during swallows. When they use a higher pillow, a closed-mouth posture is more likely, and it becomes easier for them to swallow without a tongue thrust. For most patients, sleeping on one side seems preferable. This may have etiological implications.

Yet Dewel[14] cautions that a lateral tongue thrust may develop from habitually sleeping on one side. "Gravity alone will cause a sleepily-relaxed tongue to flow into the interocclusal space between the right posterior teeth" (p. 9). When there are indications of a unilateral tongue thrust developing, Dewel suggests having the patient switch to sleeping on the other side.

ORAL SENSORY DEFICIENCY

Oral motor function is guided by oral sensation. The mouth is extremely rich in sensory innervation, rivaling the fingertips in sensitivity and discrimination. Ringel[35] states that the front of the mouth is more sensitive than the posterior portions, and that increased discrimination is found at the midline rather than in the lateral regions. The tongue appears to be more highly sensitive than the lips, and they, in turn, are more sensitive than the palate. The teeth are a significant source of sensory information, particularly important in masticatory functions. Sensation from the teeth is supplemented by proprioceptive cues from the jaw muscles and exteroception from the oral mucosa.[12]

The relative importance of the contributions to sensory feedback of proprioception and surface sensation in the tongue is not known at the present time. Sensory information is directed to the thalamus and to various cortical areas. Interconnections between sensory and motor neurons occur in the brain stem and in the cortex. Sensation and motor function are modulated reciprocally and continuously. Oral experience is both dependent on, and responsive to, the emotional and physical state of the whole organism. The complexity of sensory and motor interrelationships becomes readily apparent. The study of this area of knowledge is barely beginning.

Tests of oral sensitivity

Following are some of the tests designed to assess various oral sensory abilities:

1. *Oral stereognosis.* Small plastic forms are placed on the tongue. Without being permitted to see it or manipulate it with the fingers, the subject must identify the shape or match it with an identical form placed before him in company with other, dissimilar ones.

2. *Two-point discrimination.* Dividers are set at various degrees of separation to determine the minimum distance between the two points at which the subject is able to perceive separate sensations. Normal subjects can perceive separations of 2 mm or less at the tongue tip.

3. *Texture discrimination.* Objects representing varying degrees of smoothness or roughness are placed in the mouth, sometimes in pairs. The subject tells which of the pair is smoother.

4. *Localization.* The examiner touches a spot on the tongue or palate of the subject with an applicator or wisp of cotton, after which the subject attempts to touch the same spot.

5. *Kinesthetic pattern recognition.* The palate or tongue is stroked in varying directions and patterns, and the subject replicates them.

McDonald and Aungst[28] review a number of pertinent studies. The following are two of their conclusions:

1. There are indications that seem to support the view that the quality of oral sensory function may be related to the quality of oral motor proficiency.

2. As a measure of oral sensory function, form identification in the mouth (oral stereognosis) seems to be more promising than two-point discrimination, weight perception, localization, or texture discrimination.

Ringel[35] reviews four investigations which agree that children and adults with defective articulation have poorer form recognition ability than do normal speakers. In addition, there is evidence that measurements of oral form discrimination can differentiate between degrees of articulatory proficiency. Speakers with mild articulation problems make more errors than normal persons but fewer errors than speakers with more severe articulation problems.

Silcox[37] found no significant differences between performances of tongue thrusters and normal swallowers on oral stereognostic tasks. Bosma[10] postulates that "the definition of oral functions by their sensory elicitations may apply only to the functions in their nascent state. When stabilized in mature pattern they may acquire autonomy, like that which mature speech seems to possess. At that point, they may be little affected by variations in oral sensation."*

---

*From Bosma, J. F., editor: Second Symposium on Oral Sensation and Perception, Springfield, Ill., 1970, Charles C Thomas, Publisher, p. 553.

Relevance of tests of oral sensation

It is our opinion that none of the tests described above has real pertinence to the abilities of the patients we see daily in our practices. What do we want to know about their sensory skills? We want to know if they can tell whether their tongue is contacting, or pushing against, their teeth, lips, or palate. Do they know when their lower lip is tucked under the upper teeth? If they can perceive linguopalatal contact, can they determine which part of the tongue is touching which part of the palate? Are they capable of sensing direction and degree of movement of the tongue during swallow? Are they aware of whether they have formed a bolus or simply scattered crumbs?

The child need not be able to tell the shape of the bolus in order to swallow normally. Its weight and texture do not, as far as we know, determine whether it will promote a tongue-thrust swallow. Nor does a bolus have two points. The discriminatory abilities tested by research to date are much finer than those involved in the swallow. They have more relevance to articulation disorders than to myofunctional problems. Clinically, we have seen many patients who seem to have sensory deficiencies. Many are unable to tell when the tongue tip is raised, lowered, pointed, or rounded. After repeated practice, some still cannot place the tongue tip on the same spot on the palate twice. Others are unable to sense whether the bolus rests on the anterior or middle portion of the dorsum of the tongue. When we have worked on elevation of the posterior tongue by means of the /k/ sound, a significant number of patients have been unable to tell whether the tongue was making contact with the posterior palate. When we reach the stage in therapy where the patient is to swallow food with the lips gently touching each other, some who have swallowed with a labiodental seal previously are not able to differentiate between that kind of contact and bilabial contact.

These are the kinds of sensory discrimination for which we need tests to measure our work with myofunctional disorders. In the meantime, we continue to discover deficiencies only as the patient demonstrates an inability to carry out an exercise or assignment.

A DEVELOPMENTAL THEORY

It is evident that oral function is not a static behavior. From its earliest appearance, the twelfth week of menstrual age (Hooker,[24] cited by Bosma[12]) to its maturation in the adult, the swallow adapts to changes in anatomy, diet, and general state of the organism. This section deals with those adaptations and their relationships to the persistence or development of tongue-thrusting behavior.

Basic to our philosophy is the belief that tongue thrust is a modifiable behavior. Many writers have stated that the swallow is reflexive in nature and, as such, will not respond to therapy. Others affirm that it is partly conscious and voluntary, and that part of it can be changed through training. Again a mind-closing dichotomy rears its ugly head. The importance of this topic merits its placement at the beginning of this section. Its discussion will be followed by a section that enumerates pertinent physiological conditions in infancy that are acted on by developmental changes and describes the behavioral effects of these changes. The final section will present a discussion of several factors that might interfere with the normal evolution of the swallowing process and retard or prevent the development of a nonthrusting swallowing pattern.

Swallowing process: reflexive or voluntary?

The adult eater picks up his fork, stabs a piece of meat, and directs it toward his mouth. The mouth opens and receives the food, and the tongue directs it toward the chewing and grinding surfaces of the teeth. When it is ready for swallowing, the bolus is moved onto the dorsum of the tongue, the molars are occluded, and the tongue squeezes up against the palate, forcing the food posteriorly into the pharynx and esophagus. A man may be doing all these things while he is paying varying amounts of conscious attention to what his wife is trying to tell him. Once in a while, he directs some attention to the taste receptors on his tongue to enjoy his meal. Or he may be eating alone and devoting full attention to the tenderness and taste of a sirloin steak. A child, in a hurry to join his playmates outside, may be attending only to the important activity of keeping the stoker full of food at all times, not even stopping his chewing as he swallows.

What portion of this integrated process is accomplished at a voluntary level? What portion at solely a reflexive level? Where is the dividing line between conscious and subconscious control of coordinated muscle contractions? We submit that such a line is difficult to draw. In most instances, the grasping of the fork is a conscious act, and the pharyngeal portion of the swallow is a reflexive act. All the muscle activity between the first and last steps of eating represents a series of progressively, but variably, more subconsciously controlled phases. This concept will be delineated in some detail in Chapters 9 and 11.

A similarly progressive pattern can be seen in the development of the swallow from infancy to adulthood in the individual. It begins as a purely reflexive process and acquires complexity and conscious control as other oral functions emerge and mature. Swallowing is a survival reflex. In the developing embryo, in the newborn, and in the suckling infant, control over the swallowing system is mediated in the brain stem. In the infant, suckling, respiration, and swallowing are intimately related in function and in rhythmicity.[12] With development, control over swallowing gains independence from, and dominance over, other oral functions, including breathing. Bosma[9] states:

Postnatally, the mouth acquires autonomy and differentially progresses to the most complex and heterogeneous actions effected by our motor mechanisms. These are the results of developmental encephalization, whereby the successively acquired representations of the mouth are integrated with the maturing environmental orientation, intelligence, and emotions of the organism.*

He continues:

The maturation of feeding actions of the mouth is a process of acquisition of discriminate actions of the parts that had performed in simple synergy in the action of suckling. The lips prehend and manipulate in maneuvers which appear to integrate with their formation of the "labial gate." The mandible differentially accomplishes biting and chewing. The tongue has multiple actions of prehension relevant to biting, to placing the bolus upon the molar table, and to gathering the bolus in preparation for swallowing. Its actions of sucking, of retention of bolus, and of convergence of bolus into pharynx resemble those of the infant.*

Bosma,[12] writing further of modifications in oral activities of the developing infant, states:

The most significant developmental change, however, is in the central representations of the mouth, by which it acquires its qualitative differences of function and its capacity for voluntary sensory motor functions.

---

*From Bosma, J. F.: Evaluation of oral function of the orthodontic patient, Am. J. Orthod. **55:**578, 1969.

Its actions become varied and extensively adaptive to the physical character of the nutrients which it encounters.*

He describes this development as a cerebralization of oral muscle activity, wherein the reflex actions of the anterior oral musculature yield progressively to voluntary motions.

Thus swallowing, originally a totally reflexive process, develops into a complex, integrated voluntary-reflexive one during infancy and early childhood. Bosma,[10] in referring to the role of consciousness in the developing swallow, specifically states that some functions change postnatally only by the addition of awareness and volition. In this category he tentatively places approximation to a suckle stimulus, the suckling action itself, and the initiation of swallowing by the penetration of the bolus into the pharynx.

At least until the bolus enters into the pharynx, it is *potentially* under voluntary control. Grasping the fork, directing the food toward the mouth, biting, chewing, forming the bolus— these are learned functions, not present at birth. Watch people eating in a restaurant and you quickly perceive that they did not all learn to eat in the same way. Each of them could, with proper training, learn to eat in a different manner. Most behavioral patterns that are learned can be modified, and patterns comprising all but the very posterior stages of swallowing are no exceptions. Especially amenable to change are those imposed on the person by abnormal structures, such as eccentric occlusion, grossly enlarged tonsils, extreme overjet, overbite, or open bite.

Developmental changes in infancy and early childhood

Each of the following important alterations in physiology in the developing child will be presented in three steps. *Step a* describes the physiology of the infant; *step b,* the developmental modification(s); and *step c,* the resultant effect on behavior.

1. Oral resting posture
   a. Bosma[12] likens the tongue in the infant's mouth to a piston within a cylinder. The oral cavity is filled by the tongue, which apposes the palate along its entire length, and maintains contact with the lips anteriorly.
   b. Developmentally, the hyoid descends, lowering and retracting the tongue. The oral cavity enlarges relatively more than does the tongue.
   c. More oral space is created, and the tongue no longer completely fills the cavity. At rest, the tongue no longer contacts the lips or palate.

2. Movements of the tongue, lips, and mandible
   a. In the infant, these three oral components move synergistically, as a composite motor organ.[9] The mouth is solely concerned with suckling, approximating and orienting to the nipple, and enclosing it.
   b. The changes described in *step 1b* occur. The tongue-hyoid-larynx column descends, the facial skeleton expands, and the "masticatory space" appears.[9] The diet changes, and the teeth erupt.
   c. The mouth acquires various new functions, and the tongue, lips, and mandible achieve independent functioning. Biting, chewing, moving food, and forming a bolus, all demand that new motor patterns be learned.

3. Pathway of the bolus
   a. In infant swallows, the posterior pharyngeal wall moves forward significantly to assist the movement of the bolus into the pharynx. Lingual and palatal movements contribute less than in the older child.
   b. The tongue develops more discreet movements.
   c. The tongue and palate are displaced to a greater degree during swallow, and the pathway of the bolus is more dorsal.

4. Voluntary movement
   a. Swallowing in the infant is initiated reflexively, cued by another reflexive action, suckling.
   b. The introduction of solid foods into the diet calls for the contraction of tongue and cheek muscles (voluntary movements) to prepare the food for swallowing.
   c. The initiatory phases of the swallow consist of voluntary muscle movements.

5. Anteroposterior oral space
   a. Skeletal size is small in comparison with

---

*From Bosma, J. F.: Physiology of the mouth, pharynx, and esophagus. In Paparella, M. M., and Shumrich, D. A., editors: Otolaryngology, Philadelphia, 1973, W. B. Saunders Co., p. 365.

tongue size, and the tongue protrudes at rest.
  b. The body of the mandible increases in length, as do the maxillae.
  c. The greater anteroposterior space allows the tongue to rest more posteriorly, away from the lips, and later, from the teeth.
6. Vertical space
  a. The jaws are separated during repose, and the tongue rests in a forward position.
  b. The ramus grows, displacing the body of the mandible downward and forward.[22] The teeth erupt, and their occlusion, particularly that of the molars and incisors, increases the vertical dimension of the oral cavity.
  c. These developments provide more vertical space for the tongue, permitting it to effect a seal by squeezing up against the palate, rather than pushing against the lips or anterior teeth.
7. The pharyngeal airway
  a. The pharyngeal airway is kept open in the infant by the maintenance of a forward tongue posture.[22]
  b. The tonsils may reduce in size or be removed surgically. The hyoid descends, and the oral cavity enlarges anteroposteriorly and vertically, affording more lingual space.
  c. The airway can remain open even though the tongue is retracted.
8. Central control of swallow
  a. The composite suckling and swallowing processes are subcortically controlled.[12]
  b. The acquisition of new oral skills, such as biting and chewing, enlists cortical control.
  c. The initial phases of swallowing are voluntary. The swallowing process becomes partly voluntary and partly reflexive. The successively acquired representations of the mouth are integrated with the maturing environmental orientation, intelligence, and emotions of the organism.[9]

SUMMARY. Developmental changes during infancy and early childhood foster basic changes in the oral stages of swallowing. The tongue at rest and during swallow learns to remain relatively retracted. The refinement of muscle movements permits the development of effective tongue raising and squeezing motions, which replace the forward-thrusting patterns comprising the infant swallow.

Deterrents to the development of normal swallow patterns in infancy and early childhood

According to knowledge available at the present time, certain developmental changes in anatomy and physiology foster corresponding modifications in the resting posture and movements of the tongue. These changes are necessarily accompanied by, if not guided by, perceptual cues that are also changing. If the environment in which the tongue functions fails to develop normally along any dimension, or if the space available in the oral cavity is restricted in any other way, the thrusting pattern present during infancy may persist, even throughout adulthood. Following, albeit somewhat loosely, the order in which the developmental changes were presented earlier, we list some factors that may deter development of normal swallowing patterns.

1. The tongue grows abnormally large with respect to the size of the oral cavity, creating a crowding condition and fostering the retention of infantile lingual resting postures.

2. Solid and semisolid foods are not introduced into the diet of the child at the appropriate age, and the new motor patterns that would normally develop to accomplish the biting, chewing, and moving of food do not emerge. Apposition of the tongue, lips, and palate persists during sucking and swallowing. The disruption of developmental timing, together with the additional habit strength due to prolonged infantile feeding patterns, causes the swallowing pattern to remain unchanged when solids are introduced into the diet.

3. The initiatory phases of the swallow, due to the extension of bottle or breast feeding, remain under reflexive control. The development of voluntary muscle contractions of the tongue and cheeks is postponed.

4. Growth of the mandible and/or maxilla is inhibited or retarded, and the tongue is not afforded needed additional anteroposterior or lateral space.

5. Insufficient or delayed eruption of the incisors or molars limits the enlargement of the oral cavity in a vertical direction. The crowded tongue persists in resting and moving forward in the mouth.

6. The nasal airway is restricted in size by the

Table 8-5. Number of children diagnosed as tongue thrusters at 4 years 9 months, who were swallowing normally by the age of 8 years 2 months

Thrusters, 4 years 9 months	Age when normal swallow was acquired				Total	Percent
	5 years 8 months	6 years 7 months	7 years 5 months	8 years 2 months		
103	24	4	16	18	63	61.2

presence of obstructions, such as enlarged adenoids or swollen membranes. Enlarged tonsils partially block the oropharyngeal port. The mandible is habitually depressed and the tongue held low and forward in the mouth to facilitate mouth breathing. The tongue remains forward during swallows.

7. Genetic factors preclude normal size relationships among the mandible, maxilla, and tongue. The tongue rests and functions principally in the mandibular arch rather than in the smaller maxillary arch.

8. Oral perceptual skills are inadequate, and the normal refinement of movement required for the development of the nonthrusting swallow is not achieved.

Many of these speculative conclusions regarding possible etiologies of tongue thrust are supported by research findings. None of them has been definitively proved to be true. Evidence is substantial, however, that alterations in normal physiological development are strongly associated with the retention of the infantile swallowing pattern.

Changes in later childhood

Much of the data from the research of Hanson and Cohen[21] indicates a strong relationship between maturation in later childhood and tongue thrust. Their results will be discussed in considerable detail.

The swallowing pattern of most children undergoes a maturational transition either prior to or during the period of mixed dentition. It changes from an infantile swallow, with the tongue protruding between the upper and lower teeth, to a "normal, mature swallow," with the tongue tip assuming a position posterior to the alveolar ridge during deglutition.

High percentages of tongue thrust among preschool children are often referred to in the literature, but no incidence studies concerning children in this group have been reported. The earliest studies have been completed with children in kindergarten and first grade. In a population of 353 5- and 6-year-old children, Bell and Hale[6] found that 289 (82%) demonstrated a low, forward tongue position during swallowing. Studies by Fletcher and associates,[16] Andersen,[1] and Werlich[44] report an inverse relationship between tongue thrust and chronological age in children of all ages. Ardran and associates,[3] Baril and Moyers,[5] and Findlay and Kilpatrick[15] have demonstrated changes in the pattern of swallowing occurring as functions of growth and development. Moyers[30] describes the development of the swallow as a maturational process, dependent on dental, muscular, and neurological development. Normally this maturational process is complete by the age of 15 months, but he reports that some children retain the infantile patterns for several years. Tulley[41] writes that tongue-thrust swallows often correct spontaneously by the time permanent teeth have erupted.

Hanson and Cohen[21] found developmental changes in swallowing patterns occurring in their group of 178 children, but the children did not all develop from a tongue thrust to a normal pattern. Some of the children who were tongue thrusting at 4 years 9 months of age learned to swallow normally at some time in the period of the research, whereas others who had demonstrated normal swallow at the initial evaluation developed a thrusting pattern over the years. Table 8-5 shows, of the subjects who were found to be tongue thrusters when 4 years 9 months old, the number of children who were first seen to have acquired a normal swallowing pattern at each of the annual examinations from 5 years 8 months to 8 years 2 months of age.

Of the 103 subjects who at 4 years 9 months of age protruded the tongue into the space either between the maxillary and mandibular incisors or between the maxillary and mandibular cuspids during swallowing, 63 (61.2%) had changed to a normal pattern of swallowing by the age of 8 years 2 months. Of these 63 children, 34 had

Table 8-6. Number of children whose swallows were "normal" at 4 years 9 months, who swallowed with a tongue thrust by 8 years 2 months

Normal, 4 years 9 months	Age when tongue thrust was first manifest				Total	Percent
	5 years 8 months	6 years 7 months	7 years 5 months	8 years 2 months		
75	11	9	1	4	25	33.3

normalized their swallowing patterns between the ages of 6 years 7 months and 8 years 2 months. This is the developmental period characterized by the greatest number of missing teeth. Of this group, 18 (17.5%) of the subjects changed to a normal pattern of swallowing between 7 years 5 months and 8 years 2 months of age.

When first examined at 4 years 9 months of age, 75 of the children exhibited normal swallowing patterns. Of the 75 normal swallowers, 25 (33%) had changed to a tongue-thrusting pattern by the conclusion of the study. Table 8-6 shows the numbers of these children at the age when they were first diagnosed as having become tongue thrusters. Of the 25, 20 of the subjects began swallowing abnormally by the age of 6 years 7 months; only 5 children developed a tongue thrust during the ages of 7 years 5 months to 8 years 2 months, when the greatest number of teeth were missing.

A few of the children demonstrated swallow patterns that were completely or nearly completely stable during the five years. Others were found to be tongue thrusting at 4 years 9 months and swallowing normally at 8 years 2 months of age. Another group used a normal swallow during the first year and developed a thrusting pattern by the fifth year. A final group would be labeled "transitional thrusters": that is, these children were swallowing normally at 4 years 9 months of age, developed a tongue thrust at some time before the final year, but returned to a normal pattern by the age of 8 years 2 months. The following data show patterns of change or constancy among the 178 subjects:

NUMBER OF SUBJECTS

Group I. Consistent swallowers

1. Tongue thrust during all five years — 9
2. Normal swallow during all five years — 20

NUMBER OF SUBJECTS

3. Tongue thrust four of the five years — 33
4. Normal swallow four of the five years — 29
5. Total number of relatively consistent swallowers — 91
6. Percentage of total subjects — 51.1%

Group II. Tongue thrusters who developed normal swallows

1. Tongue thrust at 4 years 9 months; normal at 5 years 8 months, 6 years 7 months, 7 years 5 months, and 8 years 2 months — 21
2. Tongue thrust at 4-9; normal at 6-7, 7-5, and 8-2 — 29
3. Tongue thrust at 4-9; normal at 7-5, 8-2 — 46
4. Tongue thrust at 4-9; normal at 8-2 — 62
5. Tongue thrust at 4-9 and 5-8; normal at 7-5 and 8-2 — 12
6. Tongue thrust at 4-9 and 5-8; normal at 8-2 — 22
7. Tongue thrust at 6-7; normal at 7-5 and 8-2 — 22
8. Tongue thrust at 6-7; normal at 8-2 — 39
9. Tongue thrust at 4-9, 5-8, and 6-7; normal at 7-5 and 8-2 — 4
10. Tongue thrust at 4-9, 5-8, and 6-7; normal at 8-2 — 14
11. Tongue thrust at 4-9, 5-8, 6-7, and 7-5; normal at 8-2 — 10

Group III. Normal swallowers who became tongue thrusters

1. Normal swallow at 4-9; tongue thrust at 5-8, 6-7, 7-5, and 8-2 — 5

	NUMBER OF SUBJECTS
2. Normal at 4-9; tongue thrust at 6-7, 7-5, and 8-2	8
3. Normal at 4-9; tongue thrust at 7-5 and 8-2	13
4. Normal at 4-9; tongue thrust at 8-2	25

Group IV. Transitional tongue thrusters

1. Tongue thrust during fourth year of study only	1
2. Tongue thrust during third year only	8
3. Tongue thrust during second year only	5
4. Total subjects thrusting only one year	14
5. Normal swallow first, second, and fifth year; tongue thrust at least one of two intervening years	12
6. Normal first and fifth years; tongue thrust other three years	4
7. Normal first and fifth years; tongue thrust at least two of the intervening three years	9
8. Normal first and fifth years; tongue thrust at least one of the intervening three years	30*

In summary, the number of children with tongue thrust was reduced during the mixed dentition stage from 103 to 63. There was considerable variability of swallowing patterns among those who were tongue thrusters at the initial evaluation and among those who were diagnosed as normal swallowers. About half the subjects, however, displayed fairly consistent patterns throughout the forty-nine-month period. A study of individual subjects reveals that of the 114 normal swallowers found in the last year, 62 had been tongue thrusting at the age of 4 years 9 months. Over 50% had developed normal swallowing patterns without therapy.

Of the 75 children who swallowed normally at 4 years 9 months of age, 25 were swallowing with a tongue thrust at age 8 years 2 months. Another 30 had manifested a thrusting pattern at some time during the research but had re-

---

*16.9% of 178 subjects.

turned to a normal swallow by the age of 8 years 2 months.

More than half the children at 4 years 9 months of age were tongue thrusting. Evidence from the Lewis and Counihan[17] research, together with the results of incidence studies cited here seem to give some support to a developmental theory of tongue thrust, with a thrusting pattern being replaced by a nonthrusting pattern in the majority of children by the approximate age of 5 years.

Of 75 children who were swallowing normally at the age of 4 years 9 months, however, 25 began to tongue thrust during the subsequent years of the research and were still doing so at the age of 8 years 2 months. We can only conclude that tongue thrust, apparently a normal phenomenon in infancy, more often than not yields to a pattern we label as normal, and returns in a significant percentage of children during mixed dentition.

CONCLUSION

On the basis of evidence available at the present time, we believe that tongue thrust is a normal behavior in infants. At about the age of 5 or 6 years, more children appear to be swallowing without a tongue thrust than with one. If we were to describe the behavior in psychological terms, we would say that tongue thrust, when it occurs in children beyond the age of 6 years, represents either a fixation of, or a regression to, early childhood behavior. In either case, the child is demonstrating a behavior that at an earlier age was a normal pattern. Perhaps we ought to be searching for the etiology of the "normal" swallow, rather than the etiology of tongue thrust. When we combine research results with our clinical experience, we have to believe in a multiple causation theory. We are convinced of the strong interrelationships between form and function. The basic oral anatomy that a child inherits and develops determines to a great extent, for example, the habitual resting position of the tongue. The tongue learns to rest in a place and manner that offer the least physiological resistance. If the tongue rests in a low anterior position in the mouth, approximately once every minute, when a saliva swallow occurs, the tongue will probably move as little as possible to accomplish the swallow. Since any kind of swallow requires a tight seal between the tongue and some part of the mouth, this seal will probably be made anteriorly rather than superiorly. Although children do not always manifest consistency among the swallows of liquids, saliva, and food, those who do not are exceptions rather than the rule. The child who swallows saliva by pushing the tongue against the anterior teeth usually swallows liquids and foods in this manner as well.

Anything that fosters a low forward resting position of the tongue, then, can contribute to the retention or the development of a tongue-thrust swallow. Certainly mouth breathing contributes to such a resting posture. Anything that contributes to the mouth breathing may be contributing to tongue thrust. In some children allergies affecting the upper respiratory system are severe and persistent enough to make mouth breathing easier than nose breathing. Enlarged adenoids, swollen nasal membranes, and deviated septums are culpable in many children. The child with a narrow and/or high palatal arch often finds it difficult to rest the tongue in that arch and resorts to a low habitual tongue posture. A lingual crossbite, found in the Hanson and Cohen research to be significantly related to tongue thrust, may be a factor because the resulting relatively greater width of the mandible arch encourages the tongue to rest low in the mouth. Vertical crowding of the tongue may occur, such as in the children with deep overbite. Any of these factors, we believe, may in some children contribute to the abnormal resting position of the tongue and subsequent abnormal swallow. In our opinion, any of the other etiologies discussed in this chapter may contribute in certain children, and we would not want to exclude consideration of any of them as we attempt to diagnose a problem in a particular child. The significance of some of them, such as thumb sucking, is difficult to assess. Whereas it is impossible to swallow normally with the thumb in the mouth, it is also impossible to breathe through the mouth with the thumb occluding the opening. Thus, inasmuch as thumb sucking fosters proper nasal breathing, it may be of help in developing normal resting postures and swallowing.

We prefer to keep our minds open to all possible etiologies when we see individual children. George A. Kopp's organismic theory has particular pertinency to this problem, we believe. Kopp, a speech pathologist, preferred to avoid controversies regarding etiologies of speech problems based on a dichotomized "functional-organic" concept, by considering the human being as an organism consisting of a mind and body, both of which contribute to the production of normal, fluent, intelligible speech. A single anatomical structure is involved in the performance of various functions. We will paraphrase two of his concepts, substituting "swallowing" where he used the word "speech."

1. The automaticity of swallowing can be conceived of as involving various bodily processes working as an integrated whole. Since they are related, the principle of relativity (that the qualities of related things are determined by their interrelationships) can be applied. A change in the condition of any component of the system of forces conceived of as the swallowing mechanism entails a change in the unity of the entire system.

2. An important corollary of this theory is that every type of swallow that has been used has imprinted its psychomotor pattern in the organism and is subject to recall when similar organismic states prevail. There is not one swallowing pattern, but many, all subject to use when the conditions under which they were implanted recur. When we establish new habits, either developmentally or as a result of therapy, we do not erase the old patterns.

These principles are useful in our efforts to understand multiple etiology, and equally useful in planning treatment for the disorder. Any force or condition that modifies form (anatomy) potentially alters physiology and function. Conversely, function leaves its imprints on form.

REFERENCES

1. Andersen, W. S.: The relationship of the tongue-thrust syndrome to maturation and other factors, Am. J. Orthod. **49**:264, 1963.
2. Ardan, G. M., and Kemp, F. H.: A radiographic study of movements of the tongue in swallowing, Dent. Pract. **5**:8, 1955.
3. Ardan, G. M., Kemp, F. H., and Lind, J.: A cineradiographic study of bottle feeding, Br. J. Radiol. **31**:11, 1958.
4. Ballard, C. F., and Bond, E. K.: Clinical observations on the correlation between variations of the jaw form and variations of orofacial behavior, including those for articulation, Speech Path. Ther. **55**:63, October 1960.
5. Baril, C., and Moyers, R. E.: An electromyographic analysis of the temporalis muscles and certain facial muscles in thumb and finger sucking patients, J. Dent. Res. **39**:536, 1960.
6. Bell, D., and Hale, A.: Observations of tongue

thrust in pre-school children, J. Speech Hear. Disord. **28**:195, 1963.

7. Bijlstra, K. G.: Frequency of dentofacial anomalies in school children and some aetiologic factors, Trans. Eur. Orthod. Soc. **44**:231, 1958.

8. Bosma, J. F., editor: Symposium on oral sensation and perception, Springfield, Ill., 1967, Charles C Thomas, Publisher.

9. Bosma, J. F.: Evaluation of oral function of the orthodontic patient, Am. J. Orthod. **55**:578, 1969.

10. Bosma, J. F., editor: Second symposium on oral sensation and perception, Springfield, Ill., 1970, Charles C Thomas, Publisher.

11. Bosma, J. F., editor: Third symposium on oral sensation and perception, Springfield, Ill., 1972, Charles C Thomas, Publisher.

12. Bosma, J. F.: Physiology of the mouth, pharynx, and esophagus. In Paperella, M. M., and Shumrich, D. A., editors: Otolaryngology, Philadelphia, 1973, W. B. Saunders Co.

13. Carr, D. T.: Habits associated with dental anomalies, Am. J. Orthod. **31**:152, 1945.

14. Dewel, B. F.: Canine development and function, Trans. Europ. Orthod. **57**:1, 1971.

15. Findlay, I. A., and Kilpatrick, S. J.: An analysis of myographic records in swallowing in normal and abnormal subjects, J. Dent. Res. **34**:629, 1960.

16. Fletcher, S. G., Casteel, R. L., and Bradley, D. P.: Tongue-thrust swallow, speech articulation, and age, J. Speech Hear. Disord. **26**:219, 1961.

17. Fletcher, S. G.: Processes and maturation of mastication and deglutition, ASHA Reports, No. 5, p. 92, 1970.

18. Garliner, D.: Myofunctional therapy in dental practice, Brooklyn, N.Y., 1971, Bartel Dental Book Co., Inc.

19. Hanna, J. C.: Breast feeding versus bottle feeding in relation to oral habits, J. Dent. Child. **34**:243, 1967.

20. Hanson, T. E., and Hanson, M. L.: A follow-up study of longitudinal research in malocclusions and tongue-thrust, Int. J. Oral. Myol. **1**:21-28, 1975.

21. Hanson, M. L., and Cohen, M. S.: Effects of form and function on swallowing and the developing dentition, Am. J. Orthod. **64**:63, 1973.

22. Hoffman, J. A., and Hoffman, R. L.: Tongue-thrust and deglutition: some anatomical, physiological, and neurological considerations, J. Speech Hear. Disord. **30**:105, 1965.

23. Holik, F.: Relation between habitual breathing through the mouth and muscular activity of the tongue in disto-occlusion, Cesk. Stomatol. **57**:170, 1957, and Dent. Abst. **3**:266, 1958.

24. Hooker, D.: Early human fetal behavior, with a preliminary note on double simultaneous fetal stimulation, Res. Publ. Assoc. Res. Nerv. Ment. Dis. **33**:98, 1954.

25. Jann, C. R., Ward, M., and Jann, H. W.: A longitudinal study of articulation, deglutition, and malocclusion, J. Speech Hear. Disord. **29**:424, 1964.

26. Leech, H. L.: A clinical analysis of orofacial morphology and behavior of 500 patients attending an upper respiratory research clinic, Dent. Pract. **9**:57, 1958.

27. Lewis, J. A., and Counihan, R. F.: Tongue thrust in infancy, J. Speech Hear. Disord. **30**:280, 1965.

28. McDonald, E. T., and Aungst, L. F.: Studies in oral sensorimotor function. In Bosma, J. F., editor: Symposium on oral sensation and perception, Springfield, Ill., 1967, Charles C Thomas, publisher.

29. Moyers, R. E.: Handbook of orthodontics, Chicago, 1958, Year Book Medical Publishers, Inc., pp. 118-119.

30. Moyers, R. E.: Postnatal development of the orofacial musculature; patterns of orofacial growth and development, ASHA Reports, No. 6, p. 38, 1971.

31. Najera, A.: A critical evaluation of early feeding procedures, their implications on oral, facial morphology, and related factors, Thesis, St. Louis University, 1963.

32. Palmer, J. M.: Tongue thrusting: A clinical hypothesis, J. Speech Hear. Disord. **27**:323, 1962.

33. Picard, P. J.: Bottle feeding as preventive orthodontics, J. Cal. Dent. Assoc. **35**:90, 1959.

34. Ray, H. G., and Santos, H. A.: Consideration of tongue thrusting as a factor in periodontal disease, J. Periodontol. **25**:250, 1954.

35. Ringel, R. L.: Oral sensation and perception: A selective review, ASHA Reports, No. 5, 1970, p. 188.

36. Rogers, A. P.: Open-bite cases involving tongue habits, Int. J. Orthod. **13**:837, 1927.

37. Silcox, B. L.: Oral stereognosis in tongue thrust, Dissertation, University of Utah, 1969.

38. Strang, R. H. W., and Thompson, W. M.: Textbook of orthodontia, ed. 4, Philadelphia, 1958, Lea & Febiger.

39. Straub, W. J.: Malfunction of the tongue. Part I, Am. J. Orthod. **47**:596, 1960.

40. Subtelny, J. D.: Examination of current philosophies associated with swallowing behavior, Am. J. Orthod. **51**:161, 1965.

41. Tulley, W. J.: A critical appraisal of tongue thrusting, Am. J. Orthod. **55**:640, 1969.

42. Watson, R. M., Warren, V. W., and Fisher, N. D.: Nasal resistance, skeletal classification and mouth breathing in orthodontic patients, Am. J. Orthod. **54**:367, 1968.

43. Weinberg, B.: Deglutition: a review of selected topics, ASHA Reports, No. 5, p. 116, 1970.

44. Werlick, E. P.: The prevalence of variant swallowing patterns in a group of Seattle school children, Thesis, University of Washington, 1962.

Chapter 9

CONTROVERSIES

We return to a discussion of controversies raised in the introductory chapter. Incidence studies give convincing evidence that tongue thrust is a describable and real behavior.

DOES TONGUE THRUST EXIST?

Weinberg[72] offered the following opinion: Current scientific data do not provide sufficient information for specifying normal patterns of swallow as they relate to occlusion. An acceptable definition of tongue-thrust swallow and specification of tongue-thrust swallow as a distinct clinical entity have not been accomplished. Current data suggest that patterns of tongue-thrust swallow should not be regarded as atypical, abnormal, or representative of a syndrome.*

Fletcher,[17] in the same year, disagreed. After reviewing inconsistencies and conflicting opinions among writers on the topic, he concluded, "In spite of the inconsistencies noted, most clinical and experimental evidence continues to suggest that the tongue-thrust pattern of oral activity is likely a meaningful cluster of behavioral signs and as such is worthy of continued scrutiny to determine more precisely its specific characteristics and possible place in the hierarchy of oral physiology."†

There is a wide range of incidences of tongue thrust reported by investigators. Tulley[69] found only 2.7% of a large group of British children to be tongue thrusting, and Bell and Hale[8] found an incidence of 80% among 5- and 6-year-olds. Nevertheless, there is general agreement among *most* researchers regarding the percentage of tongue thrusters and regarding, as well, incidence by age of subjects.

Fletcher and colleagues[18] examined 1600 schoolchildren ranging from 6 to 18 years of age, and found some 41% to be swallowing improperly, with a marked decrease in incidence among the older children. At 6 years of age, the incidence was 52.3%; at 8 years, 38.5%; at 16 years, 20%; and at 18 years, 21%.

Andersen[2] found a lower incidence, but the declining pattern still obtained (Table 9-1).

Werlich[74] found an incidence of 30.4% in a group of 640 children. Incidence by age was: 6.6 years, 37.3%; 11.5 years, 27.6%; and 17.4 years, 26.4%.

Hanson and Cohen[24] studied a group of 178 children for a period of four years. Again, a pattern of declining incidence, similar to those found by the Werlich and Fletcher studies, was found. Percentages found were: 4 years 9 months, 57.9%; 5 years 8 months, 43.8%; 6 years 7 months, 51.7%; and 8 years 2 months, 35.4%.

A comparison of the results of the Fletcher, Werlich, and Hanson and Cohen studies is shown in Fig. 9-1. We believe that such agreement among independent incidence findings, with respect both to incidence and to the declining pattern of incidence with age, is strong evidence of the actuality of the existence of tongue thrust.

The wording used by Fletcher offers a clue as to the persistence of so many controversies. "A meaningful cluster of behavioral signs" intimates that tongue thrust is a syndrome, rather

---

*From Weinberg, B.: Deglutition: a review of selected topics, ASHA Reports, No. 5, p. 124, 1970.

†From Fletcher, S. G.: Processes and maturation of mastication and deglutition, ASHA Reports, No. 5, p. 98, 1970.

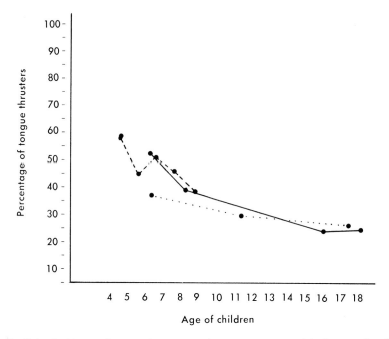

Fig. 9-1. Declining incidence of tongue thrust as age increases, as reported in three studies. Solid line denotes Fletcher and associates' 1961 study (1615 children); dotted line denotes Werlich's 1962 study (640 children); broken line denotes Hanson and Cohen's 1972 study (178 children).

Table 9-1. Incidence of tongue-thrust syndrome among 450 first-, sixth-, and twelfth-grade students*

| | Students with tongue-thrust syndrome | | Students without tongue-thrust syndrome | | |
Average age	*Number*	*Percent*	*Number*	*Percent*	*Total*
6 years 4 months	27	21.3	100	78.7	127
11 years 6 months	18	14.6	105	85.4	123
17 years 8 months	14	9.0	141	91.0	155
Total	59	14.6	346	85.4	405

*From Andersen, W. S.: The relationship of the tongue-thrust syndrome to maturation and other factors, Am. J. Orthod. **49:**264, 1963.

than a single behavioral occurrence. The high incidence reported by Bell and Hale[10] might also be attributed to their criteria for establishing the presence of tongue thrust. Their figures include subjects who demonstrate behaviors associated with tongue thrust. Traditionally orthodontists and clinicians have considered the tongue-thrust swallow to differ from the normal swallow in several ways. The normal swallower presumably forms a compact bolus and collects it in a depression in the dorsum of the tongue prior to swallowing, whereas the tongue thruster does not form such a neat bolus. The tongue thruster's chewing is considered to be abnormal. The molars are occluded in a normal swallow and unoccluded in a tongue-thrust pattern. The tongue tip is held against the front upper teeth or between the front upper and lower teeth in the tongue thruster, and is held behind the alveolar ridge in a normal swallow. In the normal swallow, the lips are immobile; the tongue thruster purses his lips and overcontracts the mentalis muscle. At the end of a swallow the tongue of a normal swallower is free of crumbs, whereas that of the tongue thruster contains scattered crumbs due to the inefficient swallow.

Two separate types of tongue-thrust patterns have been observed by some, including Moyers,[39] who described tongue thrust as being "simple" or "complex." In the former, the molars were occluded during swallows of a child with open bite. The latter was indicated when the molars were not occluded and there were marked circumoral contractions. A third pattern, which Moyers called a "retained infantile swallow," consisted of minimal occlusion (only one tooth in each quadrant) during swallowing. Chewing was difficult due to the poor occlusion and was performed largely by pressing the tongue against the palate. Extreme facial contortions were a part of this pattern.

CONCLUSION. There is general agreement among various researchers regarding (1) the incidence of tongue thrust among schoolchildren and (2) the decline in incidence as age increases. This concordance attests to the reality of the behavior. The extremely low or high incidence reported by a few investigators is probably due to varying criteria used in identifying the behavior. In Hanson's study, two definitions for tongue thrust were employed, one involving interdental placement of the tongue during swallow, and the other merely requiring contact between the tongue and anterior dentition. Results based on the latter definition included an incidence of 86.5% in children 4½ to 5 years of age, and 70.8% among 8-year-olds. At the other extreme, researchers have looked for a *syndrome* of behavioral patterns, not labeling a behavior as "tongue thrust" unless various elements of the syndrome were present. Research has found, as the following section discusses, that the only consistent aspect of tongue-thrust behavior is the thrusting of the tongue.

IS IT A NORMAL OR AN ABNORMAL BEHAVIOR?

In 1965 Hedges and co-workers[26] studied 22 children in grades six, seven, and eight, all of whom had normal dental occlusions. They concluded that, in the majority of cases, the tongue contacted the lingual surface of the maxillary incisors. According to these authors, what had been called tongue thrust was a normal pattern in children with good occlusions. They observed that children with excellent occlusions demonstrated two distinct swallowing patterns, one with teeth together and one with teeth apart. The major difference of tongue movement in these two patterns was that the tongue tip was placed more inferiorly on the maxillary incisors when the swallow occurred with the teeth apart. The implication is that tongue thrust might be a matter of degree only; it might be inferred that the lack of stability produced by the molars being unoccluded was compensated for by an increased pressure of the tongue against the teeth.

Ardran and Kemp[4] studied 250 young normal adults by observing their swallows cineradiographically. In their description of the swallows of these young adults, which they termed "normal," the tip of the tongue is said to thrust forward against the upper incisor teeth and the posterior surface of the gums. The teeth may be in apposition or slightly parted as the swallow begins.

Another traditional concept is that the tongue thruster typically rests his tongue against his front teeth, whereas the normal swallower positions the tongue more posteriorly. In 1968 Peat[45] studied 103 adult orthodontic patients to determine the habitual resting position of the tongue. It is presumed that a significant portion of these patients would be normal swallowers. He found two postural positions for the tongue: In 86.4% of his patients, the tongue tip was found to be resting against the incisors or the lips. In 61.3%, the tongue tip contacted both the upper and lower incisors. In only 13.6% was there no contact with the teeth by the tongue at rest. These studies seem to indicate that it is not abnormal for the tongue to contact the teeth either while resting or during swallowing.

Weinberg[72] reviewed the research on tongue thrust and development, and concluded that in embryonic life the developing tongue is relatively large compared to its surrounding skeleton. He noted that Scott[57] had observed this disproportionality in size between the tongue and the mandible in the fetus. At birth this condition persists, and the maxilla is in protrusive relationship to the mandible. Since the teeth have not erupted in newborn infants, the tongue frequently occupies the space between the alveolar processes, generally maintaining an oral seal with the lips during swallowing.

Moyers[38] has shown that swallow patterns change after the eruption of the deciduous teeth. The tongue may also fill gaps caused by missing incisors. During the stage of deciduous tooth eruption, the tonsils and adenoids may grow rapidly and reduce the size of the oropharyngeal port, thereby promoting tongue fronting postures at rest and during swallow. Weinberg concludes that tongue thrust in infancy is a normal behavior, but during mixed dentition, as the oral cavity becomes proportionately larger in relation to the tongue, the fronting of the tongue naturally diminishes. Tulley[68] contends that tongue-thrust behavior frequently corrects itself by the time the permanent teeth have erupted fully. Subtelny[61] agrees.

Fletcher[17] agrees that tongue thrust may be a normal pattern in infants and an abnormal one in older children and adults. He describes three conditions that might contribute to the retention of the infant type of swallow: (1) neurological incompetence, (2) insufficient anatomical change in the mouth or tongue, and (3) transitory phenomena, such as prolonged infection or missing dentition. He relates these three possible causal factors to associated sensory cues, and proposes that a disruption of these cues during critical developmental periods may well prevent a transition to a nonthrusting pattern.

The aforementioned incidence studies attest to the plausibility of this theory. All three studies found that the incidence declined fairly steadily until the end of the mixed dentition. The longitudinal study by Hanson and Cohen[24] followed a group of children through four mixed dentition years to investigate modifications in structure and function. The incidence, by age, of tongue

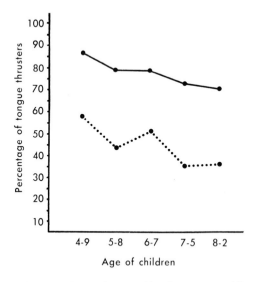

Fig. 9-2. Incidence of tongue thrust by age. Dotted line denotes tongue thrust, conservative definition (tongue protrudes between upper and lower teeth); solid line denotes tongue thrust, liberal definition (tongue contacts anterior teeth).

thrust found in the 178 children in this study is shown in Fig. 9-2. Because of differences of opinion regarding the definition of tongue thrust, two definitions were used in the evaluations: (1) a liberal one (the tongue contacts the lingual surface of the anterior teeth), and (2) a conservative definition (the tongue protrudes between the upper and lower teeth during swallows). The following percentages of tongue thrusters, according to both definitions, were found:

	Mean age				
	4-9	5-8	6-7	7-5	8-2
Conservative	57.9%	43.8%	51.7%	35.4%	35.0%
Liberal	86.5%	79.2%	79.2%	72.5%	70.8%

Of 103 tongue thrusters (conservative definition) at 4 years 9 months of age, 63 had become normal swallowers by the age of 8 years 2 months. When the more liberal definition was applied, 77 of the 154 children who had been diagnosed as tongue thrusters in the first year of the research were swallowing normally by the age of 8 years 2 months.

Some children who swallowed normally during the first year's examination became tongue thrusters during the mixed dentition period. According to the more strict definition of tongue thrust, 75 children were swallowing normally at 4 years 9 months of age. Twenty-five of these subjects were tongue thrusting at the age of 8 years 2 months. Of the 25, all but 5 began swallowing abnormally prior to the age of 6 years 7 months. Only 5, therefore, developed a tongue thrust during the mixed dentition years when the greatest number of teeth was missing. When the liberal definition was applied, 15 (54%) of 24 children who swallowed normally at 4 years 9 months were found to be tongue thrusting at the age of 8 years. This evidence suggests that fluctuations and inconsistencies in swallowing patterns are to be expected during the mixed dentition years, and that a stable pattern may be the exception, rather than the rule, at this developmental stage.

It is our contention that tongue thrust is an atypical behavior that consists of positioning the tongue against a significant portion of the lingual aspect of certain anterior or lateral teeth during rest, swallowing, and/or speech. This anteriorization of the tongue may or may not be accompanied by one or more of the behavioral patterns traditionally associated with the phenomenon. Long[33] investigated differences between the tongue-thrust and normal swallows and found a great deal of variability in the patterns. He concluded, however, that the tongue-thrust swallow appeared to be identical to the normal swallow except for the placement of the anterior portion of the tongue. Many tongue thrusters had no grimace during swallows, and many subjects who grimaced had no tongue thrust. Many tongue thrusters swallowed with their teeth together, whereas a few "normal" patients swallowed with their teeth apart. Our belief is that it is important in evaluating a child with tongue thrust to examine the total behavior and look for all the possible components. If a normal swallow can be developed by altering other aspects of the behavior, attention should be paid to them in therapy as well as to the posturing and movement of the anterior part of the tongue during swallowing. However, the inclusion of the presence or absence of molar occlusion, facial grimaces, or abnormal chewing habits, as a necessary part of the "syndrome" of tongue thrust, is not warranted.

CONCLUSION. There is strong evidence that tongue thrust is an abnormal behavior after the permanent incisors have erupted fully. In the embryo and infant, tongue thrust seems to be the normal pattern, both as a resting position and as a manner of swallowing. Behavior patterns associated with the fronting of the tongue may or may not be present in the tongue-thrusting child.

WHAT SHOULD IT BE CALLED?

We have been calling the behavior tongue thrust. This term seems to be winning general acceptance, but several other terms are still being used. We will list a few of them, along with our objections to each.

1. *Deviate swallow*. This was an interim term proposed some years ago that became submerged in the "deviate-deviant" controversy. Although we find deviate auditory canals and deviate nasal septums, we have been averse to deviate swallows.

2. *Reverse swallow*. This term conjures up unappealing pictures of food being forced forward in the mouth or even out of the mouth.

3. *Perverted swallow*. Many people object to being called perverts.

4. *Deviant deglutition*. This term has an alliterative ring to it, but it means very little to the layman and sounds a bit stilted.

5. *Visceral swallow*. This meaning of this term has never been clear to us, since all swallows ultimately lead to the viscera. Perhaps it refers to muscles not functioning under voluntary cortical control but behaving instead as do visceral muscles.

6. *Infantile swallow*. Whereas a tongue thrust is normal in infants, we object to this term for the same reason we do not like "baby talk." It tends to arouse negative feelings in the mind of the boy or girl accused of having one.

7. *Abnormal swallow*. The term is too general to be of much value.

Not that the term "tongue thrust" is without its drawbacks. Those who are unfamiliar with it often mispronounce it. When used in conjunction with another term, thumb sucking, which sometimes accompanies it, it becomes an effective tongue twister. It does, however, describe simply and effectively the behavioral problem confronting us, and we suspect that this term will outlive the other seven.

IS TONGUE THRUST RELATED TO DENTAL MALOCCLUSION?

A number of studies have found a strong relationship. In 1946 Rix[54] studied 93 children between the ages of 7 and 12 years. Sixty-one were found to be swallowing with the teeth together. Of this group, 36% had "deviant dentition." Twenty-seven swallowed with teeth apart. Eighty-one percent of this group had "deviant dentition." In the 1940s and 1950s the "teeth apart" swallows were equated with tongue thrust and the "teeth occluded" swallows with normal behavior.

In Werlich's[74] study, among those children with Class II, Division I malocclusions, 50.7% were thrusters. Among those with Class I malocclusions, children in the oldest group included only 18.2% who were tongue thrusting; in the youngest group, where the incidence was highest, only 32.6% were tongue thrusting. Among those children with open bite, 98.5% were tongue thrusters. Another significant relationship obtained between posterior crossbite and variant swallow. Of the youngest group, 68.2% were tongue thrusters, and 47.6% of the middle age group were thrusters.

Rogers[56] compared a group of tongue-thrust patients with a group of children from the public schools, some of whom had orthodontic problems and some of whom had normal occlusion. His results are reproduced in Table 9-2. The incidence of tongue thrust was high in both

Table 9-2. Tabulation of findings*

	Normal population sample	Ortho-dontic patients
Tongue thrust during deglutition	165 of 290 (56.9%)	312 of 497 (62.8%)
Deep overbite, with tongue thrust while swallowing	82 of 119 (68.9%)	156 of 277 (56.3%)
Patients showing grimace while swallowing, with no discernible tongue thrust	11 of 290 (3.7%)	46 of 497 (9.2%)
Patients showing a tongue thrust while swallowing, with no grimace	3 of 290 (1.0%)	8 of 497 (4.6%)
Class II, deep overbite, with abnormal swallowing	63 of 49 (79.7%)	98 of 156 (62.8%)
Open-bite, with abnormal swallowing	55 of 56 (98.2%)	78 of 84 (92.8%)
School pupils examined needing no orthodontic treatment	112 of 290 (38.6%)	No data
School pupils not needing orthodontic treatment and showing a normal swallow	92 of 112 (82.1%)	No data
Completely breast-fed children showing normal swallowing	2 of 4 (50.0%)	No data

*From Rogers, J. H.: Swallowing patterns of a normal population sample compared to those patients from an orthodontic practice, Am. J. Orthod. **47:**674, 1961.

groups (56.9% in the "normal" population group and 62.8% among his patients). It was particularly high among subjects with deep overbite (79.7% and 62.8% in the two respective groups). Again, subjects with open bites demonstrated a great tendency toward tongue thrust. From the normal population, 98.2%, as well as 92.8% of the orthodontic patients with open bite, demonstrated tongue thrust. Several other studies have found similarly high incidences between tongue thrust and malocclusions. That a significant relationship exists between tongue thrust and malocclusion seems to be quite well documented.

Moss in 1975[37] asserted that patients with normal occlusion show a typical pattern of muscle activity, and patients with malocclusions demonstrate muscle patterns differing from those of normal subjects. He stated, "Patients with Class II, Division I, Class II, Division 2, Class III and postural Class III malocclusions can be differentiated on the basis of their patterns of muscle activity" (p. 644).

DOES TONGUE THRUST CAUSE MALOCCLUSION?

First let us consider evidence to the contrary. Neff[40] studied 11 orthodontic patients, 6 of whom were abnormal swallowers. He found that the 6 tongue thrusters swallowed at a mean rate of 37.25 times an hour and the 5 nonthrusters at a rate of 61.4 times an hour. In his discussion he implied that whatever increase in pressure the tongue exerted against the lingual aspect of the teeth during swallows was probably offset by the decrease in frequency of swallowing in the tongue thruster. This sample, of course, is too small to draw conclusions concerning the general population.

Neff and Kydd[41] studied relationships between open bite and swallowing, and found that the thrusters with open bite withdrew their tongues earlier than did those without open bites. They concluded that the presence of tongue thrust between the dental arches indicates a more passive role of the tongue than has been reported in the literature.

Proffit,[49] who has done some of the most extensive and careful work on relationships between muscle pressures and tooth position calls attention to the stable position of the teeth most of the time in most people as evidence for some kind of equilibrium. Tooth movement that occurs when additional forces are exerted (as by orthodontic appliances, by poorly designed partial dentures, or by contacting scar tissue after surgery) is evidence that this equilibrium can be upset. He cites evidence, however, that transducer studies have consistently found maximum lingual pressures to outweigh labial pressures in subjects with normal occlusion.

Subtelny[62] studied 40 subjects to determine whether there were cause-and-effect relationships between malocclusion and tongue thrust. Group I consisted of subjects with normal occlusion; Group II, subjects with severe maxillary protrusions; Group III, subjects with severe maxillary retrusions; and Group IV, subjects with open bite. Some of his observations were as follows:

1. Some kind of anterior oral seal was found in all of the groups.

2. There was more molar occlusion among open bite subjects than among any others.

3. Only 2 of the 10 subjects in the normal occlusion group occluded molars during the major portion of deglutition.

4. In preparation for swallowing the tongue tip was positioned lingual to the lower incisors in all cases.

5. Once the dorsum of the tongue reached the posterior regions of the oral cavity, the swallowing process seemed similar and consistent in all subjects.

6. *Impression*. The tongue tip may be adapting to a specific anterior oral environment to achieve a seal during swallowing.

Subtelny confirmed our impression that it is not wise to study tongue thrust as a syndrome, since many of the characteristics that had been reported to differentiate between the behaviors of tongue thrusters and normal swallowers were found in both types of subjects. We found no evidence in a review of his research report, however, to substantiate his conclusion that functional movements of orofacial musculature structures adapt to the variables of the form of the oral environment.

Milne and Cleall[36] found evidence that tongue thrust can be a transitory phenomenon. They studied 10 males and 12 females with a mean age of 6 years 8 months. All subjects had a Class I (normal) occlusion and a normal swallow. Changes in tongue posture and function of structures were studied cinefluorographically. This was a longitudinal study, and the subjects were studied in three phases: in Phase I, the maxillary deciduous centrals were still present; in Phase II, no maxillary centrals were present, either deciduous or permanent; in Phase III, the permanent incisors were fully erupted. There was a tendency for a forward positioning of the tongue in Phase II, but the tendency was not statistically significant. The tongue tip was positioned forward in Phase II but posteriorly again in Phase III. This difference was significant at the .01 level. The same pattern obtained in speech: In general the tongue tip was positioned forward in Phase II and backward in Phase III (also significant at .01 level). The tightness of the lip seal also increased in Phase II during swallows. The occluding of the molars during swallowing was found in progressively more subjects throughout the phases of the research. In Phase I, 9 of 22 subjects occluded their molars; in Phase II, 13 of 22 occluded the molars; and in Phase III, 15 of the subjects occluded the molars during swallows. Results indicated that the increase in tongue thrusting when the maxillary

incisors were not present should be considered an adaptive measure to changes in the local environment.

Milne and Cleall[36] interpret these findings as implying that the prevalence of tongue thrust may be a normal but transient occurrence during this developmental period.

Those subjects who postured the tongue forward when the maxillary deciduous central incisors were lost, returned to their original pattern of swallowing with the eruption of the permanent incisors.

The Milne and Cleall study, of course, provides information only about those children whose occlusion was normal and whose swallowing patterns were normal before the deciduous teeth were lost. It does not shed light on the larger number of tongue thrusters found in the mixed dentition stages who, according to several incidence studies, were tongue thrusters prior to that period.

Gianelli and Goldman[21] pose a question repeated by concerned professionals the world over: After rearrangement of the teeth, what happens if the tongue-thrust habit is not eliminated? Will there be a relapse? When teeth are subjected to a tongue-thrusting force 500 to 1000 times a day—the frequency of swallowing—what will be the consequences on the attachment apparatus of mechanical retention?

We now review some opinions supporting the contention that tongue thrust causes malocclusion.

Reitan[52] affirms that in the presence of muscular balance, a well-established interdigitation aids greatly in maintaining corrected occlusion. In other cases a completely satisfactory intercuspal relationship between the arches will not prevent relapse from occurring if a strongly adverse muscular pressure exists. He maintains that muscle function must be regarded as a dominant factor.

Gianelli and Goldman[21] concur, blaming three behavior traits for the major portion of habit-related orthodontic deformities: (1) thumb sucking, (2) reverse swallow, and (3) abnormal perioral muscular habits, particularly involving the mentalis muscle.

Riedel[53] agrees, listing habits such as thumb sucking, lip biting, and tongue thrusting as causes of malocclusion. He specifically implicates tongue thrusting in the development of anterolateral open bites.

Penzer[46] states that there is sufficient clinical evidence to indicate that an abnormal swallowing pattern can adversely affect other physiological functions such as respiration, mastication, digestion, and phonation. It can also inhibit growth and development of the orofacial structures.

Begg and Kesling[9] list tongue pressure against the lingual surfaces of the anterior teeth as one of three reasons dental arches migrate anteriorly after having been moved posteriorly orthodontically.

Vogel and Deasy[70] attribute the stability of the dentition to the resistance of the supporting structures of the teeth and the magnitude, frequency, duration, and direction of forces placed upon them.

A similar comment regarding stability of dentition is offered by Dreyer,[16] who includes direct muscular forces from the lips, cheeks, and tongue among the main factors affecting resistance of teeth to movement.

Begg and Kesling[9] assert, "The only type of Class II malocclusion in which we have observed buccal teeth to return to Class II relations since using the light wire technique is the type which is associated with tongue thrusting during swallowing" (p. 648). They add that it is often necessary for tongue thrusters to wear permanent upper retention plates after orthodontic treatment, in order to prevent the upper anterior teeth from relapsing to former positions.

Posen[47] poses the question, "How does one explain the protrusive position of the incisor teeth in bimaxillary dento-alveolar protrusions?" (p. 303). He answers that evidence strongly points to a combination of weak perioral muscles and relatively normal tongue pressures. His conclusion regarding his own research is, "... there is strong evidence that the role of the tongue in determining the final position and angulation of incisor teeth is minimal *except in those patients where there is a perverted tongue position either during deglutition or at rest*" (italics ours) (p. 308).

Swinehart,[65] after studying 40 cases he had treated who had deficiencies in intercanine mandibular space, attributed the incomplete mandibular development to a lack of normal tongue pressures against the teeth. Swinehart constructed an appliance which encouraged a lower, more forward positioning of the tongue at rest within the mandibular arch. He concluded that the improved lingual function which resulted contributed greatly to the stability of the corrected mandibular form (p. 823). Sufficient

space was created in the mandibular arches of all 40 patients to allow for normal tooth alignment. He wrote, "Proper tongue function during the building of the dentition logically appears as a necessary natural force in production of the desired arch form" (p. 823).

Pressures

We have presented a number of opinions and studies opposing the concept that muscle pressures can cause malocclusion, and a few opinions supporting such a theory. We turn now to a discussion of the nature and strength of pressures acting on the dentition. The purpose of this section will be to try to answer the question: Are tongue and lip pressures of sufficient magnitude and duration to move teeth?

From the outset, our opinion is that there is no definitive answer to this question at the present time. We will give some authoritative opinions of clinicians and researchers and present reviews of pertinent research.

To determine possible relationships between tongue and lip pressures and malocclusion, we need answers to two basic questions:

1. How much pressure is required to move teeth?
2. How much pressure do the orofacial muscles exert against the dentition in normal swallowers and in tongue thrusters?

PRESSURES REQUIRED TO MOVE TEETH. Referring to pressures used by orthodontists, Gianelli and Goldman[21] state that most forces used to move teeth vary between 50 and 400 grams. "Lighter" forces are those which are generally less than 50 to 75 grams, and "heavy" forces usually represent 150-plus grams.

These same authors describe optimum forces as follows:

1. Tipping a small tooth, such as an incisor: 20 to 30 grams
2. Tipping a large tooth such as a canine: 50 to 75 grams
3. Controlled root movement of a small tooth: 50 grams
4. Controlled root movement of a large tooth: 120 to 150 grams
5. Bodily movement of a small tooth: 40 to 50 grams
6. Bodily movement of a large tooth: 150 grams
7. Extrusion: 25 to 30 grams
8. Intrusion: 15 to 50 grams

The amount of pressure required, then, varies

according to the size of the tooth and the nature and direction of the force being applied. Most of the patients we see have anterior teeth that have been tipped, rather than moved bodily, but of course in some patients the roots have also been moved. Since the incisors are the most frequently malpositioned teeth that we see in our patients, however, we should keep in mind the 20 to 30 grams of force required to accomplish their tipping.

Weinstein[73] describes research conducted by Attaway[6] and O'Meara[43] on minimum forces for moving teeth. These investigators added a 2 mm. gold onlay to either the buccal or lingual tooth surface in two separate groups of children 9 to 17 years of age. "The effect of the buccal modification was comparable to that produced by extending the cheek two millimeters by the device used to measure the stiffness or elastic quality of the cheek. . . . In effect then this protruding tooth would be subjected to an additional mean buccal force of approximately 1.68 gms."* Movement of the teeth was carefully measured with a dial indicator sensitive to 0.001 inch. In a "typical" response, the control tooth moved a total of only 0.009 inch in 52 days, whereas the premolar with the gold projection extending into the cheek moved 0.033 inch, almost 1 mm. in eight weeks, for an average rate of 0.044 inch each week.

Weinstein concludes that forces considerably below the level of those delivered by contemporary orthodontic appliances are capable of producing tooth movement.

Lear and associates[32] studied the effects of small forces of varying durations on the positions of teeth in five normal-occlusion male adults. Forces varied from 6.3 grams down to 0.5 grams, and durations were of 25 msec. to 100 msec. In four of the five subjects, "long" duration thrusts (100 msec.) of 0.9 to 1.6 grams were sufficient to displace teeth on 50% or more trials (p. 1479). As the duration of the thrust diminished, more force was required for the threshold for displacement to be reached. Nevertheless, even if relatively small forces (from 1.6 to 3.5 grams) were applied for the very short duration of 25 msec., premolars were measurably displaced. They concluded, "The displacement can be initiated by constraints similar in magnitude and direction to those that are re-

ceived by premolars from the tongue and cheeks when at rest" (p. 1481).

OROFACIAL MUSCLE PRESSURES IN TONGUE THRUSTERS AND NORMAL SWALLOWERS. Proffit and colleagues[51] studied 11 5- to 8-year-old children with malocclusion and matched them with an equal number of children with normal dentition. After conditioning the children for several days to the presence of an acrylic palatal appliance, the investigators placed the dummy plate with a similarly contoured device containing three strain-gauge pressure transducers into the arch. The transducers were placed just lingual to the maxillary central incisors and bilaterally opposite the second deciduous molars. A few involuntary saliva swallows were noted for each subject, but according to our understanding of the research report, the swallows studied by the investigators were principally command swallows of water, the subject taking a sip at a time and swallowing when the experimenter directed him to do so. Ten swallows were selected for measurement for each child. Research by Lear and Moorrees,[31] to be referred to later in this chapter, suggests that pressures involved in the swallow of liquids are much weaker than those involved in swallows of saliva or solids.

These researchers (Proffit and associates) obtained three measures for each swallow: peak pressure, pressure duration, and time-pressure integral. Peak lingual pressures ranged from 50 to 400 gm/cm² for these children. The mean peak pressure for the left transducer was 148.6 gm/cm² and for the right transducer, 137.6 gm/cm². Mean peak pressure for the center transducer was 85.9 gm/cm². For the same children, average time-pressure integrals were as follows: left, 98.6 gm/sec/cm²; right, 91.4 gm/sec/cm²; center, 48.5 gm/sec/cm². These data are typical of the child population. Pressure levels for each child were consistent from swallow to swallow. For most subjects anterior pressure was definitely less than lateral pressure.

Unfortunately, for our purposes, the mean pressures and time pressure integrals for the 6 children of the 22 who were described as tongue thrusters were not presented separately from those of the other 16 children. The means presented include data from tongue thrusters and normal swallowers. The authors do state that 4 of the tongue thrusters showed little or no lingual pressure against the anterior transducer, whereas the other 2 tongue thrusters had heavy anterior pressures—in fact, the heaviest pres-

---

*From Weinstein, A.: Minimal forces in tooth movement, Am. J. Orthod. **53:**891, 1967.

sures of any children in the group. Judging from the care taken in the research, however, and from other articles by these authors, we can accept the statement that these data are typical of the child population.

These investigators found lingual pressures in children to be quite comparable to those of young adults recorded in a similar manner. Comparative data for adults and children are presented in this article only in a figure, but the time-pressure integrals of the adults appear to us to be approximately 130 gm/sec/cm² for the right transducer; 175 gm/sec/cm² for the left transducer; and approximately 85 gm/sec/cm² for the center transducer. The adults also had greater lateral than anterior pressure.

Proffit,[49] in his review of research, concluded, regarding pressures during swallowing in children, that lip pressures are of longer duration than tongue pressures. There may be significant resting lip pressures. Typical peak pressures during swallowing were: in the maxillary incisor region, 75 ± 50 gm/cm² lingual, and 55 ± 20 gm/cm² labial; and in the maxillary molar region, 140 ± 50 gm/cm² lingual, and 30 ± 15 gm/cm² buccal.

Lear and Moorrees[31] studied 7 males, 18 to 32 years old, with normal occlusion to determine, among other things, whether teeth in normal occlusion are held in balance by opposing tongue and total cheek forces. Much of their data for the 7 subjects was presented in figure form but not in tables. Reference will be made to this research later in this chapter. They concluded that in these adult subjects, lingual forces always exceeded buccal pressures by factors varying from one and one-half to almost four when mandibular and maxillary data were combined.

Wilskie[75] investigated tongue and lip pressures during involuntary swallowing in 19 dental students. His results were as follows:

1. Mean maximum lip pressure, 22.52 gm/cm²
2. Mean maximum anterior tongue pressure, 40.77 gm/cm²
3. Mean lateral tongue pressure, 42.8 gm/cm², with anterior tongue pressure of comparable magnitude

Most subjects produced a number of pressure applications for each swallow.

Wilskie[75] found the mean maximum pressures exerted by the tip of the tongue to be 40.77 gm/cm². Toda,[66] studying tongue pressures on the anterior hard palate of 7 patients, reported a comparable mean of 51.71 gm/cm² for involuntary swallowing. Mendel[35] reported a mean tongue pressure for this area of 216 gm/cm². The tongue thrusters in this sample may account for his relatively high value. Winders[76] reported a mean anterior tongue pressure of 82.67 gm/cm².

Toda[66] studied the swallowing pressures of 15 adults, 22 to 44 years of age, of whom 11 had "good to excellent" occlusions and four had "fair" occlusions. Again, lateral and anterior pressure transducers were placed in the upper arch. Data were obtained while the subjects (1) swallowed water a sip at a time, (2) swallowed saliva, and (3) swallowed a cup of water continuously. For 7 of the subjects, a supplemental recording of spontaneous swallows was conducted while the subjects read magazines without the investigator in the room. Results reported are found in Table 9-3. It can be seen that the pressures for saliva swallows done on command exceeded those of the liquid swallows done either one at a time or continuously. It is interesting to note that the spontaneous swallows of saliva involved the least pressure of the four types of swallows. Since these data are from 7 subjects only, conclusions must be drawn carefully. The subjects were divided into subgroups according to the shape of the palate. It was observed that subjects with peaked palates tended to exert the most pressure in the anterior and lateral palatal areas, whereas the subjects with flat palates tended to exert the most pressure in the test area at the height of the palatal vault.

Toda[66] interpreted the greater pressures during the swallow of saliva as signifying that the bolus of the greater viscosity (in this case saliva) requires greater lingual pressures against the hard palate to accomplish the swallow.

Kydd and associates[28] compared tongue and lip pressures of 6 females, 14 to 20 years of age, who had undergone orthodontic treatment and had relapsed to an anterior open bite with those of 5 female control subjects who had not relapsed to an open bite. The experimental subjects were all tongue thrusters and the control subjects were nonthrusters. They found the mean tongue pressure of the relapsed group to be 285 gm/cm², and the mean tongue pressures of the controls, 123 gm/cm². They also compared the lip pressures of the subjects and found the mean upper lip pressure of the open bite subjects to be 45 gm/cm², and that of the controls, 70 gm/cm². In other words, the tongue thrusters who had relapsed to an open bite exerted more

Table 9-3. Summary of the mean swallowing pressures (pressures in units gm/cm²)*

Swallowing exercises	Anterior area of palate	Lateral area of palate	Central area of palate	Average of all exercises
Sipping water	85	84	52	74
Swallowing saliva	112	112	69	97
Drinking water	62	61	35	53
Spontaneous swallowing	52	52	20	41
Average of all test areas	86	85	52	—
Average of all measurements	—	—	—	74

*From Toda, J. M.: A study of tongue pressures exerted on the hard palate during swallowing, Thesis, University of Washington, 1961, p. 22.

than twice as much tongue pressure anteriorly, and only two thirds as much lip pressure as those whose orthodontic correction remained stable. This study also reported significant differences between the thrusters and nonthrusters in the duration of labial and lingual pressures. Mean duration of lip pressures of the thrusters was longer than that of the nonthrusters by 380 msec. Mean tongue pressure duration was longer by 300 msec.

Akamine,[1] in his master's thesis, asked whether this difference of approximately one third of a second could be of any biological or clinical significance. He explained that if differences were to be projected over a greater period of time, their significance might be more clearly assessed. Akamine therefore turned to studies of swallowing frequency and determined that an average of the different studies reported at that time was about 2500 swallows a day. According to more recent studies, this figure may be a little high. He multiplied the 1/3 second difference between the two groups by 2500 swallows and found that the tongue thrusters would be applying tongue and lip pressures against the teeth about 14 minutes longer than the nonthrusters in a 24-hour period. He then compared this 14-minute difference with his calculation of the mean of 67 minutes of the duration of all swallows for the normal population in a 24-hour period. He determined that the 14 minutes represented a 21% deviation and concluded that such a difference might be expected to be clinically significant. The value of this research is limited due to the small number of subjects, but it does bring up some interesting possibilities. The relatively heavy tongue pressures and relatively light lip pressures of the subjects who relapsed to an open bite, combined with the greater duration of the swallows of this same group, would seem to us to lend some credence to the hypothesis that tongue pressures may contribute to malocclusion.

Another study comparing pressures of patients with open bites to those of subjects with normal occlusion was done by Wallen.[71] A limitation of Wallen's research is that it was concerned with peak pressures only, which do not necessarily have any relationship to actual pressures applied by the tongue to the teeth at rest and during function. Wallen found that subjects with normal occlusion applied about twice as much tongue pressure in a vertical plane as in a horizontal plane, whereas subjects with open bite tended to apply a relatively constant pressure in all planes during swallowing.

Our own review of research concerning the frequency of swallowing in the total population includes six studies. The mean of the six is 1287 a day, or approximately one swallow per minute. We would like to ask you to examine in some depth the 1969 Lear and Moorrees[31] study with us. Lingual and buccal pressures were determined for all types of customary oral activity in seven 18- to 32-year-old university students, all of whom had normal occlusion and complete natural dentition. Daily force totals were estimated for each subject by relating the mean buccal and mean lingual force during all types of oral muscle activities to the average daily duration of those activities. Pressures studied included those of speech, mastication, deglutition, and rest. Measurements were taken in the laboratory and in the subjects' homes.

The contribution of each oral function to the total force experienced by a given region of the palatal arch was assessed by relating the mean force produced by the activity to its daily duration, producing "time average" data. Instead of reporting data on all 7 subjects in table form, the researchers presented them in bar graphs, making it somewhat difficult for us to come up with figures for the total group. They reported finding similar pressure totals for the left and right sides of all subjects save one, in whom muscle forces during speech were not symmetrical. This general symmetry of pressures prompted them to combine left and right lingual totals and left and right buccal totals, from which they calculated a ratio expressing the degree of balance between tongue and cheek forces. A close counterbalance between these forces occurred in the maxillary arches of 2 of the 7 subjects (Nos. 4 and 7). In the other subjects, lingual forces exceeded those from the cheek. For the group as a whole, lingual forces differed significantly from buccal forces, but between subjects, variations were such that the extent of maxillary-mandibular differences could not be defined.

The authors do not state why they chose to present data on subject 4 in table form, but since they did, we will present their table as a basis for discussion.

These data are evidently representative of 2 of the 7 subjects, at least to some degree, and we would not draw any generalizations on a larger population based on this one subject. Nevertheless, he is an adult male with normal dentition and occlusion.

Looking at Table 9-4, you will notice that the total gram-minutes measured by the left lingual and left buccal maxillary transducers are very similar, with the buccal pressure slightly exceeding that of the lingual. A comparison of right lingual and right buccal pressures yields a similar result. If we add the left lingual and right lingual pressures together, we get a total of 3165 gram-minutes. A combined total of left buccal and right buccal pressures is 3365 gram-minutes. When the composite muscular pressures acting on the dentition were taken into account and the time factor was computed, this subject with normal occlusion was found to be exerting more buccal than lingual pressure against his anterior teeth.

Data from the mandibular transducers are different from those in the maxillary arch. Mandibular lingual pressures greatly exceed mandibular buccal pressures. Therefore, when we combine maxillary and mandibular data and formulate a statement regarding the degree of, or lack of, balance between buccal and lingual pressures, we obtain a completely different picture than if we were to study the maxillary data alone. Since mandibular lingual pressures are much more rarely of concern to us as we work with tongue thrust, and since the architecture of the mandible so strongly favors a more stable poitioning of the dentition, it seems to us to be misleading to combine the data. Reference to the greater stability of the mandibular teeth is made by Furstman and associates[20] who explain that the rigid confinement of the mandibular periodontal ligament between the alveolar walls may account for the greater compression seen in the mandibular periodontal ligament: "The maxilla allows faster movement of teeth and also seems to display a degree of resiliency that permits a lesser degree of compression of the periodontal ligament" (p. 607). Certainly more studies of this type need to be done, and we

Table 9-4. Projected 24-hour force totals in premolar regions of subject 4 (in gram-minutes)*

Area	Speech	Chewing and swallowing food	Liquid swallows	Saliva swallows	Rest totals	Total	Lingual to buccal ratio
MAXILLARY							0.9
Left lingual	138	582	19	38	851	1628	
Right lingual	114	679	15	54	675	1537	
Left buccal	210	252	22	30	1191	1705	
Right buccal	234	262	16	23	1125	1660	
MANDIBULAR							3.8
Left lingual	210	1397	34	59	947	2647	
Right lingual	204	1436	33	66	1104	2843	
Left buccal	42	184	10	7	377	620	
Right buccal	60	165	12	13	565	815	

*From Lear, C. S. C., and Moorrees, C. F. A.: Bucco-lingual muscle force and dental arch form, Am. J. Orthod. **56:**379, 1969.

should see the raw data in order to more accurately assess the significance of this research.

From the Lear and Moorrees data on subject 4, we have calculated the percentage of daily time spent by this subject in each of the activities studied by these researchers. Totals are shown in Table 9-5.

These results have several implications for our emphasis in therapy. Although the resting pressures of the tongue for this subject were only from 0.3 to 0.8 gm/cm², the 1283 minutes spent with the tongue at rest have to be given serious consideration. In one day this subject would spend over 21 hours with the tongue in a resting position. If light forces applied over a long period of time are effective in moving teeth, and if the 14 hours minimum required by most orthodontists of their patients who are wearing headgears are adequate to produce movement, we certainly ought to spend considerable time in therapy training the patient to rest his tongue somewhere other than against the anterior teeth. In addition, of course, the resting position of the tongue will, according to our clinical experience, strongly affect the position and movement of the tongue during speech and during swallowing.

Liquid swallows, on the other hand, occupy only 0.3% of this subject's daily time. This subject's lingual pressure for swallowing liquids was from 3.7 to 4.7 grams, pressure much greater than the resting pressures, but it would be delivered very intermittently during the day. This individual spoke, they calculated, for 60 minutes each day, with lingual pressures of 1.9 to 2.3 grams each time the tongue contacted the alveolus. Lear and Moorrees combined masticatory pressures with food-swallowing pressures, which we wish they had not done, because we

would like to have seen the differences between the pressures in these two related activities. In this subject, though, the mean pressures for these activities was 6.0 to 7.0 grams, or approximately three times the amount of pressure exerted during speech. The subject spent 97 minutes of his day chewing or swallowing food, or in other words about one and one-half times the time spent in talking. If we had to weigh one activity more than the other in therapy, we would thus pay more attention to chewing and swallowing food than to correcting speech.

Our belief is, however, that all these activities are interrelated and that the resting posture of the tongue is the key determinant of the direction and force of the tongue in the other activities in which it is involved. What we need now, of course, is replication of this research, comparing children who tongue-thrust and who have malocclusions with children who have normal occlusion and normal swallowing patterns.

Research was done by McGlone and co-workers[34] to study the amount of lingual pressures against the dentition during the production of the linguoalveolar consonants /n/, /t/, /d/, /l/, and /s/. We will present here the data for the center transducer only, and not for the lateral transducer (Table 9-6). These pressures are, of course, at variance with those reported by Lear and Moorrees on subject 4, but they refer only to linguoalveolar pressures during speech. Of interest, though, is the relatively small amount of pressure involved in the production of the /s/ sound, which is probably the sound we pay most attention to when we correct the speech of a tongue thruster. We might better pay attention to those linguoalveolar sounds which are produced dentally without so much accompanying audi-

Table 9-5. Projected time spent in activities involving lingual pressures

Activity	Minutes	Percent of daily time
Speech	60	4.1
Food chewing and swallowing	97	6.7
Liquid swallows	4	0.3
Saliva swallows	12	0.8
Rest	1283	88.1
Total	1456	100.0

Table 9-6. Mean peak lingual pressures for five consonants (in gm/cm²)*

Consonant	Initial position	Final position
/n/	37.3	18.6
/t/	31.0	15.3
/d/	21.8	14.3
/l/	20.6	7.3
/s/	4.6	6.3

*Modified from McGlone, R. E., Proffit, W. R., and Christiansen, R. L.: Lingual pressures associated with alveolar consonants, J. Speech Hear. Res. **10:** 606, 1967.

tory distortion. The subjects for the research of McGlone and associates were 25 young adult males.

Proffit,[48] in his master's thesis, apparently based on the same subjects, compared anterior tongue pressures for speech with those for swallowing. He noted that during speech, pressure by the tip of the tongue was almost never greater than 25 gm/cm², and if average speech pressure had been computed, it would have been less than 10 gm/cm² for all subjects. In contrast, the average anterior lingual swallowing pressure for all patients was 40 gm/cm², and two patients had an average force of more than 100 gm/cm² against the anterior teeth during swallowing.

Although the Lear and Moorrees article does not specify whether their ''grams'' were grams per square centimeter, we assume they were. We do not know why pressures reported by these two studies differ so greatly. (Many researchers in the 1950s reported pressures in terms of pounds per square inch. Typically, lingual pressures during swallows were listed as being from 3 to 5 pounds. We have heard some clinicians cite these figures to their patients, and then compare them to the ounce or two of pressure exerted by orthodontic appliances against the teeth, unknowingly comparing measures involving pounds per square inch with grams per square centimeter. The comparison is effective in motivating patients but is not a valid one.)

In the April, 1965, issue of the *American Journal of Orthodontics* appeared an abstract of research done by Smernoff.[59] He studied 6 subjects with anterior open bites and tongue-thrust swallowing patterns. Pressures of the tongue against transducers placed directly above the mandibular incisors varied from 71.6 to 180.0 gm/cm², with a mean of 138 grams. Even these pressures represent only a maximum of approximately 6 ounces of pressure.

TRANSDUCERS AS ARTIFACTS. In 1972, Proffit[49] delivered a paper to the Australian Orthodontic Congress in Melbourne, in which he reviewed current research regarding muscle pressures and tooth positions. Proffit discussed attempts to develop transducers that would keep to a minimum the effect of artifacts on the behavior being studied. He warned that any time instrumentation is introduced into the mouth there is a possibility that the physiological activity being studied will be altered by the presence of the recording instrument. This is particularly true in the mouth when lingual pressures are to be re-

corded. Lingual patterns are likely to change to avoid the pressure transducers.

In an effort to overcome this problem, Proffit and his associates had their subjects wear a dummy lingual appliance for about 48 hours before the actual recording appliance was placed in the mouth. It is difficult, of course, to determine the extent to which the subjects accommodated to this artifact in the two-day period.

Similarly, Lear and colleagues[30] offered an opinion that the effect on lingual function of the transducer in place is unknown. They note that no transducer yet described is identical in contour to the labial, buccal, or lingual surface of the tooth. In their own research, Lear and colleagues found that changing the mass of the transducer resulted in increased lingual force. No one disagrees that measuring lingual and labial pressures accurately is a difficult task.

INTERMITTENT VERSUS CONSTANT FORCES. Brader's[11] paper on dental arch form and intraoral forces propounded some interesting hypotheses. Brader proposed a deemphasis in our thinking on functional forces and a greater emphasis on anatomical contours. He suggested that the tongue and the circumoral tissues exert forces on teeth position along a ''compound curve.'' The arch form into which the teeth are embedded can be best described as a closed elliptical curve. He presents the formula $PR = C$, when P = pressure, R = radius of the arch, and C = mathematical constant; the tighter the curve, the greater the pressure per unit area. The mathematical constant C can represent the resting potential of the tongue. This tongue energy constant C equals the constant of the cheek-lip forces (T). C equals T because the forces are in opposite directions, although they vary in value. When C equals T, a dental equilibrium results. As the radius of the curvature of the arch increases, the intraoral pressures progressively decrease. Since this radius is smallest at the anterior portion of the mandibular arch, the pressures here are the greatest and the teeth are the least stable. Then Brader draws another conclusion that we believe research has not been designed to test, which is that teeth are not moved by strong frequent pressures but by light, continuous pressures. He questions the role of tongue thrust, abnormal speech, or swallowing in contributing to the dental occlusion and postulates that perhaps lingual resting postures may be effective forces against the teeth.

Proffit[49] agrees with Brader regarding the importance of these resting postures. Light pressures are effective if they are maintained continuously or nearly so. Heavy pressures of short duration, according to Proffit, have little effect. Resting pressures are similar to orthodontic forces, whereas pressures from occlusion, speech, mastication, and swallowing are probably too short-acting to move teeth, he claims.

Gianelli and Goldman[21] also express their doubts concerning the effectiveness of brief, nonrepetitive forces to produce orthodontic tooth movement.

Many writers deny that lingual pressures such as those that occur during swallowing and speech have any effect on occlusion. They attest to the greater efficacy of light, continuous forces over stronger, intermittent forces in moving teeth. Reitan is often cited as an authority for this contention. In his chapter "Biomechanical Principles and Reactions," Reitan[52] has a section on continuous versus intermittent tooth movement. He explains:

Some practitioners would probably apply the word "intermittent" to a tooth movement of short duration as obtained with fixed appliances. However, this term may seem confusing to some readers, as the word "intermittent" was chosen many years ago to describe the use of removable appliances. It must be admitted that the words "intermittent" and "interrupted" are more or less synonymous. In the following, however, they will be used for different types of tooth movement. "Interrupted" designates a movement of short duration elicited by fixed appliances; "intermittent" is mainly employed for removable appliances.*

This type of "intermittent" pressure differs greatly from the "intermittent" lingual pressures occurring during speech and swallowing. The appliance is typically worn for several hours at a time, and then is removed for another several hours. Research on swallowing has found that saliva swallows typically occur with a frequency of once every 2 minutes to twice every minute. To draw an analogy between these two types of forces is, we believe, a mistake.

In our opinion, the conclusions of Brader and Proffit represent a dichotomization that is unwarranted at this time. Much more research is needed, particularly dealing with the total effect of combined lingual and labial resting postures

and the stronger, intermittent swallowing and chewing pressures.

Unfortunately, we have not been able to find research that measured resting pressures of the tongue against the teeth in children with tongue thrust. We have reviewed studies that have determined pressures of the tongue against the anterior palate to range from 50 to 400 gm/cm². We have cited Proffit's conclusion from his review of research to the effect that typical peak pressures during swallowing in children in the maxillary incisor region are from 25 to 125 gm/cm², lingual, and from 35 to 75 gm/cm², labial. We found that a group of patients with relapsed open bites and tongue thrust manifested much stronger lingual pressures than labial pressures when compared to a group of nonthrusters whose orthodontic correction was permanent. We found in one study that a constant pressure of only 1.68 grams was required to move teeth.

In the Lear-Moorrees[31] research, subject 4 rested the tongue against the anterior palate a total of 1283 minutes each day, with a mean of 0.67 gm/cm² of pressure. This subject was an adult with normal occlusion, with slightly more labial pressure than lingual pressure. When resting pressures were combined with all swallowing and speech pressures, the total for a 24-hour period for this subject was 1628 gram-minutes, or a mean of 1.13 gm/cm². While we await results of comprehensive pressure research on children with tongue thrust and malocclusion, we who have seen these children whose tongues are constantly against the anterior teeth, both during rest and during swallows, and especially the patients with mouth breathing or incompetent lips, or both, cannot refrain from forming some strong clinical impressions about tongue thrust and malocclusion. We offer the hypothesis that lingual pressures exerted by tongue thrusters are not strong, intermittent pressures but rather are light, variable, but very persistent, continuous ones.

Most writers refer to the pressures employed by orthodontists as light, continuous pressures. We have seen that these pressures vary from 15 to 400 gm/cm², but as Gianelli and Goldman[21] described them, lighter forces are usually from 50 to 75 gm/cm². It seems to us very possible that the only real difference between pressures exerted by the tongue of the child with a tongue-thrust swallow and those applied by the orthodontist may be in variability of force, and it may even be possible that the variable pressures are

---

*From Reitan, K.: Biomechanical principles and reactions. In Graber, T. M., editor: Current orthodontic concepts and techniques, vol. 1, Philadelphia, 1969, W. B. Saunders Co., p. 87.

more effective in moving teeth than are constant pressures. So far as we know, this theory has not been tested. At least we feel safe in saying that data available at the present time do not warrant our rejecting lingual pressures in the tongue thruster as possible contributors to malocclusion.

CAUSE-AND-EFFECT STUDIES. Studies of cause-and-effect relationships between tongue thrust and malocclusion are difficult to find in the literature. We know of only two, one of which was a study, conducted by Harvold and associates,[25] involving rhesus monkeys. An acrylic block was placed in the posterior palate of five monkeys. A matching group of monkeys was untreated. All the experimental animals developed open bites during the nine months of the experiment, along with changes in the width of the dental arch.

A related experiment in 1965 was reported by Italian researchers[42] who performed total glossectomies on ten rats. After comparing the pre-surgical and postsurgical measurements of the upper and lower jaws, the investigators found that three months after surgery the diameters of both jaws in the rats of the experimental group were smaller than those of the ten control rats.

Summary

A great percentage of the conclusions attributing changes in occlusion to function of the tongue and circumoral musculature are based on clinical judgments or on research revealing associations between form and function, with no tight control over variables. The same is true for conclusions regarding form or structure governing lingual rest position and function in swallowing and speech. The research reported by Harvold and associates on monkeys and the Italian study on rats are two exceptions. Certainly more research is needed before conclusions regarding cause-and-effect relationships between tongue thrust and malocclusion are justified.

ARE TONGUE THRUST AND MALOCCLUSION BOTH RELATED TO OTHER PHYSIOLOGICAL BEHAVIOR PATTERNS?

Hanson and Cohen[24] selected 225 children at random from birth announcement columns in a local newspaper during the year of 1962. Ages of the subjects at their first visit ranged from 4½ to 5 years. The children were evaluated at that time and at four subsequent sessions spaced approximately ten months apart. At the end of the research 178 subjects remained, including 90 girls and 88 boys. The children were studied by direct observation, cineradiographically, by orthodontists, by speech pathologists, from x-ray films, and from dental models. A complete patient history was obtained on each subject. Information included the type and duration of feeding in infancy, presence of allergies, oral habits (including speech defects), thumb or tongue sucking, lip licking or biting, mouth breathing, and dental development. The children were given perioral examinations, with particular attention to the rugae, the size and shape of the maxillary arch, the activity of the masseter and temporalis muscles, the presence of facial grimaces, and the resting position of the tongue. The status of tonsils and adenoids was also evaluated directly by the examining speech pathologist. A brief articulation test was administered, using picture stimuli to observe the subject's spontaneous production of linguo-alveolar speech sounds present in single words.

Various types of malocclusions were measured by means of the dental models. Palatal measurements were made, including palatal vault height at three anteroposterior positions, width at two points, and length from the deepest gingival margins of the central anterior teeth to a midline point along the distal transverse plane of the second premolars.

Swallows of barium-treated fruit juice and cookies were studied cinefluorographically. Throughout the study, tongue thrust was evaluated according to two definitions: a liberal definition (the tongue contacts the lingual surface of the anterior teeth) and a conservative definition (the tongue protrudes between the upper and lower teeth). Intercorrelations were computed among all the variables for each year of the study, yielding a mean of 108 significant correlations during each of the last four years of the research. Since all these correlations cannot be included here, we have selected those which we consider especially meaningful (diagnostically or etiologically) to present.

Significant correlations

The retention of a thrusting pattern through this period of mixed dentition was found to be positively correlated ($p > .05$) with the following:

1. More breast feeding
2. A narrower palate at the premolar and cuspid levels
3. Greater palatal length

4. Greater palatal height at cuspid and premolar levels
5. Less buccal crossbite
6. Greater maxillary arch circumference
7. More mouth breathing
8. Less overbite
9. More upper respiratory system allergies
10. More overjet
11. More dentalized speech sounds
12. More mentalis muscle activity during swallowing

Greater palatal height was found to be associated with the following:

1. More digit sucking
2. More upper respiratory allergies
3. More breast feeding
4. A narrower palate at the cuspid and premolar levels
5. More dentalization of the /s/ sound
6. More overjet

A narrower palate was correlated with the following:

1. More digit sucking
2. More breast feeding
3. Greater palatal height
4. More overjet

Another interesting finding pertained to the extent of movement of the hyoid bone during swallows. There was a positive correlation (.01) between this criterion and the anterior and posterior available vertical space at the maxillary level as shown on the x-ray films. This relationship is a logical one and demonstrates the involvement of the extrinsic lingual musculature in raising the tongue to the roof of the mouth when the arch is high.

Absent correlations

Significant relationships between types of anterior malocclusions and x-ray measures were few. There were none at all between open bite, anterior crossbite, or underbite in x-ray measures. In the case of overjet, significant correlations resulted only between the overjet and film measurements that included the influence of the overjet. On the other hand, amount of overjet was positively correlated with digit sucking, palatal height (as measured on dental models), and arch circumference.

Discussion

Digit sucking alone was positively correlated with four measures of palatal arch dimensions, including two measurements of height, width, and circumference, three types of malocclu-

sions, and five behavioral activities. This evidence raises doubts concerning the advisability of closing doors to any research that would explore cause-and-effect relationships in either direction. A series of significant correlations was obtained between the measurement of dental models and the measurements from lateral head films. In addition to the expected agreement on similar measures, interesting correlations were found. Palatal width, as measured on the models, correlated positively with four anteroposterior measurements (two at the mandibular level and two at the maxillary). Perhaps this means only that some palates were larger in both dimensions. On the other hand, opponents of the "function determines form" theory could argue that whatever influence the tongue might have in moving or tipping anterior segments labially, it would not be sufficient to appreciably alter relationships between palatal width and depth in this group of subjects. Supporters of this theory would in turn argue that a broad, anterior thrust could widen the arch as well as lengthen it. The meaning of the correlations involving arch circumference and palatal height and depth is also dependent on one's point of view, and any conclusions involving the role of function would be highly speculative.

Whereas the literature would lead one toward expecting to find a number of correlations between the types of malocclusion and the persistence of tongue thrust, only scattered significant correlations were found, and they were too inconsistent to be considered meaningful. These results contradict those of several researchers, and although we can offer no explanation, differences in definition of terms by various investigators may have been a factor.

Summary

We have discussed at length results from our own research. A number of factors were found to coexist to a significant degree, including oral habits, malocclusion, and anatomical and physiological measurements. In the absence of research designed to explore cause-and-effect relationships among these variables, we can only conclude that the interrelationships among them are significant enough to warrant keeping an open mind about possible contributions of each factor to the others.

SHOULD TONGUE THRUST BE TREATED?

In 1970 Shelton[58] argued against treatment of tongue thrust until more information concerning it is known. He stated that anyone treating tongue thrust is either engaging in experimentation or is working outside the realm of science.

We admit to having engaged in clinical experimentation for the past couple of decades. Progress in the field of oral myofunctional disorders has followed a pattern found in the history of other areas of the study of human behavior. Interest is aroused in a pattern of behavior, the clinician attempts to modify the behavior, and he experiments with several approaches, recording the results for each, and modifying and shaping them, or one of them, until a successful manner of treatment evolves. Research follows. We are not certain that this method is the most desirable one for obtaining knowledge, but we defer to Tolstoy: "There are times when from the imagination, rather than from reality, our wisdom should come."

WILL TONGUE THRUST CORRECT ITSELF WITH MATURATION?

According to most incidence studies, the incidence decreases progressively through the mixed dentition stage, at which point it levels off and remains fairly stable until adulthood. Research concerning modifications of swallowing patterns in adults is lacking. Prognostic information given in the above section is important in attempting to determine whether a tongue-thrust pattern in a given child is likely to be self-correcting. Of course, it is always dangerous to project information from research onto a specific child with a specific problem. Certainly, a number of children who are tongue thrusting prior to and during mixed dentition will correct themselves. The longer the clinician waits to begin treatment, the more certain he is that his treatment is definitely needed. On the other hand, he allows undesirable habits to gain in strength and risks a possible aggravation of malocclusion.

One of the questions Subtelny[62] sought to answer through research was whether muscle function adapts to altered environment. Subtelny's 40 subjects were placed in four groups of 10 each. Group I subjects had normal occlusion; Group II, severe maxillary protrusions; Group III, severe maxillary retrusions; and Group IV, open bite. Although his results describe some similarities and differences in swallows among the four groups, we found no evidence to support his conclusion that functional movements of orofacial muscular structures adapt to the variables of the form of the oral environment. Our belief is that the number of orthodontists who, from clinical experience, conclude that the function of the tongue does adapt as the physiology is altered, either as the result of normal developmental processes or in response to orthodontic treatment, is sufficient to prompt our continued research on the question. On the other hand, our experience with orthodontists in the Tucson and Salt Lake City areas, many of whom experienced years of frustration due to relapses that occurred after the physiology had been altered favorably, leads us to believe that in the majority of cases, tongue thrust in children beyond the age of 8 years is not usually self-corrective, even after orthodontic treatment is complete.

HOW CAN TONGUE THRUST BE TREATED?

There are three general approaches to the treatment of tongue thrust.

Modification of oral environment

The oral environment can be modified surgically or orthodontically. Anterior splaying of the teeth can be eliminated through surgery, and the size of the tongue can be reduced by the excision of a portion of it. The removal of grossly enlarged and inflamed tonsils provides more space for functioning of the posterior portion of the tongue. Lingual and/or labial frena can be cut to allow for greater mobility of the structures. Teeth are often removed to promote more space toward which the remaining teeth can migrate.

The orthodontist can expand the maxillary arch, creating more space for the tongue. The ability of the orthodontist to reposition teeth to produce normal arch configurations and normal occlusions seems to us to be almost limitless. In our experience, it is often preferable to precede therapy for tongue thrust by needed surgical or orthodontic procedures. For example, when the permanent maxillary central incisors are tipped labially and are separated by a significant diastema, and when there is no crowding of them by the maxillary laterals, it is helpful if the overjet can be reduced by the orthodontist prior to the beginning of myotherapy. The movement of these two teeth can be accomplished in a relatively short time (even in a matter of days in many cases), and the resultant facilitation of a natural, lips-closed, resting posture is extremely beneficial to our posture training. When mouth breathing has been present, the patient finds it much easier to condition the lips to remain closed and the tongue to rest behind the upper alveolar ridge, than he did before the teeth were moved. We have also been told by our colleagues of two children whose speech patterns and general tongue function were improved markedly after a partial glossectomy.

Mechanical restraints or reminders

Before the development of effective oral myotherapy, most orthodontists relied on "hayrakes," or "cribs," to teach the child to keep the tongue back away from the teeth (Fig. 9-3). Some orthodontists in certain parts of the United States persist in using these devices. In the areas served by our private practices, the orthodontists are almost unanimous in their rejection of this method of treatment, having experienced repeated failures throughout years of its application. Our objection to mechanical appliances is due not only to our extremely negative feelings about causing a child unnecessary pain but to our concern over the question of the permanence of the habit alteration. In most cases, tongue thrust

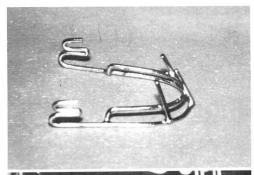

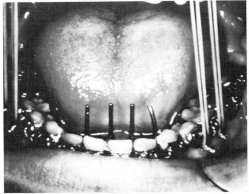

Fig. 9-3. Anti-tongue-thrust rake, **A;** in position in lower arch, **B.**

returns after the appliance is removed (Fig. 9-4). Nevertheless, we again must admit that it works for some orthodontists with some children. There are some instances when, either because of a lack of motivation on the part of the child, mental retardation, or some other extenuating circumstance, the cooperation essential for successful tongue-thrust therapy cannot be secured. In those cases we have very infrequently had to resort to the use of a crib.

Graber[23] describes the use of such an appliance for the correction of digit sucking:

After a two to three day adjustment period, most children are hardly aware of the appliance. The appliance is worn for 16 to 20 weeks in most cases. A period of three months of total absence of the finger habit is good insurance against a relapse. In most instances the habit disappears after the first week of the appliance's wear. After the three months the spurs are cut off first; three weeks later if there is no evidence of a recurrence the posterior loop extension is removed. Three weeks later the remaining palatal bar and crowns are removed.*

This seems to us to be a reasonable procedure to follow in the correction of tongue thrust as well, if such appliances are to be used. Graber, referring to the elimination of tongue thrust, notes that, depending on the severity of the open bite problem, a tongue-thrust appliance must be worn four to nine months. The best age for its use is between 5 and 10 years.

Another device, called the anti–tongue-thrust

*From Graber, T. M.: Orthodontics: principles and practice, ed. 3, Philadelphia, 1972, W. B. Saunders Co., p. 686.

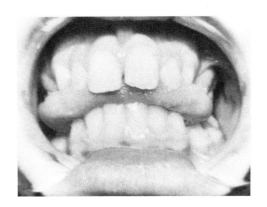

Fig. 9-4. Patient wore a hay rake 2½ years, changing thrust somewhat from anterior to bilateral pattern but correcting nothing.

device, was advertised in the *American Journal of Orthodontics* in 1965. It consisted of a small battery embedded in a plastic retainer, with two electrodes exposed where the retainer meets the upper incisors. When the tongue touches the electrodes it receives a mild shock. The originators claim that the tongue is retrained by simple Pavlovian conditioning reflex. They recommend that it be employed with children above 4 years of age and only during sleeping hours.

Myotherapy

The effectiveness of myotherapy in eliminating tongue thrust is discussed in a subsequent section. In our discussions with orthodontists from throughout the United States, we have found none who have tried mechanical restraints and myotherapy extensively and who have preferred the former. We are certain that there are some, somewhere, because there is no rule without exceptions. Certainly, myotherapy, to be effective, requires a well-trained and effective clinician. Many orthodontists have had experience with clinicians with inadequate training or capabilities and have returned to the use of cribs. Many orthodontists practice in areas where no myotherapy is available and have become effective in the use of mechanical devices. The big obstacle to any type of treatment is carry-over into the daily, distracting life of the patient. The establishment of correct postural and motor patterns at a subconscious level, we believe, is much more easily achieved by myotherapy than by any other method.

WHO SHOULD TREAT TONGUE THRUST?

1. *A dentally oriented specialist?* Of course, if the treatment is going to consist of first providing an adequate oral environment in which the tongue can function, the orthodontist or oral surgeon carries out the treatment. Many orthodontists have their assistants or dental hygienists provide oral myotherapy for their patients. These people are usually well acquainted with the structure, and with proper training can learn the function and how to modify it.

2. *A speech-oriented specialist?* The speech pathologist is well acquainted with the function involved and usually is familiar with the anatomy, although his knowledge of the developmental aspects of the maxilla, mandible, and dentition, are usually somewhat limited. His formal training should be supplemented by training in these areas.

3. *A specially trained oral myotherapist?* In November, 1972, a group of people representing the dental profession, physical therapy, and speech pathology met in San Francisco and formed the International Association of Oral Myology. The purpose of this organization is to upgrade the preparation and quality of oral myotherapists. Since the trend these days seems to be toward specialization, we see some value in a special curriculum and training format that will give the specialist adequate knowledge and experience to equip him to handle all types of abnormal oral habits better than any specialist trained in an adjunct area.

We believe the therapy can be administered successfully by any clinician who (1) knows the anatomy and physiology involved; (2) understands normal speech development, as well as developmental aspects of the teeth and surrounding structures; (3) understands normal and abnormal human behavior; (4) has had training and experience in motivating children and adults; and (5) has received adequate supervised training and experience in the field of oral myotherapy.

WHEN SHOULD THERAPY BEGIN?

Prevention is always preferable to correction. Ideally, we would be able to spot the 3- or 4-year-old child who was going to be a confirmed tongue thruster and take steps to prevent the development, or the persistence, of the abnormal patterns. About half of the preschool children who are thrusting will modify their habits without help, though some others will, according to our best knowledge, persist in tongue thrusting, but without any apparent harm to their dentition. Others at this age are swallowing abnormally and may yet develop a normal pattern before the permanent anterior dentition is complete. Few would quarrel with the precept that it is better to retrain some children whose tongue thrust would have been self-corrective than to have missed some who persisted in thrusting.

There are pros and cons to initiating therapy at each of several developmental levels.

Between 3 and 5 years of age
Pros
1. Early detection and remediation of tongue thrust may help prevent malocclusion or its aggravation.
2. Theoretically, the habit has less strength at this age and should be more responsive to therapy.

Cons

1. Motivation necessary to consistently carry out practice assignments is difficult to achieve in a very young child.
2. Some of the children will be treated unnecessarily.

During the mixed dentition years (6 to 8 years of age)

Pros

1. The diastemata and missing teeth provide a front-row view of the offending tongue during training and practice sessions. It is easy for the child to tell when he is doing an exercise improperly.
2. The boundaries for the tongue's movements are irregular and constantly changing. This encourages "scanning" behavior, which is a necessary part of relearning.
3. Children in this age group are particularly impressionable. For the right clinician, who provides the right incentives, they will do everything they are asked to do, enthusiastically.

.. This is a transitional period. Some clinicians argue that it is easier to teach a child whose oral environment is stable because of the greater consistency of sensory feedback.

2. Some tongue thrusting begins during this period of development; according to some authorities, this is due to a tendency of the tongue to want to fill gaps between the teeth. Therapy has to compete with this tendency.

After the mixed dentition years (9 to 17 years of age)

Pros

1. Although this group will present both extremes of levels of motivation, the greater number are anxious about their physical attractiveness.
2. These young people have enough foresight to strive for long-range goals, such as permanently good dental health.
3. Success in therapy can be a prerequisite for the initiation of orthodontics, and the "reward" of beginning to get the dental work done often comes to the patient immediately after therapy.

Cons

1. We have managed to fill these young people's lives with activities—homework, athletics, music lessons, paper routes, etc. They are so busy doing so many things that it is hard for them to keep their minds on such relatively uninteresting activities as lip and tongue postures and manner of swallowing.
2. They are often experiencing inner ground swells of strivings for independence and may resent the regimen of practicing.

Adulthood (18 years of age and over)

Pros

1. Almost without exception, motivation is excellent.

2. The behavioral base line is stable. Wherever the tongue rests, whatever the manner of swallowing or the nature of the oral structures, the behavior is consistent.

Cons

1. Many adult patients are very skeptical about their ability to change a habit so deeply ingrained as a tongue-thrust pattern. Their lack of confidence sometimes hinders progress in therapy.
2. Structures are relatively rigid. Palatal expansion to make more room for the resting and functioning tongue is rarely possible. The teeth do not move in response to tongue retraining, as they often do in younger subjects.

We generally have better success with patients 8 years of age and older. When a younger child is referred to us, we consider the following factors in making a determination regarding therapy:

Determining factors

1. Type of malocclusion. In ascending order of need for immediate therapy:
   a. Class I, with overjet
   b. Class II, with overjet
   c. Deep overbite
   d. Marked open bite (anterior or lateral)
2. Degree of malocclusion. If we decide against initiating therapy immediately, we take careful measurements of diastemata, overjet, open bite, or overbite, and remeasure several months later.
3. Scope of the problem. A child who habitually holds the mouth open, rests the tongue between the upper and lower teeth, speaks with a severe lisp, and consistently swallows saliva, liquid, and food with a severe tongue thrust, would be a candidate for immediate therapy. A patient who demonstrates only one or two of these behaviors would be considered a possible transitional thruster and would be asked to return in six months or so for a reevaluation.
4. Maturity of the child.
5. Attitude and degree of cooperativeness demonstrated by the parents.
6. Information supplied by the referring dentist. In cases where his records show a progressive malocclusion, we would give strong consideration to immediate treatment.
7. Structural considerations. At times it is preferable to defer therapy until other

specialists have created a more favorable environment for myotherapy. For example:

a. Nasal air blockage. Chronic mouth breathing is a serious deterrent to success in therapy and can often be successfully treated with medication or surgery.

b. An extremely narrow palatal arch. Expansion of the arch provides for a more natural resting place for the tongue, thus encouraging the habituation of a normal swallow.

c. Maxillary teeth in extreme lingual position.

d. Correctable lingual abnormalities, such as ankyloglossia or true macroglossia.

We are encouraged by the reports we receive from colleagues who are experiencing success with very young patients. We feel no reluctance to work with adults of any age. Few of them fail to habituate normal patterns.

IS TREATMENT FOR TONGUE THRUST SUCCESSFUL?

Is it possible to retrain such a deeply ingrained function? The skeptical opinion of Hoffman[27] is shared by many. They contend that swallowing is almost entirely reflexive and that successful retraining of a reflex is not likely.

Subtelny and Sakuda[63] took cineradiographic records of 8 patients with tongue thrust before therapy, after six months of therapy, and then two months after treatment. They found that the tongue usually returned to its original pattern of function. In this case, treatment consisted of the insertion of a palatal crib. Their conclusion was that the retraining of tongue function is very difficult.

In another study by Subtelny,[62] 5 subjects with "abnormal swallows," not all of whom exhibited tongue thrust, were placed in an intensive habit-therapy program in an effort to alter their swallowing patterns. Lessons were given twice a week, with each period lasting 30 minutes. Eight of the lessons were repeated in order that the program would be thorough and in order to prolong the program over a three-month period so that the subjects could again be exposed to radiation with safety. After three months of therapy, cineradiographs were made, and before-and-after-therapy records were completely analyzed. The before-and-after-therapy dental models revealed no significant changes. Two of the subjects indicated a slight increase in overjet, whereas two others indicated a comparable decrease in overjet. It was found that the subjects who exhibited tongue protrusion prior to therapy continued to protrude their tongues during swallowing after therapy. In other words, therapy failed to change swallowing patterns appreciably. Subtelny concluded that form did not seem to be appreciably altered by habit therapy. (It follows, of course, that if therapy was not successful in changing the swallowing patterns, no change in occlusion would be expected to occur.)

Before and after studies showing change

On the positive side of the issue, we will now examine some research that demonstrates that therapy for tongue thrust is effective. Most peo-

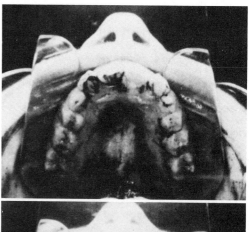

A

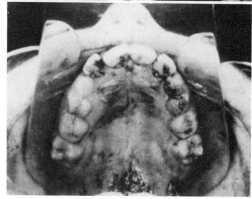

B

Fig. 9-5. A, Control subject 22, first palatogram. Judged as tongue thrust. **B,** Control subject 22, second palatogram. Judged as tongue thrust. (From Case, J. L.: Deglutition changes as a function of therapy as revealed by palatographic analysis, Thesis, University of Utah, 1968.)

ple who have worked with children with oral myofunctional disorders would agree that it is possible and even quite easy to change their swallowing patterns on a conscious level. One study designed to test this hypothesis was done by Case.[12] Case did a palatographical analysis on the effectiveness of tongue-thrust therapy. He saw 20 children with tongue thrust and 20 matched controls, also with tongue thrust. The experimental group received seven weeks of therapy for the correction of tongue thrust, and the control group received no treatment of any kind. Case sprayed the children's palates with a charcoal and chocolate mixture and had the subjects swallow saliva. Before and after swallow photographs were taken, before the seven weeks of training and after it was completed. Experienced judges made judgments of tongue thrust from the palatographs, which were presented in random order. The judges were able to differeniate the corrected swallowing patterns from the thrusting patterns consistently and reliably. The swallowing patterns of the experimental group did change significantly during the course of therapy.

In Figs. 9-5 and 9-6 are shown before-and-after photographs of a control subject and an experimental subject in Case's study. The gingival area and dentition are wiped relatively clean by the action of the tongue in both photographs of the control subject (Fig. 9-5) and in the before-therapy photograph of the experimental subject (Fig. 9-6, A). In Fig. 9-5, B, the palatal area is seen to have been cleaned of the charcoal mixture by the tongue during the swallow, whereas the gingival area and teeth retain the charcoal after the swallow.

Barrett and von Dedenroth[8] reported on the effectiveness of hypnotherapy in dealing with therapy failures. Subjects were 25 patients, 12 to 20 years of age, all of whom had failed to achieve normal swallowing patterns as a result of therapy. Twenty-one of the subjects had received orthodontic treatment and had experienced relapses. The other 4 were untreated orthodontically prior to hypnotherapy.

The subjects were in trances for 50 to 90 minutes in one to four sessions. Barrett reported that one to three years posttreatment, all patients had maintained normal swallowing habits, and no undesirable side effects were noted.

Stansell[60] studied three groups of 18 subjects each, 9½ to 14 years of age, all of whom exhibited a tongue-thrust swallow, sigmatism, and overjet. Group I received deglutition training only; Group II received only sigmatism training; and Group III received no training of any kind. Before-and-after-treatment measurements were taken from dental impressions and lateral head x-ray films. In addition, measurements were repeated three months after treatment. Stansell found that speech training alone significantly decreased overjet and that tongue-thrust therapy without speech therapy prevented an increase in overjet. Several of the control group subjects showed an increase in overjet during the treatment time. She warns that due to the growth factor, conclusions based on the results of before and after tests of any particular growing child are unreliable.

At the 1970 convention of the American Speech and Hearing Association, Overstake[44]

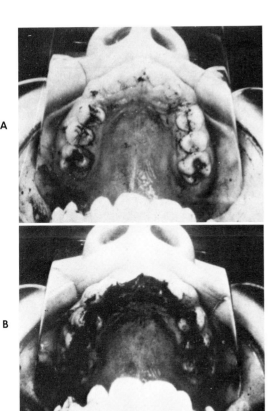

Fig. 9-6. A, Experimental subject 22, before therapy. Judged as tongue thrust. **B,** Experimental subject 22, after therapy. Judged normal. (From Case, J. L.: Deglutition changes as a function of therapy as revealed by palatographic analysis, Thesis, University of Utah, 1968.)

reported some significant research he had recently completed. He advanced two major questions in his investigation: (1) Are there reliable signs that will indicate which occurs more frequently in a given child: normal or deviant swallowing? (2) are deviant tongue-thrust swallowing, orthodontic problems of an open bite and/or overjet variety, and interdental /s/ speech defects so interrelated that swallow therapy procedures will by themselves correct deviant swallowing, cause dental open bites and/or over jets to become more normal, and correct interdental /s/ speech defects? In an effort to answer the first question, Overstake studied three groups of children 7 to 12 years of age. Group I consisted of 12 children with normal swallows; Group II, 12 tongue-thrusting children, and Group III, six former tongue thrusters who had received therapy. Overstake studied these children electromyographically. When he compared Groups I and II, he found that the tongue thrusters used significantly more masseter, suprahyoid, infrahyoid, and orbicularis oris muscle activity than did the normal swallowers. He also found certain time phase differences between the normal swallowers and the tongue thrusters. When he compared the muscle patterns of the posttreatment group with those of the other two groups, he found their patterns to compare favorably with those of the normal swallowers, with respect to both muscle energy output and temporal patterns.

A second part of this research sought to determine whether therapy for tongue thrust alone might move teeth and correct lisps. This part of the research involved 48 children, 28 of whom received swallowing therapy only and 20 of whom received speech therapy and swallowing therapy. Results of the research showed that subjects in both subgroups changed their swallowing pattern significantly in the direction of a normal pattern. In addition, after nine months of swallowing therapy only, 24 of the 28 children were using normal /s/ patterns in unguarded conversational speech. Also, in the total group of 48 children, 39 (81%) were judged by orthodontists to have manifested positive changes toward more normal dental configurations after receiving swallowing therapy. Overstake's research did not include the tight controls that Stansell had suggested were necessary. We would rather he had had the orthodontists or other qualified persons measure changes in occlusion rather than make judgments concerning them from color transparencies.

Barber and Bonus[7] tested the effectiveness of therapy in strengthening circumoral muscles of tongue-thrusting children. Subjects included 32 tongue thrusters and nine nonthrusters. Twenty of the tongue thrusters exercised their lips by the traditional method of pulling on a button placed in the labial vestibule. This they did twice a day for periods of three to six months. Initially the tongue-thrusting children exhibited weaker lips than did the control group children. Their mean "resistance score" before therapy was 16.1 oz. Children in the control group scored a mean of 27.8 oz. on the same task.

After six months of exercise the lip strength of one of the subgroups receiving therapy increased from 17.1 oz. to 119.1 oz. Children in the other subgroup improved from 16.0 to 67.2 oz. Post-treatment testing was done eighteen months after exercises were ceased, and the children were found to be retaining a mean increase of 81.6 oz. of muscle resistance over their pre-exercise strength. This represented an increase of 451.7% (p. 983).

Essentially no change in dental relationships was observed as a result of the the increase in muscle strength. The study did serve to demonstrate very conclusively, nevertheless, that circumoral muscles can be strengthened through therapy. As we state repeatedly, our aim in therapy has never been to correct malocclusions.

Long-term results

Studies cited to this point have been concerned with results after treatment or within a period of a few months after treatment. We now refer you to three studies carried out up to five years after the completion of therapy.

In 1962, Robson,[55] a Tucson orthodontist, completed a survey of Barrett's therapy program and presented the results in thesis form.

A date several years previous was arbitrarily selected. Beginning with that date, every patient who had presented himself for therapy at Barrett's office was listed until one thousand consecutive cases were compiled. Of these, 673 were located and agreed to participate in the research.

Seventeen separate items were assessed for each subject, nine of which were simply tabulated from the patient's therapy record; they included such items as associated habits, time since therapy (divided into six-month periods), age of patient, number of sessions required, how well appointments were met, cooperation during therapy as noted at the time, whether or not the patient had returned for checkups, and the therapist's evaluation of results at the conclusion of therapy. The correlation of these data with the final results of the study led to some major changes in therapy.

Primarily, the study was intended to ascertain the number of patients who continued to swallow correctly on a permanent basis and on a subconscious level. No child was found who could not swallow correctly if instructed to do so. The test employed was proposed by Dr. Joseph Fitzpatrick, speech pathologist in Denver. This test is now routinely used as a follow-up procedure some months after therapy, and consists of intermittently squirting water into the patient's mouth with a syringe or water pistol while the patient counts rapidly *in reverse*, usually from 99 toward zero. To validate the fact that this method did, in truth, reveal deviant swallowing and to sharpen the shooting eye, 200 students comprising entire fourth, sixth, and eighth grades in a district from which there had been no patient and which had no speech correction program, were thus evaluated and then given careful manual examination. In only six cases was there discrepancy between the tests.

The examiners sat side by side, one armed with a water pistol and the other with a box of tissues, while the patient sat facing them and a recorder sat behind them. A minimum of seven swallows was elicited, with opportuniity for "clearing" swallows along the way; when an examiner reached a decision, he extended one, two, or three fingers behind his back, which were noted by the recorder but which did not influence the other examiner. The categories were as follows:

1. Normal swallow. Teeth closed and no indication of lingual pressure even at extraction sites or in areas where deciduous molars had been shed and permanent teeth had not yet erupted. (This is a rather stringent expectation.)

2. Satisfactory swallow. Basically, the same as above except that some physical factor, usually malocclusion itself, prevented perfect performance, and thus the possibility of future trouble or relapse was present. Groups I and II were combined in calculating the number of successfully treated cases.

3. Anything short of the above performance was considered a therapy failure.

Space was provided in the data-gathering sheets for the recorder to note the original individual judgments of the examiners, with additional space in case of disagreement. The latter was required sixty-three times, or in 9.5% of the subjects. A softly spoken "no" from the recorder revealed this circumstance, and the patient received another volley of shots. In only 1% of the cases was there still an unresolved difference, and in each case it was settled by manual examination and discussion of the examiner's basis for judgment; however, these 7 cases were eliminated from further analysis and were not included in the totals.

History of a sucking habit was found in 368 of the 666 subjects, or approximately 55%; of these, 79.5% were successful in therapy, or slightly more than the general average. As might be expected, success dropped almost uniformly in 8% increments as additional sessions were required beyond the plan of therapy, that is, as patients were required to repeat sessions that had not been adequately mastered.

One facet of specifically dental interest was revealed. Since all these patients had been referred for therapy by dentists, the great majority by orthodontists, it is safe to assume that someone, parent or dentist, considered orthodontic treatment to be indicated. A number had already received orthodontic attention during or prior to therapy; nevertheless, in 99 patients, exactly 15%, it was thought that the malocclusion had improved, without orthodontic intervention, to the point that orthodontic treatment, in Robson's[55] opinion, was no longer essential.

Let us hasten to add that swallowing therapy is no substitute for orthodontics, and no such inference should ever be drawn. Our goal is not to straighten teeth but to correct deviations in deglutition. A spontaneously correct malocclusion is a welcome side effect but should not be expected in a given case; there were 567 cases who remained outside this group.

The relationship of success in therapy to various factors was analyzed. The results are shown in Tables 9-7 to 9-12.

One monumental result of this survey was the 146 patients in the failure group who sought free retreatment! Such an offer had been extended at the beginning of the study since it was felt that it would be an invaluable learning experience for the therapist; analysis of this group of failures served to provide considerable insight. The majority did return for at least one individual evaluation session, after which therapy was offered gratis so long as cooperation was truly outstanding. It was found that a poor attitude by the patient during the original therapy program was the basis for much of the relapse. This at-

Table 9-7. Permanency of the acquired pattern

Time since therapy	Number of cases	Number successful	Percent
Under 6 months	98	79	80.6
7 to 12 months	106	81	76.4
13 to 18 months	153	121	79.1
19 to 24 months	168	128	76.2
25 to 30 months	95	74	77.9
31 months or more	46	37	80.4
Total	666	520	78.1

Table 9-9. Therapy results relative to consecutive appointments

Appointment record	Number of cases	Number successful	Percent
Kept all appointments	338	292	86.2
Failed 1 or 2	211	166	78.6
Failed 3 or more	97	62	62.8
Did not finish therapy	20	0	00.0
Total	666	520	

Table 9-8. Success in therapy relative to age

Age at start of therapy	Number of cases	Number successful	Percent
Under 7 years	28	19	68.0
7 through 9 years	266	193	72.6
10 through 12 years	262	212	80.9
13 through 15 years	82	74	90.2
16 through 18 years	21	17	80.9
19 through 30 years	7	5	71.4
Total	666	520	78.1

Table 9-10. Results relative to cooperation as judged by the therapist during therapy

Average notation on therapy record	Number of cases	Number successful	Percent
Poor	11	3	27.3
Fair	42	26	61.9
Good (average)	118	85	72.0
Very good	234	186	79.5
Excellent	261	220	84.3
Total	666	520	

titude persisted in some patients, who were dismissed forthwith. The others were retreated, paying only for wasted sessions. No additional survey is planned to discover how successful they were.

Another master's thesis project investigating the efficacy of Barrett's therapy was carried out in 1970 by Toronto.[67] Toronto located 50 subjects, 14 to 20 years of age, all of whom had completed tongue-thrust therapy with Barrett at least five years prior to Toronto's research. He tested their swallowing of liquids, solids, and saliva and administered a squirt test similar to that described by Barrett. Following a conservative definition of tongue thrust—that is, the tongue had to be placed interdentally during swallow—only two of the children were found to be tongue thrusting (96% success rate). Following a more liberal definition—that is, the tongue contacted the lingual surface of any of the anterior teeth during swallow—there was a total of 14 thrusters (success rate 72%). An examination of the records of these patients revealed that there was movement of the teeth toward normal occlusion without orthodontic treatment in 19 of the sub-

jects. Seven of the 50 were able to avoid orthodontic treatment and now had occlusion that was essentially normal.

A similar study was done by Christofferson[13] on 25 of Hanson's patients. The investigator also chose patients who had completed tongue-thrust therapy at least five years previously. Their ages ranged from 12 to 25 years. Following the conservative definition, there were 2 tongue thrusters among the 25, when voluntary swallows were assessed. When the squirt test was applied, 2 more were shown to have a tongue-thrust pattern (success rate of 84%). Seven of the subjects had not required orthodontic treatment. Of the 7 subjects who had completed all orthodontic treatment and were no longer wearing a retainer, one had experienced some orthodontic relapse.

Conclusion

Several posttreatment studies have reported at least a 75% retention rate for manner of swallowing and at least an 86% retention rate for corrected occlusion. Two studies report on modifications in occlusion after therapy, both indicating movement of the teeth in a desired

Table 9-11. Relationship of speech defects

Speech status	Number of cases	Number successful	Percent
Normal speech	446	375	84.1
Defective speech	220	145	66.0
Concurrent speech therapy in school	56	38	68.0
Spontaneous correction of speech defect after therapy for swallow	72 (of 220 or 32.7%)	64	88.9

Table 9-12. Therapy results relative to type of swallow*

Swallow pattern	Number of cases	Number successful	Percent
1. Incisal thrust	146	125	85.6
2. Full thrust	348	266	76.4
3. Mandibular thrust	10	6	60.0
4. Bimaxillary thrust	31	27	87.1
5. Open bite	59	42	71.2
6. Closed bite	37	28	75.9
7. Unilateral thrust	9	7	77.8
8. Bilateral thrust	26	19	73.0

*See Chapter 11 for classification of types.

direction. Most speech pathologists working with the problem of tongue thrust report that the modification of the swallowing pattern and the establishment of a proper habitual rest position of the tongue greatly facilitates the correction of defective sibilant sounds in their patients. Other than Robson,[55] only one study (Overstake's[44]) reports spontaneous correction of defective sibilant sounds after therapy. More research is needed.

According to our best knowledge, in those cities, states, and areas where therapy for tongue thrust has been available for ten years or longer, nearly all the orthodontists require that their patients who are swallowing abnormally or who have other related habits receive therapy prior to or during orthodontic treatment. During the two decades it has endured in the United States, oral myotherapy has gained relatively rapid and widespread acceptance. This, we believe, is a positive indication of its worth.

REFERENCES

1. Akamine, J. S.: Tongue thrust in open bite cases: a time study of tongue and lip pressures against the anterior teeth during swallowing, Thesis, University of Washington, 1962.
2. Andersen, W. S.: The relationship of the tongue-thrust syndrome to maturation and other factors, Am. J. Orthod. **49:**264, 1963.
3. Andrews, R. G.: Tongue thrusting, J. South. Calif. Dent. Assoc. **28:**47, Feb., 1960.
4. Ardran, G. M., and Kemp, F. H.: A radiographic study of movements of the tongue in swallowing, Dent. Pract. **5:**8, April, 1955.
5. Ardran, G. M., Kemp, F. H., and Lind, J.: A cineradiographic study of bottle feeding, Br. J. Radiol. **31:**11, 1958.
6. Attaway, H. E.: A study of the buccal, lingual movement of first bicuspids under the influence of unbalanced muscular forces, Thesis, University of Nebraska, 1961.
7. Barber, T. K., and Bonus, H. W.: Dental relationships in tongue-thrusting children as affected by circumoral myofunctional exercise, J. Am. Dent. Assoc. **90:**979-988, 1975.
8. Barrett, R. H., and von Dedenroth, T. E. A.: Problems of deglutition, Am. J. Clin. Hypno. **9:**161, 1967.
9. Begg, P. R., and Kesling, P. C.: Orthodontic theory and technique, ed. 3, Philadelphia, 1977, W. B. Saunders Co.
10. Bell, D., and Hale, A.: Observations of tongue thrust in preschool children, J. Speech Hear. Disord. **28:**195, 1963.
11. Brader, A. C.: Dental arch form related with intraoral forces: PR = C, Am. J. Orthod. **61:**541, 1972.
12. Case, J. L.: Deglutition changes as a function of therapy as revealed by palatographic analysis, Thesis, University of Utah, 1968.
13. Christofferson, S.: The permanency of deglutition changes, Thesis, University of Utah, 1970.
14. Crowder, H. M.: Hypnosis in the control of tongue-thrust swallowing habit patterns, Am. J. Clin. Hypno. **8:**10, 1965.
15. Dawson, W. J.: A study of the effects of tongue depression and resultant mandibular postural change on the growth and development of the orofacial complex of rhesus monkeys, Thesis, University of California, San Francisco, 1968.
16. Dreyer, C. J.: The stability of the dentition and the integrity of its supporting structures, Am. J. Orthod. **58**(5): 433-447, 1970.
17. Fletcher, S. G.: Processes and maturation of mastication and deglutition, ASHA Reports, No. 5, p. 92, 1970.
18. Fletcher, S. G., Casteel, R. L., and Bradley, D. P.: Tongue-thrust swallow, speech articulation, and age, J. Speech Hear. Disord. **26:**219, 1961.
19. Fry, D. L.: Physiologic recording by modern in-

struments with particular reference to pressure recording, Physiol. Rev. **40:**753, 1969.

20. Furstman, L., Bernick, S., and Aldrich, D.: Differential response incident to tooth movement, Am. J. Orthod. **59:**600-607, 1971.

21. Gianelli, A. A., and Goldman, H. M.: Biological basis of orthodontics, Philadelphia, 1971, Lea & Febiger.

22. Gould, M. S. E., and Picton, D. C. A.: A study of pressures exerted by the lips and cheeks of the subjects with normal occlusion, Arch. Oral Biol. **13.**527, 1968.

23. Graber, T. M.: Orthodontics: Principles and practice, Philadelphia, 1961, W. B. Saunders Co.

24. Hanson, M.L., and Cohen, M. S.: Effects of form and function on swallowing and the developing dentition, Am. J. Orthod. **64:**63, 1973.

25. Harvold, E. P., Vargerik, K., and Chierici, G.: Primate experiment on oral sensation and dental malocclusion, Am. J. Orthod. **63:**494, 1973.

26. Hedges, R. B., McLean, D. C., and Thompson, F. A.: A cinefluorographic study of tongue patterns in function, Angle Orthod. **35:**253, 1965.

27. Hoffman, J. A., and Hoffman, R. L.: Tongue thrust and deglutition: some anatomical, physiological and neurological considerations, J. Speech Hear. Disord. **30:**105, 1965.

28. Kydd, W. L., Akamine, J. S., Mendel, R. A., and Kraus, B. S.: Tongue and lip forces exerted during deglutition in subjects with and without anterior open bite, J. Dent. Res. **43:**858, 1963.

29. Kydd, W. L., and Toda, J. M.: Tongue pressures exerted on the hard palate during swallowing, J. Am. Dent. Assoc. **65:**321, 1962.

30. Lear, C. S. C., Catz, J., Grossman, R. C., et al.: Measurment of lateral muscle forces on the dental arches, Arch. Oral Biol. **10:**669, 1965.

31. Lear, C. S. C., and Moorrees, C. F. A.: Buccolingual muscle force and dental arch form, Am. J. Orthod. **56:**379, 1969.

32. Lear, C. S. S., Jackay, J. S., and Lowe, A. A.: Threshold levels for displacement of human teeth in response to laterally directed forces, J. Dent. Res. **5:**1478-1482, 1972.

33. Long, J. M.: A cinefluorographic study of anterior tongue thrust, Am. J. Orthod. **49:**865, 1963.

34. McGlone, R. E., Proffit, W. R., and Christiansen, R. L.: Lingual pressures associated with alveolar consonants, J. Speech Hear. Res. **10:**606, 1967.

35. Mendel, R. A.: Tongue and lip forces exerted on the maxillary central incisors during swallowing, Thesis, University of Washington, 1962.

36. Milne, I. M., and Cleall, J. F.: Cinefluorographic study of functional adaptation of the oropharyngeal structures, Angle Orthod. **40:**267, 1970.

37. Moss, J. P.: Function—fact or fiction? Am. J. Orthod. **67:**625-646, 1975.

38. Moyers, R. E.: The role of musculature in orthodontic diagnosis and treatment planning. In Kraus,

B., and Reedel, R., editors: Vistas in orthodontics, Philadelphia, 1962, Lea & Febiger.

39. Moyers, R. E.: The infantile swallow, Trans. Eur. Orthod. Soc. **40:**180, 1964.

40. Neff, C. W.: Frequency of deglutition of tongue thrusters compared to a population of normal swallowers, Thesis, University of Washington, 1963.

41. Neff, C. W., and Kydd, W. L.: The open bite physiology and occlusion, Angle Orthod. **36:**351, 1966.

42. Negri, P. L., and Croce, G.: Influence of the tongue on development of the dental arches, Dent. Abst., p. 453, July, 1965.

43. O'Meara, C. S.: A study of the importance of unbalanced muscular forces on tooth position, Thesis, University of Nebraska, 1962.

44. Overstake, C. P.: An investigation of tongue-thrust swallowing and the functional relationship of deviant swallowing, orthodontic problems and speech defects (paper), American Speech and Hearing Association Convention, Denver, 1970.

45. Peat, J. H.: A cephalometric study of tongue position, Am. J. Orthod. **54:**339, 1968.

46. Penzer, V.: Chronic myo-dynamic dysphagia (paper), A.S.C.H. Annual Scientific Meeting, Miami Beach, Nov., 1970.

47. Posen, A. L.: The influence of maximum perioral and tongue force on the incisor teeth, Angle Orthod. **42(4):**285-309, 1972.

48. Proffit, W. R.: Pressures against the dentition during speech, Thesis, University of Washington, 1963.

49. Proffit, W. R.: Muscle pressures and tooth position: a review of current research (paper), Orthodontic Congress, Melbourne, 1972.

50. Proffit, W. R., et al.: Normal function: Intraoral pressures in a young adult group, J. Dent. Res. **43:**555, 1964.

51. Proffit, W. R., et al.: Linguopalatal pressure in children, Am. J. Orthod. **55:**154, 1969.

52. Reitan, K.: Biomechanical principles and reactions. In Graber, T. M., editor: Current orthodontic concepts and techniques, vol. 1, Philadelphia, 1969, W. B. Saunders Co.

53. Riedel, R. A.: Retention. In Graber, T. M., editor: Current orthodontic concepts and techniques, vol. 2, Philadelphia, 1969, W. B. Saunders Co.

54. Rix, R. E.: Deglutition and the teeth, Dent. Rec. **66:**103, May, 1946.

55. Robson, J. E.: Analytical survey of the deviate swallow therapy program in Tucson, Arizona, Thesis, University of San Francisco, 1963.

56. Rogers, J. H.: Swallowing patterns of a normal population sample compared to those patients from an orthodontic practice, Am. J. Orthod. **47:**674, 1961.

57. Scott, J. H.: The role of soft tissues in determining normal and abnormal dental occlusion, Dent. Pract. **11:**302, 1961.

58. Shelton, R. L.: Tongue what? ARSHA Bull. **5**:5, 1970.

59. Smernoff, G. N.: A preliminary study of mandibular morphology and the measurement of lingual thrusting pressures in subjects exhibiting tongue-thrust swallowing and anterior open bites, Am. J. Orthod. **51**:306, 1965.

60. Stansell, B.: Effects of deglutition training and speech training, Dissertation, University of Southern California, 1969.

61. Subtelny, J. D.: Examination of current philosophies associated with swallowing behavior, Am. J. Orthod. **51**:161, 1965.

62. Subtelny, J. D.: Malocclusions, orthodontic corrections and orofacial muscle adaptation, Angle Orthod. **40**:170, 1970.

63. Subtelny, J. D., and Sakuda, M.: Open bite: diagnosis and treatment, Am. J. Orthod. **50**:337, May, 1964.

64. Subtelny, J. D., and Subtelny, J.: Malocclusion, speech, and deglutition, Am. J. Orthod. **48**:685, 1962.

65. Swinehart, D. R.: The importance of the tongue in the development of normal occlusion, Am. J. Orthod. **36**:813-830, 1950.

66. Toda, J. M.: A study of tongue pressures exerted on the hard palate during swallowing, Thesis, University of Washington, 1961.

67. Toronto, A.: Permanent changes in swallowing habit as a result of tongue-thrust therapy prescribed by R. H. Barrett, Thesis, University of Utah, 1970.

68. Tulley, W. J.: Long-term studies of malocclusion, Trans. Eur. Orthod. Soc, **47**:256, 1961.

69. Tulley, W. J.: A critical appraisal of tongue thrusting, Am. J. Orthod. **55**:640, 1969.

70. Vogel, R. I., and Deasy, M. J.: Tooth mobility: etiology and rationale of therapy. N. Y. Dent. J. **4**(3):159-161, 1977.

71. Wallen, T. R.: Vertically directed forces and malocclusion: A new approach, J. Dent. Res. **53**:1015-1022, 1974.

72. Weinberg, B.: Deglutition: a review of selected topics, ASHA Reports, No. 5, p. 116, 1970.

73. Weinstein, A.: Minimal forces in tooth movement, Am. J. Orthod. **53**:881, 1967.

74. Werlich, E. P.: The prevalence of variant swallowing patterns in a group of Seattle school children, Thesis, University of Washington, 1962.

75. Wilskie, G. H.: Tongue and lip pressures exerted on the dentition during involuntary swallowing, Thesis, University of Washington, 1963.

76. Winders, R.: Recent findings in myometric research, Angle Orthod. **32**:38, 1962.

Chapter 10

IMPLICATIONS FOR THE DENTAL SPECIALIST

Myofunctional disorders have been considered historically to be primarily matters of orthodontic concern. Consequently, some of the resultant influences that extend into other areas of dentistry have been almost overlooked; even when noted, such after-effects have often been handled in a cursory or piecemeal fashion. A more comprehensive understanding of the situation may be achieved by pulling together some of the neglected concepts inherent in tongue thrust. We will not attempt a full harvest; merely a sampling of this fruit brings the realization that the seed is scattered into almost every specialized field of dentistry.

GENERAL DENTISTRY

The family dentist, who sees something of all areas, might well be expected to have a special awareness of the manifestations of tongue thrust. He is the dental counselor, the only dentist that some patients ever see; his potential for service to his patient is magnified accordingly.

The province of the general dentist includes the whole of the "gnathodynamic system," which approximately corresponds to the broad definition of the stomatognathic system given in Chapter 3. In other words, the general dentist should be concerned with that portion of anatomy lying between the top of the skull and the diaphragm. Although he cannot be expected to have the answer for every question that arises in this area, he is expected to know someone who does have the answer. Referral is thus a basic ingredient of general practice.

If the general practitioner ignores myofunctional disorders, at least some percentage of his patients will be condemned to suffer some of the consequences discussed in this chapter. As a minimal routine he should recognize and refer appropriate patients while the mouth is still intact, rather than waiting until it becomes necessary to repair the resultant damage.

ORAL SURGERY

The relevance of myofunction to the surgeon might seem obscure at first glance, and certainly there is a limited number of occasions when such considerations are germane. However, these few instances of overlapping jurisdiction are of such critical importance to the patient that their existence should be recognized and explained.

Our bias is beyond question regarding partial glossectomy as a solution to abnormalities of deglutition. This procedure has been employed historically in many countries and is still suggested by some adherents. Its utilization emerged from the concept of tongue thrust as being predominantly a product of macroglossia, so that reduction of the bulk of the tongue should spontaneously effect normal function.

In cases of true macroglossia such a reduction might logically seem to have merit; we have had no personal contact with such cases and thus no opportunity to observe the results. The patients that we have seen postoperatively have all involved tongues whose original size may well have been within the normal range, and the results have been unfortunate. Basic patterns of muscle movement are little altered by the surgery—the thrust remains a thrust even though the blow is delivered by a lighter instrument.

In point of fact, the thousands of patients that comprise our combined total have provided very few cases of true macroglossia. Countless others have appeared so, on superficial examination, due to abnormally fronted function and lalling posture. The repositioning inherent in therapy renders a dramatic change in this deceptive illusion of enlargement.

On the other hand, we have been privileged to observe a few tongues such as that seen in Fig. 10-1, *A*. This is a case of true macroglossia. The characteristic scalloping of the lingual margin is obvious; the imprint of each tooth is permanently embedded in the tissue. The dental structure enclosing this massive tongue is shown in Fig. 10-1, *B*. Without benefit of any type of orthodontic treatment, this 30-year-old occlu-

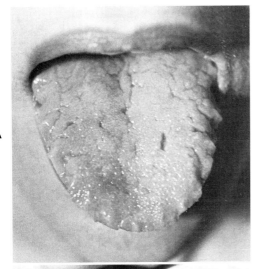

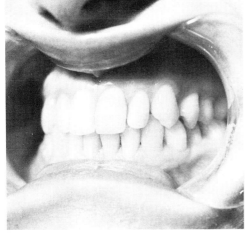

Fig. 10-1. Patient with true macroglossia. **A,** Tongue shows imprint of every tooth. **B,** Natural, untreated teeth showing no malocclusion.

sion is nearly perfect. It belongs to a speech pathologist whose articulation is flawless and who never personally required speech correction. It would appear that mere bulk is not the sinister influence that its reputation portrays, given compensatory function.

While in the surgical province, we may mention an attempt that was made to eliminate thrusting behavior by severing the genioglossus muscle. The details of this study will be discussed in Chapter 13. For now, it is sufficient to note that the researchers were disappointed in the results, although proposing that continued efforts be made in this area. We would welcome the availability of such a procedure for some patients but continue to feel that less radical measures are preferable when they can be effectively provided.

The most frequently recurring situation in which muscle dysfunction should concern the oral surgeon is that surrounding mandibular reduction, or ostectomy. The truly prognathic mandible supporting a tongue of reasonably normal size and function can produce gratifying surgical results. The same is true of the functional Class III case, once function is habilitated and the cause of the deformity removed. The aftermath can be quite opposite when no preoperative provision is made for myotherapy.

The premise is usually voiced that during the prolonged period after surgery when the mouth is wired shut, the tongue is *forced* to behave properly and thereafter adjusts itself to the altered environment. This idea harks back to the orthodontic assumption that correcting the occlusion eliminates tongue thrust. Experience indicates that both suppositions frequently prove misleading; nevertheless, the surgeon may routinely attribute relapse to noncooperation of the patient in not persevering in an ability never truly acquired by the patient. In our observation the contrast is thus striking between the patients for whom we have provided therapy prior to surgery and the resentful, angry patients who make their initial appearance postsurgically.

One of the latter is pictured in Fig. 10-2. This 20-year-old woman had a mandibular thrust and a functional Class III molar relationship. With no mention of the myofunctional disorder, she received full-banded orthodontic treatment for just over a year. Since she still had anterior crossbite, a mandibular reduction was performed and upper and lower jaws were wired together for six weeks. The slide reproduced in Fig. 10-2, *A*, was

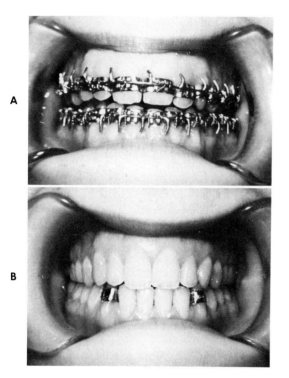

A

B

Fig. 10-2. Mandibular surgery in untreated tongue-thrust case. **A,** Relapse beginning almost immediately after mandible was freed. **B,** Stable occlusion 5 months after bands were removed.

taken exactly two weeks after the interarch wires were removed, when the young lady and her very emotional mother stormed into the clinician's office. The bite was opening with dramatic speed, and everything seemed to be disintegrating. The process began to reverse with the same surprising speed only four or five weeks after myotherapy was initiated. The bite had reclosed and the bands were removed only a month after the completion of therapy, with all teeth holding in a stable occlusion. The patient's status eight months after the initial session, or six months after she finished the therapy program, is shown in Fig. 10-2, *B.* A considerable tempest of ill feeling might have been forestalled had the force of the thrust been relieved before surgery. The tempest might have grown to a hurricane had correction not been made available swiftly.

PEDODONTICS

It is the pedodontist who should be the preventive and interceptive expert. He is often the first to see the patient, and at an age when the full range of options is still at his disposal. His is the influence that can guide and control dental development, bending aberrant tendencies back into line, rectifying faulty fundamentals, and anticipating and forestalling future problems.

Traditionally the dedication of the pedodontist has been primarily to the battle against tooth decay—repairing cavities and teaching proper prophylaxis. He has therefore tended to maintain an understandable orientation toward structure rather than function. Orthodontists once considered the dental arches almost as a set of study models, with little concern for the muscles and tissues attached to that framework. Just as the modern orthodontist has broadened the scope of his treatment plan to include environmental forces, so too the pedodontist is lifting his focus from the static tooth and gingiva, and is seeing them more accurately as mere cogs in the gyrating total mechanism that constitutes the child's mouth. He is also starting to see the mouth as only one integrant of the total child who is his patient.

Nevertheless, even if we limit our attention for the moment to a basic solicitude for tooth decay, we find myofunctional implications for the pedodontist. Dentists have frequently noted the detergent effect of saliva on oral hygiene. In normal deglutition, saliva is sucked around the teeth and through the gingival embrasures with a cleansing result. In abnormal function, this frequently repeated procedure is not only absent but in some respects is reversed, as when food particles are forced into the proximal spaces during a meal by the piston action of the tongue unmodified by a strong sucking component. Should it be proved that tongue thrusters are, in truth, more cavity-prone as a result of their dysfunction, pedodontists might well become responsive to this plight.

An extension of the foregoing is seen in the child with a problem of drooling. Emotional factors may be far more traumatic than dental aspects, for the social rejection which this child encounters may be almost constant. We have accepted into therapy a number of children at a somewhat earlier age than we might otherwise have liked, simply to ameliorate societal crises. The teacher seeking removal of a child from her classroom may have been only mildly exaggerating in her note to the parents complaining that the child "does all of her seatwork in a smelly pool of saliva." Although we cannot charge the pedodontist with responsibility for anticipating

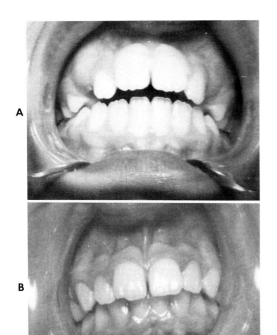

Fig. 10-3. A, Malocclusion developing from incisal thrust. **B,** Healthy occlusion after myofunctional therapy.

before the teeth got so crooked?'' It is difficult to answer such a question. Logically or not, parents expect some guidance in these matters from the pedodontist.

Some of the finest work that we have seen in the field of tongue thrust management has been contributed by pedodontists. Working in co-operation with the orthodontist and myotherapist, timing their efforts in an integrated program of prevention, they have achieved outstanding success. Except with regard to cases of congenital deformity and allied conditions, such pedodontists feel almost a sense of failure when referral for formal corrective orthodontics becomes necessary.

A case in point may be seen in Fig. 10-3, *A*. The malocclusion of this 9-year-old girl seemed to worsen despite the efforts of the pedodontist. Because of family circumstances, formal orthodontic treatment was not to be expected. However, as part of the pedodontist's custom, she was referred for correction of the swallowing abnormality. Although an upper incisor was chipped even before myotherapy could be completed, the occlusion began to improve. The status a year later, at the time she was dismissed from therapy, is shown in Fig. 10-3, *B*. Perhaps this is what pedodontics is all about.

PERIODONTICS

Although the periodontist has, in the past, believed that he had less occasion to be aware of myofunctional disorders than some of the other dental specialists involved, he probably sees more of their deleterious effects than the orthodontist, who has made them a major concern. In part this may result from the age group that the periodontist treats; many patients are beyond the age when modification of muscle patterns seems feasible. Also, malocclusion is often viewed as a result of "premature" contact, the touching of certain features of the occlusal surfaces of the two dental arches in such a manner as to prevent normal intercuspation of the teeth. Yet tongue thrust is not always a suspected factor in the etiology of these interfering occlusal contacts.

A basic technique of the periodontist is occlusal equilibration—grinding away points of premature contact and forming new inclined planes designed to guide the teeth into harmonious relation with each other. Given a mouth under the influence of normal function, this procedure can be most effective.

such occurrences, he should at least be aware of the possibilities so that he will be able to counsel the parents who are faced with this situation.

To return to more conventional aspects of pedodontics, we should note that all of the procedures listed in Chapter 3 under prevention and interception are suitable tools of the pedodontist; they need not be repeated here. Again, without duplicating the list, many of the periodontal problems sketched in the following section have pertinency for pedodontics. All in all, however, the single most dramatic preventive service which the pedodontist can provide may well be the accurate diagnosis and proper management of myofunctional disorders. As long as such dysfunctions persist they color and threaten every measure employed by the dentist. Meticulous plans are thrown awry and large amounts of time wasted when these ruinous forces remain unseen.

One of the more common laments of the parents of our teen-age patients is: "But why weren't we told of this before? We have taken this child from the age of 5 years to a dentist in whom we had great faith. Why didn't he tell us

When, on the other hand, the patient has even a mild anterior thrust, there can be unwelcome sequelae. Second molars, held out of occlusion by the interdental tongue tip, may start to super-erupt, opening the bite still more. Repeated grinding on the occlusal surfaces may lead to destruction of the second molars. At that point, first molars may begin a similar eruptive pattern. We have seen several tongue-thrusting patients who have undergone equilibration, 30 to 50 years of age, with few teeth remaining distal to the bicuspids.

We may note in passing that such patients provide a great challenge for the myotherapist. With a reduced complement of posterior teeth comes reduced proprioception, posing an additional problem in retraining. When present in the mouth, these occlusal surfaces are the telegraphic keys that transmit signals through the periodontal membrane to the neuromuscular complex and thence to outlying areas of the stomatognathic system. When degeneration and destruction are permitted for any reason, it is unfortunate. When they are encouraged, even wholly unintentionally, by grinding teeth in a dysfunctional mouth, the consequences are still more deplorable.

Perhaps more fortunate is the patient seen in Fig. 10-4. This 42-year-old woman had full-banded orthodontic treatment from her late teens into her early 20's. When her bite began to reopen, she consulted a periodontist who treated her for about one year, to the best of her recollection; she is sure that he did a full occlusal equilibration. Somewhere along the way she had a root canal procedure on one upper lateral incisor. The point is, this mouth is not the result of neglect, but the product of treatment by four or five dentists, two of whom were periodontists, but none of whom recognized even blatant tongue thrusting.

Nonetheless, the implications of tongue thrust for the periodontist reach far beyond the foregoing. It has previously been noted that degeneration and resorption of supporting alveolar bone must inevitably follow interruption of the strong intermittent pressure supplied by normal deglutition. Transferring these normal pressures from occlusal to lingual tooth surfaces, which occurs in some types of myofunctional disorders, may threaten the integrity of the temporomandibular joint itself, as discussed in Chapter 5. The synchronization of the normal condyle and articular disc movement with relation to each other and the articular eminence can

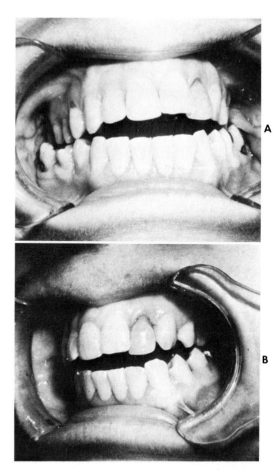

Fig. 10-4. Result of multiple failures to recognize tongue thrust. **A,** Dysfunctional mouth after both orthodontic and periodontic treatment. Molars are in crossbite, occlusion on one cusp in each quadrant. **B,** After treatment by second periodontist; evidence of root canal on upper lateral incisor.

be destroyed, thus opening the door to the manifold problems that may beset this capsule.

Various other results of the lack of sufficient and forceful occlusion have previously been discussed. They may take the form of a bilateral narrowing of the maxillary arch as the tongue drops lower in the mouth, providing less support for the upper teeth. This in turn may give rise to a unilateral crossbite, with further damage to the temporomandibular joint as the mandible swings laterally under the influence of tooth guidance.

Function is requisite to dental health. The investing tissues of nonoccluding teeth may show drastic degeneration. Thus the breakdown of gingival tissue in open bite is simply a matter of time. The vestibular surface of the gums in the mandibular incisor region may appear edematous and engorged with blood in the closed-bite deviate swallower. Bone loss due to periodontal disease renders the dentition still more vulnerable to pressure from either the tongue or lips and may thus lead to abnormal wandering of the affected teeth. ''Disuse atrophy'' of the tooth itself has been reported and does little to increase the longevity of the tooth.

''Mouth-breathing gingivitis'' has long been known; it is usually described as a chronic marginal gingivitis showing a pronounced tendency to hypertrophy or hyperplasia. The hypertrophy may be caused by edema but in most cases is a true hyperplasia. A ''mouth-breathing line'' has been described at the junction of the edematous with the normal tissue on the labial side, a line that marks the limit of the area exposed to the air when the mouth is in the rest position with lips apart. However, the gingivitis is thought to be a product not only of the drying of gingival epithelium but also of an accumulation of debris caused by lack of salivary and labial action, and bacterial growth. Cold air impinging on the exposed gingiva causes vasoconstriction and increases the susceptibility of the tissue to infection. The actual occurrence of mouth breathing is not necessary to this condition; an open-mouth rest posture accompanying deviate deglutition is sufficient cause.

PROSTHODONTICS

One of the primary concerns of the prosthodontist relative to myofunctional disorders lies in the design of proper dentures. Tremendous improvements have been made in recent years in the form and construction of these prosthetic replacements. It is thus disturbing to produce a masterpiece only to discover that each time the patient swallows the denture is dislodged, at times with a disconcerting clatter. Yet the age of these patients frequently dims the hope of modifying a lifelong subconscious pattern of deglutition. The best that the prosthodontist can do, in many cases, is to make due allowance for the orofacial malfunction and hope for the best. It may be necessary to alter the amount of freeway space; positioning of the incisors may be adjusted. After the most careful precautions, however, some problem often remains. Individual prosthodontists have shown considerable ingenuity in meeting this situation. However, when attempts have been made to reposition the mandible into a more ideal functional relationship temporomandibular symptoms have been reported in some cases.

One of the most frustrating experiences for the prosthodontist is to encounter a so-called ''floating bite.'' It is found in the older tongue thruster who has spent a lifetime without benefit of firm molar occlusion, as a result of which the dentition has deteriorated to the point that full or partial dentures are now essential. As an additional result of having no constantly repeated *pattern* of occlusion, he is now seemingly able to bite in any of a hundred positions with equal facility. Attempting to locate a logical functional posture in which to establish the prosthesis is a form of dental roulette. Even the best possible judgment may eventuate in dentures that prove intolerable to the patient, who may then begin an odyssey from dentist to dentist, seeking one who can make dentures that ''fit.''

Since myofunctional disorders contribute to early destruction of the teeth, the age at which dentures become necessary is accordingly lowered. A few patients in their twenties have been seen who were already wearing prosthetic substitutes. Several patients in their early thirties, faced with the imminent probability of having to wear dentures, have been seen in recent years. They completed therapy with varying degrees of success, but at least some of them were enabled to have their own teeth placed back in occlusion orthodontically and seemingly ward off dentures.

Since the anterior teeth are frequently the first affected, a fixed prosthesis in the incisal region is a common first step down the denture trail. The patient may then bend the prosthesis with incessant tongue pressure, and thereafter break the artificial teeth from the denture during incision. In some cases it has been necessary to construct the denture in the unattractive arch form of the original malocclusion, thus providing a ''built-in tongue thrust,'' as an escape route for the tongue and to prevent further damage to the prosthesis. Such cases make it difficult to accept the phenomenal adaptability of the tongue that is postulated by those who rely on orthodontic treatment alone to correct swallowing patterns.

An example is seen in Fig. 10-5. This patient was 29 years of age and had already managed to destroy not only her upper central incisors but two fixed prostheses in addition. Once tongue thrusting was recognized as the malefactor, the prosthodontist supplied a removable denture, with incisal edges of the replacement teeth conforming to the outline of the original open bite.

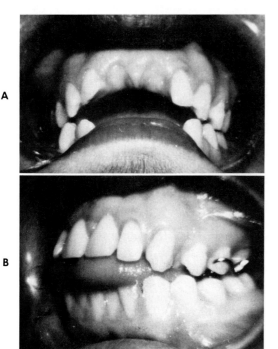

A

B

Fig. 10-5. Early loss of incisors occasioned by severe tongue thrust. **A,** Natural state of mouth with temporary prosthesis removed. **B,** Removable prosthesis in place, conforming to original malocclusion. Patient's tongue rested much of the time in this position.

The patient still displaced this denture with almost every act of swallowing, but it served its purpose until the thrusting habit could be corrected and a more attractive and comfortable reconstruction completed in the anterior region of the mouth.

The interests of all might be better served by correcting deglutition in our children, at an age when it can be done readily, and thus lighten the patient load of the prosthodontist. Considering the increase in time and trouble required of the dentist in tongue-thrust cases, the prosthodontist might feel no deprivation.

ORTHODONTICS

The orthodontic effects of tongue thrust are, of course, the most pronounced, varied, and inescapable, and the ones with which we are the most directly concerned. Of necessity, therefore, they have been mentioned or described in almost every chapter and will not be recapitulated here.

Neither is it necessary to rehash the contro-

versies that persist in the relationship between myofunction and orthodontics. Our impatience for their abatement does not impair our understanding of their roots and rationale. One's natural inclination is to abide by his original learning. Many of the orthodontists practicing today learned their basic skills from a single preceptor, a tutor who may or may not have been alert to myofunctional considerations. For the individual student there was then less variety of viewpoint, less standardization of procedures, and simply less information than are available today.

Orthodontics as a component of the dental school curriculum is a relatively recent arrangement. Even today, not all dental schools provide actual instruction in matters of deglutition. As the orthodontic course of study becomes more eclectic, divergent opinions are proved or disproved with some measure of objectivity, and controversy ebbs.

Until then, we may close this chapter as we began, by stating that myofunctional disorders are generally seen as orthodontic problems. The orthodontist is the most frequently consulted of the dental specialists. He advises the pedodontist, bands and splints teeth for the oral surgeon, and moves teeth into line for the prosthodontist, in addition to conferring with the oral myologist. Our experience convinces us that careful coordination of orthodontics and myofunctional therapy is able to achieve optimum results safely, efficiently, and certainly, with greatly reduced wear and tear on the patient, who is the important figure in the entire situation.

REFERENCES

1. Ballard, C. F., and Bond, E. K.: Clinical observations on the correlation between variations of the jaw form and variations of orofacial behavior, including those for articulation, Speech Path. Ther., pp. 55-63, Oct., 1960.
2. Graber, T. M., Orthodontics: principles and practice, ed. 2, Philadelphia, 1966, W. B. Saunders Co.
3. Leech, H. L.: A clinical analysis of orofacial morphology and behavior of 500 patients attending an upper respiratory research clinic, Dent. Pract. **9:**57, 1958.
4. Ray, H. G., and Santos, H. A.: Consideration of tongue-thrusting as a factor in periodontal disease, J. Periodontol. **25:**251-256, 1954.
5. Shore, N. A.: Occlusal equilibration and temporomandibular joint dysfunction, Philadelphia, 1959, J. B. Lippincott Co.
6. Sicher, H., and DuBrul, E. L.: Oral anatomy, ed. 6, St. Louis, 1975, The C. V. Mosby Co.

Chapter 11

NORMAL AND ABNORMAL DEGLUTITION

The most accurate method of describing an abnormal movement is to set forth precisely how it deviates from the normal act; this in turn requires a clear statement of the normal. In the case of deglutition some cloud remains over both areas. Thus we find it impossible to delineate all particulars of abnormal function and must await further study. However, we know in broad general terms the constitution of normal behavior, we may piece together a more complete picture than has heretofore been available, and since the aberrations with which we must deal are, in most cases, so different from normal behavior as to become apparent, we have some basis on which to proceed.

We should not fall into the trap of defining "normal" as "average." Some authors[4,29] have implied that once a simple majority of children swallow improperly, this behavior pattern then becomes "normal" and requires no further attention. Just because 51% of a given population performs in a certain manner does not make their behavior normal. There was a time when over half of the children experienced smallpox, but this was not considered healthy or *normal*. It appears that the incidence of malocclusion continually increases, and studies thirty years ago showed that, in the United States, half of the population had malocclusion severe enough to warrant orthodontic treatment,[12] whereas malocclusion was found in only 20% of Swedish children.[23] Crooked teeth are not "normal" in the United States and abnormal in Sweden.

NORMAL SWALLOWING

Drawing from the best available descriptions, and combining elements where necessary, we may arrive at the following composite of the swallowing act. Some elements are conjectural,

some are controversial, and some occur inconsistently; just as there are numerous "correct" ways to produce some speech sounds, so there are individual variations in orofacial behavior during deglutition. Lack of agreement arises both in some of the basic aspects common to all and in establishing normal limits beyond which the act becomes pathological.

Most authorities pick up with Magendie, who in 1813 presented the classical account of swallowing; the surprising accuracy of his work, considering the limitations of his day, has maintained for him a place in the literature. It was Magendie, for example, who established the concept of three stages in swallowing: oral, pharyngeal, and esophageal. Since this arrangement is convenient for our purposes, it will be used as part of the framework for our discussion. Several sources have stated that the oral stage is both conscious and voluntary, the pharyngeal stage conscious but involuntary, and the esophageal stage both unconscious and involuntary. Having noted this tidy arrangement, some have then ignored its implications and proceeded as if the entire process were an unconscious, involuntary, global reflex.

Swallowing as a reflex

Some examination of the description of swallowing as a "complex reflex" activity is thus necessary. Certainly it is a complex act, and there can be no dispute that portions of it are purely reflex. However, this description does not apply to all aspects of deglutition.

A reflex may be defined as the involuntary muscular contraction that results from the stimulation of a sense organ.[5] With excitation of a receptor organ, a chain of events is set in motion that must be carried on to its irrevocable conclusion. It has been noted[10] that swallowing is probably the most complex all-or-nothing reflex obtainable by peripheral nerve stimulation. But where does this reflex begin? Where are the end organs located that fire off the reflex? Most studies place them primarily in the tonsils and in the anterior and posterior pillars of the fauces, with other concentrations in the base of the tongue, the soft palate, and the posterior pharyngeal wall. A bolus reaches this region, and thus triggers the reflex, only at the *conclusion* of the oral stage of swallowing. To state that the second and third stages are reflex is quite correct, but if one wishes to initiate the reflex in the absence of food, it is first necessary to voluntarily collect saliva and voluntarily proceed through the oral stage of swallowing, after which the saliva may serve as a mechanical stimulus for the reflexive remainder. There is general agreement among authorities that the oral stage is not bound in the reflex; it is voluntary, and although it is usually unconscious, it may easily be called up to consciousness. It is doubtless performed in a *habitual* manner, but habit is quite a different proposition in terms of modification.

Even were the action a reflex, it could still be changed. It is only necessary to alter one element in the reflex arc to change the response. It may be noted also that the pupillary reaction to light, Babinski's sign, and the contraction of blood vessels are highly inaccessible reflexes on the whole; yet, using modern biofeedback procedures, or under even a relatively moderate level of hypnosis, they become accessible to alteration.

Mastication

It is well to have some picture of the oral action immediately preceding deglutition. Mastication is a complex activity in itself, but it is also voluntary although not always conscious; placing food in the mouth does not trigger a reflex, although, once initiated, it may be continued on a subcortical level. It is centrally regulated by a relatively large area in the inferior medial portion of the motor cortex, described in Chapter 5. Mastication may also be considered in three stages: incision, crushing, and trituration.

INCISION. Incision begins with a lowering and protrusion of the mandible to bring the incisal edges of the upper and lower teeth into functional relationship. This is achieved by the digastric (anterior belly), mylohyoid, geniohyoid, and external pterygoid muscles and is assisted by gravity. During incisal penetration of the food, the mandible is elevated continuously so that the incisal edges of the lower teeth contact the uppers and pass on over the lingual surfaces of the upper teeth, accomplished by combined action of the antigravity muscles—the masseter, temporalis, and internal pterygoids.

CRUSHING. The food thus ingested is placed by the tongue and cheek muscles between the occlusal surfaces of one side or the other to be crushed by the molars and bicuspids. The lips are routinely closed and all the facial muscles are subjected to strenuous exercise during forceful mastication. Dropping off the influence of the external pterygoids, which protruded the jaw in incision, crushing is accomplished similarly by a simple hingelike opening and closing of the mandible, with molars tending toward normal intercuspation on the functioning side. The condyle is set well into the fossa to brace against vertical forces that have been variously measured between 200 and 270 pounds in the molar area; pressures exerted by the incisors vary from 25 to 55 pounds.[13]

TRITURATION. Mastication proper reintroduces the external pterygoids, but in alternate rather than bilateral function—that is, the mandible is lowered and then moved laterally by contraction of the external pterygoid on the functioning side only, until the molars on this side are in cusp-to-cusp relationship as the jaw moves toward closure. The cycle is completed as the mandible slides back laterally toward centric occlusion on the functioning side. Grinding continues in this somewhat rotary fashion, with the bolus usually being shifted occasionally from one side of the dental arch to the other. Masticatory strokes are adapted to the resistance of food being chewed and are thus not necessarily uniform. There is negligible tooth-to-tooth contact during mastication, the stroke being reversed immediately at the first proprioceptive signal of impending contact.

The spatulating action of the tongue maintains the food in a fairly cohesive bolus while mixing in the mucous and salivary secretions of the sublingual and submaxillary glands, thus serving to moisten and lubricate the reduced particles. Contractions of the buccinator muscle impregnate the bolus with ptyalin and serous fluid secreted by the parotid gland. The extrinsic tongue muscles, primarily the genioglossus, act jointly with the buccinator (to a lesser degree, the orbicularis oris) to pass the bolus in and out between the occlusal surfaces in synchronization with action of the mandible until nerve endings in the mouth indicate sufficient pulverization. The sensitivity of these receptors is so precise, and differential movement of lingual muscles so versatile, that adequately prepared particles may be selected and passed back into the pharynx while the main bolus is retained for further comminution. Thus children eating soft foods may find nothing left to swallow on completion of chewing.

Oral stage of deglutition

The oral stage of deglutition is often abridged, even in the better references, to a statement that the bolus is centered on the tongue and propelled into the pharynx, as though an arm reached out from the dorsum and thrust posteriorly with a snow shovel. Yet it is this stage which requires the most careful evaluation because it is the *only* stage of deglutition with which the clinician need be directly concerned. Any abnormality that occurs is present only in this stage; once the bolus is delivered to the oropharynx, it may be consigned to its ultimate destination with a light heart.

There is general agreement that the first component of the swallowing act is to center the bolus on the dorsum of the tongue. The manner in which this is done is of vital importance to the clinician, for it is a pivotal concept in the retraining program presented herein. With tongue and mandible depressed to some degree, a sucking action pulls the bolus into a reasonably cohesive unit on the tongue.[26]

It is precisely this sucking action which must be held firmly in mind as a critical factor in initiating normal deglutition. This sucking action not only positions the bolus but to some degree *continues through the entire oral stage.* In view of some concern over facial movement during deglutition, it may also be noted that facial muscles are perforce active during bolus formation, for they are subjected to considerable stress during the production of the near-vacuum and may assist in the collection of dispersed food particles, or of saliva in the absence of food, and at least momentary closure of the lips is absolutely essential if the mouth is to be cleared. Although overt facial movement may not occur invariably, its appearance can certainly be accommodated within the limits of normal performance.

The first discrete movement preparatory to swallowing is a depression of the apex of the tongue as the bolus is moved forward in the mouth. A sucking action centers the bolus in a groove on the dorsum of the tongue; with a combined sucking and lifting action the tongue is then raised and a seal is established between the periphery of the tongue and the hard palate. The tip of the tongue at this point is most commonly on, or slightly posterior to, the incisal papilla, in which position it is able to achieve some stability; this is the free portion of the tongue—the muscles have no skeletal attachment—and to function efficiently they must therefore seek anchorage through sheer pressure against the alveolar ridge. The ingesta are completely circumscribed at this moment. The lateral margins of the tongue seal against the buccal teeth and adjacent palatal mucosa. Posteriorly, the pharyngeal portion of the tongue arches behind the bolus. The posterior pillars contract toward the midline, and the tensor-depressed soft palate moves inferiorly to seal against the tongue.[32]

Practically all the intrinsic and extrinsic muscles of the tongue, plus the suprahyoid muscles, are active as the bolus is positioned and propelled. In addition, the muscles of mastication routinely hold the teeth in firm occlusion, thereby supporting the act with increased mechanical stability, particularly with coarse food or a large bolus. However, molar occlusion is not essential to normal deglutition, for once the bolus is trapped between tongue and palate, there is less concern for what occurs in the oral cavity below the level of the seal.

Then begins the phase that has immortalized Ardran and Kemp,[1] for in almost every current description of swallowing is an echo of their analogy of toothpaste being squeezed from a tube. The bolus is subjected to pressure, primarily by contraction of the mylohyoid muscle, as the tongue presses forcefully upward in a wave of distal motion that has been characterized[22] as a "stripping wave." The apex and lateral aspects of the tongue remain fixed, preventing escape of the bolus, while the pharyngeal segment of the tongue is depressed, releasing the bolus posteriorly.

The depression of the posterior tongue follows only an instant after elevation of the apex and is the first of two such movements that occur; the entire oral stage is ordinarily completed in a fraction of a second. It is this initial lowering of the base of the tongue which allows access of the bolus to the receptor organs in the oropharynx, resulting in the firing off of the reflexive second and third stages of deglutition. Once the second stage has been initiated, it has been noted[6] that no further mechanical stimulation is necessary for the passage of the bolus.

Pharyngeal stage of deglutition

The second stage is a very rapid, highly organized sequential composite of actions. Having arrived in the oropharynx, the bolus has four possible outlets through which it might pass: back into the mouth, upward into the naso pharynx, forward into the larynx, and downward into the esophagus.[5] The first route is blocked by combined action of the tongue and anterior faucial pillars; although the pharyngeal portion of the tongue has dropped, the segment immediately anterior is still pressing the bolus backward as the intrinsic muscles of the tongue distribute the pressure, firm the tongue, and assure an adequate seal. At the same time, the isthmus of the fauces is narrowed by contraction of the palatoglossus muscle. The nasopharynx is sealed off by contraction of the levator veli palatini, lifting the velum to meet the opposing posterior pharyngeal wall, which is reciprocally approaching through contraction of the superior constrictor. The tensor veli palatini stabilize this seal, which is further reinforced a moment later by compression of the velum between the pharyngeal wall and the posterior tongue.

The protection of the airway at this point in the swallowing act has been the subject of some controversy in the past, primarily related to the function of the epiglottis; however the course of events has now been generally agreed on. Breathing is suspended as both the ventricular folds and the vocal folds are approximated, and the entire larynx is elevated and drawn slightly forward. This action combines with simultaneous pressing of the base of the tongue against the posterior pharyngeal wall to fold the epiglottis horizontally over the aditus and move the entire larynx out of the path of the bolus. Although some small portion of the bolus may penetrate under the depressed epiglottis, its further progress is blocked by the ventricular folds, and it is removed immediately by a combination of negative pressure and compression from the stripping action of the inferior constrictors. But we are getting ahead of our bolus.

As the ingesta are propelled into the oropharynx by the undulating motion of the tongue, it is sufficiently posterior to be in contact with the soft palate before the latter structure moves to close the nasopharyngeal port, as described above. As the velum touches the posterior pharyngeal wall, a second "stripping wave" is set in motion. The pharynx, which has been elevated and expanded through contraction of the stylopharyngeus and salpingopharyngeus muscles, is now squeezed from above downward through the precise sequential contraction of the fibers of the superior, middle, and inferior constrictors in order. The base of the tongue, which dropped to allow the passage of the bolus, rises from the trough of the wave as the mylohyoid tenses. The procedure is further accelerated as contraction of the hyoglossus produces a second rapid backward and downward movement of the tongue. It is concurrently with this motion that the larynx is brought up and forward, which in turn carries the anterior wall of the esophagus upward and forward through attachment to laryngeal structures. The sphincter of the upper esophagus, the cricopharyngeus muscle, relaxes simultaneously; since the posterior wall of the esophagus remains fixed, the upper portion of the tube is suddenly pulled open, with a resulting drop in air pressure. Such negative pressure speeds the bolus still more, often projecting it deep into the esophagus.

Esophageal stage of deglutition

Once in the grasp of the esophagus, the bolus is propelled by peristaltic action. The primary peristaltic wave appears to be almost a continuation of the stripping wave of the constrictors, so that the entire swallowing act, through all its stages, from original bolus formation to arrival in the stomach and reinflation of the respiratory system, is usually one continuous, synergistic, wondrously coordinated process. The peristaltic wave is preceded down the esophagus by a wave of relaxation, which facilitates progress of the bolus. This wave of relaxation also serves to relax the cardia, the orifice into the stomach, allowing passage through the cardiac valve.

ABNORMAL SWALLOWING

There has been a growing tendency to consider and label this problem as a "syndrome." This term implies a running together, a set of symptoms characteristically occurring in combination and typifying a given disorder. In the case of faulty deglutition, a number of elements comprising the syndrome have received a plurality vote: teeth apart, tongue thrust, circumoral contraction, etc.

The worth of defining a particular syndrome, aside from its curiosity value, lies in the fact that if one or two factors can be demonstrated in a given case, all other elements may be presupposed or predicted without overtly establishing them. Such, unfortunately, is not demonstrable in deviant deglutition. Efforts have been made to discredit any further investigation of the entire problem simply because the "syndrome" fell apart in selected patients. Such a framework of symptoms is not only unnecessary, it is misleading and stultifying.

It should be understood at the outset that we are not dealing here with an entity, a single "thing" such as a virus infection arising from a unitary source, causing specified damage and running a predictable course. We are dealing with thousands of entities, the diversity of nature, the individual differences that we worship in the forum and abhor in practice.

We have strayed far from original concepts. Early observers were often impressed by the endless variety of form that atypical swallowing might evince; we have tried to confine it within artificial and untenable limits. This becomes more palpable when we examine the various types, specified hereafter, and delve into problems of diagnosis. Nevertheless, some of the general physiology may be examined. It should be understood that just as normal deglutition was viewed as a general average, so deviant swallowing must also be granted leeway for multitudinous variations.

Mastication

We may refer again to the process of mastication, since differences frequently occur at this stage. The mores of society and the unrelenting efforts of parents have usually prevailed in achieving lip closure during mastication; however, the impulse of the deviant swallower is often otherwise. Wafers and pretzels are used in our offices, and king-size tissues are a boon in collecting the half of the cooky that is frequently lost during mastication. The tendency toward open lips disrupts the fine coordination required to pass the bolus back and forth over the occlusal surfaces of the teeth. The tongue tends to maul the food rather than function with the exquisite precision required in normal trituration. Instead of a cohesive bolus, the tongue allows dispersal of particles throughout the anterior portions of the mouth. The accompanying malocclusion reduces the usable segments of the dental arches, but even the remaining segments often are not efficiently utilized for comminution. Frequently there is a reported aversion to meat and other fibrous foods. When such food is taken there is a proneness, if a chunk strays into the posterior region of the mouth, to swallow it whole—perhaps the "gulping" swallow reported by several observers. One would almost suspect an unconscious realization that if the portion were returned to the anterior part of the mouth, and properly chewed, the child would be required to expend some considerable effort in getting it once more to the pharyngeal region.

Oral stage

All the aberrations with which we are concerned here ensue. At the risk of redundancy we must reiterate that *all* these factors are not necessarily present in *each* swallowing act of *every* patient. Any one of them may be absent, depending on many individual influences.

One of the most significant differences may be found in the process of bolus formation. With food or saliva tucked into every cranny of the vestibule and their lingual counterparts, it is no easy matter to prepare for deglutition; several procedures are seen. With reduced utilization of a vacuum in the anterior mouth, some children (and adults) display an inept and exaggerated sucking process, dropping the mandible excessively to increase the volume of the mouth and thus reduce the pressure, tensing the mentalis to maintain an oral seal, or, in some cases, contracting the orbicularis oris, triangularis, and other circumoral muscles while squeezing excessively with the buccinator. Others send the apex of the tongue scampering about collecting drops or particles and retracting them into the oral cavity proper. All of this accounts for much of the facial movement that has been described, and it occurs *before* the act of swallowing.

The food having been gathered lingually to the teeth, but not necessarily on the dorsum of the tongue, the "tongue thrust" occurs. With no concept of a peripheral seal, most patients employ the process of *physical displacement*, simply taking up space with their tongue that was formerly occupied by the more yielding bolus. They force the ingesta distally by sheer muscle force, primarily through excessive contraction of a probable combination of mylohyoid, geniohyoid, styloglossus, and genioglossus mucles. The chin in a few cases is lifted to secure some slight assistance from gravity during passage of

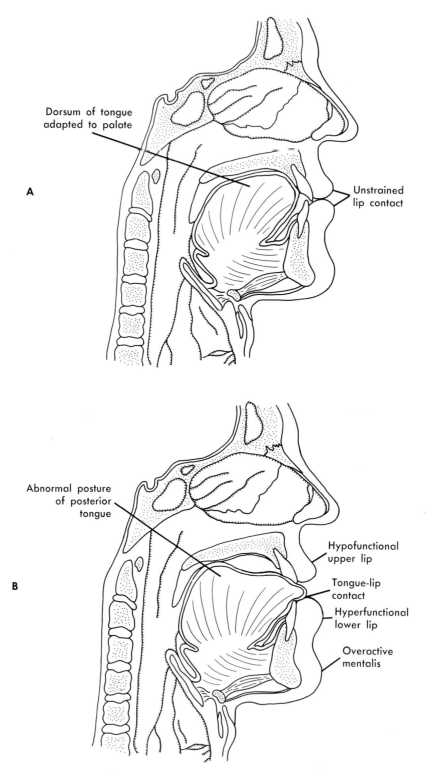

Fig. 11-1. Tongue and lip postures in deglutition. **A,** Normal swallow. **B,** Abnormal swallow.

the bolus distally. Teeth may be apart or oc-cluded, depending on the type of deviation, but tend to be apart. Lips may or may not contract excessively to resist the pressure of the tongue, depending on any number of factors such as type of deviation, status of teeth, consistency of the bolus, and how effectively it is managed. In many cases there is either discrete hyperaction of the mentalis and lower fibers of the orbicularis oris, or generalized contraction of the entire fa-cial network.

If the teeth are separated, the tongue fre-quently spreads between the occlusal surfaces as far distally as the first or second molars. Since the entire tongue is displaced forward, the pos-terior tongue moves in an anterior and superior oblique direction until pressed with some force against the palate, as indicated in Fig. 11-1, *B*. Although the contact between the tongue and palate is complete throughout the length of the soft palate, the direction of force creates a stronger seal in the area slightly anterior to the junction of the hard and soft palates. This in turn forces considerable dysfunction in the oropha-ryngeal region and near-disuse, certainly misuse, of some of the muscles normally active.

More unfavorable therapy results can prob-ably be traced to inadequate attention to the posterior musculature than to any other aspect of therapy. The apex of the tongue is forced dur-ing therapy to retreat from its interdental posi-tion, but the posterior tongue tends toward its original spot on the palate, resulting in a tense contracted tongue of impaired usefulness. In order to function at all, it escapes laterally, changing the type but not correcting the deviant pattern, since an anterior thrust has now become a bilateral thrust. Although such cases are usu-ally considered thereafter as relapses, we would rather agree with those who view such an out-come as evidence of incomplete therapy.[11]

Encountered almost as consistently as abnor-mal function in the veloglossal region is contact between tongue and lower lip or cheek. Many patients have built a *conditioned reflex* of press-ing, or at least touching, tongue to lip and find it almost impossible to swallow if not permitted such contact. One exception to the labiolingual contact usually produces a ''functional Class III'' type of malocclusion; even in this pattern there may be contact buccolingually. The apex of the tongue is thrust against the lingual surface of incisors or against the symphysis of the man-dible and basically remains within the oral cav-ity. The teeth are separated only slightly, and contraction of the external pterygoids collabo-rates with the tongue thrust in displacing the en-tire jaw forward. Pterygoid action may be an attempt to relieve some of the lingual pressure by moving the teeth out of harm's way; however, the result is usually a mandible of normal shape and proportion but with an expanded alveolar margin and a Class III posture. The lateral edges of the tongue may be forced between the teeth to lie in contact with the cheek in the molar region.

Remaining stages

The bulk of the act of deglutition is encom-passed in the second and third stages. Nothing abnormal has been demonstrated to occur in these phases, although Cleall[8] observed some jerkiness and incoordination in the finer details. For the moment, and for our purposes, it is be-lieved that we may safely ignore the pharyngeal and esophageal stages.

CLASSIFICATION OF ABNORMALITIES

We have implied what must be obvious to anyone who has closely observed a sizable sam-ple of tongue thrusters: there seem to be an in-finite number of ways to swallow wrong. And it is true that certain individual peculiarities may be present that will not be seen again through a long run of cases. Nevertheless, a few specifics may be consistently associated in combination, and having identified the pattern, we may learn to predict oral behavior even before it is demon-strated to us; we are then ready to assay some basic classification of cases. However, we may actually understand the scope of the problem more completely once the broad outline of a classification system is before us. We become more aware of specific items and proceed with more assurance when we are not jolted by the appearance of a supposedly extraneous factor. We may also avoid some conflict and confusion when we cease treating this problem as a single unified phenomenon and think instead of sepa-rate forms that may or may not have common characteristics. Moreover, there are important considerations for therapy in making some dis-tinction between types.

Proposed classification

A number of systems have been suggested in the past. Those of Tulley,[31] Straub,[28] and Moy-er[20] appeared in print, as well as one by Brauer and Holt.[7] Each classification has been based on a description of the resulting oral deformity and in some cases on the implied muscular malfunction that would suffice to create the various malformations that are observed. It is not feasible at this time to base a system on etiology, for as noted by Brauer and Holt,[7] the etiology in a given case is usually obscure and often impossible to establish.

The categories used by Barrett describe only those patterns of deglutition which result in overt harm to the dental structure. Some cases are presented in which there is reduced molar occlusion during swallowing, or a tongue posture that is lower than normal or even an observable thrust of the tongue during swallowing, and yet no associated dental impairment is apparent. It has been proposed that a category be provided for a benign, or nondeforming, deviant swallow. Such cases might instead be considered as a gradation of normal, instead of the abnormal with which we are concerned here, as long as there is no discernible damage.

Deviant deglutition is at root an orthodontic problem; it seemed logical, then, to base its classification as nearly as possible on the Angle system, the most widely accepted classification of malocclusion. Although it could not be carried beyond the first three categories, it nevertheless provides a point of departure, as may be seen in Table 11-1. Only the major headings are listed; in addition, a frequently recurring subtype is identified under each basic category.

Note that deviant swallowing may be superimposed on any type of occlusion or may be a major etiological factor, depending on the individual case. Although certain patterns of behavior are characteristic of each type, the categories are so closely adjacent that some overlapping occurs. It is best to view this system as a continuous spectrum, with slight differences in behavior sometimes leading to one or another manifestation.

Each type may then be examined, noting (1) classification of molar occlusion, (2) incisal relationship, (3) status of teeth during swallowing, (4) presence or absence of facial movement or contraction, and (5) action of the tongue. Figs. 11-2 to 11-17 depict each type and subtype.

Type 1. Incisor thrust (Fig. 11-2)

    Occlusion: Class I; may have crossbite.

    Incisors: Overjet, lowers moderately retruded.

    Teeth: Apart.

    Perioral muscles: Usually a generalized constriction of lip and cheek muscles.

    Tongue action: Pressure concentrated

Table 11-1. Classification of types of tongue thrust

			Type
Anterior thrust	Anteroposterior discrepancy		1. Incisor thrust (Angle Class I)
			2. Full thrust (Angle Class II, Division 1)
			3. Mandibular thrust (Angle Class III)
			4. Bimaxillary thrust
Lateral thrust	Vertical discrepancy		5. Open bite
			6. Closed bite
			7. Unilateral thrust
			8. Bilateral thrust

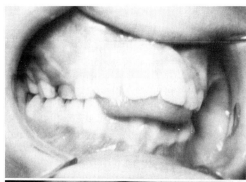

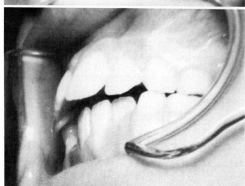

Fig. 11-2. Type 1 (incisal) swallowing abnormality. **A,** Tongue is thrust between incisors only. **B,** Malocclusion resulting from incisal thrust.

on the incisors in a wedging action, driving uppers and lowers apart antero-posteriorly.

Subtype /ls/ (Fig. 11-3)

Differentiating characteristics: Upper incisors relatively normal; lowers excessively retruded and often supererupted.

Type 2. Full thrust (Fig. 11-4)

Occlusion: Class II, Division 1.

Incisors: Marked labioversion of uppers; lowers retroclined and classically in a jumbled but direct line from cuspid to cuspid. Incisal edges contact nothing when molars are occluded.

Teeth: Apart.

Perioral muscles: Hyperactive mentalis;

lower lip on lingual surface of upper incisors.

Tongue action: ''Dispersing'' action, spread between teeth around the dental arch from approximately first molar to first molar, an exaggeration of Type 1.

Subtype /2s/ (Fig. 11-5)

Differentiating characteristic: Accompanying anterior open bite, perhaps arising from teeth occluded against tongue and causing infraeruption of all affected teeth.

Type 3. Mandibular thrust (Fig. 11-6)

Occlusion: Class III, usually in the absence of true prognathism, often re-

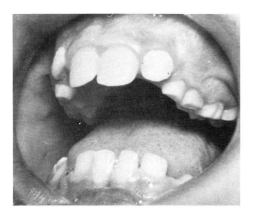

Fig. 11-3. Subtype /1s/ (variation of Type 1). Upper incisors in normal posture; lower incisors tipped lingually.

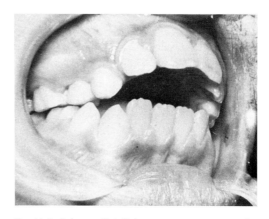

Fig. 11-5. Subtype /2s/. Subtype creates accompanying open bite.

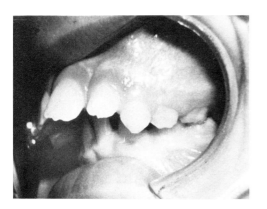

Fig. 11-4. Type 2 (full thrust) pattern. Magnitude of thrust is greater than in Type 1; thrust extends distally as far as first molars, resulting in this malocclusion.

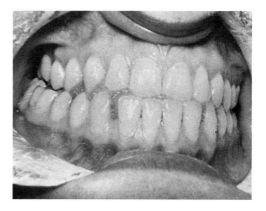

Fig. 11-6. Type 3 (mandibular) thrust. Thrust is splaying lower teeth as well as forcing mandible forward, with no apparent abnormality in growth pattern (usually the mandible, when relaxed, can be manually retruded into Class I relationship).

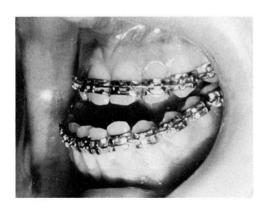

Fig. 11-7. Subtype /3s/. This variety has accompanying open bite. Note that mandibular molars are still contained within maxillary arch.

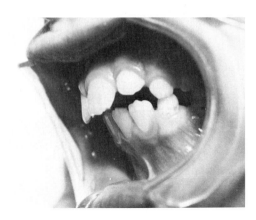

Fig. 11-9. Subtype /4s/. All incisors tipped labially in presence of Class II relationship of jaws.

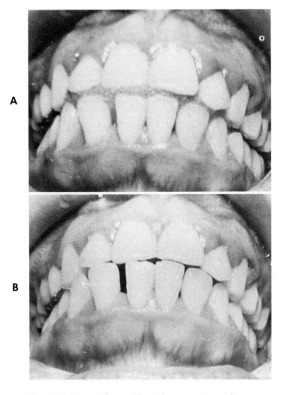

Fig. 11-8. Type 4 (bimaxillary) thrust. **A,** Lingual pressure may cause lower spacing similar to Type 3. **B,** Incisal region of both arches tipped labially.

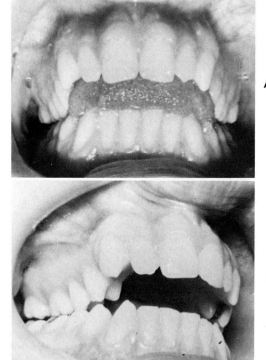

Fig. 11-10. Type 5 (open bite) thrust. **A,** Tongue protrudes in preparation for swallow. **B,** Incisal edges are parallel, with nearly normal anteroposterior relationship.

ferred to as "functional" Class III. Lower molars, usually contained within uppers, may have unilateral crossbite. (NOTE: Class III occlusion accompanying bilateral crossbite would indicate aberrant growth pattern, true macroglossia, etc. rather than tongue thrust and is thus called *true* Class III.)

Incisors: Uppers relatively normal, may have constricted upper arch; lowers protrusive, may display spacing.

Teeth: Slighty parted, although cusps may overlap a bit.

Perioral muscles: Facial grimace, particular tension in triangularis and upper fibers of orbicularis oris.

Tongue action: Apex thrust against lower incisors or symphysis of mandible.

Subtype /3s/ (Fig. 11-7)

Differentiating characteristics: Anterior open bite.

Teeth: Apart.

Perioral muscles: Similar but with strong contraction of buccinator.

Tongue action: Inversion of Type 2s, spread between incisal edges in contact with *upper* lip.

Type 4. Bimaxillary protrusion (Fig. 11-8)

Occlusion: Class I.

Incisors: Both uppers and lowers in labioversion, often some spacing of lowers.

Teeth: Apart only slightly, or closed.

Perioral muscles: Mild contraction.

Tongue action: Thrust against lingual margins of upper and lower incisal edges.

Subtype /4s/ (Fig. 11-9)

Differentiating characteristics: Class II, Division 1 occlusion. Often appears to be a basic Type 4 swallowing pattern superimposed on a different dentoskeletal structure.

Type 5. Open bite (Fig. 11-10)

Occlusion: Class I.

Incisors: Normal anteroposterior relation, both uppers and lowers infraerupted, incisal edges parallel in molar occlusion.

Teeth: Apart, close only to contact tongue; molars are upright.

Perioral muscles: Generalized moderate constriction of facial network, especially of mentalis.

Tongue action: Thrust into contact with lower lip before molars occlude.

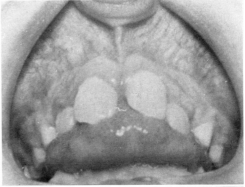

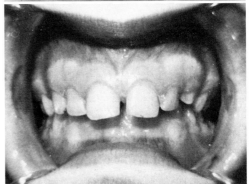

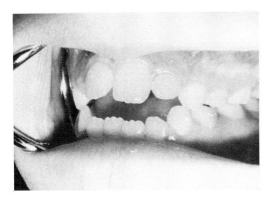

Fig. 11-11. Subtype /5s/. Incisal edges in well-defined oval, with molars usually tipped lingually.

Fig. 11-12. Type 6 (closed bite) thrust. **A,** Tongue engulfs entire lower arch in deglutition. **B,** Angle Class I molar relationship but slight protrusion of upper incisors.

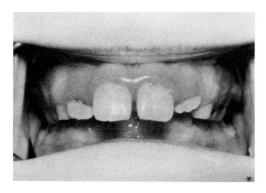

Fig. 11-13. Subtype /6s/. Lower arch is constricted in Class II relationship and almost disappears within encircling maxillary arch when teeth are occluded.

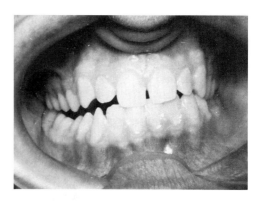

Fig. 11-15. Subtype /7s/. Thrust is focused distally from basic type.

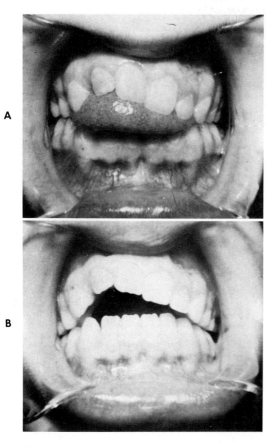

Fig. 11-14. Type 7 (unilateral) thrust. **A,** Lingual pressure centers at about right lateral incisors. **B,** Marked imbalance in resulting open bite.

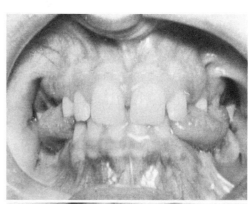
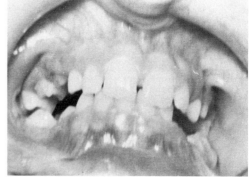

Fig. 11-16. Type 8 (bilateral) thrust. **A,** Lateral margins of tongue thrust buccally while tongue tip braces against incisors. **B,** Incisors may appear normal despite bilateral open bite in buccal region.

Subtype /5s/ (Fig. 11-11)

Differentiating characteristics: More circumscribed, constricted.

Incisors: Incisal edges form a well-defined oval when molars are occluded.

Teeth: Closed.

Perioral muscles: Strong circumoral contraction, particularly buccinator, causing constriction of both arches; all molars tipped lingually; usually overdeveloped mentalis.

Type 6. Closed bite (Fig. 11-12)

Occlusion: Class I.

Incisors: Normal relationship or slight mild overjet; both uppers and lowers may be supraerupted.

Teeth: Apart; great excursion of the mandible as it drops to allow tongue protrusion.

Perioral muscles: Little contraction.

Tongue action: Flaccid generalized protrusion.

Subtype /6s/ (Fig. 11-13)

Differentiating characteristics: Class II, Division 1 occlusion.

Incisors: Entire lower arch constricted.

Tongue action: Spread over lower arch.

Type 7. Unilateral thrust (Fig. 11-14)

Occlusion: Class I; may have crossbite on side opposite tongue thrust.

Incisors: Normal centrals; lateral incisors, cuspids, and first bicuspids on *one side only* undererupted, display unilateral open bite.

Teeth: Usually closed.

Perioral muscles: Strong generalized contraction.

Tongue action: Thrust at a 45-degree angle toward the involved cuspid. This is somewhat like a misguided Type 5.

Subtype /7s/ (Fig. 11-15)

Differentiating characteristics: Unilateral open bite distal to basic type.

Perioral muscles: Reduced contraction.

Tongue action: Thrust toward involved first or second bicuspid.

Type 8. Bilateral thrust (Fig. 11-16)

Occlusion: Class III, may be Class I in younger patients. Bilateral open bite in molar region.

Incisors: Normal relationship or slight retrusion of uppers.

Teeth: Apart; incisors may touch.

Perioral muscles: Little or no contraction.

Tongue action: Spread bilaterally between buccal teeth, often centering at the first molar but may be slightly distal or may extend as far mesially as the cuspids. Tongue tip usually braced against lower incisors in order to execute thrust.

Subtype /8s/ (Fig. 11-17)

Differentiating characteristics: Class II, Division 2 occlusion. Bilateral open bite less pronounced. Note that in Class II, Division 2, incisors are frequently supererupted, resulting in anterior *closed* bite.

It is interesting to observe the relative incidence of the various types, although this, too, must remain somewhat inexact for the moment. The results of surveying 1000 consecutive cases in Barrett's practice yielded the results shown in Table 11-2. It should be noted that these cases were simply those referred for therapy by dentists and do not necessarily reflect the relative

Table 11-2. Relative incidence of deglutory pattern of 1000 deviant swallowers

Swallowing pattern	Number	Percent
Type 1. Incisal thrust	217	21.7
Type 2. Full thrust	521	52.1
Type 3. Mandibular thrust	18	1.8
Type 4. Bimaxillary thrust	46	4.6
Type 5. Open bite	89	8.9
Type 6. Closed bite	57	5.7
Type 7. Unilateral thrust	13	1.3
Type 8. Bilateral thrust	39	3.9

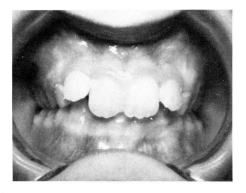

Fig. 11-17. Subtype /8s/. Rather than bilateral open bite, sides of anterior tongue carry upper laterals and cuspids, at times even bicuspids, labially or buccally. Central incisors are slightly retruded.

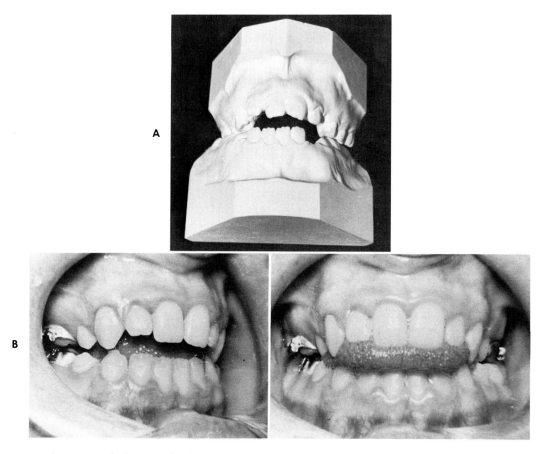

Fig. 11-18. Orthodontic results of untreated tongue thrust. **A,** Patient before treatment, showing open bite and crossbite caused by Type 7 (unilateral) thrust. Over four years in full bands were required to achieve normal occlusion. **B,** Status eight months after removal of bands. **C,** Probable basis for orthodontic relapse.

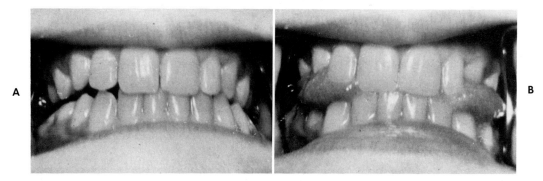

Fig. 11-19. Unhappy orthodontic effects of Type 8 thrust. **A,** Full-banded appliance for 3½ years placed all teeth in contact. Occlusion had relapsed to this point six months into retention. **B,** Tongue function that has been ignored.

incidence in the general population. For example, Type 1 may be more common than Table 11-2 would indicate, for since it is less deforming, it may be accepted by some persons without consulting a dentist. Again, some informal observations lead one to surmise that many Type 8 and some Type 7 patterns are not diagnosed even by dentists who are acutely aware of anterior thrust, and thus may also occur more frequently than indicated here.

Some of our historic differences of opinion should not be unexpected when one views a classification system such as that above, particularly those aroused by the presentation of a simplistic tongue thrust "syndrome." It may be noted that not one characteristic remains constant throughout the various types.

CONCLUSION

It is hoped that the major impression created by this chapter has been that of *variation of function*—differences in both normal and aberrant forms, with a range of behavior encompassed within each. It is also hoped that some separation has been shown between anomalous and acceptable function. Much sharper distinctions will be drawn as knowledge increases.

We would like to anticipate some reconciliation with those who have rejected all consideration of deglutition[8,29] because of the misapplication of a stereotyped syndrome concept. An unwelcome but significant portion of our practices consists of patients such as those depicted in Figs. 11-18 and 11-19. They were intelligent and physically fit children whose speech development was normal and without incident and whose orthodontic care was competent and thorough—except for recognition of tongue thrust. They deserve a better expectancy from treatment.

REFERENCES

1. Ardran, G. M., and Kemp, F. H.: A radiographic study of movements of the tongue in swallowing, Dent. Pract. 5:252-263, 1955.
2. Atkinson, M., Kramer, R., Wyman, S. M., and Ingelfinger, F. J.: The dynamics of swallowing. I. Normal pharyngeal mechanisms, J. Clin. Invest. 36:581-588, 1957.
3. Barclay, A. E.: The normal mechanism of swallowing, Br. J. Radiol. 3:534-546, 1930.
4. Bell, D., and Hale, A.: Observations of tongue thrust swallow in preschool children, J. Speech Hear. Disord. 28:195-197, 1963.
5. Best, C. H., and Taylor, N. B.: The physiological basis of medical practice, ed. 7, Baltimore, 1961, The Williams & Wilkins Co.
6. Bosma, J. F.: Deglutition: pharyngeal stage, Physiol. Rev. 37:275-300, 1957.
7. Brauer, J. S., and Holt, T. V.: Tongue thrust classification, Angle Orthod. 35:106-112, 1965.
8. Cleall, J. F.: Deglutition: a study of form and function, Am. J. Orthod. 51:566-594, 1965.
9. Code, C. F., Creamer, B., Schlegel, J. F., et al.: An atlas of esophageal motility in health and disease, Springfield, Ill., 1958, Charles C Thomas, Publisher.
10. Doty, R. W.: Influences of stimulus patterns on reflex deglutition, Am. J. Physiol. 166:142-158, 1951.
11. Harrington, R., and Breinholt, V.: The relation of oral mechanism malfunction to dental and speech development, Am. J. Orthod. 49:84-93, 1963.
12. Heath, C. W., Brouha, L., Gregory, L. W., Seltzer, C. C., Wells, F. L., and Woods, W. L.: What people are: a study of normal young men, The Grant Study, Department of Hygiene, Harvard University, Cambridge, 1945, Harvard University Press.
13. Howell, A. H., and Manly, R. S.: An electronic strain gauge for measuring oral forces, J. Dent. Res. 27:705, 1948.
14. Kydd, W. L.: Quantitative analysis of forces of the tongue, J. Dent. Res. 35:171-174, 1956.
15. Kydd, W. L.: Maximum forces exerted on the dentition by the perioral and lingual musculature, J. Am. Dent. Assoc. 55:656-651, 1957.
16. Kydd, W. L., and Toda, J. M.: Tongue pressures exerted on the hard palate during swallowing, J. Am. Dent. Assoc. 65:319-330, 1962.
17. Langley, L. L., and Cheraskin, E.: The physiological foundation of dental practice, ed. 2, St. Louis, 1956, The C. V. Mosby Co.
18. Magendie, F.: A summary of physiology, translated by John Revere, Baltimore, 1822.
19. Meader, C. L., and Muyskens, J. H.: Handbook of biolinguistics, rev. ed., Toledo, 1962, Herbert C. Weller.
20. Moyers, R. E.: · Handbook of orthodontics, Chicago, 1958, Year Book Medical Publishers, Inc.
21. Palmer, J. M., and LaRusso, D. A.: Anatomy for speech and hearing, New York, 1965, Harper & Row, Publishers.
22. Ramsey, G. H., Watson, J. S., Gramiak, R., and Weinberg, S. A.: Cinefluorographic analysis of the mechanism of swallowing, Radiology 64:498-518, 1955.
23. Seipel, C. M.: Variations in tooth position: a metric study of variations and adaptation in the deciduous and permanent dentitions, Svensk Tandalakare-Tidskrift, No. 39 supp., State Institute Human Genetics and Race Biology, Uppsala, Sweden, 1946.

24. Sicher, H., and DuBrul, E. L.: Oral anatomy, ed. 6, St. Louis, 1975, The C. V. Mosby Co.
25. Strang, R. H. W.: A textbook of orthodontia, ed. 3, Philadelphia, 1950, Lea & Febiger.
26. Strang, R. H. W., and Thompson, W. M.: A textbook of orthodontia, ed. 4, Philadelphia, 1958, Lea & Febiger.
27. Straub, W. J.: The etiology of the perverted swallowing habit, Am. J. Orthod. 37:603-610, 1951.
28. Straub, W. J.: Malfunction of the tongue, Part 1, Am. J. Orthod. 47:596-617, 1960.
29. Subtelny, J. D.: Examination of current philosophies associated with swallowing behavior, Am. J. Orthod. 51:161-182, 1965.
30. Syrop, H. M.: Motion picture studies of the mechanism of mastication and swallowing, J. Am. Dent. Assoc. 46:495-504, 1953.
31. Tulley, W. J.: Clinical types, Part II, Dent. Pract. 6:225-235, 1956.
32. Wildman, A. J., Fletcher, S. G., and Cox, B.: Patterns of deglutition, Angle Orthod. 34:271-291, 1964.

PART TWO

TREATMENT

Section **A** ☐ **FUNDAMENTALS**
Section **B** ☐ **PROCEDURES**

Chapter 12

DIAGNOSIS AND PROGNOSIS

A "diagnosis" can range from the determination of the presence or absence of abnormal behavior, to the detailed description of the history, possible etiology, consistency, severity, and scope of the problem. The person who refers the patient to the oral myologist is usually interested only in knowing whether there is a real problem, whether it is treatable, and if so, something about the prognosis. For his own purposes, however, the therapist wants more information. He bases his individualization of treatment on information derived during the initial consultation. He may compile data from his patients periodically and examine them to evaluate changes brought about by therapy. He gains important knowledge concerning etiology and prognosis by reviewing diagnostic data on large numbers of patients. Parents of children receiving therapy are taught to observe for habituation of correct patterns by distinguishing them from incorrect ones, based on characteristics listed on the original diagnostic sheet.

The complete diagnostic process should provide answers for the following seven basic questions. Answers to the first five of them will provide information to report to the referral source.

DIAGNOSTIC QUESTIONS

When a child or an adult is referred to you for diagnosis and possible treatment for tongue thrust, there are certain basic questions you will want to answer. (1) Is there really a tongue thrust? (2) If so, is it doing any harm? To the speech? To the dentition? (3) Are there any other myofunctional disorders present? (4) Is the swallow pattern consistent? (5) What treatment is indicated? (6) What structural and functional factors characterize the tongue thrust in this par-

ticular patient? (7) What type of tongue thrust is manifested?

1. *Is there really a tongue thrust?* Long[4] compared the swallows of 25 tongue thrusters and 25 normal swallowers cinefluorographically and found the only significant difference between the groups was in the placement of the anterior portion of the tongue during swallowing. Although other research has yielded significant correlations between type of swallow and various structural and functional criteria, no consistent patterns of such criteria have emerged. Except in the patients whose tongue consistently and definitively protrudes between the anterior and/or lateral upper and lower teeth, the judgment of the presence or absence of tongue thrust has to involve some subjectivity. Many people with normal dentition rest the anterior portion of the tongue against that part of the anterior teeth closest to the gingiva. The mere contact between the tongue tip and a portion of one or more of the anterior teeth during swallowing does not necessarily indicate tongue thrust. When there is significant pressure by the tip or blade of the tongue against a major portion of the area of an incisor, cuspid, or premolar, then the diagnosis of tongue thrust is warranted. Most clinicians would agree that the presence of even a severe frontal lisp, if swallowing behavior is normal, does not constitute a tongue-thrust problem.

The clinician should be wary of using the so-called Payne technique to establish the presence of tongue thrust. This "black light" may be used to assess tongue position at rest or during swallowing. A fluorescent substance is applied to the tongue, and after a swallow or a period of rest, the palatal area and teeth are illuminated to detect areas of lingual contact. Caution should be

187

exercised in the implementation of any ultraviolet or near-ultraviolet light in treatment, according to Birdsell and co-workers.[2] To avoid the possibilities of skin cancer or eye damage, both the clinician and the patient should wear safety glasses. The device should be properly designed and shielded to prevent any stray light emission.

2. *Is the tongue thrust doing any harm to the speech or to the dentition?* Until more conclusive cause-and-effect data are available, the answer to this question, in every case, has to be speculative. There is enough evidence, however, of the coexistence of tongue thrust, malocclusion, and dentalization of linguoalveolar consonants that it is important to attempt to answer this question in the diagnostic process. In our opinion, proper attention to the correction of faulty habitual tongue posturing facilitates the correction of a lisp. Most orthodontists agree that the presence of tongue thrust hinders the progress and threatens the permanence of the results of orthodontic treatment. If there is a tongue thrust, however, without an accompanying speech or occlusal problem, we see no reason to prescribe treatment for the behavior. Instead, we ask the patient and his parents or spouse to observe the occlusion carefully during the next six months to two years to determine whether there is any change in the direction of the malocclusion. If there is, they are to contact the clinician for a reevaluation.

3. *Are any other myofunctional disorders present?* These would include (a) digit sucking, (b) lip biting, (c) object biting, (d) cheek biting, (e) lip sucking, (f) lip licking, (g) leaning against the hand or fist, and (h) bruxism.

4. *Is the tongue-thrust behavior consistent?* To assess consistency of the swallowing behavior, it is advisable to observe the patient swallowing saliva, liquids, and solids, each several times. Inconsistencies among the media swallowed or among repeated swallows of the same medium might indicate a transitional pattern.

5. *Is treatment indicated?* Most of the patients seen for oral myotherapy are referred by dentists who are aware of the requirements for successful treatment of tongue thrust. Therefore most of the patients seen for an evaluation are accepted for therapy. For some, though, treatment is not advisable.

The following are some possible contraindications to therapy:

a. An extremely mild tongue thrust, with no apparent associated malocclusion or speech defect.

b. An inconsistent pattern of swallowing, with frequent normal swallows.

c. A patient who is too young or immature.

d. A negative attitude in the child toward therapy and an unwillingness to respond to the clinician's efforts to motivate.

e. Need for medical treatment before initiation of oral myotherapy. Particularly important is the elimination of structural problems impeding nasal breathing. Examples of medical steps that can alleviate mouth breathing and provide more optimal structure for therapy include a desensitization program for allergies affecting the upper respiratory system; removal of tonsils and adenoids; correction of a deviated septum; reduction of swelling of the nasal membranes; and lingual frenectomy.

f. Need for orthodontic treatment. If the palatal arch is not wide enough to provide a comfortable resting place for the tongue, and expansion is feasible, it is wise to have this done before therapy is initiated. Also, in many children who have an extreme overjet wherein the incisors are tipped labially, the orthodontist will move the upper incisors lingually with a "flipper," or orthodontic elastic. This often requires only a few weeks, and the posterior movement of these teeth makes it easier for the patient to learn to rest his lips in a proper position and to develop better breathing habits. Another problem sometimes requiring early orthodontic attention is the correction of faulty molar occlusion. It is difficult to teach a normal swallow when the patient is unable to bite down firmly and naturally at the initiation of the swallow.

g. Any significant change in manner of swallowing or reduction in malocclusion during the past year. If these changes are in the direction of normalcy, it is better to postpone therapy to see whether the habit is correcting itself. Up to approximately the eighth birthday, many children are still undergoing a change from a tongue-thrust pattern to a normal swallow.

6. *What structural and functional factors characterize tongue thrust in this patient?* It is important to see the total problem. As we study

this individual patient, the statistical significance of a given factor is of minor importance. If we are to successfully eliminate a habit, we must eradicate all its aspects.

7. *What type of tongue thrust is manifested?* By keeping in mind the many variations of tongue thrust, the clinician can avoid overlooking less obvious conditions. Also, the orofacial behavior that you observe should be compatible with your identification of thrust type.

DIAGNOSTIC PROCEDURES
Preliminary observations

We should miss no opportunity to study the child when he is in repose and unaware of our scrutiny. Since this state is not achieved often, our observations may well begin in the waiting room. A plentiful supply of comic books, toys, and other such materials should be considered a part of the diagnostic equipment. An effort should be made to engage the parent in conversation while the child remains immersed in his own affairs. A number of specifics may be garnered from this situation.

FACIAL POSTURE AT REST. The habitual resting posture of the tongue and mouth may be the most valuable bit of information the waiting room supplies; it should be carefully noted.

In the child who breathes nasally and whose lips are competent, the lips are lightly closed or only slightly parted; if extreme incisal protrusion interferes, the lower lip is in contact with the lingual surface of the upper incisors to maintain oral closure. Some care should be taken to assess the morphology of facial and dental structures and the adaptation of soft tissue to teeth. If the rest posture reflects a comfortable "best effort" at mouth closure, the child may swallow correctly. If mouth closure is achieved with obvious strain and tension in the facial muscles, it is probably phony and never occurs during school or while watching television.

Tongue thrusters tend to sit with mouth ajar. They often give the impression that there is inadequate labial tissue with which to close the mouth, but this is seldom the case.

REST POSTURE OF THE TONGUE. The published statements that there is no difference in the posture of the tongue in abnormal swallowing is simply not borne out by patients (Fig. 12-1). These investigators have been studying either normal children or tongue thrusters who were aware that they were being studied.

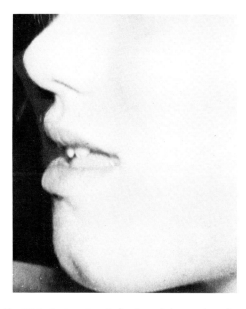

Fig. 12-1. Rest posture indicative of abnormal swallowing. Tongue, which appears to be bulging from mouth, proved to be compatible with its oral environment once tongue thrust therapy was completed.

The great majority of abnormal swallowers, including adults, rest the tongue low in the mouth. Some manage to retract the tongue within the lower arch; some allow the tongue to spread over the lower teeth; and some protrude the tongue until it is in almost constant contact with the lower lip. Parents frequently report a series of school pictures over the years, in each of which the prominent feature is the tongue.

Even if the mouth is closed in the waiting room, the posture of the tongue should be noted as soon as the patient is interviewed.

FACIAL MOVEMENT. Despite the controversy, facial movement should remain on the mental checklist. In normal swallowing it is rare if indeed it does occur, during the act of swallowing proper. Some effort should be made to observe one or two swallows covertly. In some cases a single example suffices.

ASSOCIATED PROBLEMS. Watch for signs of such habits as digit sucking, lip biting, object biting, cheek biting, lip sucking, bruxism, or lip licking. Occasionally the effects of thumb sucking are clearly manifested in the malocclusion. Notice whether the lips are smooth, chapped, or cracked. Some children display an almost continuous series of nonswallow, nonpurposive tongue protrusions.

Case history

An important part of the diagnostic procedure is the case history. It is important to know what medical, dental, or speech treatment related to this problem the child has already received. It is helpful if this information has been secured during the initial telephone conversation during which the appointment for the consultation was made, in order that appropriate communication with other specialists may be made before the consultation visit.

Detailed examination

The detailed examination can be conveniently divided into two areas: (1) examination of structures and (2) examination of function.

STRUCTURES. We will begin with the external structures and proceed posteriorly into the oral cavity.

Nose. The correlation between mouth breathing and tongue thrust warrants a layman's inspection of the nostrils, which are often reduced in size in the mouth breather, and a general determination of the symmetry of the nose.

Lips. Due to a malocclusion or merely to habit, the lower lip may rest against the cutting edge of the upper incisors in the tongue thruster. When the child requires undue effort to approximate the lips, difficulty in habituating nasal breathing will probably be encountered. Chapped or cracked lips may be an indication of habitual lip licking, another habit that contributes to the total thrusting pattern. The lips should be examined for evidences of injury or surgery. Deep lines at the corners of the mouth and inferior to the lower lip often reflect excessive circumoral muscle activity associated with swallowing. If the lips appear to be tight or deficient in tissue, the labial frena should be examined.

Teeth. The state of repair of the teeth gives important information regarding the attitudes and interest of the patient and his parents. Evidence of poor hygiene should be noted. We are interested in intraarch and interarch dental relationships. Within the upper arch, particularly, gaps from missing teeth tempt the tongue to fill them. Unusually large or numerous diastemata may also be important diagnostically. At the other extreme, excessive crowding of teeth in either arch should prompt the examiner to check carefully for discrepancy between upper and lower arch sizes. Unequal crowding or spacing between the two sides of an arch may be accompanied by asymmetrical lingual function. Since less lingual pressure is required to tip incisors than to move them "bodily," labially inclined anterior teeth should be viewed with suspicion.

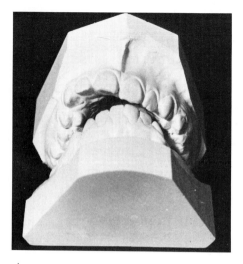

Fig. 12-2. Palate molded by thumb sucking. Upper arch shows marked asymmetry. Despite thumb habit and Class II malocclusion, no tongue thrust was present in this case.

Abnormal interarch relationships, including open bite, overjet, and overbite, should be measured, not for purposes of defining treatment, but as baselines for movement that often follows therapy and precedes orthodontic treatment. The clinician should be familiar with a classification system, such as the Angle system, since research has found prognostic differences among the various types of malocclusion. Angle Class I patients, for example, have been found to be spontaneously self-correcting with regard to malocclusion as well as to manner of swallowing, more frequently than Class II or Class III patients. Note should be taken of which teeth do not approximate sufficiently with their fellows in the opposite arch to allow them to function in biting or chewing.

Finger or thumb sucking often leaves its imprint in the anterior occlusion and in the shape of the palatal arch. The offending digit fits snugly into an anterior open bite and depression in the hard palate (Fig. 12-2).

Palatal rugae. In the normal mouth the rugae are usually restricted to a cluster in the most anterior part of the palate. The two major ridges approach laterally toward the posterior tip of the

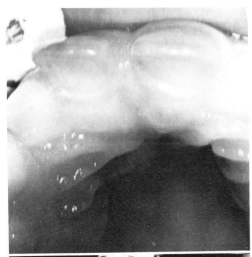

A

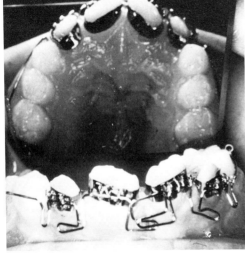

B

Fig. 12-3. Excessive number and size of rugae common in tongue thrust. **A,** In this case rugae were soft and pendulous, resembling plastic bags of jelly. More frequently they are smaller and sharper in appearance. **B,** Unusual palate. Rugae cross entire palate and extend back almost to junction of hard and soft palates.

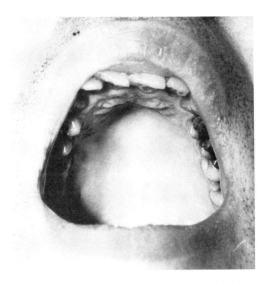

Fig. 12-4. Palate reflecting no deviation resulting from tongue thrust.

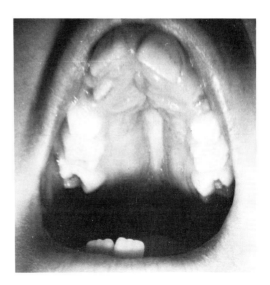

Fig. 12-5. Palate that appears never to have known lingual pressure.

incisal papilla, with lesser rugae, usually four to six in number, in parallel proximity. These rugae are said to be vestiges of the much more extensive corrugations used by some lower animals to assist in mastication; in man they are usually sparse, smooth, blunt, and rounded.

Perhaps because of throwback, because of lack of lingual pressure ironing them out, or for some more obscure reason, the palate of the abnormal swallower is frequently exceptional in

regard to the great number of rugae—dozens of pairs, in some cases—that have a sharp, deep, angular appearance. They may extend the full length of the alveolar ridges. Rugae such as those seen in Fig. 12-3, *A*, are a common accoutrement in tongue thrust; they are not thought to be usual in normal deglutition. Less common are rugae such as those depicted in Fig. 12-3, *B*.

Palatal arch. Many patients with deviant swallowing display a palatal vault that is well within

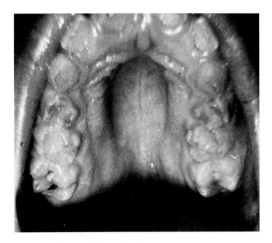

Fig. 12-6. Type of palate most commonly found with myofunctional disorders.

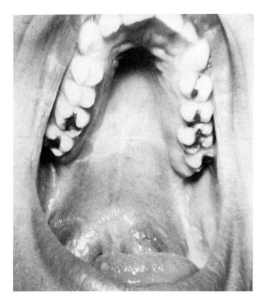

Fig. 12-7. High narrow formation with maxillary buccal segments curving lingually can also be expected with tongue thrust.

normal limits (Fig. 12-4); others have a palate that is almost diagnostic in itself. In some instances the palate may almost resemble a cleft more than a vault. The lateral gum pads may extend so far toward the midline, forming broad shelves on either side, that coaptation of the tongue to the central portion of the palate is a physical impossibility (Fig. 12-5). In other cases, such as the so-called "collapsed" upper arch, some preliminary orthodontic treatment must be

instituted before any hope of swallowing correction can be offered.

More characteristic are the palates seen in Figs. 12-6 and 12-7. The anterior region is featured by a marked indentation that is usually circular in form, whereas the posterior palate may be abnormally flat, probably from excessive pressure of the posterior tongue along the distal margin of the hard palate. It would be difficult to account for this particular palate, given normal deglutition.

Tongue. Although tongues are rarely too large or too small to permit proper functioning, an estimate of tongue size relative to the size, particularly of the upper arch, is worthwhile. If the patient can enclose the tongue effortlessly within the arch when the tip is positioned against the alveolar ridge, the tongue can usually be trained to rest in that position.

FUNCTION. Nonswallow function should be assessed. Labial, lingual, and velar muscles, along with the muscles of mastication, are examined to determine whether there is adequate strength and symmetry of movement. The patient should be able to touch the palatal rugae with the tip of the tongue when the mouth is open far enough for the front teeth to be from ½ to 1 inch apart, depending on the patient's size. Also with the mouth in an open position, the patient should be able to produce a satisfactory /k/ sound. If he is able to produce bilabial sounds in a normal manner, the lips are probably competent enough for purposes of chewing and swallowing. If the voice does not sound excessively hypernasal, the velar muscles are in all probability functioning adequately for normal swallowing.

Gag reflex. It has been the position of some, including Barrett, that those who swallow abnormally have a reduced tendency, as a group, to gag as a result of mechanical stimulation.

Actually, two separate reflexes should be differentiated here: the palatal and the pharyngeal. Stroking the soft palate should trigger the palatal reflex, causing arching of the palate. Impulses thus initiated are carried up the afferent fibers of the glossopharyngeal nerve and are conveyed to the nucleus ambiguus and thence to the levator veli palatini down the efferent limb of the vagus nerve, resulting in the sudden withdrawal of the soft palate from the stimulus. Abnormal swallowers frequently report that such stroking "tickles" but seldom evince the expected arching.

The pharyngeal reflex is different. It is elicited

most readily by pressure against the pharyngeal aspect of the posterior tongue or the posterior pharyngeal wall and is manifested by intense gagging. The afferent nerve pathways are similar to the palatal reflex, but the impulses are of greater magnitude and, if repeated, may traverse the vagus to the gastric musculature and cause vomiting. In many persons the two reflexes are bound together to the point that touching the soft palate results in gagging; in a few cases, pressure anywhere in the posterior region of the mouth produces gagging, making even routine tooth-brushing a problem.

Whereas the palatal reflex seldom occurs in tongue thrusters, the pharyngeal reflex is seen in a slightly greater percentage of patients but when found is usually less intense than normal. There appears to be a definite lowering of sensation in the oropharynx, and real "gaggers" are quite rare. Proponents of an opposite view have sought to demonstrate their ability to make tongue thrusters gag; the result has often been a manhandling assault of the pharynx, or a dental mirror thrust so far down the throat that choking and some gagging ensued. Such measures are not necessary to elicit the normal reflex.

"Anesthetic" throat, which may be secondary to mouth breathing, has been reported on occasion. It may or may not prove to be a diagnostic tool in abnormal deglutition.

Speech. A complete speech evaluation is probably unnecessary. We find that engaging the child in conversation helps to put him at ease and gives us an opportunity to check for the presence of a lisp or the dentalization of linguoalveolar sounds (/l/, /t/, /d/, /n/). Having the child count from one to twenty will reveal most obviously defective speech sounds. If any doubt concerning the normalcy of his speech remains, a formal articulation test may be administered.

Breathing. Breathing patterns should be observed. The mouth habitually held in an open position and the tongue held low in the mouth does not necessarily mean that mouth breathing is habitual, but the condition at least makes the examiner suspicious. Pay attention to audible breathing. If the noise seems to come from the throat, it may signify either congestion in the pharyngeal airway or tension accompanying breathing. If the noise comes from the nasal passages, it is indicative of restriction, through either abnormally small nares, swollen membranes, a deviated septum, or the presence of mucus.

Swallowing. We find the limitations imposed by a binary rating system to be alleviated somewhat by using a 0-1-2 rating scale for swallowing. If the tongue does not contact any part of the anterior or lateral teeth during swallow, a rating of "0" is assigned. If there is linguodental contact, but only against the lingual aspect of the anterior or lateral dentition, "1" is assigned. If the tongue protrudes beyond the cutting edge of any of the upper and lower anterior or lateral teeth, the rating is "2."

For those who insist upon an "either-or" determination or who feel uncomfortable with the suggested rating system, a pleasant alternative is offered by Poupard; writing in the text edited by Boundy and Reynolds,[1] she proposes the terms "NTS" (nontraumatic swallow) and "PTS" (possibly traumatic swallow). These terms show a nice restraint, lowering the emotional overload in some situations. Nevertheless, there are instances that find the clinician privately translating the initial unit of PTS from "possibly" to "positively."

Before checking for tongue thrust during swallowing, it is wise to look for areas of open bite, laterally as well as centrally, and diastemata in order to know the most likely area for tongue thrust to occur. Thus in the case of a unilateral open bite, rather than breaking the labial seal centrally during the swallow, the examiner would break it in the area of the open bite. We believe that it is important to assess the swallows of food, liquid, and saliva routinely.

Food swallows. We prefer to use a sugar wafer in our evaluation of food swallows. Most children like these cookies, and they afford a good opportunity to study chewing and swallowing behavior because they are relatively difficult to handle. Watch the child closely throughout the process. As the cooky is brought toward the mouth, do the head and tongue reach out to meet it? Note the size of the bite the patient takes. Watch the lips and tongue during mastication. A tendency to keep the lips open during chewing disrupts the fine coordination required to form a bolus and move it back and forth over the occlusal surfaces of the teeth. Instead of forming a cohesive bolus, the tongue allows for dispersal of particles throughout the anterior portions of the mouth. Observe whether the child swallows at various times during the masticatory process.

Ask the child not to swallow until you tell him to do so. If you will gently rest your index or third finger at the top of the larynx, which is readily palpable in most patients, and your thumb on the patient's lower lip, you can tell when the swallow is beginning by noting an upward movement of the larynx. Quickly depress the lower lip, gently but firmly. Some clinicians prefer to elevate the upper lip simultaneously. One of four patterns below can usually be readily identified by following this procedure.

1. If swallowing is normal, no movement of the mandible is detected. The teeth are closed, and the swallow is executed effortlessly with the lips parted. You get a "What's wrong with that?" look from the patient.

2. If an anterior thrust occurs, its presence is usually obvious; withdrawing the lower lip exposes the apex of the tongue between the incisors, and all doubt is erased.

3. In some cases an anterior thrust occurs, but breaking the labioglossal seal results in instant retraction of the tongue, possibly to prevent escape of the bolus. This retraction may be entirely too rapid for visual detection. However, sudden closure of the teeth accompanies tongue withdrawal, and the resulting jar transmitted through the mandible is readily felt by the fingers. The sensation is quite distinct.

4. In some cases great resistance is met when the thumb attempts to depress the lip. These patients feel that the labioglossal seal is absolutely essential to the swallowing act. Moyers,[5] in describing his "complex tongue thrust," found that separating the lips actually inhibited the swallow itself. These patients almost invariably prove to have a Type 2 swallowing pattern. Repeat this procedure two or three times to determine consistency of pattern. Timing is a critical factor in breaking the lip seal, and the novice will need experience with dozens of patients before he feels competence.

In certain patients the tongue thrust is difficult to see, either because of the quickness with which it occurs or because the dentition obscures the tongue. Most people who swallow normally do not find it difficult to swallow with the lips held wide apart. You may wish to have your patient try this; the tongue thruster will experience considerable difficulty in swallowing without bilabial or labiodental contact. One of the most difficult thrusts to observe is that found accompanying some with a deep overbite. It is always better to try to observe the thrust without introducing artifacts. However, we have found the insertion of a tongue depressor between the upper and lower first molar on one side of the mouth just prior to the swallow has diagnostic value in some cases. Most normal swallowers swallow just as efficiently with the tongue blade in place as without it; most tongue thrusters, temporarily deprived of the anterior tongue-teeth or tongue-lip seal find it difficult, if not impossible, to swallow.

Notice the tongue after the swallow of the bite of cooky. If scattered crumbs remain on the tongue, the swallow has not been efficient. This does not necessarily mean there has been a tongue thrust, but it is helpful in future reevaluations to know whether the swallow before therapy left crumbs on the tongue. If these crumbs are found only in a certain area of the tongue consistently, there is probably asymmetry in tongue function during swallowing.

After the swallow, does the patient exhibit any nonswallowing tongue protrusions, such as making an effort to clean the teeth of remaining crumbs? A tongue thrust during the swallow of food occurs only once or twice per mouthful; tongue thrust associated with the chewing of the food and tongue-thrust movements made after the swallow often add up to ten or twelve and must be dealt with in therapy.

Have the patient swallow enough times so that you can assess circumoral muscle contraction as well as masseter and temporalis contraction during the swallow. The masseter is not difficult to palpate and may be assessed by placing the back of the fingers gently against the posterior jaw. If contraction is not obvious during deglutition, the back teeth are not occluding firmly enough to provide stability for the tongue during the swallow.

Some writers have suggested that the hyoid be palpated for diagnostic purposes. Our clinical experience and research have failed to uncover any differences between the manner of hyoid movement in normal and abnormal function. Judgments based on hyoid movement must be open to question at this time.

Liquid swallows. We recommend that each patient first be tested drinking continuously. Observe the head and tongue again to see if he reaches for the glass excessively. Note any circumoral contraction and palpate the masseter. If the facial grimaces are present during swallowing, they will go away with proper swallow training, and their presence or absence will be a valuable means of checking for habituation of the proper swallow as the months go by. Observe the clearing swallow as the cup is lowered.

Saliva swallows. The procedure is the same

for saliva swallows. Have the patient gather some saliva and swallow on command. Note the gathering process. If there is considerable effort displayed by the facial muscles, and if there are indications of tongue thrust during gathering, be sure to take note. Again part the lips during swallowing.

We routinely ask our patients what their orthodontist told them about tongue thrust and about his purpose in having them come to see us. We find that sometimes the orthodontist has already given a minicourse in proper swallowing, and on all these command swallows, the patient swallows correctly. For this reason and because we have learned to trust the judgment of the referring dentist, we place less confidence in conscious attempts to swallow than in random unsolicited swallows.

Laboratory methods

For clinical purposes, we find that little is gained by routinely making x-ray films, cineradiographic studies, or dental models. When we have need for the x-ray films and models, we look at those prepared by the orthodontist. The distinguishing aspects of the swallow are not readily observable on cineradiographic films, as Hanson learned in several years of studying films on his research subjects. The dentition, in the majority of cases, effectively obscures the tongue placement and movement, and only in the teeth-apart swallowers is definitive information about the presence of tongue thrust gleaned. These cinefilms are invaluable in research, but their use in clinical diagnosis is limited. In therapy we attempt to change only the anterior portion of the swallow, and that part of the swallow is easily visible by means of the techniques described above.

Statement of diagnosis

In addition to declaring whether or not there is a tongue thrust present, the examiner should define the type of thrust and, in some manner, assess the severity and consistency of the abnormal swallow. Any special problems or positive considerations should be noted, including an estimate of the motivation of the patient. A prognostic statement is always appreciated by the referring dentist.

Recommendation

If therapy is recommended, is it going to begin soon? If the clinician sees the need for possible surgery, orthodontic treatment, or attention by any other specialist, he should so indicate. The decision concerning therapy or alternative steps to be taken by the patient or his parents should be clearly explained and substantiated by the clinician. There should be no doubt as to what steps should be taken next and by whom. If therapy seems to provide a logical precaution in a given case, to prevent malocclusion, to improve malocclusion, or to expedite the treatment for malocclusion, therapy should be initiated with gusto. It should never be entered into half-heartedly.

Summary

The competent clinician is acquainted with diagnostic patterns that relate type of malocclusion to type of tongue thrust and associated problems. The patterns help him to recall and observe all possible components of the total habit. The assessment must include a thorough examination of all aspects of the behavior, however, and not permit overgeneralizations regarding such patterns. The oral myologist need not make the diagnosis without help. The patient, the parents or spouse of the patient, the dentist, various medical specialists, and teachers are sources who should be asked to help with diagnostic information. A therapy plan based on the results of a thorough examination will not be stereotyped. Unnecessary exercises and assignments will be ruled out and pertinent ones included. This first step in treatment should not be taken hurriedly.

PROGNOSIS

A purpose in Hanson's[3] longitudinal research, which included 178 subjects, was to determine which diagnostic criteria would be related to retention of tongue thrust and which would be associated with spontaneous correction. According to incidence studies, about half of the children who are tongue thrusting at the age of 4 years will correct this habit by the age of 8 years. Children in this research who were tongue thrusting at the mean age of 4 years 9 months and were found to still be doing so at the age of 8 years 2 months (persistent thrusters) were compared with those children who were also tongue thrusters at the younger age but who had achieved a normal, nonthrusting swallowing pattern without therapy by the mean age of 8 years 2 months (temporary thrusters).

Table 12-1 presents the criteria that effectively discriminated, at four age levels, between subjects whose tongue-thrusting patterns persisted

Table 12-1. Diagnostic factors demonstrated by persistent tongue thrusters, in comparison with temporary tongue thrusters

Diagnostic factors	Statistical significance (%)			
	4 yr. 9 mo.	5 yr. 8 mo.	6 yr. 7 mo.	7 yr. 5 mo.
DIRECT OBSERVATION				
Less masseter contraction when swallowing	5.0			
Higher, narrow palate	5.0			
More lip movement during swallowing		5.0		
More dentalization of linguoalveolar sounds			5.0	
More dentalization (specifically) of /s/ sounds			2.5	
More mentalis contraction on swallowing			2.5	0.5
Larger tonsils				2.5
CINERADIOGRAPHY				
More lip movement on swallowing liquids	5.0		5.0	
More lip movement on swallowing solids				5.0
Less extension of hyoid on swallowing liquids		5.0		
Less dentalization of /d/, /z/, and /l/ sounds			2.5	5.0
More molar occlusion on swallowing liquids				5.0
CASE HISTORY				
Fewer allergies	5.0			
More digit sucking		5.0		
More mouth breathing		0.5	0.5	
DENTAL MODELS				
Greater general palatal height	1.0		2.5	
Greater palatal height in premolar region		5.0	0.5	0.5
Greater maxillary arch circumference			2.5	
Narrow maxillary arch in cusp region	5.0			
Less buccal crossbite		5.0	2.5	2.5
LATERAL HEAD FILMS (MOYERS' ANALYSIS)				
Less space from point A to SO vertical parallel to r FOP (indicates available anteroposterior space at maxillary level)	5.0			
Greater distance from SE to intersection of FOP with PM vertical (indicates available anteroposterior space at maxillary level)				5.0

through the age of 8 years and those who were swallowing normally at that age.

Of 154 subjects whose tongue contacted the lingual surface of the incisors or cuspids during swallowing at age 4 years 9 months (liberal definition of tongue thrust), 77 (50%) changed to a normal swallowing pattern by the age of 8 years 2 months. Over half of those who made that change did so after the age of 6 years 7 months. Of the 103 subjects who at 4 years 9 months of age were found to be thrusting the tongue beyond the cutting edge of the anterior teeth, 63 (61.2%) had changed to a nonthrusting pattern by the age of 8 years 2 months. Of the 63, 34 had ''normalized'' their patterns between the ages of 6 years 7 months, and 8 years 2 months. Therefore, following either definition, it appears unwise to administer therapy for tongue thrust before the age of 6 years 7 months or 7 years 5 months, unless the critical prognostic criteria have been considered.

It is significant that of 75 children who were swallowing normally at 4 years 9 months of age, only 5 children developed a tongue thrust after the age of 6 years 7 months. Although it is possible that the spaces caused by missing teeth after this age contributed to the retention of a tongue-thrust pattern in other subjects, it seems reasonable to conclude that such spaces do not frequently cause a tongue thrust to occur in subjects who previously had swallowed normally.

The greatest number of prognostically significant criteria was found at the age of 6 years 7 months. Although orthodontists occasionally see younger children, probably more than 90% of the children they examine are older than 6 years 7 months on their first visit. For many reasons this is an early enough age at which to identify a tongue-thrust pattern and attempt a prognosis regarding its permanence. Many of the children tongue thrusting at 6 years 7 months of age will change to a normal swallowing pattern during or immediately following the mixed dentition stage, according to the results of this study and others. Orthodontic work usually does not begin until after the permanent incisors have erupted, so that when the child is 6 years 7 months old, sufficient time still exists in which to correct the thrusting pattern if therapy is indicated.

Criteria that discriminate most reliably between persistent and temporary tongue thrusters are those which appeared as factors of differential diagnosis during more than one year in the study. More lip movement during swallowing, greater general palatal height, and more mouth breathing were among the characteristics that occurred repeatedly among the persistent thrusters. No pattern of diagnostic criteria was found consistently throughout the four years of the study. However, the marked decrease in the incidence of tongue thrust that occurred as the children in the study became older gives significance to the role of those diagnostic factors which occurred even inconsistently from year to year. They are important in the determination of whether to treat a child's tongue thrust or to wait for it to modify spontaneously.

SUMMARY

A complete diagnostic evaluation should include a case history and a thorough examination of oral structures and their functions in swallowing and nonswallowing activities. Observations of the patient's oral behavior are more valid when the patient is unaware that he is being observed. Random, unsolicited saliva swallows are more meaningful diagnostically than swallows done on command. Certain characteristics have been found to be important prognostically. Enlarged tonsils, a high and/or narrow palatal arch, mouth breathing, and lingual crossbite appear to be significantly associated with the retention of a thrusting pattern through the mixed dentition period of development. The total diagnostic picture serves as a basis for determining habituation, or regression, during and after treatment. Individualized therapy planning is made possible when careful attention is paid to *all* aspects of the oral behavior.

REFERENCES

1. Boundy, S. S., and Reynolds, N. J., editors: Current concepts in dental hygiene, St. Louis, 1977, The C. V. Mosby Co.
2. Birdsell, D. C., Bannon, P. J., and Webb, R. B.: Harmful effects of near ultra-violet radiation used for polymerization of a sealant and a composite resin, J. Am. Dent. Assoc. **94:**311-314, 1977.
3. Hanson, M. L., and Cohen, M. S.: Effects of form and function on swallowing and the developing dentition, Am. J. Orthod. **64:**63, 1973.
4. Long, J. M.: A cinefluorographic study of anterior tongue thrust (abst.), Am. J. Orthod. **49:**865, 1963.
5. Moyers, R. E.: Tongue problems and malocclusion, Dent. Clin. North Am., p. 529, July, 1964.

Chapter 13

A REVIEW OF TREATMENT APPROACHES

There are many ways to cope with tongue thrust. It can be ignored. The orthodontist can straighten the patient's teeth and wait for the tongue thrust to disappear when the malocclusion is corrected, or the orthodontist can fasten an appliance to the lingual aspect of the teeth to encourage the tongue to stay away from them. It can be treated surgically. Hypnosis can be employed in its treatment. Oral myotherapy is another alternative; it can be perfunctory or comprehensive, and it can be administered intensively or extended over a period of years. Some approaches combine the use of appliances with myotherapy. Still another approach combines surgery with a reminder appliance.

Representative treatment programs will be presented in this chapter. We do not affirm that the programs included are necessarily those the authors follow at the present time. They are programs that have been proposed and tried in the past.

APPLIANCE THERAPY

The use of "habit appliances" is the historic approach of dentistry to tongue thrust. They are still widely used, and oral myofunctional therapists should be able to recognize them. They come in infinitely assorted styles, a few of which will be described, together with the philosophy behind their use.

The hay rake

The hay rake appliance consists of a metal bar or wire fitted to the lingual surface of the maxillary incisors. It is usually held in place by welding the ends to metal crowns over the first permanent molars or the second deciduous molars, and is equipped with a row of prongs, usually four to six in number, welded at right angles to the bar and projecting posteriorly and downward. One example is seen in Fig. 13-1. These prongs are frequently sharpened and are positioned in such a way that the tongue may be protruded only at the expense of laceration. Some have been seen in which the prongs were placed in light contact with gum tissue above the maxillary incisors, and a loop of wire was so placed behind the teeth that protrusion of the tongue caused torquing, driving the needle points into the gums.

The entire philosophy behind the hay rake is to make tongue thrust so painful that the patient will stop the behavior. It does not teach him to swallow correctly, and the resulting patterns of deglutition may be quite bizarre. Not surprisingly, many patients learn to avoid lingual protrusion. It is now becoming common to implant the prongs in an acrylic plate that is adapted to the lingual surface. In many cases the prongs extend upward and backward from the mandibular arch, making impossible any normal function of the tongue in the anterior portion of the mouth.

The cage

The cage is an extension of the hay rake; its prongs are not sharpened but are much more numerous, usually ten to twelve, and are sometimes an inch long. The cage is welded to either the upper or lower arch, the distal ends of the wires hanging free. Although more humanitarian in concept, the cage frequently results in even greater problems. The child is asked to place his tongue within this wire cage, thus preventing lingual excursion between the teeth. Provided the child cooperates, the added resistance provided by the cage serves only to confirm and strengthen the pattern of protrusion in lingual

198

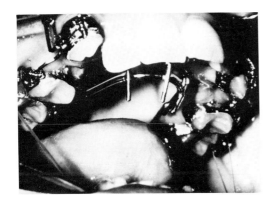

Fig. 13-1. One of many types of hay rake construction.

muscles. Regardless of whether the upper or lower arch is employed for anchorage, the cage renders marked insult to speech, since normal articulation is obviously impossible. One 14-year-old girl with a Subtype 2s swallowing pattern was seen after she had been through orthodontic treatment twice. She had worn a cage over a year, but her bite was more open than in the original malocclusion and her speech was grossly distorted. This child was dropped from therapy, to the great sorrow of all, because she had become convinced that everything was hopeless and that she was a failure; she refused to make any further effort.

The fence

Used only on the maxillary arch, the fence, also called the crib, begins as something similar to the hay rake. A heavy arch wire is fitted, in this case immediately posterior to the gums, and welded to molar crowns. A wire screen is suspended vertically from the arch wire; this screen may take the form of another piece of arch wire bent into a series of broad V shapes, the wires may crisscross, or the crib may be a thin sheet of acrylic. The tongue encounters the fence before it arrives between the teeth and is thus harmlessly contained without pain. The dentist who installs a fence should be aware that the most effective method by which to strengthen a muscle is to provide resistance for that muscle. As with the cage, the end product of a crib, once it is removed, is a tongue with an enhanced capability for tongue thrust.

Cleall[2] placed cribs in the mouths of 20 patients and then compared cinefluorographic films of each adolescent before the crib was placed with those made immediately after removal of

the crib six months later and others made after an additional two months. He found that the tongue resumed much of its original thrusting as soon as it was free of the crib, and that after two months of regained freedom it had reverted almost entirely.

Probably the best that can be said for a fence is that it interferes considerably less with speech. In combating tongue thrust, it restrains; it does not retrain.

The curtain

The curtain consists of a U-shaped sheet of acrylic that drops directly down from the palate, usually at about the cuspid region; by being somewhat posterior to the incisal ridge, it may extend a bit lower in the mouth. It is often braced by an acrylic palatal arch that in turn is held firmly in place by continuous loops of arch wire extending around the buccal surface of the molars. The reasons given for its use are the same as for the fence, but its function is somewhat different. It might actually restrain the tongue if tongue thrusters really close their teeth before swallowing; the more common sequence is: The tongue is protruded, such closure as may occur is initiated—and the curtain comes down across the dorsum of the tongue like a Spanish bit in a horse's mouth, effectively keeping the teeth apart even farther than usual.

Reminder appliances

Some orthodontists advocate the use of a "reminder appliance," rather than the more tortuous rake or crib. For example, Walker and Collins[23] suggest anchoring a transpalatal reminder wire to the maxillary cuspids. The patient is instructed to keep the tongue behind the wire when he talks, eats, and swallows.

A different type of reminder is described by Littman.[14] A pear-shaped opening, extending from the distal aspect of the canines to the mesial aspect of the second premolars, is made in an upper Hawley retainer. The patient wears this appliance at all times. He places the tongue tip in the opening, bites down on his posterior teeth, and swallows. The tongue tip is to remain in the opening after each swallow. He practices this exercise twenty-five times, three times each day. The usual treatment time is approximately three months.

Another modification of the Hawley appliance is suggested by Kaye.[11] Palatal extension loops are attached to a retainer. The loops extend inferiorly to the lingual cervical areas of the lower incisors. They reportedly restrict tongue movement only anteriorly, allowing free movement laterally and vertically. This is similar to the "fence" described earlier in this chapter, except that the Kaye appliance is removable. Kaye instructs his patients to remove it only for meals and tooth brushing. An average of six months wearing time is required for most patients to eliminate tongue thrust, according to Kaye.

The Andresen appliance

Some orthodontists advocate treatment of tongue thrust with the Andresen appliance (described in Chapter 4). This device completely encircles the lingual aspect of both dental arches, forcing the tongue away from the teeth. The patient swallows with his tongue restricted to the small space available to it. In patients with "functional" open bites, the appliance frees the teeth from the tongue's intrusive influence and allows them to erupt to a normal bite. Most writers recommend supplementing the use of the appliance with myofunctional therapy.

The Andresen appliance also can be used in the treatment of distoclusion related to tongue thrust. As the patient swallows with the appliance in position, the swallowing muscles cause the upper dental arch to move distally, while the lower arch is encouraged to move mesially, it is claimed.

The Bionator

Balters' Bionator is similar to an activator appliance, but is less bulky and allows the child to speak normally with the appliance in place. It does not cover the anterior palate, and fits loosely in the mouth. It can be worn at all times, night included, except during eating.

There are three types of Bionators: the standard (for Class II, Division 1 malocclusions), the Class III, and the open bite appliance. Essential elements for all three types are a vestibular wire and a palatal arch. Lip closure is necessary for the treatment to be effective.

The purposes of treatment, according to Graber and Neumann[10] are: (1) to promote lip closure and contact between the back of the tongue and the soft palate; (2) to enlarge the oral cavity; (3) to move the incisors into an edge-to-edge relationship; (4) to elongate the mandible, allowing for more favorable tongue resting postures; and (5) to improve relationships among the jaws, tongue, dentition, and surrounding soft tissues. The efficiency of the Balters approach has not been tested sufficiently. Although his explanations seem logical, the permanence of the restraint forced upon the tongue by the appliance is questionable.

The oral screen

Graber and Neumann[10] contend that the oral screen, primarily designed as a "lip molder," is also helpful in the correction of tongue thrust. A double screen, one on the labial aspect of the anterior teeth, the other on the lingual aspect, keeps unwanted tongue and lip pressures away from the teeth. Its most helpful contribution, in our opinion, would probably be to promote nose breathing, allowing the tongue to be trained to rest "on the spot." It is used principally on the early deciduous dentition.

Summary

One of the perplexing problems in the field of oral myofunctional disorders is that so many treatment procedures are successful with some patients. Some orthodontists today still routinely use rakes to overcome tongue thrusting. Had they not been successful with this procedure in a significant number of patients, they undoubtedly would have discarded it long ago. From discussions we have had over the years, though, we would have to conclude that those orthodontists who have had extensive experience with appliances and with myotherapy prefer the latter. Certainly the use of the appliance keeps the patient's progress more directly under the orthodontist's control. He does not have to worry about the qualifications, personality, or general effectiveness of an oral myotherapist. The appliance is concrete and stable. What, then, are its disadvantages?

Disadvantages of the anti–tongue-thrust appliance

1. It impresses many parents and children as being a type of torture device.
2. Habits developed with it in place are dependent on the cues, or feedback, it provides when the tongue is misplaced at rest or moves forward during swallowing. When the appliance is removed, these cues are withdrawn. The tongue's environment again more closely resembles its former state, when the thrusting habit was present. There is a strong tendency for old habits to return.
3. Its presence often makes proper produc-

tion of sibilant sounds very difficult. The resultant lisp is sometimes only temporary but often persists until the rake is removed. This is a source of embarrassment to the patient and can affect his social verbal behavior and his self-concept.

4. The teeth can be damaged by their use. With regard to cribs and curtains specifically, it has been noted both by Cleall[2] and by Subtelny and Sakuda[22] that the effect on the lower arch, in particular, can be unfortunate. Since these appliances withhold all lingual pressure from the anterior teeth, the frequently hyperactive lower lip is enabled to exert unopposed force on the lower arch. The mandibular teeth move lingually, and crowding often results.

A malocclusion is at all times in a state of functional equilibrium; the dangers of disturbing that balance without making compensation are clearly illustrated in this situation. The loss of precious intercuspid distance alone would result in a poor bargain even if the tongue thrust were eliminated, which is usually not the case.

We prefer the use of such an appliance only when oral myotherapy is contraindicated, such as when the patient is mentally or emotionally not equipped to carry out the assignments in a retraining program. If no myotherapy is available, the rake or crib may be better than no treatment at all. Very infrequently, it can be helpful in keeping the tongue away from the teeth until the palatal arch can be expanded enough to make myotherapy more feasible.

If such a device is used, it is helpful if the orthodontist removes it in stages, removing first the spikes but leaving some kind of crossbar in place for a time. If the crossbar can be reduced in size gradually, this is desirable.

SURGERY

We have heard reports of greatly improved tongue function, for speech as well as for swallowing, after the surgical removal of a triangular wedge from the anterior part of the tongue. In addition to this wedge, Lines and Steinhauser[13] suggest the removal of an oval segment from the central portion of the tongue, leaving the lateral margins intact but reducing the tongue in both length and width. Still another surgical procedure involves the detachment of the genioglossus muscle from the mandibular mental spines. This operation, described by McWilliams and Kent,[15] was performed on 7 patients, all with an anterior open bite and tongue thrust. The genioglossus muscle makes up the body of the tongue and is chiefly responsible for its protrusion. Measurements of protrusive tongue forces were taken twice before surgery and four times postsurgically at ten days, six weeks, three months, and six months.

They report that their patients had difficulty swallowing immediately after surgery but felt comfortable doing so 48 hours afterward. The mean lingual pressure recorded presugically was 4.83, which was reduced to 2.67 after surgery. At the six-month postsurgical recording the mean measurement was 3.22. No orthodontic treatment was instigated, and six months after surgery there were no significant changes in cephalometric and/or plastic model measurements. The authors concluded that detaching the genioglossus muscle significantly reduced the maximum protrusive tongue forces.

The use of this surgical approach as a principal means for tongue thrust and open bite correction must be questioned. The possible usefulness of genioglossus muscle detachment in conjunction with orthodontic treatment or other surgical procedures should be explored. Surgical detachment may be indicated to effect a stable result and to prevent regression.*

Recently, more and more surgery has been carried out for "pseudomesial" cases with functional Class III occlusion apparently caused by a mandibular tongue thrust. Many oral surgeons are claiming to "cure" the thrust simply by keeping the patient's mouth wired shut for six to eight weeks. They are not happy with the relapse ratio but blame endocrine imbalance or uncooperative patients for the lack of permanent success.

We appreciate the caution advised by McWilliams and Kent[15] regarding the use of surgery to alleviate tongue thrust. We of course condone surgery for patients with true marked Class III occlusions, and possibly for others with extremely abnormal oral anatomy, but not as a general procedure for the problem of abnormal swallowing.

HYPNOSIS

Barrett[1] has described the successful use of hypnotherapy with 25 "failure" patients in his own practice. He continues to use hypnotherapy

---

*From McWilliams, R. R., and Kent, J. N.: Effect on protrusive tongue force of detachment of the genioglossus muscle, J. Am. Dent. Ass. **86:**1310, June, 1973.

as an adjunct to his program, particularly for patients who present unusual motivational problems. Several other writers have described hypnotherapy they use with their patients.

In 1965 Crowder[3] listed three types of treatment—mechanical, myofunctional, and psychological—and stated that hypnosis represents the third type of treatment. His hypnotherapy typically involves a series of four appointments spaced approximately one or two weeks apart. At the first appointment impressions are taken of the malocclusion. An explanation of the therapy procedure is given to the patient and to the parents. The patient is then taught to swallow correctly, without the use of a trance. He is instructed to practice for 10 minutes, three times a day. At the second session the child is given an explanation regarding hypnosis and its role in retraining the swallowing. The child imagines a favorite television program or movie be has seen. This induction process is the "sleep-game" technique. During the third and fourth sessions a deeper trance is achieved, and strong posthypnotic suggestions are given to the patient. He is then seen at approximately two-month intervals for the next six months. At these follow-up sessions, reinforcement of the posthypnotic suggestions is given if necessary, but according to Crowder it is not often required.

A similar technique is reported by Secter,[18] who had a child visualize an unpleasant theater scene during a trance, and then through suggestion produced an association between both tongue thrusting and nail biting and the unpleasant feeling the scene aroused in her.

Lambert[12] reported a study involving 12 subjects. The subjects received an average of ten sessions involving hypnotherapy, and of the 12, 10 stopped tongue thrusting.

Palmer[16] reported on 13 patients with whom he had spent an average of 1 hour 21 minutes in a total of five sessions. His finding was that the depth of the trance was not a critical factor in success in therapy. There were no relapses found in 315 days.

Barrett's personal experience with hypnotherapy has been very positive. He does not use it routinely, however, but only with patients who have special problems and only as an adjunct to the later stages of therapy. Hanson uses hypnosis in his therapy for other types of speech and voice problems; he has tried it several times with tongue-thrust patients but prefers not to use it routinely. Both prefer the rapport gained in a simple person-to-person relationship in therapy. We have the following objections to hypnosis in therapy for oral myofunctional disorders:

1. Some subjects require several trance inductions before success is achieved. Although children of the ages of most of our patients are generally good subjects for hypnosis, it has not been easy for us to spot the difficult ones.

2. Many hypnotherapists provide little or no instruction in learning of normal function at the conscious level, prior to trance induction. The complexity of the change from a thrusting pattern to a nonthrusting one makes any expectancy of success with this procedure seem to us to be highly unrealistic.

3. Many parents have antiquated apprehensions about hypnosis. We prefer to use the time it would take to correct these impressions in motivating or training the patient.

4. There is no controlled research attesting to the efficacy of hypnotherapy for this problem.

ORAL MYOTHERAPY

In the United States the treatment approach that has gained widest acceptance is myotherapy. Walter Straub's pioneering efforts in this field were alluded to in Chapter 7. His was the earliest therapy (1) to provide a complete, step-by-step program for the correction of tongue thrust, and (2) to be published in detail and taught as a method to other professionals. It has served as a model for many programs developed subsequently.

Straub program

Faced with a lack of information from research on the relative importance of the various muscles and structures involved in the swallowing process, Straub[21] devised a comprehensive therapy program in an effort to omit no possible contributing factor. His program included speech exercises, muscle-strenthening exercises, and habituation assignments. He modified his program often. We present here a summary of one he used relatively late in his development of procedures.

Before beginning with swallow retraining, the therapist helps the patient to eliminate any harmful habits he may have, including "the leaning habit," stomach sleeping, nail biting, pencil biting, and thumb sucking. Work on the tongue-thrusting problem begins with a thorough oral and speech evaluation and an explanation of the problem and its therapy to the patient.

Lesson 1
1. The differences between normal and tongue-thrust swallowing
2. Proper elastic placement on top of tongue for placement practice
3. Proper occlusion of teeth for swallowing
4. Learning to suck when swallowing

Lesson 2
1. Tongue-popping, or clicking, exercise for placement of middle part of tongue
2. Swallowing with this part of the tongue in position
3. "Choo" exercise, with teeth together

Lesson 3
1. Explanation of rest position of tongue and teeth
2. Word exercises, involving /t/, /s/, /d/, and /n/ sounds

Lesson 4
1. "2-s" exercises—consisting of two parts: the "spot" and the "squeeze"
   a. The "spot"—tongue in position for initiating /ch/ sound, which is proper rest position for tongue
   b. The "squeeze"—tongue squeezed tightly against "spot" several times

Lesson 5
1. "4-s" exercise—placement of tongue on spot; salivation; squeeze; and swallow

Lesson 6
1. Practice of /unka/ sound to create awareness of posterior tongue
2. Practice of /k/ and /g/ sounds

Lesson 7
1. Pushing (by child) of tongue depressor upward with tongue
2. More /k/ practice

Lesson 8
1. Two types of whistling—with lips and with tongue
2. Lateral lip-stretching exercise

Lesson 9 (important for child with open bite or short upper lip)
1. Stretching of upper lip over upper teeth
2. Holding of card between closed lips

Lesson 10 (to eliminate crevice caused by overdeveloped mentalis)
1. Puffing out of lower lip by blowing against it

Lesson 11 (important for child with open bite or lateral thrust)
1. "Slurp" exercise—spread the lips wide apart; close teeth tightly together; suck air back vigorously as tongue is drawn back; then swallow

Lesson 12 (for "side thruster")
1. Swallow is accomplished with sharp instrument extending into oral area at premolar area, with care being taken to avoid touching instrument with tongue

Lesson 13
1. Swallowing of a little water by biting down and sucking the tongue up
2. "Straw-pull" exercise—child holds a straw against roof of mouth with tongue; lips and teeth are apart; he sucks and swallows
3. Practicing saying "kick" and similar words

Lesson 14
1. Yawning practice to stretch throat muscles and pull tongue into back of throat
2. Reviewing of sounds produced by tip, middle, and back of tongue

Lesson 15
1. Gargling taught, so that throat muscles will be strengthened and the tongue pulled downward and backward
2. Elimination of facial grimaces during swallow
3. Patient shown how the hyoid bone moves during swallowing

Lesson 16
1. Exercise of the uvula (raising and lowering)
2. Swallowing with fingers touching lips to check for movement during swallowing

Most oral myologists whose programs are adaptations of Straub's have shortened the part of the program devoted to formal lessons and exercises. Many continue to see the patient for rechecks during the entire period of orthodontic treatment, but few programs we have seen include as many structured lessons as his.

Abbreviated programs

Some clinicians have gone to the other extreme, providing only a brief instruction period and expecting habituation to occur spontaneously. This procedure has sometimes been used by dentists who, not having access to an oral myologist, have made at least a token effort to make their patient conscious of the importance of keeping the tongue away from the teeth. One such program is described by Whitman,[24] who first locates the "spot" with an instrument. He then places a broken-up mint on the dorsum of the tongue. The child holds the mint against the spot as he swallows. This exercise is done "constantly" for three or four days. The patient is then advised to take smaller mouthfuls of food, and to swallow the food in the same manner as he swallowed the mint. Whitman attributes this basic method to an old French dental textbook published in about 1840. In those days, he said, they used buttons, Sen-Sen, or wax instead of mints.

We have seen few children who benefited from this limited type of training. We have also attempted this kind of abbreviated therapy with patients who seemed unusually intelligent and well motivated, or who lived so far away from the clinician that further instruction was not possible. In nearly all of the cases it has not proved to be effective. Swallowing correctly is deceptively easy to teach but difficult to habituate, and many clinicians have fallen into the trap of providing too short a training period for their patients.

Phonetic placement method

Many orthodontists, including Straub, who found it impossible to provide therapy for all of their patients, turned to speech pathologists because of their familiarity with oral anatomy and physiology and their training in the modification of habits. It was natural that the speech pathologists would utilize speech principles and tongue placements and movements in their training programs. One such person was Goda.[8] His approach was to divide the therapy into five goals, as follows:

Goal 1
   The child understands the swallowing process.
Goal 2
   The tongue tip is elevated to the spot. The child repeats the /l/ sound several times, then the /t/ sound, to get the feel of the seal, and the /d/ sound. The child drills on a series of one-syllable words.
Goal 3
   Tongue-tip placement for swallowing saliva and liquids.

An appealing feature of Goda's therapy is the brief, succinct descriptions he teaches the child to remember as he swallows. For liquids and saliva, the three steps are "tongue up, tight seal, swallow." While this goal is being achieved, the child continues to perform the /t/, /d/, and /l/ word drills.

Goal 4
   The child occludes the lips and the teeth. Two new steps are introduced, and the process becomes "food in, chew food, food back, tongue up (seal), and swallow." The child drills on sentences and phrases, including the /t/, /d/, and /l/ sounds.
Goal 5
   Carry-over of tongue-tip placement for all swallows and for speech. The child is instructed to do much self-observation. Reminders are provided, and a checklist is used to ensure compliance with the assignment.

Goda states that this goal is accomplished after ten to twelve weekly meetings, which we understand include all meetings involved in reaching the five goals.

This type of approach appeals to many speech pathologists throughout the United States because of its reliance on positions and movements in speaking. There are some advantages to this type of approach. Those children who do habitually dentalize their linguoalveolar consonants often rest the tongue habitually against the teeth. Attention in therapy to proper habitual rest position and to correct production of these consonants is often complementary. The speech sounds are something the child readily understands, and they provide a good reference and reminder for him. We include attention to speech training for those clients in whom we find the speech to be defective.

There are also inherent disadvantages. Many children with tongue thrust have no accompanying speech problem and must spend considerable time on word drills needlessly. Attention to proper production of the words is often given at the expense of attention to movements and postures involved in proper swallowing. We prefer to work directly with the swallowing movements and resting postures of the oral structures, providing articulation therapy only when articulatory defects are present.

Commercially available programs

A number of clinicians have for several years been offering training courses in myotherapy. Some programs have been printed and are available commercially. We shall summarize the contents of two such programs, including one designed for use with small children.

PICTOGRAPH PROGRAM.[20] The Pictograph program includes a series of six well-structured progressive lessons leading to the establishment of a new swallowing pattern. The exercises are quite comprehensive and give considerable attention to the tongue-tip speech sounds. They are typical of exercises used in other programs throughout the country. The distinguishing feature of this program is its use of visual aids (for showing with an overhead projector) in the education of parents and teachers. Three sets of visual aids are available: (1) *The Speech Clinician Talks With Tongue Thrust Children's Parents*, (2) *The Speech Clinician Talks With Preschool Children's Parents*, and (3) *The Speech Clinician Talks With Teachers*.

Each set contains twelve or thirteen 8½ × 11 inch transparencies that present important information in cartoon fashion. Anatomical illustrations are simple, and the language should be readily understood by lay people. The lessons are printed two to a page and can be handed to the patient or parent at the end of each session. Each set of visual aids is accompanied by a list of suggested comments for the clinician to make as he gives the presentation. This program does an effective job of communicating instructions to those who are asked to help the child.

PROGRAM FOR YOUNG CHILDREN. Pierce and Warvi[17] have written a manual designed to help the myotherapist work with children between the ages of 4 and 9 years. We quote from the instructions to the therapist:

It is our intention that you use this manual as your guide in correcting the deviate swallowing pattern and that you be flexible about supplementing the program with whatever additional exercises the individual child needs for associated oral habits.

This program is designed to cover three very important stages of the therapy process: (1) to build up the muscles and movement patterns necessary for a good swallow, (2) to teach the correct swallow, and (3) to make it a habit.

Lessons 1 to 6: Muscle Training
Lessons 7 to 10: Swallow Training
Lessons 11 to 14: Habituating the Correct Swallow

It has been our experience that this program can be used successfully on the following schedule: Once a week for 10 weeks (Lessons 1 to 10); once a month for four months (Lessons 11 to 14). After completing the

14 lessons, the child should be seen at six-month intervals for two years.

We have also found that this program can be used successfully in either individual or small group therapy.*

This manual uses cartoon-type illustrations to teach and motivate the child. The lessons progress in easy steps, and the successful completion of the lessons requires several months' work. The manual is filled with motivational helps and interesting reminders for the child. After the final lessons are completed, the child is put on a maintenance type of program and is seen periodically for rechecks. He is given a special diploma when he completes the course.

This manual has been written by people who understand the needs and limitations of children. The language used is simple and entertaining.

Research has indicated that some children between the ages of 4 and 7 years will probably continue the tongue-thrust habit into adulthood. Others will spontaneously develop a nonthrusting pattern. We favor therapy for those children in this age range who (1) have severe malocclusions apparently related to tongue thrust (open bite, overjet, overbite, lingual crossbite), (2) are chronic mouth breathers and demonstrate a severe thrusting pattern, (3) reveal a progressively severe malocclusion with the passage of time, and (4) present a number of related abnormal oral habits (thumb sucking, lip biting, tongue thrust, etc.). We caution that from one third to one half of 4- and 5-year-olds who are tongue thrusting are likely to be self-corrective by the time the permanent incisors have fully erupted.

Behavior modification therapy

Behavioral psychologists have developed an approach to therapy for behavioral change that gives the child immediate, attainable rewards; many clinicians have found it to be very helpful in their work with tongue thrust and related problems. Behaviorists have defined learning principles and devised an approach based on these principles that alters behavior in a predetermined, highly structured manner. We will not discuss behavioral *theory* in this chapter but will make an effort to describe enough basic princi-

---

*From Pierce, R. B., and Warvi, V.: Swallow right: a program for the correction of the deviate swallowing pattern in young children, Huntsville, Alabama, 1973, Huntsville Rehabilitation Center, pp. 2-3.

ples and procedures to enable us to show their application in therapy for oral myofunctional problems.

CLASSICAL AND OPERANT CONDITIONING. Conditioning is the process in which a behavioral pattern is repeated enough times under certain conditions to enable an observer to predict its occurrence whenever those conditions occur. Classical conditioning is the kind you learned about in college by studying Pavlov's experiments with dogs. You will remember that by pairing the ringing of a bell with the presentation of food to dogs, he was eventually able to elicit a salivary response from the dogs by presenting the bell stimulus alone. The dogs became conditioned to salivate in response to hearing the bell ring. The ringing of the bell (the stimulus) occurred before the salivation (the response). In classical conditioning this is always the case.

Operant conditioning, on the other hand, begins with a response. The human being enters life with a number of basic responses. His body contains several systems that are not under voluntary control, and others that he is able to control at will. As the infant makes random responses, such as arm and leg movements and vocalizations, adults are often present and respond to his behavior. Consider, for example, the infant cry, which, of course, is a reflexive response, not a conditioned one. As the infant develops, however, he finds that certain things may predictably follow his crying response. His mother may enter the room, pick him up, give him a hug, and hold him for a long time. Since the mother's appearance occurs immediately after (contingent on) the infant's cry, he learns that he can make his mother appear by crying. He learns, in other words, that a certain response pattern causes changes to occur in his environment. When he uses that behavior to bring about those changes, he is "operating" on his environment, and his behavior is called "operant behavior."

In operant conditioning the response occurs first and is followed by a stimulus that encourages or discourages the repetition of the response.

REINFORCEMENT AND PUNISHMENT. When the stimulus, or change in the environment that follows the individual's response, is of such a nature that it encourages the response to be repeated in the future, the response is said to be reinforced. When the stimulus discourages the repetition of the response, it is called punishment. A given stimulus may be a punishment to one child and a reinforcer to another child, or a punishment or reinforcer to the same child under different conditions. Consider again the example of the baby crying. If he has been grossly neglected and finds that the cry brings to him the attention of his mother, he may repeat the cry even though the mother shouts at him menacingly as she approaches him. The shouting and the appearance of the mother occur simultaneously, and even though the shouting is unpleasant, it is better than not having mother with him at all. The shouting, then, becomes associated with a desired stimulus and encourages the crying response to recur. It is therefore a reinforcer, not a punishment for the crying behavior.

Positive and negative reinforcement and punishment. Positive reinforcement is the presentation of a desired stimulus contingent on a response. Examples are a smile, a nod of approval, a piece of candy, a "that's fine," or a hug. Negative reinforcement is the withdrawal of an unwanted stimulus. Examples would include the cessation of a spanking, the disappearance of a parent's scowl, the removal of a pricking pin, the exit of an unpleasant person, or release from an unwanted responsibility, such as helping with the dishes. It is important to understand the distinction between negative reinforcement and punishment. Punishment also has two forms. Both forms *discourage* the repetition of a response. One type of punishment involves the presentation of an unwanted stimulus contingent on a response. An example would be the presentation of pain. Another would be social disapproval in its many forms. Still another would be the requirement of the performance of an unpleasant task. The second type of punishment is the withdrawal of a desired stimulus, such as prohibiting certain types of play activities, "grounding" the child, or not allowing him to eat dessert. Both types of punishment diminish the probability of recurrence of the response that preceded them.

Primary and secondary reinforcers. Primary reinforcers are stimuli that feel, taste, or smell good, or are in some other way innately pleasurable, such as a push from a parent to a child in a swing, a piece of candy or stick of gum, a warm smile, a "that's good!" a movie, an affectionate squeeze. Secondary reinforcers are stimuli that can be redeemed or converted into something that is innately pleasurable. Poker chips, money, check marks on a chart, or tokens of any kind are examples. Secondary reinforcers are often preferable to primary reinforcers during therapy for the following reasons:

1. They can be presented or withdrawn, according to the response of the patient. To take candy away from a child when he makes an inappropriate response is to arouse his emotions negatively toward the clinician and the therapy; to matter-of-factly take away a token is not so painful to the child.

2. The child does not have to be hungry at the moment to want to work for a token.

3. With primary reinforcers there is always the problem of whether to give the food, for example, to the child immediately or to wait until the end of the session. Either solution produces distractions. Tokens can be given immediately after correct responses.

4. Tokens are more flexible. A certain number of tokens can represent anything the clinician and patient, or parent and child, agree they will represent.

5. A hard-working patient can be "full" before the session is over if primary reinforcers such as candy are used. This problem does not occur when tokens are presented to him.

Reinforcement schedules. A child may be reinforced each time he produces a given behavior, or he may be reinforced inconsistently. In therapy, the schedule of reinforcement used initially is often "crf" (continuous reinforcement). Each time a child produces a desired response he receives the token, plus mark, or favorable comment from the clinician. The schedule may then progress to a fixed-interval or a fixed-ratio schedule. If the child is rewarded for every second correct response or every third or fourth one, the therapist is following a fixed-interval schedule. If the presentation of the reward depends on a predetermined ratio of correct to incorrect responses, the schedule being followed is a fixed-ratio type. The next schedule to be employed as therapy progresses is often the variable one in which the stimulus is presented in random, unpredictable patterns so that the child never knows when a given response is going to be rewarded. This type of progressive change in schedule has the advantage of gradually weaning the child from those types of reinforcement schedules that he is not likely to find in everyday, outside-the-clinic living. The child who is being assisted in the elimination of a thumb-sucking habit must learn to keep the thumb out of his mouth even when there is no one else in the room but himself. The tongue thruster must learn to swallow correctly under all types of conditions, day and night, and his correct swallows are not going to be rewarded by a nod of approval after therapy has terminated.

The same principle, that of preparing the child for the reinforcement situations of everyday life by progressively making reinforcement more closely approximate what he will expect to find in daily life, should be applied in determining the type of reinforcement to be utilized. If it is necessary, in order to achieve satisfactory motivation, to use primary reinforcers such as candy or alphabet cereal at the beginning of therapy, it is wise to structure the training to include a gradual elimination of these types of reinforcers. As therapy progresses, the candy should gradually be replaced by social reinforcers. These reinforcers should then, in turn, be presented with less and less frequency, until finally the child learns to depend totally on his own awareness of his correct swallowing patterns for reinforcement. That type of reinforcement is best, in other words, which most closely approximates the types of reinforcement the child will receive in everyday life.

STEPS IN BEHAVIOR MODIFICATION. Three basic steps are involved in operant conditioning: (1) establishing base line, (2) modifying behavior, and (3) extending stimulus control.

Establishing base line. "Base line" is the starting point for therapy. It is the behavior which the patient has in his repertoire that most closely resembles the behavior the therapist wants him to habituate. A given behavioral pattern, such as a tongue-thrust swallow, may require the establishment of several related base lines, due to the complexity of the muscle interaction involved. Base line for a child who sucks his thumb might be his behavior when he is in the presence of someone who is not a member of his immediate family. He may not suck his thumb in that situation but does so in all other situations, that is, when he is alone or with members of his family. The desired behavior is the cessation of thumb sucking. His behavior when he is with nonmembers of the family is the behavior that most closely resembles the goal behavior—the complete elimination of thumb sucking. It is a place from which to begin.

Modifying behavior. Modification of behavior is often not too difficult while the patient is in the therapy situation. The behavior is "shaped" in a systematic, step-by-step manner until it conforms to the desired pattern. A shaping procedure that brings about a series of alterations in behavior, each of which brings the person nearer the ultimate goal, is called successive approximation. During this process, the appropriate reinforcers and/or punishments are used. Each step must be satisfactorily completed before the patient advances to the next step. The criteria for successfully completing each step are well defined and often expressed in terms of percentages. For example, a therapist may be helping a child to eliminate the dentalization of the linguoalveolar sounds /t/, /d/, /n/, and /l/. The child may be asked to tell a story that lasts for 5 minutes. The therapist counts the number of linguoalveolar sounds produced during the time period, and then tallies the number he produced defectively. If more than 10% were defective, the child is not allowed to proceed to the next step, which may be in this case a part of the third step, extension of stimulus control.

Extending stimulus control. It is not difficult, in most cases, for a child to understand how to swallow correctly. Basically, he is to form a seal between the tongue and the roof of the mouth, rather than between the tongue and the cheeks, lips, or teeth. The explaining can be accomplished in a relatively short time, but understanding is, of course, not the goal of therapy. The goal is to help the child make new muscle patterns so habitual that they become a part of his subconscious motor activity. This is the purpose of the third step, extension of stimulus control. We used to call this "carry-over" in speech therapy, back in the days when we called speech therapy " speech therapy." "Extension of stimulus control" is a better term because it more accurately describes the procedure involved in reaching the goal of subconscious habituation. In our opinion this step should not be considered accomplished until the myofunctional disorder has disappeared completely from the patient's behavior. This step must be equally as systematized as the preceding step. When therapy fails to be completely successful, it is most often due to a lackadaisical attitude on the part of the therapist, patient, or parent with regard to the specifics of achieving this step. This part of therapy is also the most misunderstood; many parents have the mistaken notion that once a child has learned to do something or has learned to stop doing something, failure to apply what he has learned indicates laziness, lack of motivation, or negativeness on his part. A goal-directed plan is extremely important in this stage of therapy.

The therapy program presently followed by Hanson, described in Chapter 26, contains several applications of behavior modification principles.

Cassette program

Zickefoose[25] has developed an approach to therapy utilizing tape cassettes. Instructions are recorded during the therapy sessions and taken home by the patient. This procedure, according to Zickefoose, has several advantages. It eliminates much of the misunderstanding that results when assignments are written out or merely remembered. The need for involvement of parents is lessened in practices and the use of the tape recorder is enjoyable for the young patient. Use of the tapes is continued through the habituation stage of treatment, when they are played at night. Zickefoose reports improved motivation, better parent-child interaction regarding therapy and practicing, and quicker, more satisfying results following this procedure.

Neuromuscular facilitation

Falk, Wells, and Toth[6] have developed a treatment program for tongue thrust based on procedures used by Margaret Rood. The approach is subcortical, designed to condition proper muscle tone and action by stimulating the sensory receptors. Details of the method are presented by Falk[7] in a later article.

Three types of stimulation constitute the treatment: brushing, icing, and pressure. The purpose of brushing is to reduce flaccidity of the tongue. The sides of the tongue are stroked repeatedly with a No. 6 oil paint brush, for ten seconds. The exercise results in a narrowing of the tongue and improved tonicity.

Icing consists of applying ice to the hard palate, in the area of the incisal papilla, for about ten seconds. This results in a reflexive elevation of the blade of the tongue to the area iced. Falk asserts that the focus of therapy should be to elevate the blade of the tongue, rather than its tip, as advocated by most clinicians.

Light pressure is applied to the dorsal and inferior surfaces of the tongue with the rounded end of a cocktail stick. The tongue is held in a relaxed position as the clinician taps the anterior part of the tongue in a rapid, alternating manner. The result is a posterior movement of the tongue, according to Falk. Pressure to the lateral aspects of the tongue is applied in some patients to supplement the brushing exercise. Pressures are applied for only a few seconds.

Patients are instructed to carry out the above procedures before each meal and at least two other times in addition, for a total of five or six practice sessions a day. Sessions are brief, requiring only a minute or two. The regimen is typically continued for six months. Except for occasional attention to specific needs of individual patients, such as strengthening of the muscles of mastication, these procedures comprise the whole of Falk's treatment. He tested its effectiveness with an experimental group of eleven patients[6] and found that all subjects experienced a reduction in severity of anterior malocclusions during the six months of therapy. Nine of the eleven demonstrated no regression during that period. There was no control group in this study.

In a subsequent study, however, Falk[7] compared this type of treatment with a more traditional approach to tongue thrust. Two clinicians, both trained in procedures advocated by Daniel Garliner *and* the Falk et al., method, were each assigned two groups of five patients each, ages eight to twelve years. Each clinician treated five subjects with each approach. The subjects received six months of training.

Serial dental models were made before treatment, after three and six months of treatment, and six months following termination of therapy. Fourteen orthodontists judged the dental models in pairs, indicating whether one of the pair was "same," "better," or "worse" than the other. In addition, each judge indicated on a seven-point equal-appearing-intervals scale the amount of improvement each subject had made during the six-month course of treatment.

Both groups were judged as having made significant improvement toward normal occlusion following treatment. To a statistically significant degree:

1. Subjects treated with neuromuscular facilitation were more improved after three months of training than were subjects receiving treatment utilizing the Garliner approach
2. A similar significant difference in improvement favoring the Falk treatment group was found after six months of treatment
3. No significant regression in dentition was found in either group after six months following treatment

KINESIOLOGY

We should take cognizance of some of the concepts presented under the general heading of kinesiology. Special applications of this field, specifically of a dental nature, have been appearing with regularity. Since kinesiology is customarily considered to be the study of muscles and muscular movement, it behooves the oral myologist to be aware of these developments.

Among the leading spokesman for this aspect of kinesiology have been Goodhart,[9] a chiropractor; Eversaul,[4] a psychologist; Diamond, a physician; and dentists such as May, Mittelman, and others. Fryman, an osteopathic physician who practices and teaches *cranial osteopathy,* might be considered a part of this movement.

While kinesiological procedures are often presented as an adjunct to oral myotherapy (or vice versa), they are sometimes proposed as the sole requirement for remediation. Suggested procedures, in addition to those designed to elevate the tongue and correct tongue thrust, include others to improve jaw relationships, to remove muscle spasm, to strengthen or weaken muscle reaction, to eliminate the gag reflex, to increase the range of mouth opening, and to change the fatigue rate in muscles throughout the body. For example, any muscle can be shown to fatigue more quickly if a few grains of refined sugar or other noxious substance is placed in the mouth. The same effect is shown even if the sugar, or a cigarette, is merely held in the hand rather than the mouth.

Another application of the foregoing is found in *therapy localization.* This is a diagnostic method in which the patient is asked to touch his fingertips to a suspected problem area, a TMJ, for example; should dysfunction be present, any muscle group in the arm or leg which has previously tested at normal strength will now show less resistance or will fatigue more quickly.

Remediation in basic kinesiology consists primarily of muscle manipulation. In cranial osteopathy it is achieved by adjusting the supposedly immovable bones of the skull.

There is also some reliance on "temple tapping." This is a procedure wherein the clinician offers a suggestion while tapping the patient's temple sharply and rapidly with fingertips; the suggestion is then rephrased while tapping the opposite temple. The effect of the suggestion or command is then manifested by the patient; for example, for a time thereafter he no longer gags when mechanically stimulated to do so.

BIOFEEDBACK

Attempts to utilize biofeedback for the correction of oral myofunctional problems have been made in some quarters. When conventional equipment has been pressed into this service, the results have generally been disappointing. However, Shepard[19] has developed an instrument specifically designed for this purpose.

Shepard came to dentistry from an engineering background, and after twenty years in pedodontics returned to his original interest and designed the Bio-My Master. His latest refinement is seen in Fig. 13-2, the Bio-My Master II. This is a six-channel instrument with both surface and intraoral probes. The surface probe may be positioned over any basic muscle for either diagnostic or therapeutic use; it is also able to reveal differences in strength between upper and lower fibers of the orbicularis oris.

The intraoral probe monitors tongue position, supplying the patient and clinician with both visual and auditory feedback. The visual display consists of the palatal arch and maxillary teeth; as the tongue contacts the palate or teeth, or when teeth occlude, corresponding diodes light up on the display. At the same time, each location is represented by a different tone, providing auditory feedback.

Shepard suggests many applications of the in-strument, but does not propose it as the sole means of remediation. Rather, he utilizes a full program of muscle retraining, measured, motivated, and expedited by the use of the machine. He has also developed an instrument called the Bio-My Satellite, described in Chapter 23, to assist in subconscious habit-strengthening of acquired patterns.

SUMMARY

Many treatment approaches have been reported by qualified people to be successful in treating oral myofunctional disorders. We have reviewed some of them, including the use of appliances, surgery, hypnosis, abbreviated therapy, prolonged therapy, and behavior modification therapy. Patients sometimes present special problems that warrant the choice of a nontherapy approach, either as a substitute for, or as a supplement to, myotherapy. Most patients, though, can be most effectively treated by applying sound principles of motivation and learning in a well-planned but flexible therapy program. We have discussed behavioral modification at length. Some clinicians are opposed to the philosophy of using extrinsic rewards to

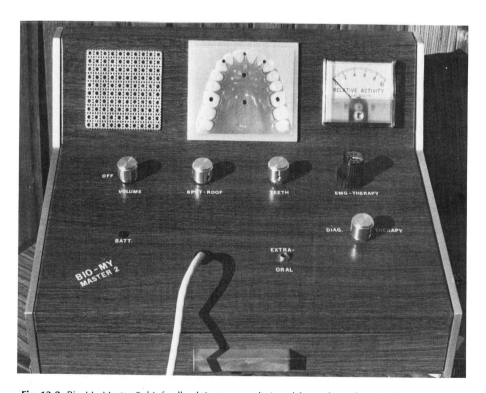

Fig. 13-2. Bio-My Master 2, biofeedback instrument designed for oral myofunctional rehabilitation.

achieve motivation in patients. Others find them helpful with certain patients, and still others routinely use them effectively.

There are many programs and approaches to therapy that we have excluded from this chapter. A beginning clinician often yields to the pressure to adopt either the program he *first* learns about or the one whose advocate has the most persuasive personality. Our advice is to consider the following questions in evaluating a particular program:

1. Does every exercise and assignment have a specific purpose?
2. Is there any unnecessary duplication of exercises?
3. Is the succession of skills planned so that each new step builds on previous ones?
4. Is it adaptable to the needs of patients of all ages?
5. Does it allow for periodic reevaluations of the patient's progress?
6. Does it include proper emphasis on resting postures of orofacial muscle?
7. Are appropriate motivational procedures included?
8. Does it provide for necessary feedback to the patient, his parents, and the therapist, so that each can objectively know of the patient's progress?
9. Does it include attention to all related orofacial habits?

The development of treatment methods in this field has paralleled that of other sciences dealing with the modification of human behavior. Before methods are adequately tested and compared, years or even decades are spent in clinical experimentation and development. Programs are adopted by many clinicians merely because they exist, or because their developers are respected or are simply effective salesmen. Certainly we are at the stage when relative effectiveness of various approaches needs to be scientifically determined.

REFERENCES

1. Barrett, R. H., and von Dedenroth, T. E. A.: Problems of deglutition, Am. J. Clin. Hypno. **9:**161, 1967.
2. Cleall, J. F.: Deglutition: a study of form and function, Am. J. Orthod. **51:**566, 1965.
3. Crowder, H. M.: Hypnosis in the control of tongue thrust swallowing habit patterns, Am. J. Clin. Hypno. **8:**10, 1965.
4. Eversaul, G. A.: Biofeedback and kinesiology: technologies for preventive dentistry, J. Am. Soc. Prevent. Dent. **6:**19-23, 1976.
5. Falk, M. L., Delaney, J. R., and Litt, R. L.: Comparison of selected cortical-level and reflexive-level treatment programs for establishing normal deglutition patterns. Unpublished paper.
6. Falk, M. L., Wells, M., and Toth, S.: A subcortical approach to swallow pattern therapy, Am. J. Orthod. **70:**419-422, 1976.
7. Falk, M. L.: Treatment of deviant swallow patterns with neuromuscular facilitation, Int. J. Oral Myology **3:**27-29, 1977.
8. Goda, S.: The role of the speech pathologist in the correction of tongue thrust, Am. J. Orthod. **54:** 852, 1968.
9. Goodhart, G. J.: Kinesiology and dentistry, J. Am. Soc. Prevent. Dent. **6:**16-18, 1976.
10. Graber, T. M., and Neuman, B.: Removable orthodontic appliances, Philadelphia, 1977, W. B. Saunders Co.
11. Kaye, S. R.: Modified appliance to control tongue-thrust, Dental Survey, pp. 24-25, Aug., 1973.
12. Lambert, C. G.: Hypnotherapy in control of tongue thrust occurring during perverted swallowing, Abst. Am. J. Orthod. **45:**869, 1959.
13. Lines, P. A., and Steinhauser, E. W.: Diagnosis and treatment planning in surgical orthodontic therapy, Am. J. Orthod. **66:**378, 1974.
14. Littman, J. Y.: A practical approach to the tongue-thrust problem, J. Pract. Orthod. **2:**138, March, 1968.
15. McWilliams, R. R., and Kent, J. N.: Effect on protrusive tongue force of detachment of the genioglossus muscle, J. Am. Dent. Assoc. **86:**1310, June, 1973.
16. Palmer, G. L.: The effectiveness of post-hypnotic suggestion upon control of the tongue-thrust habit in relation to trance depth, Abst. Am. J. Orthod. **47:**228, 1961.
17. Pierce, R. B., and Warvi, V.: Swallow right, Huntsville, Ala., 1973, Huntsville Rehabilitation Center.
18. Secter, L. L.: Tongue thrust and nail biting simultaneously treated during hypnosis: a case report, Am. J. Clin. Hypno. **4:**51, 1961.
19. Shepard, R. S.: Personal communications.
20. The speech clinician talks series, Boulder, Colo., (P.O. Box 2099), Pictograph Corporation.
21. Straub, W. J.: Malfunction of the tongue, Part III, Am. J. Orthod. **48:**486, 1962.
22. Subtelny, J. D., and Sakuda, M.: Open bite: diagnosis and treatment, Am. J. Orthod. **50:**337, 1964.
23. Walker, R. V., and Collins, T. A.: Surgery or orthodontics—a philosophy of approach, Dent. Clin. North Am. **15:**771, 1971.
24. Whitman, C. L.: Correction of oral habits, Dent. Clin. North Am., p. 541, 1964.
25. Zickefoose, W. E.: Personal communications.

Chapter 14

OTHER ORAL HABITS

The profession of oral myology originally grew out of a concern solely for tongue thrusting. After the "pernicious habit" of tongue thrusting was identified as a faulty manner of deglutition, it became logical to look at function rather than confining attention to structure. However, this pursuit so dominated the attention of clinicians that other harmful oral habits were ignored. Unfortunately, this narrow view still persists in some quarters. The present-day oral myologist should be prepared to recognize and treat any counterproductive function of the orofacial musculature.

GENERAL CONSIDERATIONS
Types of habits

A complete and useful list of oral habits was formulated by E. T. Klein[9] over a quarter of a century ago. It is reproduced with some deletions:

A. *Intraoral habits*
1. Thumb sucking
2. Finger sucking
3. Tongue sucking
4. Lip sucking
5. Cheek sucking
6. Blanket sucking
7. Nail biting
8. Lip biting
9. Tongue biting
10. Mouth breathing
B. *Extraoral habits*
1. Chin propping
2. Face leaning on hand
3. Abnormal pillowing positions
4. Habitual sleeping on one side of the face

To Klein's list could be added bruxing, lip licking, tongue rubbing (rubbing the tongue in an up-and-down motion on the lingual surfaces of the incisors), and many others. Chapter 16 will be devoted to digit and tongue sucking, comprising the first three items on the list; the balance will be discussed in this chapter.

ETIOLOGIES

The etiology of other oral habits appears to be similar to that of tongue thrust, in that both behaviors have been observed in fetuses and both are very prevalent in infancy. A review of etiologies by Gellin[5] refers to three studies, involving a total of over 3,800 children, which agree in finding about 50% of infants and preschool children to be engaged in "extra-nutrition" sucking. Our efforts to determine etiology need to be directed toward discovering why certain children *persist* in the habits beyond the age when other children discontinue them.

Proposed causes of oral habits may be divided into three categories: physiological, emotional, and conditioned learning.

Physiological causes

Enlarged adenoids, a deviated septum, swollen nasal turbinates, nasal polyps, and other physiological conditions often lead to mouth breathing, an undesirable habit in itself and an important factor in tongue thrust. Faulty occlusion may lead to an habitual open-mouth position and to abnormal chewing habits. Rabuck[20] explains how premature occlusal contacts can result in bruxism. When normal compensatory movements fail to produce a comfortable closure, reflex mechanisms are activated which result in painful muscle spasm. The patient, in an effort to avoid the pain, moves the jaw from one premature contact to another and frequently develops a bruxing habit.

Emotional causes

With the exception of mouth-breathing, most oral habits are probably caused and/or perpetuated by emotional disturbances. Any condition or stimulus which upsets a child's sense of security or sense of worth may produce tensions which result in oral habits. This topic is the basis for several books, and will not be dealt with in great depth in this chapter. Examples of such factors are:

Excessive parental demands, related to cleanliness, mature behavior, and accepting responsibilities

Inconsistency within behavior of either parent, or between the parents

The birth of a sibling

An abnormally high ratio of negative to positive verbal and nonverbal input from parents

Teasing, criticism, or physical abuse from siblings

Rejection from parents, siblings, or peers

Forced inhibition of normal avenues of expression for anxieties and fears

Repeated or prolonged separation from one or both parents

Frequent moves from one locale to another

Gorelick[7] found a statistically significantly greater number of foster children between the ages of 6 and 10, and 11 and 15, to be sucking their thumbs than his private patients. He concluded that the greater incidence was due to the general insecurity found in the foster children.

The mouth, an early and perdurable zone of pleasure, is a natural resource for the child or adult seeking relief from anxiety. Its stimulation with a finger or thumb, tongue, fingernail, blanket, pacifier, or cigarette is a universal tranquilizer.

Learning

Oral habits may be randomly learned behaviors. A cheek may accidentally wedge between the upper and lower canines as the person listens during a conversation. It may relieve some of the uneasiness experienced when one is being looked at very intently. The act of cheek biting is thus reinforced and is likely to be repeated during a subsequent, similar experience. Faulty sleeping postures would seem to be the products of selective reinforcement. This third type of cause is not, of course, separable from the first two. An act may be repeated to bring about a

desired physiological or emotional state, either to avoid an unwanted stimulus, or to secure a wanted one.

Research into etiology of oral habits is extremely difficult to do. Relationships among various behaviors, and between them and physical and emotional factors are studied extensively, but without the essential design and controls that would enable the researcher to conclude that A caused B. The implausibility of holding several factors constant in human subjects in order to isolate a given behavior for study is so well known that any elaboration on it would be superfluous. When we are confronted with a patient with an oral habit, we try to consider all the possible contributors to the problem and do our best to eliminate or modify whatever factors we can.

INFLUENCES ON SPEECH

It is obviously difficult to talk while sucking one's thumb, biting one's lower lip, bruxing, chewing on a pencil, or sucking one's tongue. Thus, oral habits may directly inhibit speech production. A less direct relationship between oral habits and speech may be found when the two behaviors are linked to a common cause, such as insecurity or general tensions in the home. The number of interrelationships among these three phenomena, speech problems, oral habits, and emotional problems, is limitless. A few of them are presented in the following paragraphs.

Oral habits may produce malocclusions and physiological alterations which, in turn, may have an effect on speech. Thumbsucking can restrict the width of the arch, making sibilant sounds difficult to produce. A number of case studies are presented by Dunlap and Streicher[3] to demonstrate that lateral lisps often result from oral habits. One student was found to be keeping his little finger under his tongue persistently and consistently. Another held his index finger under his tongue and held it in place by turning the tongue over to hold it between his teeth. Still another held a lock of hair in her mouth across the top of the tongue. Other cases were described, and the authors proposed a theory based on 1,200 cases. The substance of the theory is as follows.

Vegetative oral movements occur prenatally. Postnatally developed speech functions have to coexist with the earlier appearing, more important responses. An efficient oral mechanism functions in both areas effectively. The introduction into the system of abnormal stimuli, whether in the form of external objects, or of a malpositioned tongue or finger, interferes with normal development processes, and speech development is hindered. A common problem among these patients is a lateral lisp. At times the lisp is not present while the habit is occurring, but is evident when the finger or foreign object is removed.

The presence of a lateral lisp in children whose palatal clefts were closed surgically at an early age is common. The resultant narrowing of the palatal arch makes it difficult for the tongue to accomplish the lateral linguoalveolar and linguodental seal, so a substitute, defective phoneme is emitted. A narrowing of the arch resulting from habits often has the same effect on the sibilants.

Mouth breathing can produce a short, incompetent upper lip, which yields its function in the production of bilabial sounds to the upper incisors.

One-sided habits, such as jaw-leaning, object sucking, and sleeping postures can result in asymmetries which require compensatory movements for speech production. Some persons succeed in their efforts, and others accept approximations that fall short of producing acoustically normal speech.

ORAL HABITS AND MALOCCLUSIONS

Davidian[2] asserts that pressures upon the mandible of the fetus can affect the size and shape of the jaw in the adult. The fetus' arm may be placed under the mandible in such a way as to inhibit growth. Insufficient amniotic fluid diminishes the amount of protection afforded the growing structures and may produce abnormalities in the face.

In the young child, persistent, vigorous thumbsucking can tilt the maxillary incisors labially and/or laterally. The mandibular incisors may be tipped lingually as well. Leaning on a fist may inhibit the growth of the mandible. Bilateral pressure against the mandible produced by leaning on both hands at once may, in addition to restricting the forward mandibular growth, result in a bilateral crossbite in the molar regions.[2] Fluhrer stated:

Chin leaning will cause the bite to be closed if the pressure is exerted on the underside of the chin, and the writer has observed at least a dozen skulls which illustrate this deformity. The anterior one-half of these

mandibles is bent upward, graphically revealing the effects of this pressure.*

Biting or licking the lower lip can cause a forward shifting of the upper incisors.

Gellin[5] contends that thumbsucking has a deleterious effect on children with "poor" bites, but has little or no effect on the "good" bites. Gellin refers to a study by Benjamin,[1] which found definite correlations between malocclusion, in primary and permanent teeth, and thumbsucking.

Warren[25] observed 100 eleven-year-olds in Denmark to determine habitual mentalis muscle function, then examined their occlusions, He found that 67% of the patients with malocclusions showed a marked mentalis muscle function, whereas in only 7% did the muscle remain passive. Among patients whose occlusion was normal, the figures were almost reversed; in only 5% was the mentalis muscle active, and in 62%, passive. Of the 100, 31 children had active mentalis function; 90% of the 31 had malocclusions. Ninety-two percent of the 39 patients with a passive mentalis muscle had no malocclusion.

Posen[18] studied maximum lip and tongue forces in 135 subjects aged 8 to 18 years, and drew several conclusions regarding tongue and lip functions and malocclusions. One of these related to Class II, Division 2. He stated:

The evidence is strong that it is the significantly great lip force that is a contributing factor, or indeed the main cause for the central incisors assuming this lingual inclination.

The maxillary lateral incisors are forced to assume a more labial position because they are squeezed between the deciduous canines and the lingually erupted central incisors.

The evidence presented so far seems to indicate rather strongly that in Class II, Division 2 and in some types of Class I the incisors are positioned lingually as a result of the activity of a strong perioral musculature.†

Posen's findings also implicated lip habits in the development of bimaxillary dentoalveolar protrusions. In this case the habit is an habitual lips-apart posture. Patients with this habit con-

---

*From Fluhrer, A. V.: Some original investigations into pressure habits as etiological factors in dentofacial abnormalities, Pacific Coast Soc. Orthod., 1957.

†From Posen, A. L.: The influence of maximum perioral and tongue force on the incisor teeth, Angle Orthod. **42:**285-309, 1972.

sistently exhibited a low maximum lip pressure. The absence of contant lip pressure on the anterior teeth allows them to migrate forward, and severe periodontal problems may occur at a relatively young age.

Gingold[6] attributes open bite to digit sucking, lip sucking, or tongue thrusting; crowding and rotation of anterior teeth to nail biting; overjet to tongue thrust, mouth breathing, lip biting, or lip sucking; incisor crowding or lingual inclination to excessive habitual neck and head postures. Gingold's plea is to eliminate these deleterious habits early as a preventive measure.

SPECIFIC ORAL HABITS
Mouth breathing

CAUSES. The causes of mouth breathing were described above. Basically, any impairment of the nasal airway can cause oral respiration. It is not the result of indolence. In some patients, the antigravity muscles in the tongue and jaw have not developed adequately, so that resting tonus is not equal to the task of maintaining normal elevation and allowing effortless lip closure. These patients may continue to breathe nasally even with the mouth ajar; whether or not breath passes through the oral cavity, both dentition and deglutition suffer.

EFFECTS. A comprehensive review of literature on mouth breathing leads any reader to conclude that this habit does not have a friend in the world. No one has anything good to say about mouth breathing. Its causes and effects are quite well known by the lay public. Our discussion will be limited to its relevance to occlusion. Typical beliefs among dentists regarding malocclusions resulting from mouth breathing are summarized by Sood and Verma.[24] (1) The upper incisors are protruded and spaced, due to the loss of the molding effect of the closed lips. (2) The upper arch is narrowed, due to the loss of the molding effect of the tongue. (3) The maxilla becomes V shaped, due to the contraction of the buccal segments and the protrusion of the anterior teeth.

The observations of Sood and Verma have been tested experimentally by Paul and Nanda,[16] who analyzed dental models of 100 15- to 20-year-old males, equally divided into mouth breathers and nasal breathers. They found significant differences in maxillary arch dimensions and in anterior occlusions between the two groups. Maxillary arch width was less in the mouth breathers. The authors postulated that

this lengthening resulted from the contraction of the width of the arch. Although the palatal arches in the mouth breathers appeared to be lower, no significant difference between groups was found.

Both overjet and overbite were more prevalent in the mouth-breathing subjects, and in both cases the difference was highly significant ($P <$ .001). Seventy-four percent of the mouth breathers had a Class II malocclusion.

The findings of Paul and Nanda contradicted those of Linder-Aronson[10] and Backstrom,[12] who found no significant differences in overjet, overbite, or arch width between groups of nose breathers and mouth breathers. A later study by Linder-Aronson, however, obtained results essentially in agreement with those of Paul and Nanda.[11] This research dealt primarily with nasal airflow and adenoidal tissue, and found that children with large adenoids had low nasal airflow, as would be expected. Linder-Aronson also found that children with large adenoids held the tongue habitually low in the mouth. Significant relationships were found between large adenoids and a narrow upper arch, crossbite or a tendency to crossbite, and retroclined lower and upper incisors. Linder-Aronson attributed the retroclined upper incisors to be due to the influence of the muscles of the upper lip when the mouth was held open.

Another study by Nanda and colleagues[14] was conducted on 2,500 2- to 6-year-old children in Lucknow, India. Mouth breathing was found in 27.3% of the children. Relationships between the presence of tongue thrust and mouth breathing were not reported, but children having both habits were found to have fewer Class I and more Class III occlusions. There was no significant difference between these children and children with no oral habits with respect to the incidence of Class II occlusions.

Ricketts[22] found underdevelopment of the oral musculature and varying degrees of distoclusion in 85% of the children with mouth breathing he studied.

Watson, Warren, and Fischer[26] found no relationships between the presence of mouth breathing and skeletal classification in 20 orthodontic patients with mouth breathing.

As usual, in studies concerned with human subjects, research findings relating mouth breathing to occlusion are inconsistent. One of the most important reasons for the inconsistency is the subjectiveness involved in labeling a subject as *either* a mouth breather *or* a nose breather. In reality, most people are either *predominantly* one or the other, and methods for determining the *degree* of mouth or nose breathing are subjective, even when considered, and are rarely even considered.

Nevertheless, the preponderance of studies has found significant relationships between mouth breathing and structural characteristics of the oral cavity. Subjects who habitually breathe through the mouth tend to have narrow maxillary arches; crossbites in the molar area; either overjet or retroclined upper and lower incisors; overbite or open bite, and something other than a Class I occlusion. The presence or direction of cause and effect relationships have not been determined, but most writers implicate mouth breathing as a causative factor in oral structural abnormalities.

TREATMENT

Therapy. The oral myologist should be trained to make a determination, after obtaining a case history and examining the oral cavity, of whether a referral to a medical doctor for further evaluation is necessary. If the clinician concludes that the habit may be only functional, he should help the patient eliminate the problem as a first step in treatment of tongue thrust. If not, referral to an ear-nose-throat specialist, or an allergist, is necessary. Most patients who habitually mouth breathe can now be successfully treated by surgery, medication, or desensitization measures. Either in the absence of the need for medical treatment, or following such treatment, the patient proceeds more effectively to establish nasal breathing with help from a therapist. Specific suggestions for promoting habitual lip closure are given throughout most of the remaining chapters of this book.

Mechanical devices. A number of devices have been developed to aid in establishing nasal breathing. Several of these are described in Chapter 13. Devices often prescribed are: (1) an oral screen; (2) the Andresen appliance; (3) the Bionator; and (4) the "anti-snore" mask (see Chapter 25).

The difficulty with these devices comes when the patient *stops* using them. If the "weaning" can be done gradually, chances of success are greater. If their use is discontinued abruptly, a return to old habits frequently occurs. Nearly all our referring dentists use them only as a last device, when all other approaches have failed, if at all.

Bruxism

Bruxism is usually defined as any nonfunctional grinding or clenching of teeth. "Nonfunctional" refers to the vegetative functions, of course, because bruxism may well be serving some psychological function. The loud noises produced by bruxing during sleep often cannot be reproduced by the same person during waking hours, which is indicative of the great amount of force being applied to the biting and chewing surfaces of the teeth. In other patients, the grinding occurs without any noise, and the patient is unaware that he has the habit.

The incidence of bruxism, as reported by Reding, Rubright, and Zimmerman,[21] is 5.1% in the 16- to 36-year age group, and 15% in the 3- to 17-year group.

CAUSES. The habit is most frequently attributed to psychogenic factors or to local irritating factors or combinations of the two. Psychologically, the bruxer may be expressing anger, hostility, or tension.

An excellent summary of the problem of bruxism is written by Meklas,[13] who lists several *local* factors in bruxing:

1. Discrepancies between centric relation and occlusion
2. Tipped or otherwise malposed teeth
3. High restorations
4. Chronic inflammation of the periodontal membrane
5. Differences in or uneven eruption of teeth
6. Presence of unusually steep cusps
7. Tight occlusion
8. Overcarving of restorations
9. Rough or chipped enamel or restorations

The bruxing, then, represents an effort of the patient to alleviate pain, discomfort, or pressures caused by dental irregularities.

EFFECTS. Symptoms of bruxing include: (1) nonmasticatory occlusal wear; (2) soreness and/or sensitiveness of the teeth; (3) loose teeth due to periodontal damage; (4) muscle fatigue, spasm, or pain; (5) cheek, lip, or tongue biting; and (6) headaches.[19]

TREATMENT. Treatment methods vary, but dentists agree that the first step is to try to determine what factors are contributing to the persistence of the habit. Any remediable local factors should be taken care of first. Various appliances are constructed to preclude harmful dental contacts. Direct instructions to the patient are given, such as resting with the lips together and the teeth slightly apart. As in the treatment of mouth breathing, suggestions for relaxation and proper resting postures of the teeth and tongue may be given while the patient is going to sleep or during sleep. Hypnosis has been found to be helpful with several of our own patients. Some clinicians use ''negative practice,'' wherein the patients grind their teeth several times a day consciously. It is relatively easy to achieve temporary improvement in bruxing patients, but relapses are common. If repeated failure in therapy occurs with a patient, referral for a psychological or psychiatric evaluation is in order.

Lip habits

The four conditions that we wish to address in this section include lip malposture, lip and cheek biting, lip licking, and lip sucking.

MALPOSTURE OF THE LIPS

Causes. The causes of lip malposture trace directly to lip nonfunction in mouth breathing, and lip malfunction in deglutition, plus a few inborn jaw relationships, such as extreme upper or lower protrusion, which impel the lips in improper directions.

Effects. The lips exercise an optimal molding effect on the upper and lower teeth when they rest together habitually with moderate tonus and avoid involvement in any biting and sucking habits. Normally the lower lip at rest covers the lower one third or one fourth of the crowns of the upper incisors.[23] Most harmful lip habits are those of the lower lip. However, when the upper lip is short, habitual lip closure is difficult and may contribute to functional (chewing, swallowing, speech) and nonfunctional contacts between the lower lip and upper teeth. Instead of exerting a light, constant pressure against the labial surfaces of the anterior maxillary teeth as it normally does, the lower lip pushes against the lingual surfaces, and is often implicated as the principal etiological factor in labially tipped upper incisors.

Treatment. If the anterior malocclusion is so severe as to preclude habituation of lip closure at rest, ask the orthodontist whether it is possible to move the maxillary incisors toward normal positions as either a first step in treatment of the total orthodontic problem, or as a temporary procedure before total treatment procedures are initiated. If the upper lip is short and passive, have the patient do some stretching and strengthening exercises several times each day. Chapter 17 is devoted almost entirely to the strengthening and reposturing of lips.

LIP AND CHEEK BITING. Lip biting and cheek biting are relatively infrequent habits, at least to a pathological extent. Biting with sufficient force to displace teeth becomes painful. It is a common reaction to certain types of stress even in the well-ordered mouth, on a periodic basis. Unfortunately, a few patients do persist to the point of habit formation, to the detriment of their teeth.

These are usually among the less difficult habits to displace. Once the causes and effects have been explained to the patient, it remains only to call up to consciousness the instances of habitual occurrence. For the lip biter, this is often possible by keeping the exterior of the lip well coated with a lubricating ointment or paste. The cheek biter often has a shelf of buccal tissue that forms and hardens from incessant nibbling; a thin sheet of polyethylene plastic placed in the buccal vestibule allows the shelf to resorb while preventing further cheek biting.

This fibrous buccal ridge of the true cheek biter is readily apparent. Some lateral tongue thrusts are misdiagnosed as cheek biting when in reality the tongue is the guilty agent. These patients display a smooth, normal inner surface of the cheek, even at the site of the posterior open bite.

LIP LICKING. Lip licking is vexingly self-perpetuating and self-enlarging. While it is occasionally the result of chronic nervousness, in most cases it is another product of mouth breathing. As described in earlier chapters, breath fanning in and out over the lip (usually the lower lip) parches and chaps the vermillion portion. In an effort to alleviate the resulting discomfort, the tongue coats the lip with saliva. The drying saliva encourages further chapping, but also extends the affected area somewhat below the vermillion line. The excursion of the tongue must necessarily increase accordingly, but never quite catches up to the progressing outer boundary of the red, sore, traumatized tissue.

The primary treatment, of course, is to institute a closed-mouth resting posture. In the interim, as with lip biting, it is helpful to keep the entire outer surface of the lip constantly coated with a cream or unguent.

LIP SUCKING. Lip sucking is often an advanced stage of lip licking. Once the tongue has reached a comfortable limit of protrusion, the alternative of sucking the lip into the mouth is discovered. Once this is established on a habitual level, the evidence is unpleasantly obvious: the lower lip is not only chapped and discolored, but is marked by an angry red semicircle dipping down toward the mentalis.

It is generally impossible to even begin procedures for mouth closure until this habit is disrupted: the instant that the mouth closes, the lower lip darts between the teeth.

Consistent with our therapy for other oral habits, we prefer to avoid the use of appliances as much as possible. Lip sucking drives us to such recourse at times, calling forth an oral screen. The acrylic type, made to fit the individual mouth by a dentist, is to be preferred; the plastic translation described in Chapter 21 is less likely to be retained in the mouth, but it is usually satisfactory.

As in the two preceding conditions, it is essential that the lower lip be kept well lubricated on a 24-hour basis; otherwise, the chapped status of the lip creates an intolerable sensation, the screen is yanked out, and lip sucking is resumed.

Nail biting

INCIDENCE. This habit, according to an oft-quoted study by Wechsler,[27] is found in about 43% of adolescents and 25% of college students. It is unusual in children under the age of 3, and is found in about one-third of the children from age 6 to the beginning of adolescence. There is a sharp drop in incidence at the age of 16, to about 19%. Approximately 10% of adults bite their nails, according to Pennington.[17]

EFFECTS. Whereas it may be possible for damage to the gingiva and teeth to result, usually the only physical damage is to the nails themselves and the soft tissue surrounding the nails. Because it is not a socially accepted habit, its chief damage may be psychological rather than physical in nature. It is quite possible that it is the chronological successor to thumbsucking as a sign of insecurity or nervous tension.

Because of its rather common occurrence in children, the identification of nail biting as a *problem* depends on its effects on the subject. If it is a source of embarrassment to the child or the child's parents, or is causing some physical damage, a logical specialist to refer to is the oral myologist.

TREATMENT. A review of treatment procedures is presented by Nunn and Azrin.[15] These include negative practice, operant conditioning, and psychotherapy. According to Nunn and Azrin, none of the procedures has been generally effective in eliminating nail biting. The authors' "habit reversal program" consists of the following series of procedures:

1. Clients are trained to heighten their awareness of the nature of their problem.
2. They are then taught activities which are incompatible with nail biting, such as manicuring them, then grasping an object firmly or clenching the fist when tempted to bite the nails.
3. In motivational discussions the undesirable personal and social results of nail biting are reviewed. The support of family members and peers is enlisted to help provide reinforcement for proper behavior.
4. The clients imagine themselves in situations in which they would be likely to engage in nail biting, and demonstrate the use of the incompatible activities in those imagined situations.
5. The clients seek out situations where nail biting is likely, and practice the competing activities.
6. The clients inspect their hands and nails nightly and repair any roughness or peeling of the cuticles.

This program was given to thirteen patients, ranging from 11 to 38 years of age, all of whom had bitten their nails for at least eight years. All thirteen eliminated the nail biting within one month after beginning treatment. Only two of the clients demonstrated any relapse during a 16-week period following treatment, and these two clients each had only one incidence of nail biting during that time.

Since we know of no other approach claiming comparable success with nail biters, we recommend that the reader try the Nunn and Azrin procedure.

SUMMARY

The terms "oral myologist," "oral myofunctional therapist," and "orofacial muscle imbalance" are misleading if the only function of the clinician is to correct a tongue thrust. Early in the development of a private practice, nearly all referrals are for tongue thrust treatment, with a few for elimination of thumbsucking. As the clinician inquires of his patients concerning the existence of other oral habits and treats them, he begins to receive referrals for a wide variety of habit disorders, even a few having nothing to do with the mouth. If he decides another oral habit does in fact exist and is causing harm to teeth, tissues, or emotions, the application of certain principles is recommended:

1. Determine whether any etiological factors still persist. If so, deal with them as effectively as possible.
2. Be alert for signs of insecurity and tensions in the patient. Consider your own training, competencies, and limitations in making decisions to treat or refer to another professional.
3. Explain to the patient and parents the advantages and disadvantages of mechanical devices in eliminating oral habits.
4. Provide a means for the patient to give you regular feedback on progress.
5. Select types and schedules of reinforcement appropriate to the age and needs of the patient.

REFERENCES

1. Benjamin, L. S.: Nonnutritive sucking and dental malocclusion in deciduous and permanent teeth of the Rhesus monkey, Child Dev. **33**:29-35, 1962.
2. Davidian, C.: A study of oral and learning habits and their physiological effects uppon the growing face and dentition. Thesis, University of Southern California, 1957.
3. Dunlap and Streicher Institute of Speech and Hearing: A new theory based on oral habits as causal factors—speech development, Monograph, 1970.
4. Fluhrer, A. V.: Some original investigations into pressure habits as etiological factors in dentofacial abnormalities, Pacific Coast Soc. Orthod., 1957.
5. Gellin, M. E.: Management of patients with deleterious habits, J. Dent. Child. **31**:274-283, 1964.
6. Gingold, N. L.: Oral habits and preventive orthodontics, N.Y. J. Dent. **44**:148-149.
7. Gorelick, L.: Thumbsucking in foster children, a comparative study. N.Y. J. Dent. **20**:422, 1954.
8. Holick, F.: Relation between habitual breathing through the mouth and muscular activity of the tongue in distoclusion, Cesk. Stomat. **57**:170-180, 1957.
9. Klein, E. T.: Pressure habits, etiological factors in malocclusion, Am. J. Orthod. **38**:569-587, 1952.
10. Linder-Aronson, S.: Adenoids: their effect on mode of breathing and nasal airflow, and their re-

lationship to characteristics of the facial skeleton and the dentition, Acta Otolaryngol. Suppl. 265, 1970.
11. Linder-Aronson, S.: Effects of adenoidectomy on dentition and nasopharynx, Am. J. Orthod. **65**:1-15, 1974.
12. Linder-Aronson, S., and Backstrom, A.: A comparison between mouth and nose breathers with respect to occlusion and facial dimension; a biometric study, Odont. Revy. **11**:343-376, 1961.
13. Meklas, J. F.: Bruxism—diagnosis and treatment, J. Acad. Gen. Dent. **19**:31-36, 1971.
14. Nanda, R. S., Khan, I., and Anana, R.: Effect of oral habits on the occlusion in preschool children, J. Dent. Child. **37**:449-452, 1972.
15. Nunn, R. G., and Azrin, N. H.: Eliminating nailbiting by the habit reversal procedure, Behav. Res. Ther. **14**:65-67, 1976.
16. Paul, J. L., and Nanda, R. S.: Effect of mouth breathing on dental occlusion, Angle Orthod. **43**:201-206, 1973.
17. Pennington, L. A.: Incidence of nailbiting among adults, Am. J. Psychiat. **102**:241, 1945.
18. Posen, A. L.: The influence of maximum perioral and tongue force on the incisor teeth, Angle Orthod. **42**:285-309, 1972.
19. Prince, R.: Bruxism, occlusion and migraine, Anglo-Cont. Dent. Soc., Feb., 1971.
20. Rabuck, R. H.: Occlusal imbalance and concomitant oral habits, Unpublished Thesis, University of Texas Dental School, 1971.
21. Reding, G. R., Rubright, W. C., and Zimmerman, S. O.: Incidence of bruxism, J. Dent. Res. **45**:1198-1205, 1966.
22. Ricketts, R. M.: Respiratory obstruction syndrome, Am. J. Orthod. **51**:495-515, 1968.
23. Schlare, R., and Leeds, D.: The trapped lower lip, Brit. Dent. J. **102**:398-403, 1957.
24. Sood, S., and Verma, S.: Mouth habits—mouth breathing, J. Indian Dent. Assoc. **38**:132-135, 1966.
25. Warren, E.: Simultaneous ocurrence of certain muscle habits and malocclusion, Am. J. Orthod. **45**:356-370, 1959.
26. Watson, R. M., Warren, D. W., and Fischer, N. D.: Nasal resistance, skeletal classification and mouth breathing in orthodontic patients, Am. J. Orthod. **54**:367-379, 1968.
27. Wechsler, D.: The incidence and significance of nailbiting in children, Psychoanal. Rev. **18**:201, 1931.

Chapter 15

PHILOSOPHY OF TREATMENT

The most important elements in any therapy program are the philosophy on which it is based and the attitude of the therapist that is reflected by that philosophy. It may develop that the reader will wish to modify many of the procedures that will be presented in the balance of this volume; if he knows why he is changing it and how this change relates to the ultimate goal, and if he makes the adjustments with the proper attitude, he can only be successful. The specific techniques that will be set forth are merely those with which the writers feel comfortable; they may adapt poorly to the personality of a different clinician. They are meant to achieve a certain purpose; it is the goal that is important, and these techniques will be some of the possible courses by which it may be reached. They in no way exclude alternate routes.

A PSYCHOPHYSIOLOGICAL APPROACH

It is prudent to have a map of the region before entering the therapeutic area. A brief overview of the entire program that will be presented in detail in subsequent chapters will therefore be made available. With some grasp of the progression involved, the reader may find the individual sections to be more meaningful. Then, too, a number of factors that are thought to be important to the success of this program have not always been incorporated into some of the traditional approaches to tongue thrust.

Orientation of clinician

The goal of therapy, of whatever sort, is to modify the behavior of the patient; if we did not wish to bring about change, there would be no point in treating the case. What these changes are, specifically and in some detail, must be

ever in the therapist's mind. However, it has been considered undesirable to pour children into a mold, to force their conformity to a set standard; instead, we have been trained to meet the patient where he is, to assess his present abilities, and to proceed from there. After assessing a number of tongue thrusters, it became evident that their "present abilities" bore little resemblance to normal deglutition in any given particular. For a time thereafter, the components of normal swallowing were scrutinized instead. It was found that a basic group of abilities is essential to this act, that these abilities are lacking almost *in toto* in tongue thrusters, and that once these skills are acquired, regardless of what else the patient might or might not be capable, some hope appears of establishing normal function. The program presented here is thus oriented toward the goal, not the origin; whatever the original swallowing type, or the status of the patient, we wish to achieve *normal* deglutition, and we move as directly as possible toward that end.

It should certainly not be inferred from this that every assignment hereafter described is given to every patient. The clinician must be alert, knowledgable, and sufficiently flexible to adapt the program to fit the specific needs and abilities of the individual patient. Only minimal requirements are included, but it is generally found that most patients are deficient, at least to some degree, in almost every requisite skill.

Both formal and informal studies have indicated that the success ratio drops as treatment is prolonged. Accordingly, we would like to disencumber the program of all nonessentials. Unless a procedure makes a direct and positive contribution to the habituation of normal deglutition, it is better not assigned.

Cooperation of patient

The foregoing also implies a certain degree of authoritarianism; although this approach may be contrary to our training and inclination, it has been found necessary. These changes must be wrought, quickly and exactly, before the effort and enthusiasm of the child begin to deteriorate. Only the child himself can implement these changes; the function of parent and therapist is to instruct, support, and supervise, but any further efforts would have little effect on the neuromuscular system of the patient.

The clinician should not assume a responsibility he cannot discharge. The child is clearly apprised of the rules before the game starts. Thereafter, if the patient returns after a week of practice and demonstrates that he has not made a sincere and thoroughgoing effort, he is immediately sent home to repeat the work correctly. A second reflection of the same attitude may bring dismissal from therapy. The child is always welcome to return—when he decides he *wants* to complete the project. The instant the clinician accepts an obviously disinterested response, he has, in effect, advised the child, "Never mind, I will see that you learn to swallow correctly even if you make no effort." The clinician cannot accept this responsibility.

The operant word in this situation is "effort." Many patients encounter *difficulty* in some aspect of therapy; the program may require twice its planned duration before mastery is achieved. This is to be expected, and the clinician should be willing to make any allowance and provide extra assistance as indicated in support of a patient who is having trouble but honestly *trying* to make progress. In all therapy, we are simply striving to make some compromise with nature; nature drives a harsh bargain at times.

In actuality, this "tough" attitude has been found to be entirely in the patient's best interests. If it is not vitally important that the patient learn to swallow correctly, the program should never be started in the first place. If it is essential, the therapist's assignment is to see that the job is done. When uncooperative patients have been continued in therapy week after week, the result invariably has been stagnation of attitude, nil progress, and eventual failure. On the other hand, it has almost never happened that a child dismissed for lack of effort has not later returned with a new appreciation of the importance of cooperation and thus completed therapy. It is believed that the clinician best discharges his fuction with the prodigal rather than the dropout.

The fuel on which patients operate best is a blend of praise, kindness, and approbation. Even a mild display of effort should be stoked with this combustible compound. However, children have the marvelous ability to "read our muscles." They recognize instantly when praise is undeserved and tend to exploit the situation. A phony "sweetness and light" attitude by the therapist may easily produce a negative effect.

Nevertheless, praise need not be restricted to specific behavior. In the beginning, before the child has had an opportunity to perform a praiseworthy act, it is possible to confer approbation for color of eyes, neatness of dress, etc. During oral examination, it is better to replace perfunctory grunts with some display of elation at even the most commonplace lingual ability—not that the average person could not do these things, but you are delighted to observe them in a tongue thruster. Let the child see at the outset that you are prepared to warmly reward the effort he expends and reflect the assumption that *of course* he will do well, and he is oriented toward success. For emphasis, he has already been advised that anything short of his best efforts will not be accepted; if praise is fuel for the patient, his cooperation and adherence to instruction, as enforced rather inflexibly by the clinician, is the propellant that drives the therapy program.

In the rare instances in which suspension from therapy becomes necessary, the attitude of the clinician will, of course, reflect some sorrow, regret, and disappointment: we expected better things of the patient, we have demanded nothing that he could not do easily had he cared to do so, and we are infringing on only a very brief segment of his life. If he has not made the little effort required to complete these things, he would obviously not have completed the more difficult things ahead, leaving the clinician no choice in the matter—which is the simple truth. We are certain that if the child ever decides he wants to learn to swallow correctly, and gain its attendant benefits, he can do so readily; nothing could please us more than a telephone call saying that he wishes to complete therapy. Until then, the therapist is powerless, deprived of any chance to help the patient.

Needless to say, rejoicing is boundless when the child does return—but he understands that the rules have not changed. If matters are properly handled from the first, this situation arises very infrequently: a hundred or more patients complete therapy routinely in our practices before it becomes necessary to suspend someone. Again, if handled properly, not one in ten fails to return with an improved attitude. The very rare case who does not return could probably never have been coaxed or coerced through therapy in any event. This type of tongue thrust is probably the only one for which there is no known cure.

Age of patients

The question of the age of a patient was discussed at some length in Chapter 9. A few supplemental details are worthy of note.

In line with good preventive dentistry, we would like to see retraining completed at the youngest possible age. However, as noted earlier, it is not certain that all these threatened youngsters will even require later therapy, since so many changes occur spontaneously during the early stages of mixed dentition. Hanson and Cohen's research, reported in Chapter 12, provides some basis for predicting the retention of tongue thrust. It can be helpful information after the age of 5 years.

Maintaining the position that in most cases there is no commanding reason for undue haste in this matter, we believe that a wait-and-see attitude may logically be adopted at least until the age of 7 years. Thereafter, individual circumstances may influence proper timing. Physically, it is safer to have the upper central incisors erupted beyond the midpoint in their growth, given an anterior tongue thrust, although a few children with late dental development have succeeded during an "open door" stage. It may prove still more unwise to treat while the deciduous centrals are still present, for relapse might then be invited during the period of edentulous anterior spacing. Naturally, such considerations are governed by the state of posterior teeth in the case of bilateral thrust.

Psychological factors are the major determinant, however. Simple execution of certain oral maneuvers, because the mother or the clinician instructs the child to do so, would have little permanent effect. Unless the child can bring some understanding to this project, performing the assignments with some awareness of what the exercise is expected to accomplish and the necessity for doing so, we could hardly aspire to subconscious modification. Furthermore, un-

less the child has experienced at least a year of school regimen, he is ill prepared to carry out specific directions on a routine basis even if he is cooperative and well motivated initially. Some degree of emotional maturity will be required in any event, and a few unfortunate children reach a rather advanced age before achieving the necessary stability.

Exceptions to the foregoing are made routinely when the child's articulation is grossly distorted.

In the absence of a related speech defect, we prefer to see children at approximately 8 years of age, and certainly before the age of 10 years. Even though there may by then be obvious resultant damage to the occlusion, experience leads us to expect some definite spontaneous improvement in dental alignment in this age range, once muscle function is rendered normal. We can find no valid justification for the policy, proposed by some authors,[2] of deliberately postponing therapy until the age of puberty. The time for prevention is by then past, leaving formal corrective orthodontics as the patient's only recourse.

Handicapped patients

Some notice should be taken herein of the deviant swallower who is further afflicted with an unrelated handicap. Depending on the nature and extent of the disability, he may or may not be a logical candidate for retraining.

A number of children with moderate to severe mental retardation have been referred with the expectation of receiving some benefit from therapy. Unfortunately, such therapy has seldom proved fruitful. Although there is great variation from one individual to the next, it has occasionally been possible to accomplish some of the more routine mechanical aspects implicit in the first stages of therapy. However, lasting improvement has seldom occurred. The lack of mental and emotional maturity previously discussed has imposed the same unrelenting limitation at some point in the program, providing yet another regrettable failure situation for the child. It would seem a kindness in most cases to avoid subjecting the child to almost certain frustration.

Many physically handicapped children have shown quite different results of therapy. It has been our pleasant duty to supply swallowing therapy for children who were totally blind and some who were nearly so, as well as for deaf children. As a rule, these youngsters had accepted their handicap and were not allowing it to affect their life unduly. They found the requirements of therapy quite simple compared to some of their other tasks, and their success was even more gratifying to the therapist after observing the martyred attitude that many "normal" patients bring to therapy. Although it was obviously necessary to adapt many details of the program to the individual situation, no insurmountable problem was encountered with these children.

An area of great need, of course, lies in the field of cerebral palsy. Here again, individual circumstances differ too greatly to allow for meaningful generalities. Some of the foregoing concepts may serve as guidelines, however. If intelligence is impaired, feeding would probably continue to be a lengthy, tiring process. The child whose problem consists primarily of muscular involvement might profit greatly from a modified version of the program presented below.

One of the guiding principles of this approach is the concept of *fragmentation,* the process of breaking down a total act into its component elements, bringing concentration to bear on these submovements, thus developing a selectivity in the individual muscles for the desired function and accordingly a sense of contrast between this and the original movement. The parts into which the act of deglutition is broken remain relatively large in the case of the average patient; they require further subdivision for the cerebral palsied child, but it is believed that the basic outline is here and that the therapist skilled in this field might thereby achieve quicker positive results than by attacking gross function. Since we have never been obliged to work out the necessary details, no specifics of such a program or the results of its application can be supplied.

Outline of therapy

We view the program detailed in the following chapters as a rational psychophysiological approach aimed at establishing as routine those patterns of muscle movement employed in normal deglutition. Since swallowing is a complex act, requiring the coordination of many muscle groups, it is no more logical to propose modification of the intact total function than to require a child with multiple articulation problems to correct them all at one time. The gross synergy is thus broken up into segments for therapeutic purposes, the fragmentation process described above, and the patient is required to be concerned only with certain aspects of the problem at any given time. Accordingly, no attempt at normal deglutition is expected or even desirable during the early stages of therapy, since such an effort could only be a distortion of truly normal function. Probably the two most important contributions that the program herein has to offer are (1) a specific technique for rendering necessary changes in subconscious behavior quickly and (2) this concept of disassembling the motor—rather than tinkering with external adjustments and accessories, actually taking it apart, machining down some pieces and replacing others, then reassembling into a smoother-running apparatus.

The various portions that comprise the assignments are thus specific elements of the normal swallowing act, and are referred to as "steps" in therapy; in no sense is this term intended to be interchangeable with "weeks." The length of time required to master and perfect any given portion of the technique naturally varies with the ability of the patient, the amount of effort the patient expends in practice, and the attitude brought to this practice. The patient of average ability, properly motivated, can master each of these areas in approximately one week, during which he is expected to practice several brief sessions *under parental supervision* each day. Without motivation, as indicated, no amount of drill or change in exercises is likely to alter the original subconscious manner of deglutition.

It is possible to group the different segments of therapy into eight major areas, one devoted to muscles of the facial network, and the remainder to concerns of deglutition as such. The implication is that the average patient is thus able to complete the formal program in eight weeks. However, in actuality, the length of treatment time, as with the specific procedures employed, must of necessity be modified from case to case in order to meet the specific requirements of the individual patient. As implied above, the greater the speed with which therapy can be completed, the greater the possibility of maintaining enthusiasm and thus permanency of result.

It develops that a lower limit to this haste is imposed by the human neuromuscular system; when practice sessions have been further abridged, or elements omitted, the result has usually been the repetition of the entire program at a later date. If the patient does not require the time and effort prescribed in this program, he probably has no thoroughgoing pattern of deviation; only orthodontic correction, a few lip exercises, or a pat on the head might be required. If he truly needs therapy, every aspect must be perfected, not simply to the point where the patient is *able* to execute it, which he should be capable of before he ever leaves the therapy room, but to the degree that it is performed *effortlessly* and with little thought required.

The initial interview is a rather lengthy indoctrination session, during which the case history is compiled, the problem is explained to child and parent, the benefits of therapy and the hazards of failure are sharply contrasted, the necessary rules are clearly established, and a brief overview of the entire program is presented for orientation purposes. A full and careful evaluation is made of the patient and his problem, his orofacial structures, his abilities, and his deficits. Examination is made for labial weakness or malposture, and the necessity for corrective exercises is weighed. When extensive work will be required in the area of lip exercises, as it usually is, the balance of the session is devoted entirely to this end. When lips are a less vital consideration, the first step of the seven that comprise the therapy program for deglutition proper is presented, with minor lip exercises distributed over the first two or three sessions.

The initial segment of the swallowing program thus is frequently held in abeyance for one week, during which lips receive full attention. It is thereafter possible to concentrate with less interruption on swallowing itself. The goal of the first step is to establish a foundation on which each of the following portions can be built. Specifically, the habitual labioglossal seal displayed in deviant deglutition must be broken, molar occlusion initiated, and an active sucking component blended into the swallowing act, by means of a single exercise designed to establish normal posture for the *tip* of the tongue.

The second step includes exercises to strengthen the musculature that serves to elevate and support anterior tongue segments, as well as exercises that tend to position the entire anterior tongue for normal swallowing; some labial exercising usually continues. Additionally, procedures are begun at this time to modify the habitual oral resting posture.

The third step is devoted almost exclusively to efforts to reposition the posterior tongue—the crux of therapy in most cases. Any necessary adjustments are made in the exercises of the previous step, and these exercises are continued, usually at a reduced level.

Not until the fourth step is the patient expected to execute a complete swallow in a normal manner. Each component movement is examined and integrated into a total pattern of eating and drinking, and exercises are assigned that tend to reduce the amount of effort required to utilize this new pattern.

The fifth step is an intensive effort to establish the newly acquired ability as a conscious *habit*, and various devices (nonmechanical) are employed to this end. Some work also continues in the oropharyngeal area, strengthening correct function in this region.

Once normal swallowing is occurring routinely on a conscious level, it is necessary to complete the process by making the correct habit subconscious and thus permanent. This is the entire focus of the sixth step, with procedures employed during both waking and sleeping hours. It is at this point that hypnosis may be used effectively, but it is not the procedure of choice.

The seventh step completes the routine formal aspect of therapy. Tests are applied to determine the thoroughness of the subconscious habit. Renewed consideration is given at this point to the physiological rest position, although attention is never allowed to wander too far from this item throughout therapy.

At the conclusion of the formal program, a recheck period is started that may extend over eight to ten months. The first recheck is made only three or four weeks after the last therapy session, and then the period between checks is lengthened to as much as three months if the new pattern appears to be establishing roots. Patients are not considered to be dismissed from therapy until at least one recheck is adequately passed after a three-month lapse to the complete satisfaction of clinician and patient.

COOPERATION OF CLINICIAN AND DENTIST

A program such as that sketched above can flourish only in the congenial atmosphere of dental agreement. The individual responsibilities of both therapist and dentist that serve to foster this necessary climate will be presented. These facets have arisen and have been resolved in our practices; modifications may be required to meet the reader's particular circumstances.

Responsibility of dentist

REFERRALS. The great majority of patients seen by the clinician will have been referred by a dentist, primarily an orthodontist or pedodontist, as part of a program to prevent or correct malocclusion. The manner in which this referral is made can make a critical difference in therapy. If the dentist proposes therapy in a disparaging or even casual manner, it is perhaps better not to make the referral at all; the patient can bring little specific knowledge to the situation, and if therapy seems unimportant to the dentist, the patient can only judge by this estimate. Patients often pursue the matter no further or do so only tentatively. As a group, they prove in therapy to be hopeless from the start. Thus if the dentist cannot wholeheartedly endorse both the program and the clinician, he should turn to other procedures or seek a change in personnel.

This program is based squarely on the motivation of the patient; the dentist must assume responsibility for at least a share of this incentive. The orthodontist sees patients fail in treatment when they do not cooperate, despite the mechanical forces of appliances; the therapist has no appliance—only the nervous system of the patient.

When referral is made in a positive manner, reflecting a supposition of certainty that the program will be completed, or better yet, is stated as a requirement for the completion of orthodontic treatment, this certitude is then reflected by the patient, and the difference is dramatic. There is then no question of *whether* therapy will be completed or not, and only the assumption of success remains. An orthodontist would scarcely cement bands over carious teeth; prior restoration of the teeth is simply a routine requirement. Learning to swallow correctly is well placed in the same category as a routine prerequisite.

We are in no way attempting to be highhanded in this matter. If it is not essential that the patient undergo therapy, we have already stated that he should not be referred in the first place; if it is important, the dentist who does not support the therapist is only impairing his own treatment. On the rare occasions when it has been necessary to suspend a patient from

therapy, the patient has sometimes returned to the orthodontist and sought treatment anyway. Those who were accepted on this basis by the orthodontist have been almost the only patients who have not returned to complete therapy. They have reportedly been miserable orthodontic patients, and in a few cases the orthodontist eventually removed the appliance and dropped them from treatment also.

TIMING OF THERAPY. At what point in the orthodontic program should deglutition be corrected? Cases have been reported in which patients were tossed back and forth between clinician and dentist in a deplorable fashion, the dentist believing that his treatment will be prolonged or impaired until adverse pressures are relieved, the clinician believing as strongly that his work cannot be effective until orthodontic procedures have established a more normal environment for the tongue.

A few specific factors are operating in this situation, and if they are recognized and evaluated in a given case, a sound decision is usually made. This result often requires some consultation between clinician and dentist, but the latter should realize that the primary program is his and that he therefore owes some cooperation in the matter. The final decision is his, but he and, of course, the clinician should not assume indiscriminately that all patients can be managed identically in deglutition therapy.

As a general rule, it has been found advantageous to complete therapy before orthodontic appliances are installed. The pathway of the clinician is thus kept more free of obstruction, particularly in not being required to dodge around shifts in the orthodontic program. The postponement of dental correction often improves the patient's motivation to complete therapy promptly. Advantages accrue to the patient also, since he is permitted to receive kinesthetic clues from his own oral tissues without distraction or reliance on the artificial environment of appliances. In fact, it is usually necessary to remove upper retainers during all practice sessions in order to allow direct contact of the tongue with alveolar and palatal tissues.

From the dental point of view, it is worth noting that, given prior correction of deglutition, the appliance is working at peak efficiency throughout treatment, the entire procedure is completed as quickly as possible, and the resulting fringe benefits in economy of chair time, stable dentition, shortened retention period, etc. are fully achieved. A large majority of patients have achieved satisfactory progress when allowed to complete the swallowing program and to pass the first recheck before dental changes are made. Normal deglutition is then reinforced and consolidated during orthodontic treatment, and any tendency to regress can be observed and eliminated while the appliance is still in place.

In certain patients, however, the upper arch may be so constricted as to prevent anything resembling normal tongue posture or function. In others, upper incisors may be far too protrusive to allow adequate facial behavior, or a congenital anomaly unassociated with deglutition may present an obstacle. For all these patients, the orthodontist should make definite changes before suggesting modifications of the swallowing pattern.

In a small number of cases, it has appeared to the orthodontist that his efforts would be to no avail if certain pressures were not first eliminated. A compromise arrangement has then been planned; therapy has been initiated but with the understanding by the dentist and patient that only "first aid" measures would be applied. Such improvement as was possible under the circumstances has been made, orthodontic treatment could then more readily bring about change in the structure, and swallowing therapy has thereafter been completed in a second series of sessions. Clinician and dentist must obviously work together rather closely in these cases.

It has been found repeatedly that once swallowing therapy is started, it should be allowed to progress without dental interruption until the formal program is completed and at least the first recheck has been passed satisfactorily. If bands are suddenly installed halfway through therapy or four bicuspids are extracted, it is usually necessary to drop therapy for a time, wait until equilibrium has been reestablished, and start over again; this delay does not improve the attitude of anyone in the situation. If this point is understood, interruption can be readily eliminated as a problem. Similar consideration should be given to those patients whose therapy is being applied during the course of orthodontic treatment; the dentist should arrange to refer the patient during a time when no major changes in the appliance are necessary. He can check for loose bands and maintain the status quo for a visit or two, but if instead he has clamped down the tie wires or applied other strong pressure, he can hardly expect the patient to be practicing the exaggeratedly firm molar occlusion demanded in therapy. The clinician likewise should be alert not to initiate therapy until the bands have been in place for a month or more and are no longer a strange feature in the mouth.

Obligations of clinician

The clinician must accept primary accountability for much of this program. The dentist should feel no threat to his professional standing but instead should experience some satisfaction in providing superior care for his patient, since he provides the cooperation outlined above. Nevertheless, in the usual setting the clinician is at the helm once embarked on matters of deglutition. A few areas of special responsibility should be noted.

PREPARATION. First of all, the clinician should have some actual preparation to deal with this problem. Much friction has originated when otherwise well-grounded people attack faulty deglutition without the necessary tools. We continue to be perturbed by the suggestion that we train a fellow worker "over lunch," as well as by the mail-order request for a brief note divulging the program. The futility of this approach should be obvious.

A speech pathologist is expected to have had specific study and experience with every speech defect he attempts to correct. He should have the same background in abnormal deglutition if he accepts tongue-thrust patients. The oral myologist of whatever background should be expected to know dental terminology and to function comfortably in dental discussion. He should have studied and perfected *some* program of therapy for faulty deglutition with which he can feel effective. The impression that tongue thrust is a minor problem, requiring minimal skill and knowledge to correct, has been a historically damaging fallacy as difficult to rectify as faulty deglutition itself.

SUPPORT OF THE DENTIST. The clinician usually receives cooperation to the same degree that he gives it. He should know and honor the treatment philosophy of every referring dentist. The clinician should be scrupulous in any necessary discussion with patients to reflect only admiration for whatever treatment the dentist is employing. The clinician is not qualified to judge dental techniques and should make it a rule to avoid doing so. If a remark is necessary, it should imply enthusiastic support of the dentist;

the patient must approve of him, or another dentist would have been consulted.

We must also expect a degree of courage if the dental philosophy is fundamentally incompatible with the clinician's views. This is no place for pretense; if no easy working relationship can be established between clinician and dentist, only damage to the patient can result. The clinician should either have a frank discussion with the dentist, withdraw from the situation, or make such adjustment as may be necessary to prevent hampering a single patient's dental program. Some adaptability is required when referrals are received from several dentists using different methods; the clinician should be adequately responsive.

REPORTS. One of the most effective devices by which the clinician can assure the smooth operation of this program is to keep the dentist informed as to the progress of each patient. This task need not be burdensome. Forms can be mimeographed or printed (Appendix 1) that require only that the clinician sit down with the records approximately every two weeks and in a minimal time fill in the necessary blanks. Two forms are suggested—one on white paper for use during active therapy, and the other, designed for the recheck period, on colored paper.

After a patient has been seen two or three times, thus providing the therapist with some basis for judgment, the first report is sent. The dentist is then aware that the patient has actually started therapy, and by comparing the number of sessions with the attained step in the program, he can determine what progress is being made. Patient cooperation and prognosis are easily noted, and space is allotted for additional remarks where appropriate. It frequently develops that the clinician gains certain insights concerning the patient or his parents that might prove valuable to the dentist; they should be reported. This is not meant to be an alibi slot for the presentation of negative factors only; special abilities, or approaches which seem particularly effective, are more meaningful for the dentist.

This form can also be used to advise the dentist of any necessary delay before initiating therapy. If a tonsillectomy is required, a sucking habit is to be eliminated, or any other preliminary procedure is indicated, the dentist should be appraised of the situation in order to plan his own schedule. The body of the report form is then crossed off and the appropriate note inserted.

After the first recheck has been successfully completed, the colored form is mailed. The mere presence of this sheet in the patient's folder indicates to the dentist that therapy has been finished and normal function should be expected. If he observes anything to the contrary during dental treatment, he can so advise the clinician. The form indicates the approximate date of the next recheck, but the dentist may wish the patient to return prior to that time if any regression is noted and the recheck is still some time in the future.

Succeeding rechecks are similarly reported until such time as the patient is dismissed. The latter event may deserve a singing telegram but is customarily confined to the blank portion of the colored form.

CONCLUSION

This chapter has attempted to set forth some of the realities of oral myofunctional correction. It has also presented an abbreviated outline of the therapy program to follow.

The overriding principle that we have tried to enunciate is that of cooperation. Everyone in the situation—patient, parent, dentist, and clinician—must not only direct his individual efforts toward the common goal but blend those efforts into a unified endeavor that moves without friction or interruption to its destination. Most children derive their attitudes from parental influences, and most parents are swayed by professional guidance. Thus it is the dentist and the clinician who must be most acutely aware and responsive.

When full cooperation can be woven into a therapy program based on sound physiological precepts, properly directed and faithfully executed, functions that have been described as irremediable may be swiftly altered.

REFERENCES

1. Hanson, M. L.: Some suggestions for more effective therapy for tongue thrust, J. Speech Hear. Disord. **32:**75-79, 1967.
2. Mason, R. M., and Proffit, W. R.: The tongue thrust controversy: background and recommendations, J. Speech Hear. Disord. **39:**115-132, 1974.
3. Moyers, R. E.: Tongue problems and malocclusion, Dent. Clin. North Am., pp. 529-539, July, 1964.
4. Rogers, J. H.: Swallowing patterns of a normal population sample compared to those of patients from an orthodontic practice, Am. J. Orthod. **46:**674-689, 1961.

Chapter 16

SUCKING HABITS

The first procedure required by many patients will be a method to control a sucking habit. The great majority will involve a problem digit or two, but an occasional unfortunate will be sucking their tongue. Accordingly, we will give these issues our immediate attention.

It is our feeling that any nonnutritive sucking habit should be under a reasonable measure of control before any attempt is made to solve other oral problems. There may thus be a hiatus of several weeks between the first two appointments. For this reason, and because not all patients suck their thumb, we will postpone until the next chapter a discussion of our usual intake procedures. The continuity of the basic program will be improved by this delay.

It seems that everyone has an answer to sucking habits, ranging from the unfounded horror of the Freudians at even raising the question, to the barbed "crib" still welded in place by a few impatient dentists. Somewhere between must lie reason.

Even this middle ground is fairly well populated, however, and the futility of reviewing all the proposals that have been made soon becomes evident. We have tried a dozen or more procedures, have read dozens of books and articles on the subject, and have managed, one way or another, to achieve the elimination of sucking habits in several hundred patients over the years. Some of the basic concepts thus derived, and techniques consistent with these premises, will be outlined. It should be stated at the outset that these procedures, none of which are claimed as original, have been remarkably successful when acceptable to parents and patients. They have generally been so accepted, and no damage or untoward aftermath has yet been demonstrated. In fact, definite emotional gains have

at times appeared to stem from successful mastery of this situation.

GENERAL ORIENTATION

It is strongly felt that the therapist should not rush in and begin tossing techniques about until he has acquired some genuine understanding of what is involved and of the guiding principles that serve as the skeleton of the methods being employed. For one thing, success in this venture will depend in large part on the extent to which you are accepted as an authority on the subject. With any given patient who retains a sucking habit there have been lay efforts in wide variety, and over a period of years, before he has appeared for swallowing therapy. You must offer *professional* guidance.

The one factor that then appears to have the greatest influence on his entire program is the *confidence* of the therapist who attempts to utilize it. If you feel unsure of your ability to work with this problem, refer the patient to someone in whom you have greater faith. In some areas, unfortunately, this approach would not necessarily be in the best interests of your patient. There remains the concept, discussed later, that sucking is a sacred right of the individual. Where one or two men holding this theory have dominated the local professions, clinicians are looked at askance if they even approach a sucking habit. To the contrary, any therapist who is adequately prepared for his profession, or any dentist, should be capable of competent guidance in this area.

A number of people have been observed, however, who did not thoroughly understand why they were making certain suggestions, how these suggestions were expected to operate, or what some of their ramifications might be. Not only are these people prone to error, but they also transmit their own feelings of insecurity to the patient, report an understandable lack of success, but tend to blame the technique rather than their lack of preparation.

Since, therefore, comprehension breeds confidence, and confidence success, let us examine some of the pertinent details. Should your background in this area be superior to ours, you will be able to scan this section with even greater confidence and self-satisfaction.

Etiology in tongue-thrust cases

The incidence of sucking habits among deviant swallowers is rather high, as was reported earlier. As hinted in Chapter 8, there may be influences imposed on the infant by his swallowing abnormality that impel him toward a sucking habit.

Perhaps the strongest instinct of the neonate is for sucking; pictures have now been circulated of fetuses sucking their thumb in utero. When the infant is required to suck vigorously in nursing, including the sucking element required to position the bolus in normal deglutition, the physiological need is met and the infant may sleep in happy exhaustion.

When, however, an abnormality in deglutition is instituted, reducing the requirement for sucking, or a rapid feeding process is presented in which sucking has a nonsurvival connotation, the infant is left without normal means by which to satisfy a basic need: his stomach is filled, but not his sucking instinct. We could only expect the normal baby to resort to fingers, tongue, or lip for supplemental gratification. He has little choice, in reality. He may be mildly and momentarily emotionaly disturbed at the necessity for accepting a substitute brand with an unknown label, but he probably loses very little sleep in cursing parents, bemoaning his fate, or planning revenge.

Since his supplemental sucking thereafter plays such a major and fundamental role, satisfying an essential craving, it should also not be surprising to find that the habit may persist far beyond the age when normal swallowers have dispensed with such activity. Observe that infants who swallow normally, but who inherit a greater-than-average need for sucking, may also institute a similar habit as something of a sideline; by 3 or 4 years of age they simply drop it. The truly emotionally disturbed may take refuge in a sucking habit; it is frequently of sudden onset beyond the age of 1 year. For the deviant swallower, his sucking habit is established as a flourishing venture at or soon after birth and often persists into the later stages of childhood. A surprising number of persons who are no longer children find themselves incapable of sleeping through the night without recourse to their preferred digit.

The continuance of this habit may be more emotionally traumatic than its elimination, in many cases. The child who is subjected to ceaseless harassment by his family as an indirect reaction to his sucking habit, who uses his habit as a weapon against parents, or who dares not contemplate slumber parties or a friend "sleeping over" because he lives in dread that his habit will be discovered by his peers is being warped and harmed in ways other than dental.

It is further to be expected that the teenagers in this group have the greatest difficulty in unseating their unconscious impulses, despised though the habit be. It is interesting to note that some of these older patients, after tremendous exertions to cooperate with the new program and conquer their habit, will so rationalize the situation and rearrange their memories that when questioned at the end of the recheck period concerning possible recurrence, will vow that they never *really* sucked their thumb; they only thought they did.

Boundaries of competence

Before going further, we should explicitly set and define the limits of the population for which these techniques are intended. We seek to entice no one from the psychotherapist's couch; to the contrary, we routinely refer patients to a psychologist when such referral is indicated.

The procedures herewith proposed are employed with reasonably "normal," fairly stable young adults and children down to the age of 6 years, who are in average physical health but who swallow improperly. They are not appropriate for children below the age of reason, for the acutely ill, for the emotionally disturbed patient, or the patient who is severely limited mentally. Indeed, we should not be working with such a patient in the area of deglutition, failing some exceptional circumstance.

The patient with any unusual need should be in the hands of someone competent to deal with such a condition. Note, however, that the existence of a stark and solitary sucking habit, unsupported by other positive and confirming data, does not indicate emotional disturbance, especially in this delimited group. In fact, we are a bit surprised when the tongue thruster does *not* have a sucking habit, notwithstanding its indulgence only in sleep or while he is immersed in television, at the stage usually seen by the clinician.

Emotional concomitants

Now that we have observed some of the side issues that are germane to this topic, let us look directly at the emotional effects that are attributed to cessation of sucking habits. Counselors, in discussing sucking habits, often become more emotionally disturbed than the patients over whom they fret. This is not to imply that there are no emotional overtones in this problem. Of course there are, and we should be aware of them. We should not overgeneralize them, however, but rather we should put them in perspective appropriate to their nature and origin.

Scanning the furor over sucking habits in medical, dental, and psychological literature confirms the impression that the basic controversy revolves about this one point: the effect of cessation on the personality of the patient.

As a general observation, we may note the growing accumulation of evidence that human emotions do not actually function in the closed system, which, hypothetical construct though it always was, has been accepted by many workers as verified and gospel. That is, the personality does not necessarily duplicate the seething teakettle, so that if the spout is pinched shut, the lid blows off. It might then be conceivable that one could stop sucking his thumb and not turn immediately to masturbation, bed-wetting, or other compensatory behavior. Certainly the use of force and coercion can have a deleterious effect, regardless of the context in which it is applied. The emotional reaction may be to the method, however, rather than to the modification of behavior thus enforced.

Naturally, sucking fills an unconscious emotional need, even if inefficiently, or the child would long since have stopped. In a few cases, true enough, the habit does persist through sheer inertia. Even excluding the latter, the emotional elements affecting these patients are generally of a superficial, tacked-on nature, acquired through mere association over a period of time, rather than the original basis for the habit. For example, an infant falls asleep repeatedly while sucking his thumb—because he feels an unsatisfied

instinctive need to suck on something—and eventually, through *association* of recurrent common aspects of the situation, sucking becomes a part of rest, so that even with a feeling of fatigue the thumb pops into the mouth. The small child is punished, and while he lies in his room sucking his thumb (perhaps for a physiological reason) and ponders the ills of the world, the thumb begins to symbolize refuge from woe, consolation when wounded, and many other things of an emotional nature conjoined by circumstance but less than causative.

Thus the patient will now be required to undergo some emotional reorganization. He will need to find other ways in which to react to some conditions; in other words, he will be asked to mature a bit. The need for sucking is usually outgrown by the age of 2 or 3 years. People who do not suck their thumb grow weary, are injured, and meet frustrations; they sleep, weep, curse, and kick, as the occasion demands, with no feeling of an overwhelming need to suck. Our patient will be asked to make similar adjustments. He will require assistance, guidance, and support in order to do so; we intend to supply them. He will be allowed the time and opportunity to work out his own solutions to the problem—but only if he sincerely wants to do so. We ask merely the chance to help him.

Wiles that do not work

It should not be necessary to insert this section, for the procedures listed below should be obvious in their futility. Yet they are hardy, time-honored specimens and do not easily die, especially after receiving the transfusion supplied by an occasional seeming success. They live also because, as with many lay solutions, they appear easy and logical on the surface. However, they are beset by hidden flaws that can only damage the sound management of a deep-seated sucking habit. Their true nature was long ago exposed, but this knowledge is still far from universal.

Therefore let us examine and dispose of them. There should be no possibility that the therapist would not understand the fallacies that entangle and mislead; parents also should be helped to understand that if these devices were truly capable of success, they surely would have demonstrated results before the age at which we see the patient.

BRIBERY. This is the most common ploy with the older child and may still be in effect when you see the child, or new bribes may be in the planning stage, by either parents or child.

Bribery puts a new value on any bad habit, and most children are capable of recognizing a good thing when they see it. The bribe is usually negotiated like a contract, with specified time periods: "If you don't suck your fingers for one entire month (or two, or more), I'll buy you a new bicycle." The child scrupulously avoids being caught in the sucking act for the required period, gets the bicycle, and rides it around the block, realizing all the way the price he has paid for it; having earned it, he parks the bicycle, sits down, and sucks his fingers. Any new offers?

When a time period is not set, the bicycle loses luster daily, the task appears more and more hopeless, and the child is driven back to his fingers in despair. His sense of failure is assuaged somewhat by sucking, and the habit gains additional strength.

Rewards in any form of worldly goods are strongly discouraged during the period when we are attempting to eliminate sucking behavior. Cold though the prospect may be, we are asking the child to find reward within himself—in self-mastery, advanced maturity, increased confidence, a sense of freedom from enslavement to his habit, even pretty teeth. In the daily life of the child, these rewards are less abstract than they appear. They are also permanent.

Should the parent feel overwhelmed by gratitude and approval at the conclusion of the project and wish to bestow a spontaneous gift on the child, well and good. But no carrots should be dangled in the interim.

PUNISHMENT. Certainly the oldest, most frequent, and earliest answer to sucking is punishment. It probably also comes in the greatest variety of forms, from simple, crude physical bruises, through more subtle refinements of agony and oppression, to outright parental rejection. It is difficult to understand the concern of some workers over presumed trauma resulting from elimination of sucking when its mere continuation proves to be the source of such real and constant emotional persecution.

An occasional child does avoid the torture by stopping the sucking habit. He is the one who then turns to other means of emotional fulfillment, usually in the form of some other habit that is even less acceptable than sucking, so that parents frequently wish they could then trade back to the original habit. The parents should hardly expect otherwise, for they have allowed the child no other recourse nor provided a better solution.

Furthermore, anyone who has worked with stutterers understands the mechanics of *secondary gain*. Although punishment is not pleasant, it does at least provide parental attention, a scarce commodity in the lives of some children. It also provides a convenient cloak for other failures in daily life. Thus, if the child persists in sucking, he receives attention and is excused from certain other obligations; he may decide the price is right.

If for no other reason, punishment should be avoided because it provides a specific and intensified *need* for sucking. Even at the threat of retaliatory action, the thumb sucker flies to his thumb for solace. The greater the punishment, the stronger and more ingrained becomes the desire to suck. Another vicious circle is complete.

We will insist during the following procedures that parents exercise some restraint in this regard. If inadvertent instances of sucking occur, the parents should feel sympathy for the child who is trying to stop, they should express regret that the project is proving difficult, and they should display affection and approval of their child as a person and admiration for his efforts. There is broad scope for responses short of ridicule, shame, or castigation.

A clear distinction should be drawn for parents between punishment for sucking behavior and *discipline*. Nothing that has been said here should be construed to imply that the child's other activities should not be held within some definite boundaries. Otherwise we may build a greater problem than we destroy. We are definitely not asking that all restraint be removed from this child's life; if he truly misbehaves, he should be penalized.

In this regard, note that it is simply not possible to *love* a child too much; it is readily possible to overindulge him. Overindulgence is not healthy and is certainly not love; it is indifference to the child's future well-being and is thus antithetical to love. When it is easier to tolerate misbehavior than to correct it, the child can only assume, usually correctly, that his parents care very little about him. The insecurity that results from parental rejection pays the rent for many psychologists and attorneys. In fact, establishing a rigid program of sound discipline may be the kindest service we can render to certain children, as we shall see in a moment.

GIMMICKS. It is difficult to find a more suitable

title than "gimmicks," for this section covers such a wide range of physical devices purporting to be quick and easy methods of "breaking the habit" but usually proving instead to be something-for-nothing snares for the unwary, the indolent, or the poorly informed.

These devices usually begin with the evil-smelling or vile-tasting solution that is painted on the child's thumb. A tolerance is quickly developed for these products much as learning to eat red-hots or olives, after which the child may enjoy licking off his thumb before sucking it. In quite a similar vein is the application of cayenne pepper to the child's fingers. Once the child has then rubbed sleepy eyes with these fingers, and screamed for an hour thereafter, most parents relent and allow the child to drop off sucking freshly washed fingers.

This failure often leads to the "old sock" routine: one of father's wool socks is tied over the hand at bedtime, hopefully making the thumb unavailable. If possible, the sock is worked off the hand as the light goes off. If not, or when the sock is retied just short of tourniquet status, a hole is forced in the sock, one way or another, and the precious digit, in one sweeping motion, darts through the hole and into the mouth.

Another favorite is the projecting stick. Preferably, a tongue depressor is cut in half, or any available substitute may be used. It is attached to the thumb, splintwise, with adhesive tape, a goodly portion protruding beyond the end of the thumb. As the thumb approaches the mouth, the stick makes prior contact, brusing the lips, stabbing the palate, or choking the child if it is injected too far before the mouth is closed. The child's allegiance is quickly switched to a different digit, its desirability augmented by the recent oral wound, and the aptitude for sucking grows in stature.

At this point, desperation measures may be brought to bear. Arms are tied to the bed or bound to the body; the child's body may be wrapped tightly in a sheet, arms at sides, in an effective straightjacket. One frantic physician, at the end of his tether, splinted both arms of his avidly sucking, switch-hitting son, and then dared him to find an out; as incredible as it still seems, the boy managed to suck his toe.

As generally employed, we can only include the dental "crib" in this category, as well as the metal bar or other contraption welded into the mouth to make sucking painful or impossible. Dentists deny vehemently that they ever place

such devices without explaining the necessity to the child and gaining his approval. The number of children who then proceed to break the crib out of their mouth, often at the cost of considerable pain, or bide their time until the crib is removed before resuming their sucking habit, or express other indications that they are submitting to this procedure with less than enthusiasm, leaves some doubt as to the advisability of this approach.

In reviewing the "gimmick" approach, we should be aware of the fact that these devices are basically merely ornamented forms of punishment; beneath the paint and bandages, they remain as crude as a hit in the head.

CORRECTIVE PROCEDURES

Prospects for success are brightened considerably if both parents are present for this interview. Fathers may be expendable, but mother is essential in all but a few unusual situations, since much of our program will be based on her understanding, acceptance, and cooperation.

A small deception is also requisite, in that the patient must have no knowledge of what is discussed at the initial portion of the conference; as far as he is concerned, you are simply compiling case history material and visiting for a longer time than necessary. His turn will come. The session is customarily handled in three segments: parent conference, a private interview with the patient, and a joint gathering with child and parents.

Although it may appear that we are overdoing this program a bit, taking unnecessary precautions and asking an excessive amount of routine from child and parent, it is felt to be justified. No ill can befall the child on this regimen except for a tragic sense of failure if our program falls short. When this procedure is carried out fully, it is adequate to the task of transferring some very deep-seated tendencies to more socially acceptable outlets. Part measures and shortcuts have frequently proved deficient.

Parent conference

Sufficient information is elicited from parents to form a general opinion of the child's personality and the family situation. The program is then explained to mother as succinctly as possible while still assuring that she understands all vital aspects.

When more than one child in the family has a sucking habit, it is far better to take them one at a time if possible. Rarely has this program proved fully effective as a group project. In the case of twins, or siblings of near the same age who share a room, and given a sturdy mother, it has occasionally been feasible to complete this program on a two-child basis. It is not recommended.

You may win the mother's instant approbation by a semblance of removing guilt from her influence, so that the lack of a sucking element in abnormal deglutition may be pointed out. However, since we wish her to feel some responsibility in this program, we will avoid discussion of the strong-arm tactics she has used to eliminate the sucking habit.

MATERNAL PROGRAM. In most cases we will ask that the mother serves as a life raft for the period when the child is floundering in deprivation for the first three or four weeks. She will be asked to increase her overt expression of affection and attention during this time. This is the arrangement of which the child should not be aware, so that it falls as manna from heaven, with no requirement that he vie for attention.

Specifically, to satisfy this function, the mother will be asked to (1) make herself available to her child at all times during the coming month; (2) provide her child with a few minutes daily when they are absolutely alone and the mother actually holds the child in her arms; and (3) at least twice daily, she is to openly display attention or affection which is *in addition* to that usually displayed.

The first requirement—that the mother arrange to be at home and available to her child—may be received as a sentence to jail. When the mother is employed in a job outside the home, this requirement poses a problem, and some provision for latitude must often be made. In all other situations we are rather rigid on this point; if the welfare of her child is not sufficiently important to justify her absence from a tea and a few bridge games, you are probably defeated in any event, and the child may have a legitimate basis for sucking his thumb.

The second proviso, that the mother arrange for a private "close time" with the child each day, may also require some planning when there are other children in the home. Assist her in thinking this point through before going on. The father may feel most useful here, in that he may be able to keep the others occupied and distracted while the mother steals away with her "problem child." Alternatively, the children may return from school at different times, younger siblings may go to bed earlier, or there may be some other time that can be found. This problem can always be worked out when there is a willingness to do so.

With younger children, the mother is expected to actually hold the child on her lap during this brief period; should the child be larger than the mother, she should at least sit very close, with an arm around the child, or otherwise maintain physical contact.

The additional attention and affection need be nothing dramatic, only consistent, overt, and unsolicited by the child. Not that we oppose something on a grander scale, except when it might startle the child if it is unprecedented. Simple pecks on the cheek are acceptable as a daily diet.

MATERNAL ATTITUDES. This is the time to ascertain the discipline program in the home and to discuss it on the basis just outlined. You should be sure that the mother understands that she is not being inhibited when a genuine misdeed occurs.

You should also assuage her guilt feelings arising from the prospect of neglecting her other children during this period. If one child became ill, she would feel no compulsion to take the others to the hospital. For the moment, this child has a special need; the others will have their turn as necessary.

We remind her, as we will point out later to the child, that no one is perfect; we expect an occasional failure along the way. If the expectation were for instant and total success, we would probably never succeed.

We also ask that no deadline be set for completion of this project. Once a date is circled on the calendar, it becomes a menace creeping ever closer; the tension thus generated might be sufficient cause for thumb sucking.

Alternate approach

In rare instances, a child is found who has been so smothered with attention that an additional layer would suffocate him. The program just discussed would then be highly inappropriate. For this child we may fill a desperate need by outlining a schedule of discipline, for both child and parents—often extending to grandparents and aunts and uncles.

It is fortunate that such cases are presented infrequently, for the prognosis is never as good. The type of parent who instigates this situation, or permits it, is not easily dissuaded. Occasionally, however, one sane member of the family has been crying for support, and you may enlist in his or her cause with some effect.

It is generally not possible to speak candidly with these parents, for they cannot accept what you are saying. The obvious results of their overprotection should be commented on as tactfully as possible, and the requirements for good discipline specified.

You can list independent activities that are appropriate to the child's age and suggest that they be made available, for immaturity may be marked. You can note the benefits of assigning daily tasks and of withholding approval until the job is satisfactorily completed.

Telling these parents that they cannot live their child's life is a meaningless abstraction. Instead, you might present them with the ridiculous picture of the parents attempting to insert themselves into the lineup of the game in which their child is supposed to play. They cannot bat for him or run for him. The parents' role is that of umpire—the arbiter who calls the fouls and who decides when the child is safe or out. The referee has an essential function; chaos would ensue without him.

Just as an umpire never changes a decision, once pronounced, so, too, the parent cannot descend to a child's role and enter into an argument over a decision once made. When a trip to the store is forbidden by the parent, the jaunt is out. Should the child defy instructions, he is punished. The parent tells the child to pick up his clothes, once, and may remind him once; if the clothes are not then picked up, the child must suffer the consequenes. This is only realistic. When the child learns that he need only complain, weep, or procrastinate to reverse the orders, discipline is a myth, the child is emotionally crippled, his security is undermined, his future is jeopardized, and his parents are remiss.

Although this fact may sail over the parents' heads on into space, you may be permitted to point out that the basic ingredient in any discipline program is *consistency:* agreement between parents as to what is right and what is wrong, and an inevitability in the child's day-to-day experience, so that he finds that the same things are right or wrong tomorrow as yesterday. Parents should decide where they wish to draw the line, but a line should be drawn. The difficult part is to keep the line fairly straight, so that it does not waver unduly.

If you are fortunate enough to put some of these points across, you should proceed with your original project. Observe the parents' reaction closely. You have no right to badger these people. If signs of resentment appear, confess that you are out of your depth and suggest that they discuss their problem with their pediatrician. You are certainly then obligated to contact the physician and present your observations before he is attacked by the parents.

Conference with patient

Once the mother has agreed to accept the role that you have specified, she is left to ruminate on the wisdom of her decision while you get acquainted with the child in a different room. Your chat with the patient is usually brief but is probably the single most decisive and critical facet of this entire program.

The goals of this interview will be to acquaint the child with your posture and province in this matter, to construct a relationship with him as friends engaging a common problem, and, most vital of all, to sign him to a verbal contract to play on your team, eliciting an oral statement of his desire to eliminate his sucking habit. This statement and desire must not be influenced by the physical presence of his parents.

There are definite advantages to making this discussion between therapist and patient private. The presence of a parent inhibits certain responses, dilutes and delays the establishment of rapport, and casts some doubt on the validity of the expressions of opinion offered by the child. When he peers across at a threatening parent and realizes the probable consequence of appearing less than jubilant at the prospect of symbolic amputation of his thumb, why should we bother to ask for his reaction?

We attempt first of all to remove some of the stigma with which the child feels branded: we daily see tongue thrusters older than he who still suck their thumb. We also define our services as assistance, not coercion; if he does not want our help, we will simply stop and go home, and nobody will be mad at anyone.

The therapist is warned never to take lightly, or to take for granted, the response of even the older child when this subject is broached in private. It may seem obvious that the patient would wish to be freed of his addiction to sucking; nevertheless, it is a continuing aspect of behavior, a fact of life—he *does* suck his thumb.

He does so despite prolonged efforts by those about him to effect the demise of the habit. He therefore tends to be defensive to the degree that he has been opposed by his parents. Any act that we thus cherish, and guard against onslaught, we must justify both to ourselves and to others. The naive therapist who approaches a child with the attitude that *of course* the child wishes help with this problem, may be shaken by a flat statement such as: "No, I don't want to quit. I'm just the kind of girl who sucks her thumb." She thereby effectively restricts the therapist's area of mobility: where do you go from there?

It is safer to scout this terrain rather gingerly at first, approaching it obliquely. Some children readily see the direction in which we are moving and spontaneously voice their desire for help or begin to withdraw in preparation for an attack. Should the child sincerely ask for assistance, the interview is closed, and we get on with the project. In many cases the child will require some guidance in finding his way out of the protective shell that he has built around his habit. Should it develop that in reality the child has no intention whatever of relinquishing his habit, you must abide by your word, stop all efforts to pressure or persuade him, and report to the parents that it appears illogical at this time to attempt elimination of sucking, that they must accept this circumstance for the moment, and that as soon as the child experiences a change of attitude, you stand ready to help in every possible way.

The latter situation has arisen infrequently and has often appeared to be a test devised by a skeptical child to prove the sincerity of the therapist. In no case to date has a period of more than two weeks elapsed before the child has called to ask that he be allowed to return for help.

When the child verbalizes the desire to stop his sucking habit, he has, in effect, signed an oral pledge of his cooperation and voluntary efforts. He should, of course, be warmly praised for this decision, returned to the room where mother awaits, and given detailed instructions and explanations covering the balance of the program.

Joint session

You will start with a much better attitude on the part of all concerned if you succeed in the immediate transfer of the child's guilt feelings to some other entity. By pointing out the inaccessible nature of the subconscious, and then placing the blame for continued sucking on these subconscious impulses, you have rendered some absolution, freed the child and parent of part of the load, and to this extent lowered the need for sucking.

Specificity is again the keystone, our unseen ally. These people should be informed not only as to what to do but *how* to do it. The confidence gained through precise knowledge increases greatly the probability that the procedures will be properly put to use. When the family remains unsure of some of the details, they often omit portions in fear of making an error.

There are four specific elements that the child should incorporate into a daily routine. He is to (1) suck on a piece of paraffin during periods of inactivity, (2) sleep with an elastic bandage on his arm, (3) have a piece of adhesive tape on the tastiest finger, and (4) keep score daily on his successes and failures.

PARAFFIN. A number of benefits are gained from the use of paraffin. Even its prospect removes at the outset much of the threat that the child faces in foregoing his thumb: he may yet salvage something from his loss. It does satisfy to some degree any residual urge for sucking activity but places it in a different context: it is acceptable to parents and therefore requires no defensive underpinning, is not really as soul-filling as the finger, is more trouble to find and soften, and consequently is gradually dropped. However, it strikes a pleasant note at the start, provides an alternative, and thus improves the frame of mind with which the child approaches the other requirements.

Bubble gum and things of a different consistency from paraffin have proved to be of little use; the child tends to push them into the buccal vestibule and suck his thumb. The pliable yet firm effect of just-warm paraffin makes a critical difference. The wax tubes or bottles filled with colored liquid and sold at the candy counter are ideal: they require no cutting, taste better, are the correct consistency, and are much more desirable to the child. However, they are frequently unavailable in the summer, when they melt unless refrigerated; they reappear in the fall, with the many varieties shaped into lips, noses, and even giant thumbs, which are a necessary part of Halloween. It is helpful to buy them by the carton when they are in plentiful supply and store them up against the lean periods.

When wax bottles are not to be found, second

choice is probably a sheet of utility wax. It is available, hopefully in a bright color, at the dental supply. You may present a ¼-inch layer to the parent, or to the child if he is old enough to wield a knife in safety. Strips ½ inch wide can be sliced and then folded over two or three times until the optimum bulk is discovered.

Should it be impractical to supply either of these types of wax, parents may be asked to buy a box of household wax (plain paraffin) at the market and cut it into cubes. Cutting this wax is more difficult, since it must be warmed to make cutting possible but melts if it becomes too warm. Whatever is used, it should be stored at home at room temperature, for it will require further warming in the child's mouth before it reaches a peak of satisfaction.

In rare instances, children have refused the wax as a substitute, disliking the taste or the idea, although cooperating thoroughly with the remainder of the program. When television or boredom has then occasioned some return to the thumb, they become distraught with their failure. Although it does nothing to alleviate the urge to suck and seems a poor second choice, some type of glove has often proved helpful. For girls, a pair of inexpensive but frilly white gloves may be purchased at the variety store and worn during periods of danger. Boys would naturally prefer to wear boxing gloves for television watching, but if they are not at hand, work gloves or cowboy gauntlets may suffice. Should the tempter be a digit on the left hand, a baseball glove may also serve.

BANDAGE. The parent should be instructed with exactitude as to applying the elastic bandage. The type that is 2 inches wide is most satisfactory, but if a wider one is already in the medicine chest, it may be used. In reality, it is not necessary to pull the bandage tightly enough to decrease circulation in the fingers; simply having it there, sufficiently snug to prevent its falling off, is all that is required. You should insist, however, that the pins holding the bandage in place be of a size that the child can open with one hand. We wish to assign all possible responsibility to the child, and he should certainly remove the pins and roll the bandage off his arm each morning without unnecessary assistance.

When the child displays no preference between thumbs, using both hands alternately, it is usually necessary to place a bandage on each arm. One elastic bandage may cover a small child's arm with only half its length, leaving a second half for the other arm.

ADHESIVE TAPE. A roll of standard adhesive tape, ½ inch wide, is preferred. Wider tape may be cut to size if it is already on hand. However, plastic backing of any type should be avoided because it is simply too smooth; it is not startlingly different from the texture of a moist thumb, and its vaunted waterproof character robs it of any potential for stool-pigeon duty. The paper-backed variety sold in a dispensing roll works well and usually provides a ready reflection in the morning of any nocturnal sucking.

It is also essential that this tape not be wrapped around the thumb in a continuous spiral that immobilizes the thumb. One small piece is placed over the nail and a separate one around the thumb above the middle joint. When two fingers are sucked, they must not be bound together, but four pieces of tape are used, one over each nail and one above the first knuckle of each finger. We wish to avoid, as much as possible, any sensation of being bound or disabled.

The child should understand from the outset that the purpose of the bandage and tape is not to *force* him to stop sucking, for he can still do so. The bandage is elastic so that he can bend his arm, scratch his head, fix his pillow, or suck his thumb. These items are merely designed to send messages to his subconscious mind when his conscious mind—the part that is really *him*—is lost in sleep and so unable to control the thumb.

In the few rare cases in which children may develop a skin rash in response to adhesive tape, they should try the nonallergenic variety. On occasion patients have been asked to obtain a bottle of make-believe nail polish, available at many drugstores and toy stores. Instead of using the tape at night, the girls manicure the nail that they habitually suck, and the boys paint a "pirate flag" on the nail. They then place their hand under their pillow as they fall asleep, the girls thus putting their thumb in a "jewel box" and the boys "locking up the pirate." If sucking occurs during the night, the polish is quickly dissolved and disappears—that is, the jewel is stolen, or the pirate wins this engagement.

CALENDAR. A sample calendar is shown in Appendix 1; it is to be mimeographed on full sheets of paper. Again, personal involvement is greatly increased by requiring the child to complete the form by filling in the numbers, etc. Older children are asked to obtain a standard calendar for this purpose. In either case, it further stimulates the child's efforts to realize that the record of his progress, being compiled daily on the calendar, will be returned later for the therapist's appraisal.

Each morning the child should inspect the tape before removing it, and keep score on himself for the preceding 24 hours. If, to the best of his knowledge, he has not sucked his thumb since yesterday morning, he places a check mark (√) for that day on the calendar. Zeros were once used for this symbol; however, to a schoolchild a zero means total failure, and the implication was harmfully incongruous for some children. When sucking has occurred, the symbol used is an "X," large enough to cover the entire number on the calendar. When ten check marks have been achieved, after the last previous X, the child is instructed to telephone the therapist to report success, receive additional instructions, and make an appointment to begin swallowing therapy. In other words, we are asking that sucking be stopped for only ten days as the criterion for success.

This ten-day requirement would certainly be inadequate to accept as an indication of permanency if no further contact with the patient were planned. However, this is only the beginning. When the child *feels* that he has conquered this problem, the heady wine of success keeps him going for a time; after all, he succeeded on his own! Once victory is achieved and is duly reported to the therapist, the child will be coming for therapy each week. The first transaction after he is seated each week will be a question concerning his continued status as an ex-thumb sucker and a restatement of the therapist's gratification with his performance; thus it would be a betrayal of himself to find it necessary, later, to confess his desertion from these ranks.

Some children inscribe additional comments on the calendar, venting their frustration with X's or their joy or surprise with a check mark. The final success may be noted by a row of exclamation points. One mature 9-year-old, who had been under considerable pressure at home because of her sucking habit, obtained a stack of 3 by 5 inch cards, dated one for each day throughout the program, and wrote a sentence or two on each one concerning her feelings, hopes, and predictions. She started with three days of failure, managed to hold out for 24 hours, slipped again, and then never sucked her thumb again. Excerpts from her "diary" show the following,

including the original spelling:

Oct. 20: This is the day it was started. At night I sucked my thumb. I didn't have the Ace bandage or tap yet. I used the wax, it worked fine.

Oct. 21: I sucked the thumb on the arm which wasn't wraped. Moms going to wrap the other arm. These morning my sister saw me start to suck my right thumb (the thumb with the tap) but before it was in me mouth I took it out. (I was asleep.) That shows it works.

Oct. 22: This morning neither taps had stain, but I have forgotten to suck the wax. Today when I was watching TV, I put the wax around a marble, it made it easier to suck and it lasted longer. But the second time the wax broke up.

Oct. 23: So far I am doing fine. I had trouble when I forgot to suck the wax. . . .

Oct. 24: I get to put a check. I don't have trouble at night. I never do it at night. But the day, when I get home from school I sometimes do it. Last night we watch a movie about two hours long. I didn't do it once. When I got home from church I did it. . . .

Oct. 25: I get another check. I think I am on the way to ten checks. . . . .

Oct. 29: Today I have four checks. Mom said she'd get me an ice cream soda when I got five checks. Tomorrow she will get me a soda.

It can be seen from her comments that after three days of failure she was still able to feel that she was "doing fine." The reason is that she had been led to expect initial difficulties, allowance having been made for human frailty; she knew that she was making progress in working out readjustments and that no demand had been made that she complete the project before she was capable of doing so. She had several siblings, but her parents, skeptical at first, furnished their support in excellent fashion; obviously, they missed the point about interim bribery.

Some children, especially older ones, do receive great reinforcement of their resolve if they are able to telephone the therapist once or twice, usually at bedtime. The therapist should never resent these calls for help; we invite them. A few words of approbation, reflecting your approval of the child as a person and your confidence in his ability to succeed, can prevent some disheartening failures.

When the child calls to report his successful attainment of ten consecutive check marks, he receives a lavish drenching in praise; a few kind words should be reserved for the parent also. The child and then the parent are instructed to begin deceleration and descent: the elastic bandage is omitted; after two nights, only the adhesive tape over the nail is used, omitting the other piece, for two additional nights; thereafter, nothing—unless the child wishes to continue sucking wax for a time. The latter contingency arises occasionally and may well be permitted; it falls of its own weight in a week or two, as the child's confidence becomes solidified. However, the bandage and tape must come off on schedule. We do not wish the child to build such a dependency on them that he feels incapable of resisting his thumb without them.

Time is usually allowed for this gradual unwrapping to be completed before the child is scheduled to return. He should continue to keep score on the calendar, and if any relapse occurs, he should immediately restore the last item that was removed from his arm or finger. If all goes well, he returns bearing a much-used calendar and receives further adulation for his efforts, the calendar is enshrined for posterity in a special folder in the therapist's filing cabinet, and the child's momentum is carried over into therapy.

When therapy is not scheduled to begin at once, the period of abstention is increased from ten days to two weeks, and after the complete withdrawal of tape and bandage crutches, the child returns his calendar in person, as above, for the the same memorial ceremonies.

TONGUE SUCKING

It is rare indeed when a child with a sucking habit does not quench his craving by "milking" his thumb, finger, or two fingers. Each item specified in this chapter, up to this point, applies with equal uniformity regardless of the digital recourse that the patient elects. Exceptional patients, unfortunately, prefer their tongue. This complicates the problem, since it is difficult to bandage the tongue. Nevertheless, tongue sucking is fully as proficient in destroying recently acquired improvements in deglutition and must as certainly be eliminated before normal function can be expected to prevail.

This problem is often as frustrating for the therapist as for the patient. It has a repulsive appearance, a damaging consequence, and a resistive nature. Saddest of all, no pat answer can be supplied at this time, and there is no truly effective counterstroke or humane plan for retaliation. Wax becomes a turncoat, enticing the tongue into the characteristic protruded, interdental posture from which the tongue continues to provide comfort while the paraffin merely rides the dorsum, the epitome of futility.

The child should be interviewed prior to the parent conference, if possible, to determine if it is even advisable to attempt elimination of tongue sucking at this time. The gravity of the situation should be explained to the patient: it is not conceivable that a normal pattern of deglutition could even be established, much less maintained, as long as this habit persists. Attitudes should be probed and powers of persuasion focused. Only a sincere and abiding desire on the part of the patient will suffice.

Should it appear feasible to begin, the parent program is put into effect as above. As for the child, only the calendar remains of our previous procedures. Even an oral screen has little value: the mandible is dropped, the tongue is protruded, and sucking proceeds. The only alternative appears to be the "antisnore mask" described in Chapter 25. When the child will accept this device as help, rather than coercion, there is some hope of eventual triumph. It is necessary to lower and then pump the mandible in order to suck the tongue in a satisfying manner; this action is inhibited by the mask and can be produced only with voluntary effort.

It is necessary to wear the mask during periods of physical inactivity throughout the day, as well as at night. No compensatory sucking sensation can be provided. It is a "cold turkey" approach, and it does not always succeed.

Chapter 17

STEP 1:
LIP EXERCISES

With all of the preceding chapters duly mastered, it is now appropriate to face the basic issue: how can deglutition be corrected? What specific procedures may be employed and what is their probable effect? In the same manner that therapy is divided into segments for the benefit of the patient, so for the reader we may now consider these individual steps one by one and how best to achieve them.

PRELIMINARY REMARKS
Professional attitude

The keynote to the success or failure of therapy, whatever its nature, is often sounded at the instant the patient steps into the therapist's office. He should enter a professional office and be treated in a professional manner by a therapist of professional appearance in whom he can confidently and confidentially place his trust. Ostentation is unnecessary and often harmful, and the same may be said for excessive dignity; there is no substitute for proper, intelligent, assured conduct reflecting genuine interest in the patient's well-being. It is helpful if the therapist acquires the ability to communicate in accurate but lay terminology; patients may be impressed by polysyllables, but they seldom respond well to them. The goal should be a display of open, friendly dignity.

Role of observer

Every patient who gains the threshold of this lair of efficient charm must be accompanied by an observer. With children, at least one parent must be present at each session, unless there is an acute emotional conflict operating; in this case, some other near relative, with whom the child will spend a major portion of his time outside of school, may serve instead. However, nursemaids, neighbors, and distant grandmothers often make poor surrogates and are seldom accepted. In most cases, even adults are required to bring someone along—a spouse, sibling, or even their own child.

We who have been taught the "horrors" of allowing the parent inside the therapy room may find this requirement difficult to accept. Nevertheless, there is sound rationale behind it. First, it is physically impossible for the patient to observe his own behavior in detail during some of the exercises, even with a mirror; a second party, oriented during the therapy session, can easily do so. The observer would have little concept of what is involved, what to look for, or how to evaluate the home practice if he were not present during the actual session.

Second, the lifelong pattern of muscle movement *feels* most comfortable and right to the patient. After starting an exercise or a meal with the new pattern, it is quite easy to drift back to the accustomed manner, thereby serving to reinforce still further the undesirable habit. An observer can detect this tendency quickly.

Finally, and sufficient in itself, is the moral support thus gained. It is a rare child, pushed into his room with the parent's admonition to "go practice," who will do so with goodwill. Attitude is all-important in this project, and the dramatic difference when parents are informed, interested, and supportive is the factor that usually tips the balance to the new pattern.

Patients are advised of this requirement when they make their first appointment. It is clarified at the time of their first session.

The child is made to feel responsible for his own progress: no one can practice for him. The parent can help, as the therapist can, but we cannot force the patient to swallow correctly; that is his job. Therapy is directed almost entirely toward the child during every session, with parents merely observing and asking occasional questions. Progress is reported by the child, not the parent. Telephone calls are invited, in case of uncertainty about assignments or to report specific accomplishments, but from the child, not the parent. Strong personal involvement of the patient is the *sine qua non*—under someone else's watchful eye.

Routine of first appointment

At the first appointment, patients are customarily greeted in the waiting room, which provides an opportunity for a few brief general observations and the establishment of some initial lines of communication between therapist and patient. After a look at their teeth, and a casual inquiry into their school or current interests, the patients are left in the waiting room, surrounded by toys and comic books. The parents are then plied with coffee, questions, and good advice in another room.

Adult patients, of course, are not excluded in this way, but the frequency with which emotional problems must be discussed, the high incidence of persisting sucking habits, the confused family situation in some cases, and the need to indoctrinate some parents, all militate against having the child present during this phase. The therapist will also be provided with an opportunity to assess the parent.

The first appointment must cover a number of aspects and is therefore rather lengthy. It can be managed as a 90-minute session, roughly divided into three 30-minute portions: (1) case history and parent orientation, (2) initial interview with the patient, and (3) oral examination and assignment of the first exercise.

PARENTAL PROCEDURES
Compiling the history form

The case history forms we use are shown in Appendix 1. Although much more comprehensive forms are customarily employed for speech defects *per se,* a shorter format has been found to encompass all essential data for deglutition cases and is more convenient and usable. The content should, of course, be modified to meet the desires of the individual therapist; the forms

shown have been frequently changed to include items of momentary interest. The form used by Barrett can be mimeographed on standard 5 × 8 inch cards, for which file cabinets are easily found. Space is provided to make a brief note after each session; the reverse side can be used for comments during the recheck period, and all information is thus available at a glance.

Whatever else the form may encompass, it should provide specific information on a few hurdles that may be expected in therapy and on several complete barriers to therapy. They will be discussed in the order in which they occur on Barrett's form.

TONSILS AND ADENOIDS. The patients we have seen divide almost evenly between those who have had their tonsils and adenoids removed and those who have not. Regardless of whether or not this surgery has been performed, the therapist should be alerted to a careful appraisal of the situation when examining the patient. Occasionally, muscle impairment results from tonsillectomies and is revealed by imbalance in velar movement; most of our problems, however, stem from tonsils still *in situ.*

Nasal breathing will be an absolute necessity at the conclusion of therapy if the child is to maintain a normal rest posture and thereby the newly acquired pattern of deglutition. Nasal blockage from hypertrophied adenoids would obviously nullify the entire program, and therapy in such cases should thus be delayed until such blockage is removed. An adequate judgment may usually be made on the basis of the patient's voice quality; if in doubt, complete the first session with the understanding that a medical examination will be performed prior to the second session.

Ideally, if tonsils are present, they should be in healthy condition. However, infected tonsils appear to pose less of a threat than sheer bulk. It will be necessary during therapy to retract the posterior tongue into the faucial region. Far less pain than would be expected is encountered from lingual pressure on tonsils bearing pustules; however, when tonsils are enlarged to the point of impinging on the uvula, or meeting on the midline, it is not logical to expect the patient to further restrict the airway by pressing them backward.

Enlarged tonsils are chronic with some children, and since speech or dental considerations may not allow time for natural resorption, surgical removal should be discussed with the patient's pediatrician or otolaryngologist. Speech pathologists of even moderate longevity will recall the great difficulties presented by the child who has been allowed to retain hypertrophied tonsils and adenoids to the point of relinquishing velar control, is operated on just before choking to death, and thereafter displays the nasality of a cleft palate.

Tongue-thrust therapy will be of doubtful value in the presence of enlarged tonsils; the tonsils should be removed or therapy should be delayed.

ALLERGIES. Problems such as hay fever, sinusitis, asthma, bronchiectasis, and chronic bronchitis all jeopardize the prospect for successful correction. The reason is the same as with adenoids: the patient must be able to acquire an easy oral rest posture that features a closed mouth and nasal breathing.

Although some mild, often undiagnosed, nasal stuffiness is frequently reported, it can usually be controlled with proper medication and the deterrent thus removed. Many deviant swallowers mouth-breathe from habit rather than necessity, and so do not have as severe a problem as it seems. Others have only one or two episodes, recurrent at almost the same date each year, and therapy can be worked around or between these times.

These circumstances, whatever their nature, should be analyzed before therapy is undertaken. Patient and parent should realize the significance of this factor. In less than 1% of patients, it is futile to begin therapy because of nasal congestion so complete and so continuous that relapse to the original swallowing pattern is almost certain. Regardless of what the parent has reported, it is good practice to ask the patient to close his mouth and keep it closed for a minute or two. Many do so with no indication of stress or discomfort.

EMOTIONAL STATUS. Some idea should be elicited concerning the patient's personality, customary reactions, attitudes, etc. Parents are not always the most accurate judges in this respect, but insight is often obtained just by listening to the parent's appraisal. Any emotional crises should be discussed, and notation made of nail biting, enuresis, or other similar indicators.

It may eventuate that the parent who seeks straight teeth for a child may also be the one who wants every "advantage" for the darling child or who distrusts or resents the private, independent activities by which children practice their true

vocation of being children. The shock is reduced through repetition when one finds again and again children who, after an intense and restrictive day at school, go for ballet lessons on Monday and Thursday, are tutored on Tuesday and Friday, have a music lesson on Wednesday, and attend religious school on Saturday, leaving the mother innocently asking for a Sunday appointment to work in therapy. We decline such cases, partly because of the obvious futility and partly because it is thought to be not in the best interest of the child to add yet another pressure. It is also mortifying to finish second to a *pas de chat*.

SUCKING HABIT. This is the point at which the previous chapter began. As noted there, attention shifts entirely to the sucking habit once its presence is verified. The next four or five items on the history form are completed, after which the sucking program is presented. Some weeks later, when the habit has been eliminated, we resume at this point and proceed with therapy. The same procedure is followed when we discover the need for a frenectomy, a tonsillectomy, an incompatible orthodontic phase, etc.

It may suffice at this point to note that any sucking habit is incompatible with the maintenance of normal deglutition; therefore, no patient is ever permitted to begin swallowing therapy until the sucking habit is stopped and appears to be under permanent control. This requirement is without qualification and includes those patients, most frequent, in fact, in whom the sucking occurs "only a little bit at night." The most difficult aspect of training a new swallowing pattern will be to alter behavior during sleep; if a finger enters the mouth at night, even briefly, it stimulates the flow of saliva, depresses the tongue, and subconsciously results in the immediate resumption of the original malfunction.

OTHER CONDITIONS. We are primarily concerned here with discovering any throat surgery (other than tonsillectomy), mouth injury, such as falling on a stick and puncturing the velum, or other condition that might cause impairment of the musculature. Cut lips and other trauma to the anterior or exterior structures rarely make a difference. However, if a muscle imbalance or inability is encountered later, it is well to know its basis. We dislike surprises in therapy.

We may also note at this point any birth injury, prematurity, or severe illness that might have significance or a continuing influence. It would be interesting to learn the percentage of premature infants who develop abnormal swallows: the number who appear for therapy seems disproportionately large. Although this impression may be erroneous, it would not be difficult to account for a heightened incidence.

INFANT FEEDING PROGRAM. Our beliefs on the subject of infant feeding were set forth in Chapter 8, and the item is presently allowed to remain on the history form merely for its curiosity value and as a springboard for discussion in case the parent wishes to delve into etiology. Many related items have been incorporated in the past but were deleted when it became obvious that most could be answered before the question was asked. For example, the occurrence of colic was almost universal, with projectile vomiting a frequent corollary.

There are indications that thrusters accept new foods with alacrity, depending on the consistency of the food. They appear to discriminate texture better than flavor; they tend to reject meats and fibrous vegetables, which would be more difficult to swallow with a tongue thrust, but assent to any soft or mushy food.

AGE OF WALKING AND TALKING. The ages at which the patient walked and talked seldom have any direct pertinency but may give some idea of native coordination. This item is also a recheck device, since the parent will sometimes remember in this context an accident or frenectomy that was overlooked on the earlier question.

ORTHODONTIC PLANS. As noted in Chapter 15, it is essential that therapy be properly coordinated with any existing or proposed dental treatment. Specifically what that program will consist of should be ascertained and proper notation made at this time, including extraction or appliance dates, etc. It is well for the patient to understand the planned sequence of events, for he can then jog the memory of the dentist or therapist who starts to stray from the plan. If a conflict in timing is apparent, an immediate call to the orthodontist is in order, delayed only until the clinician has examined the patient's mouth and is prepared to answer questions.

Parent orientation

The balance of the history card is left blank for the moment, pending oral examination. Instead, any parental questions that will not be covered later may be answered now. Etiology is discussed only at the parent's insistence, and always with regard for uncertainties involved. The parent's role in therapy is usually clarified simply by implication, but if there appears to be

unwillingness to assume it, or if there is any antagonism, the situation should be resolved immediately before the child is caught in a crossfire. It may be suggested that a different clinician might be more acceptable, or that therapy might be postponed until circumstances appear more favorable. The parent may wish to wait until further inquiry can be made into the legitimacy of this project, particularly if the referring dentist has not been explicit, since the parent may feel sure that children did not swallow improperly when he or she was a child. Talk it over, but keep it gentle: no one wins an argument.

TIMING OF THERAPY. The time requirements for this project should be discussed, and an agreement reached that there will be an uninterrupted period of time, approximately two months, in which therapy can be completed, barring illness and the unforeseen. School holidays of a week or more may prove a problem, as do summer vacations, etc. It is often effectual to arrange for the first four steps to be accomplished before such a break; a few days of review thereafter and the patient is ready to make further progress. Once the total swallow has been assembled, and work is progressing on habituation, *any* delay frequently results in disintegration of the new pattern, repetition of some of the earlier exercises, and resentment on the part of the patient that we can ill afford. Although we cannot always mold events to our desire, the patient should understand the factors involved.

FEES. This is also the time to discuss fees and their payment. The importance of the recheck period should be stressed; parents should never consider this a two-month project but should be led from the first to view it more in the nature of a one-year program, incorporating an active treatment period and a longer follow-up phase, both of indefinite duration.

GROUP THERAPY. Infrequently there are three or four thrusters in the same family, or two who live next door to two others. In such cases parents may inquire into mass correction.

It was briefly noted in Chapter 15 that no truly effective plan for group therapy in tongue thrust is known to us. Doubtless one could be devised, but it would require a specialized setting and arrangements. In practical experience, even three siblings rarely complete the program as a group, and this arrangement is now discouraged when proposed. One child always seems to be out of step with the others, requiring a splinter session that usually evolves into a separate program. Two siblings are routinely treated jointly; however, even this arrangement does not always work out. The advantages, when it does prove feasible, are considerable: half the trips to the office, half the work for the parent, and far less than half the cost under our program. A small additional fee for each session is made for a second child; whereas some sessions will require extra time, some are completed almost as quickly with two as with one. It is possible to allow one child to mark time for a week while the other catches up, if only two are involved, although this circumstance should not be repeated: inevitably, the attitude of the better child deteriorates, and both may end in failure. On the other hand, some carefree youngsters have actually appeared to do a more thorough job when competing with an older sibling than could otherwise have been expected. Care should be taken in this situation, however, to mute the competitive aspects.

In this connection, we should consider the recurrent case of the tongue-thrusting parent who wishes to undergo therapy with the child. This arrangement has been tried repeatedly and found to be inadvisable. Parents should retain their supervisory role until the child is safely finished; thereafter, if the parent is genuinely interested, the program can be pursued on a ''separate but equal'' basis.

PROLOGUE FOR THE PATIENT

Attention is shifted entirely to the patient, once he joins the therapist in the consultation room. Even information you wish to fall on the parent's ears is now directed toward the patient. Younger children, especially, should not be allowed to sit and squirm and sigh while side discussions are carried on. The child enters and immediately comes to center stage.

Purposes and procedures

Whereas there are a number of specific objectives in conducting this interview, there are also some indirect general purposes behind it. In the first place, it allows the patient to become acquainted with the clinician, to form a judgment of what to expect, and to lay the basis for the interpersonal relationship to follow. Hopefully, the clinician will thus be alert to convey the proper image and initiate the proper attitudes. Also, as the patient enters the room he is frequently nervous, skeptical, and insecure as regards this entire project—hardly a frame of mind conducive to efficient therapy. The therapist should be actively aware of this situation and prepared to deal with it. Then, too, the clinician is here provided an opportunity to study the patient, to observe reactions, and to prepare himself before being committed to a definite plan of action.

There are five specific objectives: (1) to place the patient's habit in an acceptable context; (2) to explain the consequences if therapy is not done; (3) to provide an overview of what the program will comprise, so that the initial steps will have some frame of reference within which the patient can understand the exercises he will be asked to do; (4) to explain the rules that will apply throughout therapy; and (5) to secure a verbal commitment to therapy from the patient.

Implications of tongue thrust

Children who are merely told by a dentist that they swallow abnormally have little concept of the implications. To some of them it makes little difference anyway: they have been eating well and feeling no pain from the condition. Others, however, because the parent was shocked and disturbed by the diagnosis, and because they are now being brought to a strange specialist, or simply because they do not understand the situation, build some rather horrible concepts of this plague from which they suffer. Guilt or shame is a common reaction. It is safer to dispel this attitude at once, remove them from the realm of the freak, and make them welcome.

Consequences with and without therapy

The patient has the obvious choice: he can undertake therapy, or decide *not* to do so. He should be able to make this choice intelligently. Explaining sequelae serves to further reassure the patient, clarifies the condition in everyone's mind, and is the most powerful motivating force available for immediate application. The therapist should prepare himself with a set of plaster study models showing teeth in normal occlusion; a greatly oversized model that is more intriguing to children is available commercially. (See Appendix 2.) Models of actual malocclusions caused by deviant deglutition should also be at hand, including a particularly horrendous Type 2, as well as some small object of approximately 3 ounces in weight. Two concepts are stressed at this time: the disadvantages of molar super-eruption when teeth are not occluded in normal deglutition, and the futility of orthodontic treatment if the present dysfunction is allowed to remain. Be specific in contrasting the 1 to 4 ounces of force per tooth, which is all the orthodontist requires to straighten teeth, with the vastly greater total of adverse pressures applied in tongue thrusting. The powerful thrust of the tongue, multiplied by the frequency of swallowing over a 24-hour period, is sufficient in itself to maintain some types of oral deformity. When this force is augmented by an abnormal resting posture that inflicts a lighter but more constant impeding force, similar in magnitude to an orthodontic appliance, the effect of the appliance is sharply reduced or even nullified. Orthodontic treatment time is thus needlessly prolonged, and relapse after treatment is almost assured.

Overview of therapy

It is unfair to all concerned to pop patients into a therapy room and begin assigning exercises when they have no conception of what they are doing, or why. Furthermore, it is frequently useless. Having learned *why* therapy is important from the preceding section, it is well to supply some outline of *what* will be done. The concept of step-by-step progress is emphasized, a warning is voiced about expecting perfection of execution on the first try, and the parent is restrained from demanding an immediate change in the patient's swallowing behavior: the initial exercises are designed to train muscles, not transfer food from the oral cavity to the stomach.

No effort is made to specify what each step will consist of; rather, explain that there will be individual segments, that these segments will later be assembled into a total configuration of swallowing, and that exercises will then be provided to assist in making the new pattern habitual.

Rules of therapy

Stating in advance exactly what you will expect of the patient during therapy has a double advantage: it increases chances that the work will be properly done, and precludes or reduces to a minimum later conflict between child and parent. There is no substitute for specificity in making assignments throughout therapy. The number of times the patient is to practice each day and the number of times he is to repeat an exercise at each practice period should be assigned exactly, never in round numbers or "a few times." A printed card or sheet should accompany every exercise, stating this information and setting forth as well the exact manner in which the exercise should be done. Remember

that the patient is in a strange setting, assailed by many strange ideas and demands; it is easy to forget details later. Also, not being trained clinicians, patients and parents are prone to an unbelievable number of honest mistakes, even excluding the "easier way" the patient frequently discovers. Therefore spell out in detail, even before therapy begins, those items which will apply generally.

Several authorities have found that repeated, brief exercise periods achieve more than prolonged ones, yield a result seemingly out of proportion to the effort expended, and enable the muscles to maintain the achievement with little further practice. Hellebrandt and Houtz[1] found improved muscle strength after exercise sessions so short as to preclude anything other than *learning*. Certainly tongue-thrust patients have the requisite muscles, with the potential for normal function; they need only to fulfill this potential to the point of obviating conscious thought and effort. They tend to do so, incidentally, with a willingness that is directly proportional to the brevity of practice periods. It is also important that there be adequate rest periods between practice sessions. There is a physiological need for rest, if the desired coordination is to be maintained, and this need is sometimes more immediate than would appear logical. Moreover, habituation of the newly acquired pattern appears easier when practice is distributed through the day rather than reserved for an intense period in the evening.

In view of the foregoing, and after considerable trial and error in establishing the briefest possible practice that would still give the desired result, patients are requested to practice the exercises that comprise the first three or four steps of therapy on the basis of three periods per day, separated by rest periods of at least 2 hours. Each practice period is expected to be of only a few minutes' duration. If practice is a lengthy ordeal, something is wrong: the patient is exercising improperly or is seeking sympathy. Children are requested to phone the therapist if the exercises prove long or difficult. Success is greatest when the program goes quickly and smoothly to conclusion.

The necessity for practicing under supervision is explained to every patient but is stressed most strongly with the early adolescents. For older children and adults, such supervision is not necessary at *every* practice period, but there should be some daily evaluation of their performance.

The physiological basis for demanding such observation should be clearly understood by both patient and observer; if they can see that it is necessary, there is less probability of friction over this issue. In the first place, it is not possible to observe the anterior portion of one's own palatal vault in a mirror, short of a periscope arrangement that would interfere with tongue function. Thus the patient cannot adequately rely on self-observation. Also, there is reduced sense of position in the tongue. Sense of position arises primarily from points of muscle attachment to bone or cartilage, a condition that is lacking in the anterior tongue. As long as we are able to touch a point in our mouth with our tongue, and identify what we are touching, we are secure in our knowledge of tongue position. The hard palate, however, tends to be uncharted territory, and even adults frequently miss by a considerable margin a given spot in this region. The reader may think back to his last dental appointment and recall the difficulty encountered in keeping his tongue out of the dentist's way: with the most cooperative patient, the dental assistant strives valiantly to prevent the dentist from drilling into the tongue.

The clinician is warned specifically about the teenagers who have arrived at the point of knowing *everything*. These patients tend to lock the door of their room to prevent the parent's observation, return after a week to demonstrate that they have rehearsed some exercise unrelated to the one assigned, but are indignant when this fact is pointed out. The therapist soon becomes familiar with the wail from the parent, "Well, she *said* she was doing it right." This situation should be forestalled.

The cardinal rule, of course, is that the patient must cooperate. He should be apprised of this before he ever begins actual therapy. We are not asking that he perform above his ability, only that he make an honest effort. However, he must accept the responsibility for his performance. If he is truly unable to achieve a given objective in the allotted time, we will be patient in assisting him. If he avoids practice periods or does them in a slovenly fashion, he will simply be dropped from therapy until a hoped-for change in attitude.

Verbal commitment of the patient

The verbal commitment of the patient seems to be of sufficient importance to warrant its own notation. After all the foregoing is explained to the patient, he is given a chance to speak up. His opinion is invited, as are any comments or questions he may have. If any indications of reluctance appear, which is rare, they are probed a bit. If they are found to be genuine, he also may be asked to consider a delay in starting therapy until he is sure he wishes to participate properly. If he overtly voices the desire to begin therapy, his wishes are complied with at once.

THERAPY PROCEDURES

Under the usual routine, a move is now made from a consultation room to a therapy room. This move not only permits the patient to stretch and awaken from the foregoing conversation, which was primarily a listening situation for the patient, but also serves to orient him toward a *working* environment. Although the entire procedure can easily be conducted in a single room, there are definite advantages, and a more professional atmosphere, in providing separate rooms.

Therapy room

After experience with a common therapy room that accommodated patients of all ages, we can now recommend even further subdivision of the floor plan to provide a separate therapy room for younger patients. This room can be supplied with juvenile furniture and otherwise equipped to help the child to be interested and secure, as well as to maintain maximum attention. The youngster is not impelled to twist the knobs off the audiometer if it is safely ensconced in the adult's room, and the dignity of the teenager is not threatened by his being in the same room with "kid stuff." It should go without saying that stark-white cabinets and instruments of forbidding appearance should never be employed.

Although little in the way of special equipment is required for this work, a few suggestions may smooth the way. A large mirror adjacent to the therapy table is certainly convenient; however, there are marked advantages if the patient sits directly across the table from the therapist, rather than beside him; both communication and observation are enhanced. Yet this arrangement requires a swiveling movement to use the mirror, which places strain on some of the muscles of the throat and mouth; it may therefore be advisable to supply a smaller mirror as well. A hand mirror or a makeup mirror equipped with a stand may be used, or a special mirror constructed so that it stands upright on a wooden base may be used. It can be pushed aside when not in use.

A small portable light will be required. Although many styles are available, a standard penlight is usually quite satisfactory, provided it has a positive "on-off" action; some types refuse to remain on.

The major problem often lies in the plumbing: a washbasin or other ready source of water, both hot and cold, will be essential in the later steps of therapy.

Of course, plenty of facial tissue, always within easy reach, forms the prudent underpinning of therapy.

Peripheral examination

The oral abilities and disabilities of the patient must be carefully assessed. Such techniques as the clinician may wish to apply may be used, but they should include the evaluation of some specific irregularities to which the tongue thruster is prone. A penlight and a tongue depressor are adequate to this task.

GENERAL CONCERNS. It is well to check the gag reflex at once, working the depressor slowly back on the tongue and stopping at the first sign that the patient will truly gag. Be sure to observe the tonsils while you are in the neighborhood. A general incoordination of the tongue is frequently noted, especially if a speech defect is present, but lingual ability may range up to a high degree of coordination in some cases. When the tongue is protruded to touch the edge of a depressor, some imbalance of the musculature is occasionally found, the tongue consistently missing its mark to right or left. This imbalance does not always accompany unilateral thrust.

Many tongue thrusters cannot form a well-defined point with the tip of their tongue, having instead a rather bulbous aspect. They may also have difficulty in touching the tip of their tongue to the corners of their opened mouth, touching instead with the side of the tongue.

In any event, the range of motion of the tongue should be observed, both vertically and laterally. It often appears that there is little differentiated movement of the tongue, that it is a mere appendage of the jaw and works only when accompanied by movement of the mandible. Few patients with an abnormal swallow are able to open their mouth, protrude their tongue slightly, then lift the tongue into contact with their upper lip, and still keep the mouth open; they cannot get their tongue and lower teeth to part company.

Speech can be adequately evaluated for the moment by asking the patient to count aloud from one to eleven. However, the therapist's eye, as well as ear, should be attuned; at this point, we are less concerned with auditory effect than with possible interdental production of consonants. When speech is defective, the patient is advised at once that correct speech is essential before he can be dismissed from therapy.

The physical structure of the mouth should be studied, including lip morphology, occlusion of the teeth, conformation of the palate, etc. If any physical barrier to therapy is apparent, such as an upper arch nearing collapse, or upper incisors so protrusive as to prevent lip closure even with effort, a conference with the orthodontist is indicated, as discussed in the previous chapter, before proceeding with therapy.

RESTRICTED TONGUE LIFT. A spot behind the incisal papilla should be stimulated with the tongue depressor and the patient asked to touch this spot with the tip of his tongue; this ability will be requisite. Patients are occasionally found who are incapable of touching the tip of their tongue to any point on the palate, at least on a voluntary basis. When this situation is discovered, it obviously becomes necessary to devote some preliminary time to the acquisition of this ability.

Since at least two publications have proposed a technique to combat this condition that is not only futile but often damaging, the clinician should recall a basic characteristic of muscles: the tendency to oppose force. It has been suggested that if the patient has difficulty in lifting the tongue, the therapist place a tongue depressor under the tongue and assist in lifting. Such a procedure causes the tongue to press *down* against the depressor, strengthening the tendency we are trying to reverse. If, instead, the depressor is placed *on top* of the tongue, and gentle pressure is exerted, the tongue will tend to resist by lifting, so that at least the muscles will be properly innervated; there is then some hope of success. It sometimes helps to stimulate the tip of the tongue and the palate alternately.

In these cases of restricted ability, the parent is usually asked to select a tablespoon at home, preferably one with a flat handle. The spoon should be held by the bowl and the handle laid on the child's tongue. The parent should be warned to use almost no pressure at first, allowing the child to succeed in lifting the tongue against the handle. If this is done several times daily, and the resistance is gradually increased, a marked increase is usually noticed in tongue strength. When the child is able to press upward fairly firmly, the parent should suddenly retract the spoon; the tongue usually continues on up into the palatal vault. They should continue working in this way until the child is easily able to touch his tongue to various spots on the palate when the parent stimulates these places with the spoon handle. This goal can usually be reached in a week. It is a necessary preliminary in only a few cases, but the first step of the formal program should never be attempted until it is accomplished. Of course, the parent can always be sent home with a quantity of tongue depressors if the tablespoon idea seems objectionable.

LINGUAL FRENUM. The status of the lingual frenum should also be noted. Only in rare cases is an abnormality present. It is not unusual to discover frena that appear short or that extend somewhat farther anterior on the tongue than we might wish. However, the frenum is normally a rather diaphanous affair, and even if the tissue is of fairly solid texture, there is remarkable elasticity as a rule, making it possible to stretch the frenum to permit normal tongue movement.

In those few cases in which the frenum is continuous to the tip of the tongue, or attachment extends up to the gingival line, frenectomy is indicated. There is also a type of frenum, found only occasionally, in which the tissue is tough and fibrous and has little similarity to a membrane; instead, it appears to be two tapered cords, like two cones standing upright on their bases, tying the tongue to the floor of the mouth. The potential for stretching these cords is seemingly small, and surgical removal is usually necessary. Bear in mind that oral surgery is never to be taken lightly. "Clipping the tongue" sounds simple, and in the newborn it is, but in the older patient the chance of postsurgical infection is high. There must also be some ensuing cicatrix; patients have been seen for whom repeated "tongue clips" have been performed to correct an unrelated speech defect, with a resulting mass of scar tissue more immovable and more disabling than the original frenum.

If frenectomy is unavoidable, therapy must obviously be delayed until this procedure has been completed. If it appears necessary and possible to stretch the frenum into usable condition, exercises to accomplish this stretching should be assigned and routine therapy similarly postponed. In most cases, results are obtained in a week or two if the patient is instructed in forceful tongue "popping." This exercise will be necessary in any event later in therapy and is explained in detail in Chapter 19.

TEMPOROMANDIBULAR JOINT. It is advisable to make some cursory evaluation of the status of the TMJ. You will have noted the extent and symmetry of jaw opening in the course of intraoral examination. A gentle palpation of three areas, the masseter, the temporalis, and over the joint itself, will reveal any clicking or painful area. A direct question concerning chronic headache, earache, or other facial discomfort will complete this section and usually suffices to expose any serious problem existing at this time.

Other preliminaries

Pertinent information gleaned from the peripheral examination should be noted on the history form. It should be an easy matter at this point to classify the type of swallowing deviation presented by the patient. If you keep a photographic record of patients, this is the time for intraoral picture-taking. The balance of this session is ordinarily concentrated on the needs of the facial muscles. However, should this patient prove to be one of the rare cases who has no need for any form of lip exercises, as with some Type 8 (bilateral) thrusts, we would move directly to Step 2 (Chapter 18) and eliminate further consideration of lips.

It does not seem conceivable that it should be necessary to present yet more lip exercises; we have had an abundant supply in many forms and sources. Still, the needs in this particular situation are somewhat specialized, some readers will not be acquainted with the literature in this area, and many others would be required to do considerable sifting. Thus a small number of the exercises that have appeared to be effective in tongue thrust will be offered. Many others that are not listed might serve as well. You might even succeed in developing an absolutely new exercise.

Recall the composition and effect of the "buccinator mechanism" described in Chapter 6, and the nature and requirements of normal rest posture; they establish the goals that lip exercises must meet and surpass if function is to be normal and correction permanent.

In many cases the integrity of the buccinator mechanism has been destroyed; rearrangement of the facial musculature regarding both posture and strength is necessary if this essential force is to be reestablished. Exercises that reposition do not necessarily strengthen, and it thus becomes advisable to give our attention to each aspect individually.

Angle observed rather early that when lips close in normal alignment, the lower lip rests against the labial surface of the *upper* incisors, covering approximately one third of this surface, and that therefore it is the upper teeth, rather than the lower, that establish the curve of the lower lip. This phenomenon becomes more relevant for us when we note that the converse is equally true; it is primarily the lower lip that establishes the curve of the upper teeth. The upper lip impinges on root structure and alveolar process and thus affects gross alignment; the lower lip gains leverage from its location against the free end of the tooth, increasing greatly its potential in this function. As with any bilateral function, however, maximum effect is the product of reciprocity between the opposing members; in this case, such beneficial interaction is available only when the upper and lower lips are in actual contact.

As a general concept, we should keep in mind that we are not dealing with congenitally deformed structures in this pursuit. Muscles and connective tissue are basically normal and adequate; they have simply been led into faulty development. Certain muscles have been overdeveloped, whereas others have been allowed to remain latent, often in a most contrary fashion. Nevertheless, the potential for normal posture and function is inherent in the lips, and we seek only to establish their capacities, to gain a more typical balance between antagonists. Hence we may logically and realistically hope to weaken some muscles, strengthen others, and arrange the tissues of the lips in a fulfillment of their native growth pattern. We cannot add or subtract a single cell in the process, so that concepts of "growing more lip" or "reducing the bulk" are chimerical impressions, not genuine actualities.

TESTING THE NEED

Little or no testing is required to determine the need for changes in lip posture, for it is apparent through observation. You will have gained this information during the patient interview. The need for shifts in lip strength is frequently less obvious, and some criterion should therefore be available as a yardstick.

The Bio-My Master, the biofeedback machine described in Chapter 13, has an extraoral circuit designed to measure the relative potential of many of the individual facial muscles. A separate machine from the same manufacturer is capable

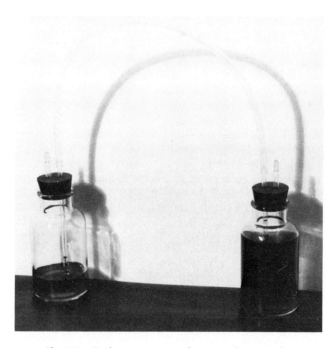

Fig. 17-1. Oral manometer used to assess lip strength.

of converting such potentials into pounds-per-square-inch measurements, which is more meaningful for research as well as for assessing progress in therapy.

Clinicians often have pet devices by which to assess such abilities, and, again, the oral manometer presented here is certainly not unique or indispensible; it has proved helpful to some people and is offered in case you have no procedure that you prefer, or in case adequate directions for the production of this device or something similar have not been found elsewhere. Should you have access to a manufactured manometer, your problem is solved. The homemade version described below is probably more realistic for the average therapist.

The device itself is pictured in Fig. 17-1. Its construction is expedited by having a friend in the chemistry department, but it may be built by the average person with only occasional laceration of the hands.

There may be some problems in locating the right bottles; those pictured are sold in the housewares section by some stores, or you may be able to cultivate a druggist to the point that he will supply you with usable substitutes. Some that originally contained Lilly brand pharma-ceuticals (other companies may also use them) are clear glass bottles a fraction over 5 inches high, flattened on the sides to facilitate compact storage, and hold approximately 200 capsules of average size. Most drugstores save a few empties. These bottles are fairly sturdy, a stopper of the necessary type fits well, and they have an adequate capacity for our purpose. The model made of brown tinted glass should be avoided. The fragile jars for which the stopper is designed hold far too little to be useful and are much too easily broken by youngsters.

From the medical supply house, you will require two No. 10 two-hole black rubber stoppers, two ¼-inch connectors of the type used to splice rubber tubing, a length of ¼-inch glass tubing, and 4 or 5 feet of ¼-inch *clear* plastic tubing. It is well to be adamant in demanding that the latter be clear, not the brown, opaque tubing that is more readily available but that robs our finished product of much of its appeal. Should the medical supply have no clear tubing in stock, it may often be found at hardware stores, refrigeration companies, where it is used to transport refrigerant between parts in some equipment, or even at foreign car dealers, who use it for gas lines.

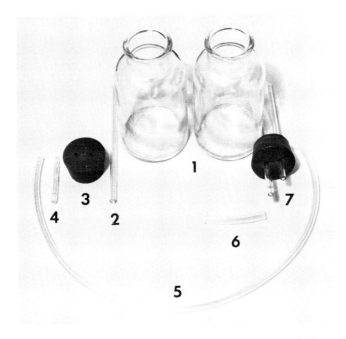

Fig. 17-2. Components of manometer. *1,* Bottles with 1¾-inch mouth; *2,* ¼-inch glass tubing cut to size; *3,* rubber stopper, No. 10, two-hole; *4,* connector; *5,* clear plastic tubing; *6,* mouthpiece cut from plastic tubing; *7,* assembled stopper.

The glass tubing usually comes in 3-foot lengths. It is probably most easily cut in the average office by using a three-cornered file. Lay the tubing on a flat surface, press the file at the desired cutting point, and rotate the tubing until it is scored around the entire circumference. The tubing will then snap off where it has been scored.

The various components are shown in Fig. 17-2, ready for assembly. The glass tubing has been cut to extend through the stopper for approximately 1 inch but still clear the bottom of the bottle by only about ¼ inch when the stopper is seated in place. Forcing the tube through the stopper is the only difficult task; both must be coated with glycerin or kept entirely under water to reduce friction between rubber and glass; once either becomes dry, it is well-nigh impossible to proceed. Also, the stopper must be pressed over the tube in a precisely vertical manner, for the glass will break, excising a portion of the hand, if lateral pressure is applied. A towel spread over the bottom of a filled basin prevents slipping of the glass tube.

The connector need only be inserted a portion of the way through the other hole in the stopper, sufficiently to hold it firmly in place. Two feet or a bit less of the plastic tubing is then used to connect the projecting inch of the two glass tubes. Some of the remaining plastic tubing is cut into 3-inch lengths to form mouthpieces.

One bottle is filled somewhat less than full with water, to which various combinations of food coloring may be added. The stoppers are fitted into the bottles, and a mouthpiece is placed lightly over the connector on the full bottle. Blowing through the mouthpiece forces the water into the other bottle, and the mouthpiece can then be switched to the other connector and the liquid returned to the original side. The mouthpiece can be sterilized and used again later. A covered jar of sterile mouthpieces should be kept at hand.

Testing with such a "blow bottle" is an intriguing procedure for most children, regardless of age. Parents have even requested permission to try it, and some children demand to be tested on each visit. Part of the enjoyment is in watching the colored water move through the plastic tubing, and when the latter is replaced with opaque tubing, or when brown bottles are used, some motivation is lost.

There are advantages to using the manometer over some of the other procedures that have been suggested. It is a motivational ploy, serving to strike a pleasant note at the outset of therapy. It also reflects the muscle force *in function*, rather than the static potential.

In using this device to assess lip strength, it is only necessary to count the number of breaths required to transfer the contents from one bottle to the other. Lips of normal strength are able to seal easily about a tube of this size, preventing the escape of any breath, and even the 7-year-olds have adequate vital capacity to complete this process in a single breath. In order to avoid lip exercises, or to earn permission to terminate those already assigned, the patient should accordingly demonstrate the ability to transfer the entire contents from one side to the other, using only one exhalation. He should be instructed not to attempt to blast the water over with an initial explosion of breath: a long, steady breath is far more effective. In addition, since we are not assessing digital power, no use of fingers to reinforce the lip seal is permitted.

In most cases, much of the breath will be found to escape around the mouthpiece, there being insufficient lip strength to maintain an effective seal. Any leakage of this type indicates a need for strengthening exercises.

Some patients have lips so weak that they are incapable of building up sufficient air pressure to hoist the water even to the midpoint in the plastic tube; to avoid frustration, it may occasionally be advisable for the therapist to blow part of the water over, allowing the patient to complete the task. Once the plastic tube is filled, there is a siphoning effect that continues until the bottles are equally filled; a finger must be placed over the connector on the receiving bottle, between breaths, if such siphoning is to be avoided. The number of breaths required for completion may be noted, and weekly progress in lip development is thus reflected as the number is reduced to one.

STRENGTHENING EXERCISES

Blowing balloons, as a means of strengthening lip closure, was once considered the panacea; in the present instance this exercise has been found somewhat deficient. Most tongue thrusters manipulate back pressure with tongue and teeth, relieving their lips of the expected strain and resulting in damage equaling the questionable benefit. We should be able to supply more effective measures, although balloons may serve as a supplement in a few selected cases.

Keep in mind the principle that one very efficient means of strengthening a muscle is to apply *resistance*. If we wish to enhance the ability of the orbicularis oris, the basic provision that we have for sealing the oral aperture, we should provide an opposing force tending to open the lips. This effect is what we hope to produce with devices such as buttons and a plastic jug.

We should state at the outset our reservations concerning strengthening exercises. There appears to be far too much emphasis in some quarters on strengthening the lips and far too little attention to *repositioning* and stimulating normal lip *function*. Also, unless some care is taken, exercises designed to strengthen one muscle, such as the orbicularis oris, may in reality fortify an antagonist, for example, the mentalis. While some invigoration is often necessary, we tend to play down the brute force aspects.

BUTTON EXERCISE. Whereas many lip exercises are not enjoyable, the button exercise has the added advantage of ready acceptance by most patients. It attacks the problem directly, and results are usually seen quickly and in full measure.

The patient is asked to secure two buttons of equal size but preferably of different colors. They should be about as large as a nickel but many range from the size of a dime to that of a quarter. A piece of string 7 or 8 feet long is then obtained, each end of the string being threaded in and out of a button. The ends of the string are tied together, and the buttons are pulled apart until the doubled string is stretched between

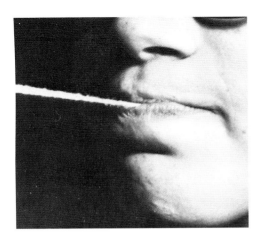

Fig. 17-3. Labial tug-of-war.

them, as seen in Fig. 17-3. The only remaining need is for an opponent, for a labial tug-of-war is to ensue. Seated on opposite sides of a table, to prevent more violent conflict, each contestant places a button on the labial surface of his incisors, holding it in place solely by closing his lips; sanitation is improved if they remember who gets the blue button each time. On signal, they are then to lean *slowly* away from each other; the string refuses to stretch, and before long, someone loses a button. The winner is usually awarded his opponent's button—right in the face.

It is considered foul play to brace the lips and jerk the head back suddenly, thus popping the button from the opponent's mouth. Turning the head to the side, thus sliding the button in the corner of the mouth and gaining reinforcement from solid tissue, is likewise frowned on. We seek a steady pull directly backward.

It can be seen that the button is attempting to open the lips and effect its escape; only forceful application of the orbicularis oris is available to thwart it. This force is exactly what we set out to administer.

This exercise is usually best assigned as a "fun" exercise. Therefore no set number of repetitions is specified. The enjoyment is reduced if fancy ornamental buttons are used; they can mangle the lips as they pop free. Smooth standard buttons are harmless.

Adults feel some restraint about engaging in this activity. For them, it is best to advise the use of a single button placed on a shorter string; the patient can place the button identically and simply resist the force of his own fingers as they pull on the string.

PLASTIC JUG. For the "only child" whose parents are somewhat less than fun-loving, thereby reducing the field of contenders, a similar effect may be achieved with the plastic-jug exercise. A 1-gallon jug, preferably the clear plastic type in which distilled water or swimming pool acid is frequently dispensed, is obtained if possible. If not, the opaque version containing household bleach is acceptable. Again, a button of the above description is placed on a much shorter string, and in this case the other end of the string is tied to the handle of the jug.

The jug is placed on the floor with a bit of water inside, and the cap is securely tightened. The patient bends over and grasps the button with his lips, as shown in Fig. 17-4, and the container is lifted and lowered twenty times. Each

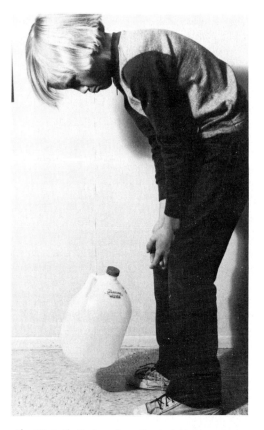

Fig. 17-4. Plastic-jug alternative to labial tug-of-war.

cularis oris; the proclivity of the thruster is to tense an already overdeveloped mentalis, forcing his lower lip against his incisors to the detriment of both, again failing to bring his upper lip into the desired function. This error can be avoided by requiring that the lips be protruded and retracted while they are held in forceful occlusion; the result is rather fishlike.

CHIP PULLUP. A far more acceptable method of stimulating bilabial opposition can be supplied through the use of poker chips. These require a small hole in the center, easily accomplished with an electric drill. Household string—not thread or waxed kite string—is cut into pieces approximately 2 feet in length. One end of the string is tied to a paper clip or something similar, the other end threaded through the hole in two or three of the chips.

The patient is to place the free end of the string behind his teeth and hold it with his tongue (a ready tongue-thrust skill), and then place his hands behind his back and bend over at the waist until his face is parallel with the floor and the string hangs perpendicularly between, as in Fig. 17-5. He should then *open* his lips and stretch them as far down the string as possible, grasp with his lips, hoist a section of the string up to his teeth, maintain it there until he can transfer the string to the dorsum of his tongue, and again stretch his lips down to harvest more string. This process continues until the top chip is lifted into contact with his lips.

Not only does this exercise strengthen bilabial opposition, but it provides a start on the repositioning of everted lips and the stretching of foreshortened upper lips. It furnishes the means for an incremental progression; as ability increases, additional chips are added until the weight reaches or exceeds one ounce. Depending on the weight of the product sold in your area, that translates into a stack of chips somewhere between five and twelve. When too many chips are strung at the first, the lips slide repeatedly over the same bit of string in a frustrating demonstration of weakness. A similar inability may result, however, when the string is too small or is wet where it touches the lips; dry string of an average size is more logical.

This exercise is also subject to faulty execution. When the assigned manner of execution seems difficult, the tongue thruster is inclined to lift his head until it is fairly upright, despite his tilted torso; in this posture he can attain the goal with relative ease by scraping the string over his

day, more water is added to the jug, until the patient gradually acquires the ability to lift a half gallon with his lips. This attainment is hypothetical with some patients, but a definite increase in lip strength is nevertheless registered.

The patient should not attempt to continue lifting to the point of standing upright, since there is no provision to withstand stress in that position. His face should remain more or less parallel with the floor. Lifting the jug only 6 or 8 inches will suffice.

BILABIAL OPPOSITION. Resistance can be supplied, of course, simply by pitting one lip against the other and squeezing the lips in a forceful exaggeration of lip closure. This exercise is less pleasant and thus less easily accepted by the patient. Nevertheless, there are times when it may seem advantageous to suggest that the patient form a routine of doing this exercise repeatedly throughout the day during compatible activities.

Care must be taken that there is a true pursing of the lips resulting from contraction of the orbi-

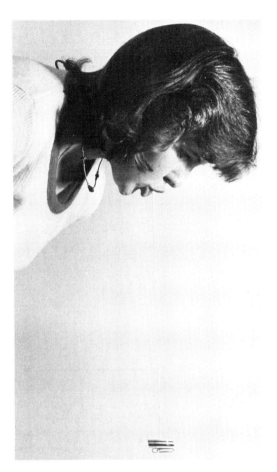

Fig. 17-5. Chip pullup. String is tied to paper clip, then threaded through holes drilled in chips.

lower lip with his upper teeth, leaving his upper lip a nonclosed, nonfunctioning knot under his nose. It remains a very profitable exercise when properly done.

The clinician should supply the materials, of course. A hank of string 30 or 40 feet in length can be stripped from a ball and placed in a plastic, self-locking sandwich bag, along with the required number of chips and even the cotton rolls to be described below. Buttons for the tug-of-war may also be included. The specified quantity of string is ample for both the tug-of-war and the pullup exercises, even allowing for periodic replacement.

MECHANICAL STIMULATORS. Many years ago, A. P. Rogers designed an "orbicularis oris exerciser." It consisted of flattened prongs that fitted into the oral vestibule and included a rod that projected through the lips, ending in a finger loop. The patient merely resisted the pressure as this device was pulled and relaxed, turned and manipulated.

Some dentists have suggested a hybridization of this device in connection with a form of oral shield. A plastic screen replaces the prongs, the rod and finger loop remain, and the patient tugs at the shield while resisting with his lips.

There would doubtless be some benefit to be derived from these exercisers if it were possible to provide one for each patient; however, speech clinicians would be hard put to produce even one. Even so, these devices are pictured as rather large affairs, filling much of the vestibular space; they would then extend beyond tissues that are governed by the orbicularis oris, stimulating other components of the facial network that are not necessary, or necessarily desirable, for our purposes. A simple button on a string may be more efficient, even if less elegant.

One possible alternative is on the market, a labial muscle exerciser (Appendix 2). It is made in a standard size that fits most lips, and it can be supplied to the individual patient without excessive cost. One advantage would seem to be the flipper that fits on the outside of the lower lip and that is supposed to deactivate the mentalis while stress is supplied to the orbicularis oris.

REPOSITIONING EXERCISES

When we consider modification of lip posture, we turn completely from the concept of *resistance* that guided us in the previous section. Quite to the contrary, the goal now is to stretch and *relax* muscle fibers, so that some reduction of the state of tonus that has maintained the previous posture may combine with the slight increase in tonus that strengthening exercises have achieved in antagonist muscles. Thus the balance is shifted sufficiently to effect some change of the position in which labial tissues are held when the supporting musculature finds a point of equilibrium: the physiological rest position.

At this time the clinician does not strive to prevail on the patient to close his mouth; the effort is toward making it *possible* for him to do so, effortlessly. It is believed that much of the hopelessness that has so frequently been reported in efforts to achieve a closed-mouth resting posture can be obviated by careful attention to this aspect of the problem. The mechanics of the antagonistic nature of muscle function is frequently discussed but less often applied; the contraction of a given muscle is more obvious and dramatic than the relaxation of its antagonist, which permits such action. Strengthening oral closure is of definite assistance, but it is doubly effective if it is accompanied by a positive reduction in nonclosure.

There are nine "muscles of facial expression" that comprise the facial network, in addition to the orbicularis oris. These ten muscles are intricately interwoven, to the point that a stimulus in any one of them finds an echo throughout the system. Directly or indirectly, every one of them interconnects at some point with the orbicularis oris and serves as an antagonist. In other words, every muscle in the oronasal region of the face tends to open the mouth, with the exception of the orbicularis oris, which alone closes it.

We must now wear down the opposition somewhat. Abnormal deglutition is manifested not only by a flaccid orbicularis oris but by a customary hypertonicity in the muscles that oppose oral closure. Some authorities have despaired of such hypertonicity, feeling that it resulted from pressures in the environment, anxiety, tension, anger, etc. Although these factors may have an influence, and should certainly be discussed when daily life appears to be generating undue pressures, it develops in most cases that emotion is secondary to mechanics in this specific area.

HOT SALT WATER. It was noted long ago by A. P. Rogers, among others, that the proper application of hot salt water has a salubrious effect on hypertonicity. It tends to increase the blood supply, quickly and markedly, to the area it bathes, as it promotes relaxation of vasoconstrictors, thus stimulating circulation. The warmth itself is relaxing, the increased blood supply speeds the modification of tissue, and if the orbicularis oris remains in contraction while other fibers are stretched, our cause is greatly advanced.

Two or three times daily, depending on individual need, the patient should place 4 or 5 ounces of water in a glass, as hot as possible short of oral discomfort, into which a teaspoon of salt is stirred. A mouthful is then forced outward against the cheeks, allowing these structures to relax completely; the water is held in place for a few seconds and then slowly withdrawn into the mouth proper, but with a feeling of still further relaxation rather than by forceful contraction of the buccinator. Continue in this way, alternately forcing the water from buccal to oral space until the cheeks have been fully distended five times.

With a second mouthful, slowly force the water in similar fashion behind the upper lip, gradually building the pressure until the upper lip is rounded out to its fullest extent. The water is transferred from oral to vestibular space an additional five times, after which the lower lip is subjected to the same procedure with a third portion of the water. Thereafter, the remaining water is used in alternate quantities behind the upper and lower lip. A preponderance may be assigned to one lip or the other if the need is apparent, but both lips should receive attention.

When the upper lip has become short and thick, very little water can be forced behind it at first, and the patient should take careful aim at a sink or washbasin, since his initial efforts may result in a spray of salt water. Similarly, the mentalis, if overdeveloped in its usual manner, tends to contract with any oral activity, leaving only a small rim of lip that may be expanded. The refractory lip must then be further stretched concurrently by means of other exercises.

The use of hot salt water is a valuable exercise in itself. However, it may well be made a preliminary for any other exercise chosen for the purpose of stretching and relaxing muscle fiber and surrounding tissue.

FORCED-AIR VERSION. It may be found useful to establish a routine of performing much the same action as outlined above, except that mere breath replaces the water. The patient forces air behind the most rebellious lip, holds it for a moment, and then releases it. He is to do this several times, after which both lips are inflated simultaneously and the breath held in place for the duration of a slow count to 10. This entire procedure should consume only a minute but should be repeated at intervals throughout the day.

LIPSTICK EXERCISE. The lipstick exercise must be given an alias when presented to boys, who will accept it as the "overlap" exercise, but it is simply an exaggeration of the action used in applying lipstick. It is a remarkably effective exercise for the short, thick or everted upper lip.

Immediately after the salt water procedure, the patient is asked to pull his upper lip down over his upper teeth as far as possible and hold it there. The lower lip is then lapped over the upper lip and stretched upward as far as possible; this maneuver may require digital assistance at first. The lower lip is then contracted firmly against the upper lip and the mandible slowly dropped, thus massaging the upper lip forcefully downward with the lower lip.

This exercise is repeated five times and is to be done at least three or four times daily. On each occasion one additional overlap is attempted until the upper lip is being massaged downward fifteen or twenty times at every practice period. The use of hot salt water should precede this exercise as often as possible, but no opportunity should be lost to practice simply because the water is unavailable.

After three weeks of the lipstick exercise as a steady diet, the upper lip often appears to have grown downward a considerable distance. Actually it has not, of course, but the tissues have been redistributed in a gratifying manner.

BILABIAL GYMNASTICS. When lip closure is accomplished only with an obvious strain in the facial network, it often helps to have the patient "mug" repeatedly during the day. He should observe his face with a mirror while doing so, and pause occasionally to rest, but 5-minute periods should be devoted to this undertaking.

The basic idea is to contract the orbicularis oris and then, using only facial muscles, distort the mouth into as many contortions as possible. The lips should be pulled as far to the right as possible, and then to the left. They should be worked up and down, then in a clockwise circle as large as possible, then counterclockwise, etc.

When fatigue sets in, he can open his mouth and stretch it laterally with his fingers, first with only index fingers, and then with two fingers, pulling the lips buccally. While doing so he should not resist the manual strain with facial muscles but should allow the latter to remain passive.

He may then resume grimacing, attempting to stretch every muscle in his face while maintaining a closed mouth.

COTTON ROLLS. It is often surprising how long we can mulishly pursue a difficult path before we notice the smooth road beside us. Thus it was that many onerous and expensive methods were for years employed to achieve results that we now find can be garnered easily and effectively through the use of simple cotton dental rolls (Fig. 17-6). They are found at almost any dental supply store and come in assorted sizes, but they are usually packaged 2000 per carton. It is best to buy the 1½-inch length in both size 2 and size 3. The latter is often prewrapped in groups of twenty-five within the box, and many pleasant hours can be spent in wrapping the size 2 rolls into similar bundles of twenty-five. This amount allows for the use of one each day for a three-week period, plus the four that fall on the floor and get dirty.

These rolls are used to form a "lip bumper" behind the offending lip. Since they have an outside covering of gauze, which disturbs some pa-

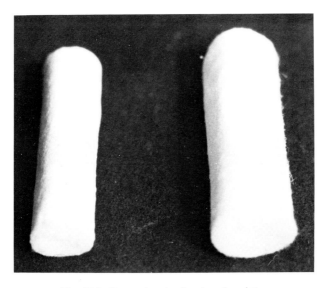

Fig. 17-6. Cotton dental rolls, sizes 2 and 3.

tients because dry gauze scrapes against their teeth, they should be dampened before use, rendering them softer and more acceptable. If the taste of disinfectant is unpleasant, the child is allowed to dip them in lemonade or a similar beverage. Also, it is politic to advise pinching the ends before use, creating a tapered terminal less likely to gouge the lip.

Many more size 2 rolls will be used, since most children can manage only this smaller mass. Older patients will require the larger size 3, although sometimes it is prudent to supply a few small ones for use the first three or four days until the larger size can be accommodated more easily. Note that they are of a consistency somewhere between that of the hard and soft tissues; they are sufficiently firm to influence soft tissue alignment but far too yielding to displace teeth or to render anything other than a helpful effect.

Cotton rolls are indicated for grossly everted lips, for the short or retruded upper lip that does not seem to be responsive to other exercises, for the lower lip that has difficulty in surmounting the edge of protruding upper incisors, and for the obviously overdeveloped mentalis muscle that continues to exist as an unsightly knob on the chin below a deeply creased mentolabial sulcus. In the last instance, cotton should be brought into use rather quickly.

Here, again, the result will be much more marked and immediate if hot salt water is used prior to insertion of the dental roll. As a typical example, the patient may perform the salt water exercise when a period of calm is imminent, then do the "lipstick" exercise for a time, and then pop a cotton roll behind the indicated lip, keeping it there for an hour. Either lip may be so influenced, although this procedure is used most frequently to stretch and deenergize the mentalis.

In a few extreme cases the orthodontist has been persuaded to install a much more fixed and rigid bumper that has taken the form of a piece of heavy arch wire shaped roughly to the contour of the lower arch. Other short pieces of this wire are then spaced around the central portion at right angles and welded in place, in order to support a band of acrylic that forms the body of the appliance. The ends of the semicircle of wire are then secured to orthodontic bands placed on mandibular buccal teeth so that the acrylic bumper is held slightly anterior to incisors.

When the patient is not currently wearing a full-band appliance, it is necessary to go back at least as far as the first molars; otherwise, attachment may be made to bicuspid bands. When the appliance has been worn for even a month or more, there has been obvious and gratifying stretching of hyperactive mentalis muscles, especially those with a seemingly high attachment. Whereas such an appliance may also yield beneficial orthodontic results, its use has thus far been rather limited.

In some few cases, cotton rolls may again be called on during the recheck period. When lips continue to flare apart in repose, they may be redirected into contact by inserting a cotton roll in the vestibule. This added hurdle provides a beneficial exaggeration of lip occlusion and may be essential when original benefits have been wasted through nonclosure.

CONCLUSION

Lip exercises are routinely assigned as the first step in the program and continue at a reduced level through the second, third, and even fourth steps. This should not limit their use thereafter, whenever a need rises to the surface, on the final step of therapy or at any time during the recheck period.

Such exercises may also be of great help to the orthodontist in the absence of any tongue-thrust problem. Many patients develop abnormal facial posture because of factors unrelated to deglutition: congenital bone structure, prolonged nasal obstruction, malocclusions of various etiologies, etc. The need for restoration of an optimum balance in the facial network may remain after dental treatment. In this regard, the problem and its solution are quite analogous to the thruster's.

Many pseudothrusters need *only* lip exercises to correct their appearance of abnormal deglutition. They almost certainly include a number of the type who "grow out of it" or who are readily "corrected" by holding a mint on their tongue. A fairly sizable group has been referred for swallowing therapy who were found on close examination to be swallowing in a basically normal manner. It has usually been possible to assign an intensive schedule of lip exercises, often including also some strengthening of the antigravity muscles; these cultivated abilities were then transferred as necessary to resting posture and to the act of deglutition, and the entire formal program was avoided.

R. H. BARRETT
SPEECH PATHOLOGIST
TELEPHONE 793-1101

LIP EXERCISES

At least three times each day, please do the following:

1. Pump HOT SALT WATER back and forth behind .... lip 4 or 5 times, spit it out and repeat. Use ½ glass water.

2. Immediately do the "overlap" exercise ....times. Pull upper lip down over teeth, overlap lower lip as FAR as possible, firmly massage upper lip DOWN with lower.

3. Using breath instead of water, FORCE air behind .... lip as firmly as you can. Do this repeatedly during the day.

At least once daily:

1. Do BUTTON tug-of-war as directed. Do not "jerk" button, or turn head to side, or bite the string.

2. Do chip PULLUP exercise, making sure that your UPPER lip does half the work.

3. Hold cotton behind .... lip for at least one hour.

These should help you BUTTON YOUR LIP!

A

	HOT SALT WATER	OVERLAP			BREATH		BUTTON	PULLUP	COTTON
1st DAY									
2nd DAY									
3rd DAY									
4th DAY									
5th DAY									
6th DAY									
7th DAY									

B

Fig. 17-7. Practice card specifying lip exercises. **A,** Assignment can be tailored to individual need. **B,** Chart on reverse side of practice card.

ASSIGNMENT

These exercises have appeared to be the most useful ones in this program. Their assignment should be tailored to the individual dysfunctions of the patient (Fig. 17-7). Provision may be made for all the common needs by combining them in various ways. Some patients require them all, some need none, and a few demand improvisation to meet an unusual situation. Additional exercises can be outlined on a separate card or sheet, with the number of repetitions specifically assigned.

The practice cards for each step are printed on different colored paper, which appears to make them more intriguing, adds to the suspense when the patient guesses each week as to the color of the next one, and hopefully is yet another detail increasing motivation. So, too, with the chart (Fig. 17-7) printed on the back of the card or given on a separate sheet. Each practice period

at home should be checked off when completed and the card returned for inspection at the next appointment.

Questions are invited from both patient and observer before they are dismissed, and the patient is urged to telephone if there is any confusion or uncertainty regarding the exercise after he arrives home.

The patient's progress is noted on the history card, with special attention to any unusual procedures that were required. Some type of uniform grading system may also be devised, and the patient should be made aware of this codification; the child with a good record may dislike spoiling it. The grading system need be nothing elaborate; if everything has gone exactly according to the usual routine, the notation may simply read, "Excellent through 1st." Here's hoping it was.

Chapter 18

STEP 2: FOUNDATION OF DEGLUTITION

The therapist should experience some relief and reassurance when the patient returns for his second appointment: if that lengthy first step did not deter him, all that follows should be relatively easy. Be not lulled, however; he may only be coming back to find out what happened the first time.

At this session we will begin working on deglutition proper. Our goal will be to instill some basic principles that have pertinence throughout the remainder of therapy. In most cases, this is completed in a half-hour session.

EVALUATION OF PREVIOUS WEEK

Nothing can be done at any session until the results of the previous step are examined. The scope of human ingenuity was never more clearly demonstrated than in the gamut of errors that are routinely recorded in the performance of these relatively simple exercises. A number of the more prevalent problems will be identified; however, the therapist should remain alert for any possibility.

Practice routine

First, discover whether a routine for practice has been established at home, what this schedule is, and how well the patient has adhered to it. Some slight leeway is permitted this first time, depending on the number of days since the previous session; ideally, it should be a full week. If only six days have elapsed, missing one or two practice periods is undesirable; even if it has been seven or eight days, missing three or four periods at home sounds ominous. The child who has been punctual in practice but has had difficulties in performing the assignment deserves our sympathetic assistance; he usually requires only some additional time and supportive measures to succeed. The child who has simply not practiced demands reevaluation.

When numerous practice periods have been missed, or if the parent reports any conflict or resentment concerning practice, a brief chat with the patient is in order. Try to establish the cause of the trouble, listening carefully to the child's side of the story. It may seem best to rearrange the observation personnel, or to tactfully suggest that the other parent become interested in this project. Sometimes a simple misunderstanding has caused needless woe.

If practice periods are in conflict with some other cherished activity, such as Little League or dancing class, you may try to assist in rescheduling appointments or practice times—but only with the understanding that therapy must remain paramount: if learning to swallow correctly is not the most important thing in life for these few brief weeks, then we are all wasting our time, and therapy should be postponed until it can receive the necessary attention. We would never achieve a subconscious change in swallowing behavior without the sincere, wholehearted desire of the patient. When such cooperation is lacking, the time to stop is now, immediately, before further trouble develops. If the child openly agrees that he is disinterested, we abide by his decision and suspend therapy. If he evinces any uncertainty, we can send him home to think about it and talk it over for a week; we will be very disappointed if he decides to stop, but we will not force him one way or the other. The alternatives were clearly presented on his first visit. We make an appointment for the following week and ask him to call and cancel if that is his wish.

When the child has merely been careless or forgetful about practice, we explain that we have made this program as short and easy as possible. We have left out everything we could, and are asking only the *least* amount of practice that will accomplish the job at hand. The little that remains must be done consistently. Sending him home to repeat the entire week usually gets the point across. This matter was discussed in Chapter 15.

Execution of exercises

Troublesome cases are fortunately rare. More commonly, the routine has been worked out and carefully followed. In any case, the manner in which the exercises have been performed should be demonstrated by the patient. The role of the observer will have been less essential with lip exercises than with the intraoral requirements of the future, but even honest mistakes do happen. Moral support also contributes.

HOT SALT WATER. Few children develop an addiction to hot salt water. In the more deplorable cases, tepid water laced with three or four specks of salt has been swished briefly through the labial vestibule.

Simulating water by forcing breath behind each lip will provide our first clue as to how things have gone. Even in this brief time, breath should penetrate lower behind or around the mentalis and create a fuller distension of the upper lip.

OVERLAP. When properly done, the lower lip should extend up an appreciable distance over the body of the upper lip, and the latter should blanch from the squeezing action as the lower lip slowly decends. Two common errors occur. Either the lower lip fails to surmount the vermillion line of the upper, or is protruded upward and then allowed to fall quickly back with only incidental contact with the upper lip. Nothing has been accomplished in either case, and the patient is still at square one.

TUG-OF-WAR. We have tried to forestall the most prevalent errors with the instructions printed on the practice card. Nevertheless, it is difficult to contain the resourcefulness of some patients; it is safer to observe a demonstration.

PULLUP EXERCISE. Problems with the pullup exercise are infinite in variety, but usually of a minor nature and almost wholly self-inflicted. It provides a ready source of sympathy. The most common errors are in failure to increase beyond two the number of chips, or in adding all the chips at once, or in *chewing* the string into the mouth despite the printed warning. More often it has assumed the proportions of a timed competition at home with a surprising roster of competitors.

DENTAL ROLL. Problems with the cotton roll are rare. They generally are an outgrowth of the time period during which the cotton is to be used. When life is interesting, alternate days may provide only minimal time for this project. In an attempt to clear the conscience, the roll may be inserted at bedtime; minutes after sleep arrives, the roll is riding atop the lower lip, the picture of futility. Cotton is of value only during a waking hour, when involuntary muscle contractions wedge it down behind the mentalis bundle, stretching the fibers and freeing the lip.

Blasé mothers

There is one other problem that does occasionally arise and that may be discussed at this time. It originates with the mother who is bored with the entire procedure before it even starts and often finds the child a bother in general.

With some consistency, this mother brings a magazine or picks one up in the waiting room to read during therapy. This attitude is easily transmitted to the child, and the therapist may quickly find that he is talking to himself. Seeking to relieve the mother of the journal so that she will not be encumbered is usually futile: she will keep it, thank you. It is often more effective to key your attention on the mother for a time; when she starts to read, simply stop talking and look at her expectantly until the silence gets her attention. Each time she starts to read, stop talking. As a last resort, dismiss the child and discuss the situation with the mother, pointing out frankly the effect of her attitude. If there is a personality conflict with the therapist, you should offer to refer her elsewhere, or some other member of the family might be able to generate a bit more enthusiasm. If she must read, provide her with this paragraph that you are now reading. In any event, this situation should be resolved in some manner before going further with therapy. When it has been ignored, the result has invariably been later failure and a still more unpleasant state of affairs.

PROCEDURES

After all problems have been resolved relating to lip exercises, we may assemble the items required for our first assault on deglutition; a cup of water, a tissue finger cot, and a supply of small elastics, approximately twenty to thirty, placed in a coin envelope or small plastic container.

RUBBER BANDS. The elastics used in this exercise are obtained from a dental supply firm (Appendix 2) or through your friendly corner orthodontist. They are called No. 6 thick-walled elastics, or simply "crossbite" elastics, since they are primarily used between the occlusal surfaces to apply lateral force in correcting crossbite. They are therefore made of live latex and are somewhat expensive; their cost per patient, however, is microscopic, their sharp edges supply a definite stimulus to both tongue and rugae, and thus they are preferred. Much less expensive bands are available; they are made of synthetics, are softer and so less easily perceived, and are usually oval rather than round, thus requiring additional maneuvering to position on the tongue. Some therapists have preferred broken bits of sugarless mints because they have even sharper edges. However, the candy is often allowed to creep over onto the dorsum of the tongue, where it cannot be observed, and an erroneous pattern is thereby encouraged.

A word may also be in order concerning the possibility that the patient will ingest some of these elastics; they are quite harmless. Perhaps we are fortunate, but although thousands of our patients have used such elastics, not one has ever choked, aspirated an elastic, or suffered harm in any way except to the dignity.

EXTRANEOUS FACIAL MOVEMENT. Before introducing the first exercise, it is well to have the patient take sips of water and observe his face in the mirror during two or three swallows; it is easy thereafter to point out the excessive facial movement that is usually present during the act. As the patient watches the relaxed face of the therapist during deglutition, it becomes apparent to him that there is an easier way, a better method, and that he is merely being asked to replace an effortful habit with a comfortable, relaxed substitute, characterized by greater efficiency with less work. This is usually contrary to the original expectation and is an additional motivating device. Of course, if the patient is one of the rare ones who displays no facial movement, this step is omitted.

LABIOGLOSSAL SEAL. While therapist and patient are engaged in the foregoing, it is also suggested that the therapist depress the patient's lower lip at the instant he swallows, allowing the patient to see his tongue as it projects between the teeth. Subsequently it is possible for the patient to feel, with careful attention, the contact of tongue to lip, or in lateral thrusts, of tongue to buccal surface. It is essential that the patient recognize this invariable contact, which is in the nature of a conditioned response in tongue thrust. If any reflex movement is present during the oral stage of deglutition it is this automatic contact of tongue to lip or cheek, a condition that is constant in the fetus, frequent in the older infant, but normally eliminated by the eruption of the teeth.

However, this reflex is readily changed: we simply remove the trigger by forbidding lip closure during the practice of *any* exercise throughout the entire course of therapy. Perhaps it would be possible to learn to swallow correctly with lips closed during practice, although this is doubtful. It would require tremendous concentration and effort by the patient to prevent resumption of the tongue-lip contact. Many unsuspected malfunctions would be concealed by closed lips, leaving patient, observer, and clinician unaware of their occurrence. It would be inestimably more difficult for the patient to acquire the sensation of sucking required in normal deglutition, or for the therapist to be sure that such a sucking action even occurred. The writers have observed clinicians who stress relaxed lip closure during practice, pleading with a child to suck food onto his tongue, or to suck up and back as he swallowed, while the frustrated child sat and stared, with no comprehension of what the therapist was talking about, having no specific, concrete experience with such function.

All this frustration can be obviated by the simple expedient of requiring that the lower lip be firmly retracted during every aspect of therapy. It is believed that many past efforts to retrain deglutition have gone aground on this particular shoal. Naturally, we do not expect the patient to swallow forever after with his lips apart; this practice device is confined to therapy, and once therapy is concluded the lips are to be closed. However, if the patient masters an entire new pattern of deglutition, in which the lips are immobilized and permitted no function, it is not surprising, after therapy, to discover that lips are closed easily, with no effort and with no extraneous movement—and with not one moment of therapy wasted on this achievement.

As we have seen, depressing the lip often appears to inhibit swallowing, specifically because the abnormal lip-tongue contact has become an integral aspect of swallowing. However, this impression is deceptive: no patient has yet been found who really could *not* swallow with lips apart. Many youngsters require a bit of convincing on this score, and at first it is frequently necessary for them to forcibly hold their lower lip down with their fingers. Within a matter of hours, at most, they discover that they possess facial muscles—primarily the triangularis and inferior depressor labii, with occasional help, not always welcome, from the risorius—that are able to accomplish this maneuver quite adequately.

In any event, the patients are required to rehearse swallowing with lips apart until assistance from the fingers is no longer necessary before they attempt the first formal exercise. The necessity of this approach is explained, the fact is noted that we will never embarrass them by requesting that they practice in public, and they are assured that we will expect swallowing with closed lips at the conclusion of therapy.

Initial exercise

The foundation of all that is to follow is laid in this exercise; it has even been quoted as being the entire therapy program. Although somewhat less comprehensive than that, it does incorporate a number of subfunctions that we wish to change. In addition to eliminating labial involvement, it is directed toward three specific goals: (1) to assure firm molar occlusion, (2) to position the *tip* of the tongue for normal deglutition, and (3) to provide a clear concept of sucking as an essential ingredient of this act.

MOLAR OCCLUSION. The clinician has already discussed with the patient, during the interview earlier, the fact that his teeth are habitually apart as he swallows. With the mirror he has observed his tongue protruding between his teeth, maintaining this condition. He can now study his sensory pattern and his appearance in the mirror as he closes his teeth firmly and retracts his lips. He should contrast this image with the look and feel as he protrudes his jaw, biting in edge-to-edge contact. He will have a strong impulse to protrude his jaw in a moment, when he is asked to press his tongue upward, and he should be aware in advance that doing so is improper.

TONGUE TIP POSITION. If we are to establish a physiologically sound and efficient pattern, the tip of the tongue must be positioned exactly, not simply "held up." If the tip is positioned a bit low, it speedily relapses forward to its original

posture. If the tip is lifted a bit too high, it later tends to curl back in an impossible conformation for deglutition, and at best results in an effortful exaggeration of the desired function. If the tip is located, as explained in Chapter 11, immediately posterior to the incisal papilla, it gains the mechanical advantage of being able to press firmly against alveolar bone, anchoring the free end of the tongue and permitting forceful action by the remaining segments.

It is a good idea to make a simple line drawing on the coin envelope or the back of the practice card, showing the mouth in sagittal section and indicating the desired point of contact; the drawing clarifies the instructions for the observer and remains as a reference later at home. A drawing as uncomplicated as that in Fig. 18-1 will suffice.

Once the parent or other observer is clear on this point, it should be identified for the patient. Dentists can use an amalgam plugger for this purpose but should be careful not to elicit pain, or the dentist may merely press the desired spot with his finger. This is a special prerogative of the dentist, who is free to grope about in people's mouths barehanded with impunity. No such privilege is conferred on the speech clinician; be his hands ever so sterile, some discomfort and aversion are occasioned if he places a single digit in the patient's mouth. The parent will remain far

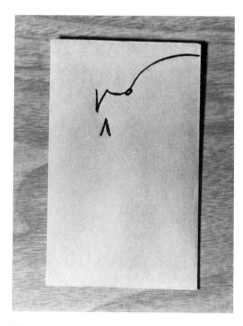

Fig. 18-1. Sagittal section drawn on coin envelope.

more calm and cool if the clinician employs a tissue finger cot. The parent's feeling of well-being will be further enhanced if the clinician is a bit obvious about disposing of the cot at the end of the session—as with tongue depressors, which should be broken loudly in half after use. Incidentally, avoid the thick brown cots that look like fingers cut from a rubber glove; they are quite unwieldy.

If the child appears timid or fearful, it is usually expeditious to merely touch the rugae with your finger and ask the child to tip his head forward against your finger; he can then stop before it hurts, although he often continues until it is more painful for the therapist than the patient.

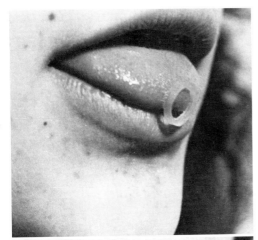

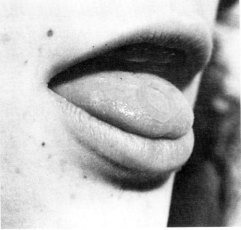

Fig. 18-2. Positioning of elastic on tongue. **A,** When moistened with saliva, elastic may be correctly placed on apex of tongue. **B,** Elastic placed too far back. Nothing normal can result from this placement.

Once the proper spot has been established, the patient is advised that this spot is where we wish the rubber band to press. However, similar care must be taken to place the elastic in the proper position on the tongue. One fallacy, among many, in having a child hold a candy mint or an elastic band on his tongue in order to retrain deglutition is that it is invariably placed on *top* of the tongue, resulting in an *upward* pressure of the blade of the tongue and eventual curling back of the tongue, or the mint is slid back on the dorsum of the tongue while the tip returns to its interdental posture in contact with the lip. Either result is quite at variance with what we are seeking to establish here.

The elastic must be placed on the very tip of the tongue, standing vertically as though encircling the tip, as seen in Fig. 18-2, *A*. The instant the elastic tips back onto the dorsum, it is too far back. It should be demonstrated to the patient that the elastic will remain in place, however precarious it may appear, particularly if it is first placed in the mouth and dampened with saliva. With the elastic in this position on the tongue, and then lifted to the exact location on the rugae, the tongue is encouraged to push *forward* somewhat as it has been accustomed to do, but in a respectable neighborhood. This action is the one we seek.

Correct positioning should be explained before the exercise is attempted so that the observer may know what to look for. Show the incisal papilla in the patient's mouth, demonstrating that if the elastic slips forward, it will begin to cover this little ridge, or else the "pink bump" will turn white, indicating that the elastic is too far forward. If the elastic is back too far, even slightly, it tends to disappear. With some low, flat palates, it is possible to see the elastic even when it is raised too much, but in any case we wish to see only the front edge of the elastic positioned immediately posterior to the incisal papilla, as shown in Fig. 18-3, *A*.

SUCKING. The subject of sucking has been adequately discussed in previous chapters. At this point, let it suffice to say that we wish the patient to acquire a strong, definite sucking component in deglutition. In order that it may be clearly established in the patient's nervous system, every swallow executed for practice during the first few weeks is accompanied by a loud, positive "slurp." When we say, "suck up," we mean it! No one in the situation—child, parent, or clinician—is left in doubt as to whether the

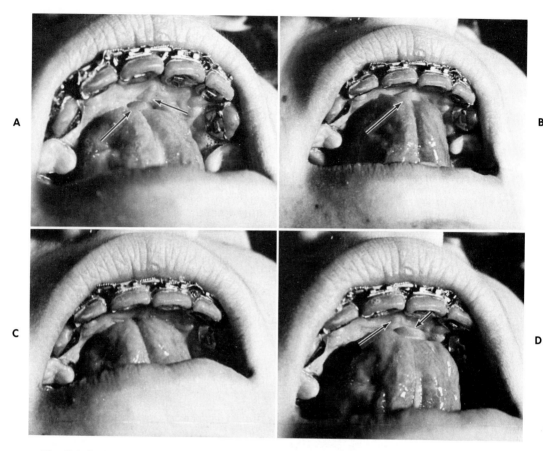

Fig. 18-3. Positioning of elastic on palate. **A,** Correct position: front rim of elastic can be seen precisely at posterior end of incisal papilla. Latter retains its normally pink coloration. **B,** Too far forward: incisal papilla is partially covered. **C,** Too far distal: front rim of elastic is no longer visible. **D,** Elastic is placed to one side, creating undesirable influence on exercise.

sucking action has occurred, since it is startlingly obvious. As previously seen, this type of exercise would not be possible with closed lips, and certainly, we are not encouraging the child to slurp his food later. This action is another practice device that will soon be modified to a discreet silence and that would be impossible once therapy is completed, but it provides the patient with a definite image of deglutition accompanied by negative pressure in the mouth. It is easy to achieve and thoroughly enjoyed by most patients, regardless of age.

TOTAL EXERCISE. The total exercise is as follows: with elastic on the tip of tongue, lift elastic into position on the rugal ridge; close teeth in molar occlusion; check mentally to make sure that elastic has not slipped as teeth were closed;

keeping lips apart throughout, "slurp" and swallow as one continuous action; lower tongue to observe that the elastic has not slipped back.

The therapist should demonstrate the entire exercise and then assist the patient in doing it, first stimulating the "rubber band spot" afresh. It may be necessary for the clinician to assist by holding the patient's lower lip down with one thumb. If possible, the patient should repeat the exercise two or three times, allowing the observer to function. If the patient finds it impossible to swallow without closing the lower lip, allow him to go home and practice as previously stated, holding his lip with his fingers. Before bedtime he should be able to execute the entire exercise.

ASSIGNMENT. Practice is limited for the first three

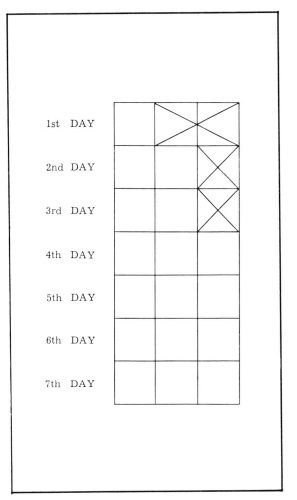

2

R. H. BARRETT
SPEECH PATHOLOGIST

TELEPHONE 793-1101

Remember, KEEP YOUR LOWER LIP DOWN. Lips must NEVER be closed for ANY exercise until the very last session.

It is important that you do this exercise exactly as you were shown. Place elastic on tip of tongue in proper position, then slowly lift tongue until elastic is pressed against the correct spot behind your upper gums. LET SOMEONE CHECK to be sure it is in the right place. If it is, then:

1. Bite your back TEETH together.
2. Notice that ELASTIC is still in place.
3. "SLURP" and SWALLOW.

TAKE TIME to think of each step, for each one must be correct.

Take tongue DOWN after each swallow.

Here is your practice schedule:

ONCE today, and do ONLY SIX swallows.

Tomorrow and the next day, TWICE each day, SIX SWALLOWS each time.

After that, THREE TIMES each day (at least two hours between sessions) and do TWELVE SWALLOWS each time.

GOOD LUCK!

| 1st DAY |
| 2nd DAY |
| 3rd DAY |
| 4th DAY |
| 5th DAY |
| 6th DAY |
| 7th DAY |

A   **B**

Fig. 18-4. A, Practice card. **B,** Chart on reverse of practice card.

days, ostensibly to avoid soreness. Many patients could practice more intensively from the first day, but several other considerations enter into this assignment. When patients are not adequately warned, they will occasionally go home and do an entire week of practice in the first hour; in this case a genuine and painful soreness is assured, making any practice done for several days thereafter a gross distortion. We are asking for muscle movements that are quite different from any the patient has previously performed; the effect of overexertion is usually perceived as a sore throat or as soreness along the inferior border of the mandible just below the condyle. Parents have even run to the physician, expecting a diagnosis of mumps.

Excessive practice can thus be harmful at this

stage but is also unnecessary. As we saw, brief practice is often best. When the exercise is performed a few times, and then allowed to "steep in the nervous system" for a time, a certain amount of learning occurs. When the exercise is attempted thereafter, fewer inappropriate movements are made, and it is thus done with greater precision and less effort. The end product far surpasses the excessive repetition of an exercise that deteriorates with each execution. Furthermore, and perhaps most important, when the patient is allowed to work into this regimen gradually, he does so with a much better will and a greatly improved attitude.

The assignment is made as in the practice card (Fig. 18-4, A). This first exercise is never varied, incidentally, whereas some of the ensuing cards may be modified drastically. If the patient is prepared to undertake therapy, he can accomplish this exercise with reasonable ease. No substitute has been found that will render so many changes in equal time. Primarily, it remains intact because it has never been found *necessary* to change.

It is common practice to reduce the hot salt water and overlap exercises to a once-a-day level for this next week and the one following. Accordingly, all lip exercises would be assigned at this rate. However, the needs of the patient govern this and repetition more than once daily may be asked, especially in areas of greater need.

We should reiterate that not every patient requires the full assemblage of lip exercises. When only minor toning or stretching is indicated, we may begin with Step 2, enriched by only some essential lip maneuvers. Care should be taken not to become overly optimistic in this regard; we are not serving the best interests of our patient by omitting elements for which he has a legitimate need.

REFERENCES

1. Hellebrandt, F. A., and Houtz, S. J.: Mechanisms of muscle training in man: experimental demonstration of the overload principle, Phys. Ther. Rev. **36:**371-383, 1956.
2. Rose, D. L., Radzyminski, S. F., and Beatty, R. R.: Effects of brief maximal exercise on the strength of the quadriceps femoris, Arch. Phys. Med. Rehab. **38:**157-164, 1957.

Chapter 19

STEP 3:
POTENTIAL OF ANTERIOR TONGUE

Our primary field of action on this step will be the anterior segment of the tongue. Some reinforcement of antigravity muscles will also be provided. After this session, every new exercise that we assign will be designed to strengthen or reposition posterior tongue and velopharyngeal elements, unless unusual problems arise.

We will also be initiating measures to modify the oral resting posture. Everything can usually be accomplished in a half-hour session.

EVALUATION OF PREVIOUS STEP

As always, our first concern is the manner in which the previous exercise was performed at home. Troublesome cases are fortunately rare, but confirm that the practice schedule has been carefully followed.

Omitting the elastic, ask the child to open his mouth and lift his tongue to the proper spot, as though the elastic were in place. The tip should go directly to the desired place. Many times, in an effort to make very sure that the tongue is sufficiently back, the tip will land somewhat posterior to the correct spot and slide immediately into correct position; this is perfectly acceptable. If the tip goes to the wrong place, particularly if it is placed forward or gropes about in search of refuge, it is immediately obvious that something has gone astray. Either the practice has not been done as faithfully as reported, or the elastic has not been used, or lips have not remained apart, or the parent has not bothered to observe. The culprit should be identified.

Regardless of where the tongue is placed, ask the patient to complete the exercise, still without using an elastic. Each element of the exercise should be definite and precise: teeth closed,

lower lip depressed, and a dynamic slurp blended with the swallow. You may feel genuine confidence when the child protrudes his tongue immediately afterward, so that you may examine the nonexistent rubber band. The therapist should not be alarmed if, during swallowing, a bit of ventral tongue appears, particularly in patients with open bite. As long as the tip remains anchored, performance is satisfactory; we will attend to the remainder of the anterior tongue at this session.

TOOTH CLOSURE. It rarely happens that the teeth are not occluded for this exercise. Those who fail in this are usually patients who are wearing bands, and questioning will reveal that the orthodontist has inadvertently retied them during the week, making occlusion temporarily painful. Review the situation with the dentist.

Failing such an excuse, allowing the teeth to remain apart could only indicate a very unconcerned attitude by both patient and observer. The matter should be discussed and the importance of molar occlusion reemphasized.

More frequently, an error in this regard takes the form of biting with jaw protruded, which is useless for our purposes. Since proper closure is required on almost an automatic basis for the third step, this step must be repeated.

LIP CLOSURE. Mistakes in this area are usually manifested in one of two ways: the lips are held apart in preparation but are closed for an instant during swallowing or the upper lip is excessively elevated while the lower lip is allowed to lift into contact with upper incisors—and tongue—during the act of swallowing. Either of these mistakes is fatal to our purposes. As stated earlier, there is no patient who *cannot* keep his lower lip out of the way; there are a number who *think* they cannot.

The patient who has practiced with closed lips has greatly increased his problem. At the instant of deglutition, his tongue has slid down toward his lip almost inevitably, further strengthening this tendency. At least, he has demonstrated considerable lingual agility in retrieving elastics, or else has swallowed a number of them. Nevertheless, we are at a standstill until he convinces himself that his lower lip is an unnecessary adjunct. The parent should be convinced of this fact first, however, for this situation arises most often with the child who wishes to conserve his effort but at the same time gain extra attention; he has usually played on the parent's sympathy with telling effect by his dramatic, seemingly excruciating efforts to swallow without closing his lips. Few tears need be shed for him.

It should be borne in mind throughout that we are discussing the ''normal'' patient: those with physical or emotional handicaps, of course, receive due allowance for their disability. Therapy must be tailored very carefully for these latter patients.

SUCKING. Failure in sucking is rare. Nevertheless, it is such a foreign concept to some patients that despite all the emphasis given during the first step, they return without a visible or an auditory trace of a sucking component. If they are not actively slurping, it is safe to assume that they are merely continuing their original malfunction. It would be futile to proceed until changes are wrought.

SWALLOWING. It came as quite a shock to discover that children, after a full session of work and discussion on *swallowing* at their last appointment, will occasionally go home and do every aspect of the exercise with meticulous care —but never swallow once during practice. Perhaps through fear of swallowing an elastic, or misunderstanding, or sheer absentmindedness, they work through the exercise up to and including a mighty slurp, and then protrude a tongue still dripping with saliva. It is therefore wise, when asking a patient of any age to demonstrate how he has practiced, for the therapist to place the back of one or two fingers against the patient's larynx to feel its definitive lift and drop during actual deglutition.

The observer should also be instructed in this maneuver if it becomes necessary. He can feel his own throat during any type of swallow and should expect to feel something similar from the patient's larynx during practice. However, once this problem becomes a matter of open discussion, it usually evaporates.

LIP EXERCISES. Whatever the regimen of labial maneuvers that was assigned last week, evaluation is now in order. Whether a preliminary week has been devoted exclusively to this aspect or only a few exercises were included with the second step, it is usual to continue them for another week or two.

However, assure yourself that they are actually being done. Discuss any points of difficulty, ask for a demonstration when indicated, answer any questions that have arisen, and encourage the patient to persevere in his endeavors.

SUMMARY. The pattern of success in therapy is set in the patient's response to this week's assignment and in your reaction to his response. If things have gone well and every detail is accounted for, be lavish in your praise of both patient and observer; you must supply the basic enthusiasm. If errors have occurred but the patient has made an honest effort, add sympathy to your enthusiasm and praise those parts which have been done correctly. However, be unrelenting in your requirement that a certain level of proficiency be achieved before moving on. If any aspect of practice is below this level, send the patient home to repeat the exercise correctly, making sure first that he understands his error.

Thus, if he has not practiced routinely, has had the elastic in the wrong position, has failed to keep teeth closed or lips apart, did not slurp vigorously, did not actually swallow, or made any other obvious mistake—or even if he is able to perform the entire exercise correctly but it still appears awkward or effortful—an additional week in which to perfect the exercise is necessary. Two consecutive weeks of failure at any point in the program usually indicate that therapy should be suspended.

If life is good and fate is kind, you are now ready to introduce the exercises of the third step. They will consist of three separate exercises, designed to (1) strengthen the lifting potential of anterior tongue musculature, (2) position the entire blade of the tongue for normal deglutition, and (3) reinforce molar occlusion. An introduction to normal resting posture of the tongue and lips will consume much of this session. Although this assignment may appear to be heavy, actual time required for home practice is little more than last week.

TONGUE-LIFTING EXERCISE

Youngsters—the ones who swallow correctly—frequently learn to "pop" their tongue at an early age, and by 8 or 9 years of age are almost able to break glassware with this explosive accomplishment. Children who swallow improperly seem not to engage in such activity, possibly because it is more difficult for them in that it would require muscle function for which they are not prepared. In any event, few deviant swallowers are found who are capable of forceful tongue popping, and yet this attainment is a rewarding and necessary one for our patient.

A distinction should be made at once between the loud, vigorous "popping" to which we refer, and the flaccid, retruded, relatively quiet, and usually rapid "clucking" of the tongue; the latter has no pertinency for us. Clucking is accomplished mainly by the extrinsic tongue muscles working within a limited scope and without sufficient force to appreciably increase muscle strength. Popping, on the other hand, utilizes both extrinsic and intrinsic muscles working through a greater range of movement and is, in effect, a ready-made resistance exercise for the tongue. The resistance is supplied by the hard palate, which for our purposes is pushing *down* against the tongue, thus working in opposition to the forcefully lifting tongue and increasing tongue strength.

The criteria for satisfactory popping are that the tongue be *sucked* firmly against the hard palate, with the tip approximately on the "rubber band spot," the edges sealed airtight, and the mandible lowered, resulting in the forceful stretching of the lingual frenum, as seen in Fig. 19-1. Simply tensing the styloglossus, *pushing* the tongue against the palate, will not achieve this result, and as we have noted, neither will clucking. The desired posture of the tongue in popping, incidentally, is quite analogous to tongue posture during the oral stage of normal deglutition. In performing this exercise we are not only strengthening the ability to swallow correctly but creating a specific image that has direct carry-over on the fifth step of therapy.

Learning this exercise is usually not difficult for the patient. Merely watching the therapist's performance and then checking his own behavior in the mirror is often sufficient. If this approach does not succeed, ask the patient to cluck his tongue three times. This series of three clucks is then repeated twice, with the last cluck being made *very hard*. The result is usually a fair approximation of what we are after, although the tongue may thrust forward, the blade completely out of the mouth, on the first few "hard" ones.

The futility of asking a tongue thruster to suck up on his tongue is clearly demonstrated here. Normal swallowers do so with alacrity; the thruster pushes his tongue up with sheer muscle force, strains the muscles ever tighter, curls his tongue back, and goes through a series of effortful contortions, trying to make the frenum appear, but he demonstrates no concept of *sucking* his tongue against his palate.

We do not expect performance of a very high quality at this point; that comes with practice. The floor of the mouth may become quite sore at the inferior attachment of the frenum if the patient has never previously done this sucking maneuver; however, this soreness usually occurs only on the day after the therapy session and is easily worked out simply by popping a few more times, as cruel as this may sound.

The number of daily repetitions of this exercise that you will assign varies widely, according to the ability of the patient. A daily routine of 100 "pops" is instituted if this skill is noticeably deficient. This situation is the most common one. If he demonstrates some proficiency, a lesser number may be assigned, but in every case at least twenty-five or thirty should be done daily.

Adults are not required to actually pop; the benefit is secured, of course, by sucking the

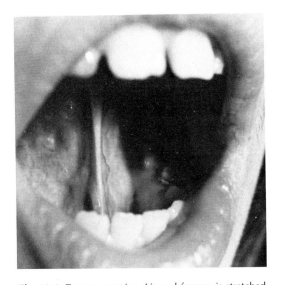

Fig. 19-1. Tongue popping. Lingual frenum is stretched as mandible is lowered.

tongue firmly against the palate, not by the noisy retraction from this position, so that if they simply relax after preparing to pop, they will achieve the purpose. This idea is not easily sold to children, who exert the necessary effort only to gain the reward of a loud noise. It would be poor policy in any event to allow silent practice for a child; the parent would never know if he were doing the exercise, or if he were doing it correctly, and consequently it would not be done.

Older children can observe their practice with a mirror, thus relieving the observer. The parent should check the younger ones daily to make sure that the mouth is open and the frenum truly stretched. All are expected to practice at intervals throughout the day rather than utilize formal practice periods for this purpose.

In case of complete inability to perform this exercise, refer to the discussion of peripheral examination in Chapter 17 and request the parent to use a tongue depressor or tablespoon, as outlined for the child who cannot lift his tongue. Do not proceed with the balance of this session, except for lip exercises. Allow at least one week for the patient to gain ability to position his tongue for popping. There would be no hope of achieving normal deglutition without effortless competence in this exercise.

POSITIONING OF BLADE OF TONGUE

The following exercise reinforces the strengthening of lifting muscles in the anterior tongue and positions not merely the tip but the entire anterior segment into an acceptable posture for normal deglutition. This exercise may be attempted with *two* elastics, placed as in Fig. 19-2. One elastic is placed on the tip of the tongue, just as in the initial exercise, whereas the second is laid on the dorsal surface some distance back.

The placement of this second elastic is somewhat arbitrary. The distance from the tip of the tongue varies, of course, depending on the size and age of the tongue; it ranges from ½ to 1 inch or more. Have the patient drop his jaw and protrude his tongue gently, so that the tongue remains fairly flaccid; if you touch or tap the tongue at approximately the desired site, the usual reaction is to lift the tongue tip, forming a depression across the dorsum laterally. The elastic should lie on the posterior "hillside" thus formed, with its front edge at the bottom of the "valley." This point is not constant, but it serves well enough in most cases.

It is necessary to instruct both patient and observer in the placement of the elastic. It is of great assistance, therefore, if you can identify some permanent feature of the dorsal surface to serve as a marker. Often the median groove ends

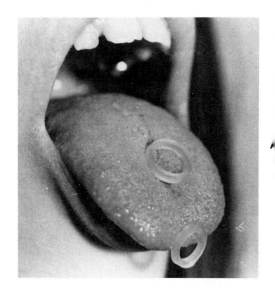

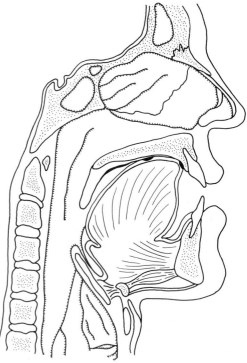

Fig. 19-2. Two-elastic exercise. **A,** Elastics are positioned correctly on tongue. **B,** Correct placement in palate.

at approximately the desired location of the front rim of the elastic; in some cases, smaller grooves helpfully branch off from the median groove, or there may be an odd-shaped papilla that stands out, a pit, a small scar, etc. Something definite should be found and the position of the elastic in relation to the landmark defined.

The exercise should be performed as follows: position the dorsal elastic first, to avoid knocking off the front one, and then place the other elastic on the tip of the tongue; lift the front elastic to the upper alveolar ridge, just as in the initial exercise; close teeth firmly to stabilize the mandible, after which the posterior elastic is pressed against the palate; with lower lip depressed, slurp and swallow. If the anterior segment of the tongue is held in place throughout, the dorsal elastic will remain in its original position; if the tongue makes any thrusting movement, the back elastic is lodged against the uvula, entangled in a tonsil, or swallowed.

As with each exercise in this program, it is beneficial to lower the tongue after each execution and pause for a second or two. Allowing the musculature to relax momentarily, so that each performance of the exercise is a completed act, lends facility later to the discrete instances of deglutition.

A paucity of saliva is often encountered midway through the practice session. When the lateral margins of the tongue must be released in an effort to find moisture, the distal elastic is also held less firmly and the chance of failure increases. It is therefore advisable to suggest the use of sugarless chewing gum, sour fruit drops, or other stimulants.

MOLAR OCCLUSION

It is advantageous to provide some specific task for the antigravity muscles, for a marked lack of tonus is usually found in tongue thrusters. Although these muscles have functioned to some degree in chewing, tongue thrusters frequently avoid virgorous chewing. The usual pattern is to allow antigravity muscles to remain slack during rest, eliminating the state of tonus that supports a closed-mouth posture. The great majority have never employed these muscles in deglutition. It would thus be less than logical to expect normal ability from the masseter, temporalis, and internal pterygoid.

This is true even in patients with an open bite who have occluded the teeth in swallowing. They have closed against an *anterior* movement

of the tongue; when we now alter tongue function to provide a firm *vertical* pressure, the usual reaction is to lower the mandible. Therefore, we must cultivate the ability to maintain firm occlusion in the presence of the lingual pressures generated by the preceding exercise.

It is not required, nor is it necessarily desirable, that the antigravity muscles resist strenuous pressure for a prolonged period; swallowing is a brief activity, and the goal should be to maintain the mandibular stability against a sharp, quick pressing of tongue to palate. Such a pressure is created in the forceful production of a /t/ sound. By combining this sound with palpable tension in the masseter, we are able to exaggerate both elements in the desired combination.

The patient is taught to locate the masseter with his fingers. He is to bite with sufficient force so that even during the production of a very energetic /t/ he can detect *no* movement of the masseter with his fingers. It is usual on the first few attempts for the masseter to disappear completely at the instant the tongue touches the palate. Thereafter comes a stage in which the masseter obviously jumps as the /t/ sound is made; this action results from the mandible tending to drop in response to pressure from the posterior tongue but being quickly restrained by renewed tension in the antigravity muscles. Once sufficient tension is maintained to eliminate this "bounce" in the masseter, most patients are able to do this exercise with some dispatch; however, many report that it feels as though they have a toothache in every molar for a day or two. This change is probably healthy, for the stomatognathic system is constructed to function best under just these circumstances.

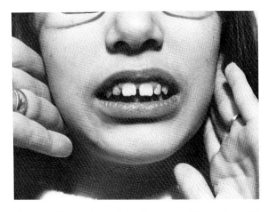

Fig. 19-3. Patient in position for /t/ ("tee") exercise, with parent feeling one side.

Some children will place most of the effort in a prolonged vowel following an indifferent /t/ sound, resulting in an ear-shattering "tEEE-EE." The vowel contributes nothing—except motivation.

The observer must be warned to allow the patient to feel the masseter, on one side at least, during practice at home (Fig. 19-3); feedback is supplied through the fingers, allowing the patient to judge his performance more accurately and therefore to make necessary adjustments as needed. The oversolicitous parent who claps the child's face between the palms for assurance of what is going on robs the child of this valuable feedback.

RESTING POSITION

We must now attack the most insidious force threatening the success of this program: physiological resting posture. The extent of its influence on normal deglutition cannot be stated too strongly. Posture is the foundation of function; every muscle movement is influenced, to a greater or lesser degree, by the posture from which the movement began and to which it returns. Once deglutition has been retrained, the physiological resting position of the various structures involved forms the single greatest determinant of either continued normal function or eventual relapse.

Characteristics of rest position

Although the minimum level of action potential in the muscle is found during the rest position, we must not consider this state as one of absolute rest. Rather, slight contraction, supplied throughout by the tonus mechanism, maintains the structures in a given alignment. It represents a state of equilibrium between opposing muscles, and between muscles and the force of gravity.

The orofacial rest position is not a constant posture from one individual to the next, nor is it a static condition within the individual. It is a variable relationship influenced by numerous factors. Muscle tonus, and thus placement, varies with body posture, activity of the moment, age, pathological conditions, etc. It is certainly responsive to function and to the overall development of the musculature. Our problem may be complicated by the fact that the muscles with which we are here concerned are innervated by the seventh cranial nerve. This nerve has connections with the hypothalamus and is closely associated with the autonomic nervous system; thus we find a ready reflection of emotional states in the muscle fibers of the lips.

LIP COMPETENCE. The term "lip competence" arises often in any consideration of orofacial rest and should therefore be clearly understood. It does not refer to the ability of the lips to achieve a certain task. Instead, it is a morphological term, having reference to sufficiency. It implies a balance between soft tissue and bone, so that when muscle tonus maintains the mandible in a normal rest position, tonus in the labial muscles holds the lips in contact.

Lips may be separated by dropping the mandible, which does not imply incompetent lips. However, if resting tonus of the lips is not sufficient to maintain easy contact of the lips when the mandible is properly placed, the lips are said to be incompetent.

A similar usage is found in a description of the oropharynx. Either an underdeveloped velum or, what occurs more frequently, the failure of the tonus in mandibular and lingual muscles to support the tongue in contact with the resting velum, may be referred to as "posterior oral incompetence."

NORMAL POSTURE. Before we can hope to achieve normal posture, we must define it. We touched on it briefly in Chapter 12 while discussing diagnostic procedures. Authorities vary somewhat in opinion, possibly because postures vary greatly. Some of the finer points of distinction are immaterial to the present purpose; we need not interject ourselves into the dispute over exact distance in millimeters between tongue tip and palatal plane. We must certainly take issue with those who report *no* significant difference between normal orofacial rest posture and that of tongue thrusters. Not only is there a difference, but there is a *critical* disparity between the limit of normality and the posture displayed by almost every patient with truly abnormal deglutition.

Again, we must synthesize. There is fairly general agreement that the mandible, in ideal physiological rest position, is maintained by tonus in the antigravity muscles to provide a distance of some 2 to 4 mm. between the occlusal surfaces—the freeway space discussed earlier. Tonus in labial muscles should provide an easy but constant contact of upper and lower lip. There have been recent research indications of a mild static pressure of lips to teeth, resulting from a continuous negative intraoral pressure.

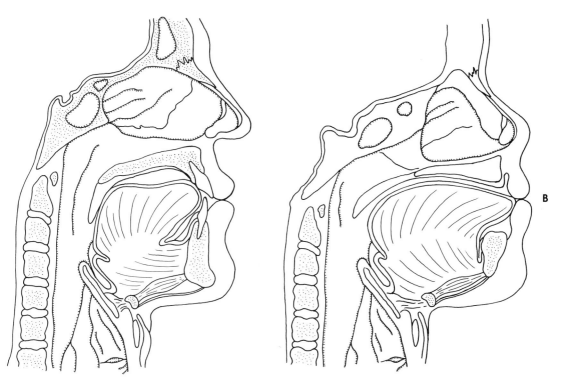

Fig. 19-4. Tongue and lips in rest position. **A,** Usual posture after the age of tooth eruption. **B,** Infant rest posture.

Tonus in the lingual muscles should supply a convexity to the tongue corresponding to, and only slightly less than, the curve of the palatal vault. The tip of the tongue is contained within the dental arches and it either may be elevated and retracted somewhat from the teeth or may contact a point anywhere from the incisal edge of the lower incisors (no great distance from the rugae, when the mouth is closed) to the upper alveolar ridge. The rounded dorsum is a slight distance below the hard palate, with the posterior segment in contact with the velum (Fig. 19-4, *A*).

We need be concerned only with the foregoing essentials. In function, the lips come together before the teeth as the teeth move into occlusion. There is a certain amount of redundant height in the lips in comparison to dentoalveolar height, making it an effortless task, for example, to chew with closed lips even during low excursions of the mandible. From such a resting posture, and with normal structure, it can be seen that swallowing saliva would require only mild contraction of the antigravity group to close the freeway

space, that the lips provide an existing seal to assist in sucking the bolus onto the already poised and elevated dorsum, and that minimal effort is required throughout this function.

An illustration of infant rest posture (Fig. 19-4, *B*) may be noted in passing. There is a great redundancy in the lips, causing a marked pursing, or protrusion of the lips if the mandible is elevated. The tongue fills the entire oral cavity; neither teeth nor alveolar bone has yet developed, so that the tongue overlies the lower gums in contact with lips.

ABNORMAL POSTURE. Compare the foregoing description of normal position with Fig. 19-5, *A*, which is a representation of the rest posture displayed habitually by the girl shown in Fig. 19-5, *B*. It would be difficult to find a place for such aberrations within the normal range, and yet this is only an average example of tongue-thrust rest posture.

Customarily, the mandible is dropped, some patients lending the impression that tonus is totally absent in the antigravity musculature. The tongue lies flat in the floor of the mouth; it shows

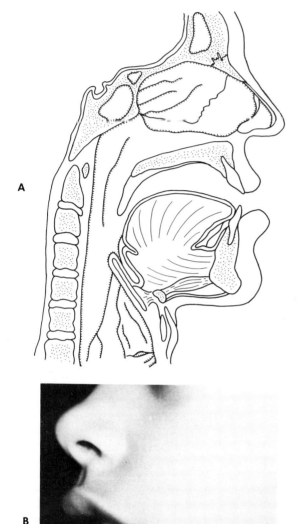

Fig. 19-5. Predominant rest position of tongue-thrust patients. **A,** Graphic rendition of basic abnormalities. **B,** Oral posture of typical case.

little or no lateral convexity, and its tip contacts the lingual surface of the lower incisors or, in some cases, extends anterior to the teeth, making contact with the lower lip. Distance between lips is not measured in millimeters but in major fractions of an inch. The lower lip is characteristically everted; the upper lip is retracted and has a short, thick, nonfunctional appearance. Even with the teeth in occlusion, there is often a noticeable lip incompetence; however, the lowered mandible may lead to this judgment prematurely. Even so, a difficult conscious contraction of the orbicularis oris is usually required in order to maintain lip closure.

Swallowing anything in a normal manner from such a posture would require rigorous revisions and adjustments. It is not to be expected that the majority of swallows, being unconscious, would receive the benefit of such effortful realignment. Rather, the unconscious tendency is to revert to a manner of deglutition that is peculiarly suited to the existing position of the organs.

Note that one frequent instruction for deviant swallowers has been to allow the tongue to lie relaxed in the oral cavity, so that it will not thrust during deglutition! Although such a directive was never less necessary, it is nonetheless anathema for normal deglutition.

Achieving normal posture

Some conclusions may be drawn from the foregoing. We found that posture is the basis for function and that normal function in deglutition is actually the *easiest* response, given normal posture. However, regardless of the therapy that has been supplied to this point, normal function becomes an effortful response; the two aspects are simply incompatible. On the other hand, if we now achieve normal rest posture, we can expect tremendous reinforcement merely from the status of the structures.

FUNDAMENTALS. There has been a tendency to expect that normal deglutition, of itself, would lead to a normal resting position. It now appears that this expectation is no more logical than the hope that articulation drill will modify deglutition: it is a matter of working down to basics, of understanding what comes first and tracing actual effects from proper causes.

Barring deformity and pathological conditions, it is nevertheless possible to bring about the required changes in muscle tonus that result in normal posture. This premise, too, has been questioned, particularly in England and by those

R. H. BARRETT

SPEECH PATHOLOGIST

TELEPHONE 793-1101

1. POP your tongue at least .... times daily. Go SLOWLY, suck up on your tongue and pull down HARD, then REST at least 2 seconds before the next POP. Watch for the "curtain" under your tongue.

2. Practice the 2 elastic exercise 3 times every day. Do 12 swallows each time.

3. Finish each practice period by doing TEE six times. Put your finger tips on your jaw, bite until you feel the muscle jump out, say "tee" HARD without letting the muscle move. Always feel one side YOUR-SELF.

4. Once each day, after you practice, place an elastic on the tip of your tongue and hold it in position for ten minutes. This is where your tongue should rest ALL THE TIME when not in use, so gradually increase to 30 minutes daily.

No LUCK this week! — WORK a little!

		TWO ELASTIC	TEE	TWO ELASTIC	TEE	TWO ELASTIC	TEE	REST POSITION	POPS
1st	DAY								
2nd	DAY								
3rd	DAY								
4th	DAY								
5th	DAY								
6th	DAY								
7th	DAY								

Fig. 19-6. A, Assignment card for step 3. **B,** Chart on on reverse side of practice card.

who accepted Angle's sorrowful observation that "very few have sufficient character and persistence to overcome it."

Normal deglutition will not be accomplished by pleadings or commands, nor by the mere exercising of muscles. Nor is it necessarily a by-product of unaided orthodontic correction of the structures. Certainly it will not result from taping the lips closed or from using other coercive means of *forcing* the structure into alignment. It must be achieved by *reeducating the neuromuscular system* to a new pattern of behavior. It must thus be performed voluntarily by the patient, who alone could implement such an undertaking.

There must first of all be the physical potential for such posture, which has now been provided, true enough, during the course of lip exercises and by the first elements inherent in the therapy program itself. These exercises were designed, however, not merely to rehearse the minimum requirements for normal rest but to *exaggerate* these demands to the point that the desired posture becomes routine and effortless: antigravity muscles are being strengthened and subjected to great strain; labial tissues and muscles have been strengthened and repositioned, the goal of exercises being *overocclusion* of the lips; and lifting potential in the tongue is being vastly increased by positioning it originally even *higher* than normally required. We will remember also that these structures were designed and developed over the centuries to perform precisely what we now demand; we are not asking anything for which there is no prototype inherent in the neuromuscular system.

The patient having attained the physical ability, we now request his voluntary cooperation in making the adaptations permanent. *Exaggeration of normal function* should continue as a basic ingredient. The athlete practices with lead ingots in his shoes or belt, and the baseball player swings a weighted bat, not because they intend to perform in this way in actual competition, but because rehearsing an exaggeration makes normal function more efficient and effortless. Thus the freeway space should be temporarily eliminated, teeth actually touching in repose. The tongue tip should be elevated to the rugose ridge and the entire anterior segment of the tongue held in contact with the palate. We will soon ask that contact of the lips be more forceful than normal for a period.

However, the concept remains that of *rest;* the patient is instructed to avoid forceful occlusion of the teeth, pressing the tongue aloft, and squeezing the lips together as a maintained posture. The medicine works best when taken in moderate doses, not drained in a single draught.

METHODOLOGY. We must now consider how the goal is to be achieved. Given a motivated patient who has been thoroughly instructed as to why and what the project entails, it is still not realistic to expect that henceforth he will be able, even with some effort, to hold to the desired pattern in repose. It must be rehearsed, brought up to consciousness time after time, and thereby established as an automatic pattern. We will begin slowly, gradually increasing demands as the patient gains proficiency. Even so, the assignments are always minimal; doing more than asked is helpful, whereas doing less is disastrous.

For his initial sally, we will merely ask that the patient hold an elastic on the tip of his tongue, positioned as in the first exercise, for 10 minutes each day at the conclusion of one of the practice sessions. This period is to gradually increase to 30 minutes daily by the time he returns next week, and later still more positive measures will be assigned.

It has been found that resolve is greatly strengthened and awareness made far more acute when a daily record is kept of this activity (Fig. 19-6, *A*). Accordingly, the chart shown in Fig. 19-6, *B*, is brought into use. Although this requirement does not guarantee the daily fulfillment of the assignment, it does enhance the likelihood of compliance.

Chapter 20

STEP 4:
POSTERIOR TONGUE

The fourth step of therapy, although of great importance in this program, is accomplished in a relatively brief time using present methods; it should be completed easily in a half-hour session.

This will be the final week of routine muscle exercises; in the next step we will be concerned with the total act of deglutition. Therefore, we continue each of the exercises previously assigned, in order to have them readily available when needed. The amount of time devoted to the former exercises will depend on the degree of skill with which the patient executes them at this session.

EVALUATION OF PREVIOUS WEEK

Examine each of the exercises that were assigned the previous week. As you observe the patient's performance of these exercises, remember for a moment that he brings them with pride, sparkling with his best efforts, almost as a gift for your appreciation. This is no time for urbanity; he deserves all the enthusiastic praise you can give in return. Even if he has not reached the level of perfection toward which you aimed him, minimize the gap and join in his elation.

Unfortunately, there are always the obvious few who enter with downcast eyes and who have not practiced or have done so with less than gusto. We must reserve *our* best efforts for them.

TONGUE POPPING. Have the patient "pop" his tongue five or six times in succession. Observe both speed and manner of performance. If he does the pops quickly, he has probably rushed through practice at home in order to get it behind him and has profited little. If the pops become successively weaker, he probably has not practiced at all. If he has done them properly, he becomes stronger as he goes along.

Note that we judge on the basis not only of loudness but also of the vigor with which this exercise is done. We seek firm muscle action; even though there may be little resulting noise, if the pops are spaced and are obviously done in a proper manner, we can ask no more. It is possible to produce a fairly loud noise by using the middle portion of the tongue, with jaw nearly closed and no tension on the frenum; this movement has little value in deglutition.

The therapist should make a mental note at this time of what will be required during the coming week. If the patient has acquired average ability, forty to fifty pops a day may be assigned, with the information that many people must continue the full 100 each day for another week. If the patient has done an outstanding job, or had already acquired this ability, he may be asked to do only twenty-five a day. If little progress is noted as the result of practice last week, 100 *or more* each day will be necessary, with the understanding that it is simply impossible to accomplish the next session without great skill in popping.

You may wish to warn the patient at this time of what is to come next week: that he will, in effect, be doing all the exercises at the same instant. Thus, should he find it necessary to struggle to do any one part, something else will slip and the entire swallow collapse; there will be too many things to think about to allow concentration on any one part. Therefore, even if every exercise has been done perfectly, we must keep at least a few of each one going this week so that all of them can be done almost without thought.

Moreover, the popping muscles go directly from the exercise into the new swallow: the patient will be required to hold a mouthful of water in the same manner and swallow it off the top of his tongue. Given any weakness, and with the lower lip held down, things might get a bit moist when the tongue is moved for swallowing.

TWO-ELASTIC EXERCISE. Without actually using elastics, ask the patient to demonstrate the two elastic exercise. Note whether the lip remains out of the way and, of paramount importance, whether any portion of the tongue is against or between the teeth during swallowing.

If this exercise has been done with any degree of accuracy, it should look quite good at this stage. Again, make sure that the patient actually *swallows*. If lips are closed, he has simply been rehearsing his original thrust. If anything else has gone awry, the tongue will be in evidence as he swallows.

When all the exercises appear to be poorly done, the patient should repeat the entire week. If everything seems in order, except that the lateral margins of the tongue are evident between the teeth during the two-elastic swallow, the patient may prefer to save a week by doing a bit of extra practice: he can perform eight to ten swallows with the two elastics at each practice period, in addition to the regular assignment, and stay on schedule. This regiment is not to be expected of some patients. If the exercise has been done faithfully and well, it is usually sufficient to require only four or five repetitions at each practice period for the coming week.

In very rare cases it has not seemed possible to retract the entire blade of the tongue until the posterior segment has been moved out of the way. All exercises for the anterior tongue are suspended, and the new exercise in this fourth step is practiced for one week, after which another week is inserted and the two-elastic exercise resumed while continuing the fourth step.

/T/ EXERCISE. Ask the patient to demonstrate the /t/ exercise without giving him any further clue. His first move is often significant: if his fingers fly to his jaw, you have some assurance that he has practiced correctly. Very little else can go wrong with an exercise so simple. He has either done it or he has not. In rare cases, children will still be trying to bite incisal edges rather than molars.

Whereas the patient was permitted to rest

after making each /t/ sound in his practice at home, he should now be able to tense the masseter and produce three explosive /t/ sounds without a flicker of masseter movement. If he can do so, it will be required at each practice session during the next week. Otherwise, he should work toward this end.

The masseter is a paired muscle and should thus be identical on the two sides. Occasionally, however, there will be a marked imbalance in the size of this muscle. Inquiry frequently reveals that *all* chewing activity occurs on the preferred side, often because of poor alignment of the teeth on the opposite side. It is sometimes helpful to encourage chewing on the unused side to prevent imbalance in the facial appearance as well.

REST POSTURE. Assure yourself that the establishment of normal rest posture has been properly begun, and that an elastic has actually been held in position. Some children will have spent the time chewing it, snapping it against teeth with fingers, or otherwise using it as an oral toy. Others will offer protestations that they have held their tongue in place, but they did not use the elastic.

For the latter, explain that the elastic serves a genuine purpose. When the bare tongue is lifted, and conscious attention is attracted elsewhere, the tongue may fall, with no bell being rung or other signal rocket fired off in the patient's nervous system: his tongue has spent its life in this lower region and feels perfectly at home there. The tongue may consequently remain down during the entire time, lifting again just before attention is returned to it. The elastic, however, stimulates both the tip of the tongue and the palate, effectively pinning them together. Should the tongue fall, the unconscious reaction is to restore contact, given any reasonable attitude on the part of the patient.

The patient having gained some familiarity with these upper elevations, we will ask that the elastic remain in place for at least 30 minutes each day during the next week, but with special attention to keeping the lips closed while doing so.

LIP EXERCISES. A rather thorough survey of lip responses should be made at this time. When previous steps have been repeated, or when for any reason a period of three weeks or more has elapsed since lip exercises were assigned—and they have been faithfully practiced—it is usually safe to suggest that they be discontinued forthwith. Should an obvious deficit still persist, renewed effort must be expended this week in order to complete this aspect quickly.

REPOSITIONING OF POSTERIOR TONGUE

The repositioning of the posterior tongue has been a neglected area in most therapy programs, and yet it seems to be of critical importance to those workers who have observed the dysfunction involved. The reader is referred to p. 175 and to Fig. 11-1, *B*, for a review of what is considered abnormal in this region.

RATIONALE. Specifically, the posterior segment of the tongue tends upward and forward in deviant swallowing, pressing most firmly against the posterior edge of the hard palate rather than the lower margin of the velum. Merely lifting the front of the tongue, then, results in contraction of the entire tongue; in an effort to flatten the tongue into a usable posture for swallowing, the lateral margins are forced between the teeth. Thus the type of deviation is changed, perhaps, but an abnormal pattern of deglutition remains.

It is therefore necessary to retract the posterior segment of the tongue into a more normal and functional alignment, leaving working room for the anterior portions. When this action is properly done, the complete synergy of normal deglutition becomes a comfortable, efficient, effortless procedure, one that is amenable to subconscious carry-over.

Again, it would be of no avail to instruct any patient to "hold the back of the tongue down" when he swallows. He would have no means by which to understand such instruction, much less follow it, and some bizarre behavior can thus ensue. Rather, the patient must be supplied with a specific and identifiable posture that he can maintain *during swallowing*. This task seems feasible only when we isolate this single factor and establish it as a routine ability; this positive element may then be blended into the total act with success and dependability.

This approach also obviates any need for attention to the central portions of the tongue; if the front is properly stabilized, and the posterior is retracted into functional alignment, the string is stretched, and what lies between must conform. It seemed logical at one time to begin therapy with attention to the back of the tongue and gradually work forward, placing the various portions of the tongue into the desired posture. It

was found, however, that the posterior positioning was the most difficult to accomplish for most patients, and that even when they succeeded, they gained a rather tenuous hold on this ability, with the result that it was almost always necessary to return to posterior exercises for an additional week before a complete swallow could be properly executed. Time and effort now seem to be used more economically by waiting until the other elements are completed, and then quickly incorporating the newly won posterior position into the total pattern as soon as it is learned.

EXPLANATION OF EXERCISE. It is particularly important that the patient understand what he is attempting to do in this exercise, and why. Later in this session, the phenomenon of losing time through hurry will be explained to the patient; the therapist may take an injection of his own advice at this point. *Take time* to explain in some detail the problem that is involved and what can be done about it, so that the patient will be enabled to achieve this exercise quickly and with some degree of intelligence. When the bare exercise is thrown at the patient, he and the therapist are both befuddled.

In reading over transcriptions of taped sessions, we were a bit surprised at first by the number of seemingly repetitious instructions. However, these repetitions have probably come about through necessity. Patients are not experts in this work and usually have a meager background with which to comprehend what we are telling them, nor do they have a tape recording to which they can refer when they get home, although this possibility has been considered. The instructions have been tried in many styles and combinations, and when the results were disappointing, the instructions have been changed. Individual therapists will certainly use phraseology that is appropriate to their own personality; the point is, we are not trying to impress parents but to achieve a response from the patient. He usually has only a foggy notion of what is expected; hence, after you have explained in adequate detail what you wish him to do, explain it one more time.

A series of pictures showing the posterior tongue in various postures might be of value here. We rely on our hands to depict the various structures and movements. The fingers of one hand are arched to resemble the hard palate, the palm bent downward to represent the velum.

The other hand impersonates the tongue. With younger children, a hand puppet over the "tongue" holds attention, clarifies the concept you are trying to instill, and motivates. Two pieces of bright red cloth can be sewn together to fit tightly over the therapist's hand, and a face can be made with buttons and yarn, as shown in Fig. 20-1.

It is explained to the patient that the back of the tongue must press *somewhere* in order to complete the swallowing act. He is asked to remember this fact while the oral structures simulated by the hand are clarified. He is made aware of the location of the uvula, and some time is spent in identifying this intriguing appendage. Some children have no idea what the uvula is, and many others think that it is their tonsils. Most languages have a common term, such as the "little bell," the "little tongue," or the "little grape" (the actual translation of uvula), that is understood on a national scale; the English language has none.

In any event, the child is made to understand that the uvula will be the "target" for this week. Whereas in actual fact the posterior tongue will press somewhat superior to this place, better results are obtained when the patient has a mental image of aiming at a lower mark.

Explain that the back of the tongue must press downward and backward in order to accomplish the valving required in normal swallowing. When the tongue is thrust either forward or lat-

erally, the posterior segment is discouraged or prevented from making its downward flight, since it cannot go in both directions at the same time. It then becomes necessary for the back of the tongue to curl upward, seeking an accessible contact. Given the steep elevation of the velum, and the attachment of extrinsic tongue muscles, the resulting lift is usually extensive, placing the pressure point near the junction of the hard and soft palates.

In an appreciable number of patients, this upward positioning of the posterior tongue has blocked the easy ingestion of small particles, such as pills, that tend to remain on the dorsum throughout a series of swallowing efforts by younger children. Increased age usually solves this problem, although it may provide some basis for the frequent rejection of meat and fibrous vegetables by tongue-thrusting youngsters.

Explain that at this stage in therapy both the front and back of the tongue would move upward, making for a contracted tongue that would have difficulty in swallowing anything. However, if the posterior segment can be moved downward and backward this week, the tongue will be "downhill," so that food almost falls into the stomach. Stress the ease with which he can be expected to swallow next week. Clarify for the parent the fact that this maneuver will be the hinge on which the entire project turns—that when the posterior tongue is repositioned, the

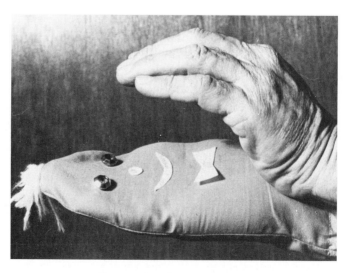

Fig. 20-1. Hand-puppet tongue.

remaining tongue can do no wrong, having gained room to function without impairing teeth in any way.

Once the patient clearly understands what is expected of him, he should attempt the exercise. Being committed to speech therapy, we employ a speech sound by which to draw the tongue into the desired position. The /k/ sound is ordinarily produced by the back of the tongue as it presses the palate anywhere from the molar region to the lower margin of the velum. However, when three fingers are placed vertically between the upper and lower incisors, the /k/ sound then produced aligns the posterior tongue in much the same area where it should function in degutition. Producing the sound also allows the patient to discriminate the coveted position; a definite area of his anatomy is stimulated. He will then be asked to maintain the tongue in this posture—and to swallow, He can succeed in this properly only if his fingers remain between his teeth.

Since it is almost never possible for the patient to swallow on his initial attempts, he will need some assistance in achieving this action. The parent will also need to observe both the correct and incorrect positions. Therefore, fill a syringe with tepid water and, standing behind the patient, have him tilt his head backward at a sharp angle. The observer may stand alongside the therapist and see what transpires.

First, ask the patient to open his mouth only slightly and swallow, using only the back of the tongue. He can usually do so easily, and it is quite apparent that the back of the tongue is thrust upward against the palate. Having identified its accustomed point of contact for the observer, now ask the patient to open his mouth wider and place three fingers between his teeth. Place a *few drops* of water toward the back of the tongue, and it will be seen that the back of the tongue drops markedly, to the lower margin of the velum, usually, in an effort to maintain contact and seal the water out of the pharynx.

If the water is permitted to seep low enough, it will trigger a spontaneous swallow; the posterior tongue is withdrawn from the velum, admitting the water to the pharynx, the velum is elevated slightly, and the posterior tongue slams firmly into the oropharynx to complete the swallow. If no swallow occurs, ask the patient to say "ah" gently; this dirty trick results in retraction of the velum, permitting the water to descend into the pharynx and assuring deglutition. The patient is presented with a choice: he can choke, or he can

swallow; since no one ever chokes, unless too much water is present in the mouth, the alternative occurs uniformly. The observer is enabled to see the contrast in tongue position.

Thereafter, the patient is asked to swallow another tiny amount of water, and then swallow a second time immediately afterward, still with head back and fingers in place; the musculature will almost spontaneously "echo" this second swallow. After two or three times, in which the patient is given an opportunity to identify the movements involved, ask him to take a small sip from a cup of lukewarm water and repeat the above procedure. He should encounter no difficulty in doing so at this point; he would almost certainly have choked had he tried it originally. The latter procedure has been tried with disastrous results for both therapist and patient: with therapist peering down into the patient's mouth, the geyser erupts, drenching everyone. This problem can be avoided by the judicious use of a syringe.

ASSIGNMENT. Having ascertained that the patient is able to swallow small sips from a cup with safety and precision, the therapist need not pursue the matter further during the therapy session. He is allowed to go home and practice this procedure until he no longer needs to use water, a level of competence that should be reached on the first day. Thereafter, he is not allowed to use water for the assigned practice periods; the water induces him to swallow almost involuntarily, whereas we require this ability on a voluntary basis. Water is permitted *in advance* of the practice period, to reestablish the sensation in tongue and throat; however, producing the /k/ sound impels the tongue into the same posture employed in holding the water, and if he swallows quickly, before the tongue can drift away from the /k/ position, swallowing becomes fairly easy.

Warn against saying the word "kay" or the syllable "kuh." Any vowel tends to pull the back of the tongue forward from its contact in producing the consonant /k/ sound, thereby making a difficult task even harder.

The observer is cautioned to feel the patient's larynx occasionally, to assure that swallowing actually occurs, and is also asked to keep an eye on the patient's fingers; it is easy to allow the three fingers to collapse to the height of only two fingers, or even one. Children with a missing cuspid are prone to tuck one finger into the edentulous space, allowing some mouth closure and

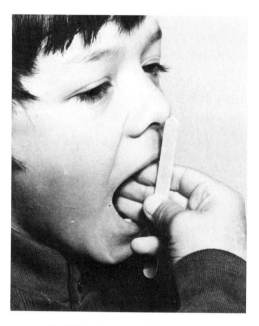

Fig. 20-2. Execution of /k/ exercise.

thereby a return to the original behavior with this exercise. Small wooden blocks were tried in lieu of fingers; the usual reaction was to bite with sufficient force on the block to stabilize the muscles, force the posterior tongue up to its original position, and swallow in the accustomed manner. With the patient's own precious fingers in jeopardy, this error is prevented.

It is possible to purchase boxes of 1000 flat coffee stirrers, similar to Popsicle sticks, from restaurant supply or ice cream companies. It has seemed advisable to wrap a number of these sticks in a tissue and send them home for routine use. One of them can be placed behind the first knuckle of the fingers and held in place by the thumb (Fig. 20-2); thus the oral opening is assured. If the patient truly has three fingers between the teeth, and truly swallows, whatever his tongue does will be the best that he is able to do at the time. Whereas the posterior tongue will strain upward at first, it begins to drop downward in a day or two, so that the exercise becomes much easier.

The usual routine is to keep this exercise in line with the previous ones and assign twelve /k/ swallows at each practice period at home. The

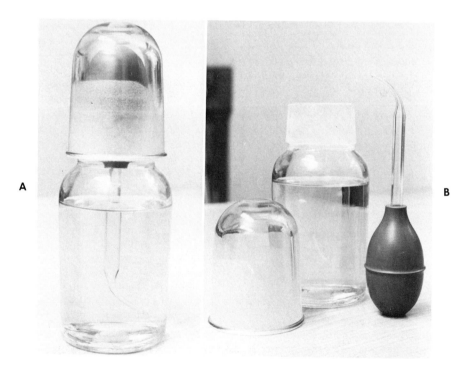

Fig. 20-3. Ziegler eye flushing bottle. **A,** Sterilizing position. **B,** Ready for use.

R. H. BARRETT
SPEECH PATHOLOGIST
TELEPHONE 793-1101

Practice **THREE TIMES** each day.
Each time, please do the following:
1. The 2 elastic swallow .... times.
2. Do the **TEE** exercise .... times.
3. Practice the "K" swallow .... times.
   a. Three fingers between the teeth.
   b. Make the "K" sound.
   c. **FREEZE** in that position and swallow as quickly as possible.
   d. Using water does **NOT** count.
Also pop your tongue .... times.
Once daily, hold elastic in position for a half hour while keeping lips **CLOSED**.

◄●►

The night before your next visit, try the complete new swallow:
1. Teeth together like **TEE**.
2. Lower lip **DOWN**.
3. Front of tongue up like 2 elastics.
4. Remember the **FEEL** of "K" swallows, and pull the back of tongue into that position.
5. Suck up on tongue as you did when you **POPPED** your tongue.
6. **SWALLOW!**

Lips must not go together, no tongue may peek out. Do not "slurp" but suck up and back on your tongue.

Success comes in **CANS** (failure comes in **CAN'TS**)

	1	2	3	1	2	3	1	2	3	REST POSITION	POPS
1st DAY											
2nd DAY											
3rd DAY											
4th DAY											
5th DAY											
6th DAY											
7th DAY											

Fig. 20-4. A, Assignment card for step 4. **B,** Chart for home practice.

uncommon patient who is able to execute this maneuver easily, without using water to "prime the pump," may be allowed to do only ten, whereas those patients who exhibit unusual disability in this function are required to practice more, dropping back to twelve swallows once their performance smooths out.

This exercise proves to be relatively simple when the patient approaches the practice period calmly and without haste. He should sit with head erect but relaxed, collect a drop or two of saliva, place three fingers between his teeth, make a /k/ sound, and swallow promptly. He should then remove his fingers, close his mouth, and allow the musculature to relax for a moment before attempting the next swallow. With older patients, producing the /k/ sound becomes a matter of choice after a time: if they are able to position the posterior segment of the tongue and swallow easily with fingers in place, making a /k/ sound becomes superfluous. However, it is usually of great assistance and reinforces the identity of the correct position.

SYRINGE. It is advisable for the therapist to avail himself of a syringe of some type; in addition to its value in this session, it will have other uses later in the program. Several types are available; however, some are less convenient than others, and there is no provision for sterilization of some types in the average speech clinic. One easy solution to this problem is shown in Fig. 20-3. It is an "eye flushing bottle" or "irrigator kit," available at most medical supply firms. The bottle can be filled with a strong solution of benzalkonium chloride (Zephiran chloride) or other germicide of adequate strength. Avoid any alcohol-base preparation; it will react with the rubber bulb of the syringe and cause a very unpleasant taste. Zephiran chloride is purchased at the drugstore. It may be bought in concentrate and mixed with water according to directions, or it is available in a much more expensive ready-mixed solution. It is odorless and tasteless, completely harmless when properly used, and in strong solution will sterilize the syringe in a few minutes. The excess may be rinsed away under the water faucet at time of use. Many similar products are available from medical and dental supply companies and may be preferred by an individual clinician.

A sample assignment card for step 4 and a chart for home practice are shown in Fig. 20-4.

Chapter 21

STEP 5:
COORDINATING THE TOTAL SWALLOW

Step 5 constitutes the first major test for everyone. If clinician, patient, and observer have been uniformly successful to this point, it should be no great task to combine the various abilities that the patient has gained and to achieve the rudimentary execution of normal deglutition.

This appointment may also provide a stern test of the patience of the clinician. This session is rather lengthy at best; it can be, at worst, a severely frustrating session for all. On the average, however, it is quite rewarding, and the patient may go away from it glowing and giddy with success. It requires careful management, about 45 minutes of time, and a therapist who is unhurried, confident, and perceptive.

In addition to helping the patient gain some ability to eat and drink normally, we will also supply a few procedures designed to strengthen and further refine the velopharyngeal contributions to deglutition.

Before the repast is spread before the patient, a detailed appraisal of his preparation for the present assignment is indispensable; despair and defeat are assured if the component exercises have not been mastered almost to the point of automaticity. We could hardly consign him to the conflict unarmed.

EVALUATION OF PREVIOUS WEEK

Despite the most careful instruction, errors in any of the previously assigned exercises may still be found. The two-elastic swallow may have degenerated; it may have seemed (to the patient) unnecessary to continue the /t/ exercise; tongue popping may be obviously too weak to hope for normal function—all in addition to the roster of mistakes exhibited in the /k/ sound exercise. If the latter appears to be executed perfectly, it is reasonable to attempt the merger of all exercises into the complete swallowing act. To the sharp eye, errors in any aspect are soon apparent. If any single element appears weak or effortful, the patient is not ready for this session and should be allowed extra time to prepare.

Of primary concern, at this point, is the behavior of the posterior tongue; problems in other areas have been dealt with above. Examine carefully the manner in which /k/ swallows have been performed. Trouble usually takes one of the following forms, any one of which portends a dismal future when the stage of habit formation is reached.

USE OF FINGERS. The most common mistake is in the manner in which the fingers are used. Sometimes three fingers are properly placed as the exercise is begun, but at the moment of swallowing, the lips contract, fingers collapse to a height of only one or two, and the posterior tongue continues into the upper reaches. More commonly, fingers have not been employed in any way: because they have proved bothersome, the teeth are merely parted ¼ inch, an indifferent /k/ sound is proffered, and the posterior tongue does exactly what it has always done. Considering the previous session, the therapist may justifiably question whether he is speaking the same language as the patient and observer.

USE OF WATER. Next in frequency is the patient who found the use of water so beneficial that he became an addict. He has assured his parent that it is impossible to swallow without water, and that with water, he is doing the same thing anyway; he thus finds it still impossibie to perform

285

this exercise on a voluntary basis. Work with this patient until both he and his parent are convinced of the feasibility of the required movements. Then reassign the entire previous week as though he had never done the exercise—which in fact he has not.

FAILURE TO SWALLOW. Failure to swallow is usually the fault of the observer. Patients will occasionally be genuinely convinced that they are swallowing, when in truth they are simply producing a pharyngeal contraction or emitting a grunt. Incidentally, there is no *noise* inherent in actual deglutition; although some children do swallow, and then emit a sympathy-inducing moan, any sound accompanying the swallow should be scrutinized suspiciously. Of course, unless this exercise has culminated in a genuine swallow, nothing has been accomplished, and the problem is treated as in the previous paragraph.

FAILURE TO PRACTICE. There is always the occasional patient who arrives with an air of total candor, knowing in his heart that he has done little or nothing during the past week, whose parent is guilty of complicity, and who waits for the therapist to detect his perfidy. Failure to practice is usually apparent rather quickly but may remain disguised until later in the session. The therapist should be alert not to accept implicitly assurances of faithfulness; when it becomes obvious that the expected abilities are not present, it is more effective with many patients to state as a fact your knowledge of the deception. Don't ask, tell; there is less likelihood of future transgression.

MOMENT OF TRUTH

Having assured yourself that the posterior segment of the tongue is behaving readily in the desired fashion, a complete performance of normal deglutition should be attempted. The initial evaluation will be easier for everyone if nothing is placed in the patient's mouth.

Combining the elements

Although it is not essential for the patient to have attempted the suggestion on the bottom of the fourth practice card (Fig. 20-4, *A*), it is usually helpful if this composite process has been subjected to experimentation at home and then allowed to reverberate through the patient's nervous system for a time. Regardless of this situation, the individual actions that you seek should be spelled out and demonstrated. When the patient attempts to duplicate your example,

each step in the progression should be judged rather harshly, with particular attention to any tendency of the middle portion of the tongue to move laterally during actual deglutition. This tendency can only indicate failure of the posterior tongue to remain in the desired position. The criterion at this point is not simply that the patient be *able* to execute the complete pattern but that he can do so easily. Effortful performance is usually centered in a single weak element, this weak factor must be strengthened before moving on.

It is sometimes clear at once that it will not be possible to complete this session. However, it is advisable to continue through the stage of positioning a liquid bolus. Should trapping a bolus also prove troublesome, or if further strengthening of the anterior seal seems necessary, practice of these aspects can be incorporated into the home program during the delay.

If anything reasonable results from the patient's endeavors to swallow correctly, secure a cup of tepid water and fill a syringe from this. Ask the patient to cup his tongue, place a few drops of water in this depression, lift it into the two-elastic position, occlude the molars, depress the lower lip, concentrate on the sensory pattern of the /k/ sound exercise, suck up on his tongue as though preparing to *pop* it (no slurp hereafter), and swallow the water. Tapping the dorsum of the tongue with the syringe will usually result in the desired cupping when the patient cannot do this cupping voluntarily. The presence of even a few drops of water on the tongue requires a more efficient execution of the entire process than does the "dry run" previously attempted; errors become more obvious rather quickly. Repeat this procedure several times until it is done with dispatch and the patient has a clear image of what is involved.

Anterior seal

We now confront the most difficult aspect of this session, and the one requiring the greatest skill, patience, and assistance from the therapist. The tongue thruster has little concept of how to approach normal deglutition, since the entire process of bolus formation and positioning is foreign to him. We noted earlier that this fact has been overlooked entirely in some therapy programs and has been made the exclusive focus of others. It is an essential prerequisite but is nevertheless only a preliminary phase of the total synergism.

Although some patients grasp this operation

quickly and with little effort, this is not the place to save time or cut corners: if the process is improperly done on the initial efforts, the mistake is perpetuated repeatedly on succeeding attempts. It is thus more economical of time and tears to supply the patient with almost a muscle-by-muscle description of what is expected, clearly demonstrated by the therapist, who makes sure that understanding is imparted before the patient is permitted to go astray. Overconfidence in this matter leads to the fighting of many unnecessary battles.

A small quantity of water, perhaps a half teaspoon, is placed under the patient's tongue. He will be asked to move this water to the top of his tongue and seal it in position against the palate, so that he might hope thereafter to swallow it correctly. It is advisable to place the water under his tongue with a syringe; if he attempts to sip it from the cup, one or more mishaps may occur. For example, he may obtain either too much water or none, his tongue may automatically go forward to meet the rim of the cup and then remain fixed against his lower lip, or he may swallow the water improperly at the instant it enters his mouth. Hence many extraneous and unnecessary factors may be brought into the situation.

Once the water is in place, it is necessary to close the lips in order to create the negative pressure that draws the water onto the dorsum of the tongue. Thrusters frequently fail to seal their lips at this point, since no negative pressure is required in deviant swallowing. If lips are closed, they are often drawn in between the teeth; the tongue can thus remain in contact with the labial surface, and the patient is stuck at that point or simply swallows in his habitual manner. For such a patient, suggest that he close his teeth prior to sealing his lips.

When the lips are closed, the procedure is simplified if the head is tilted forward, which maintains the water in an accessible location in the forepart of the mouth. This temporary expedient is required only on the first few attempts, as a rule. With the head erect, the water tends to trickle back into the throat and descend prematurely when not expertly managed.

The anterior tongue should now be lowered to the floor of the mouth. To be more explicit, ask the patient to touch the tip to the inside of his lower teeth, so that he knows when he has arrived. The tongue is thus removed from the palate, allowing the water to ascend in advance of the tongue; when the tongue remains elevated,

and the patient then attempts to suck up the water, the periphery of the tongue seals *out* the water, nullifying the entire project. This mistake constantly recurs.

With everything in position, the water should now be *sucked* to the roof of the mouth. Since this sensation is an unaccustomed one, some specific image should be supplied.

Have the patient smack his lips firmly and then start a second smack while keeping his lips closed. Have him note the feeling in his mouth, for this sensation is the one we want. Perhaps failure comes most frequently at this point. The patient will drop the velum, sealing off the oral cavity, and take great breaths of air nasally. In a mistaken effort to suck up the water, he will tense every facial and oral muscle, trying somehow to force the water up physically. Contortions are great, and often unique, as the patient attempts to relate what he has just heard to what he is experiencing in his mouth. It is occasionally necessary to allow him to get rid of the water in any way, and then use a soda straw to enhance this concept; place one end of the straw in his mouth and have him suck, and then pinch the other end of the straw with your fingers and have him continue sucking. Release the pinched end of the straw occasionally, observing the sudden rush of air through the straw when proper suction is being applied.

When the water has been drawn against the palate, suction should continue as the tongue is sucked up also, sealing the water in position as we originally set out to do. Several errors may occur in this maneuver. For example, the water may be allowed to fall back to the bottom before the tongue is elevated. More commonly, because of lack of experience with oral sucking in the present context, the tongue is simply lifted through muscle contraction and pushed with brute force against the palate; the water cascades down over this rigid tongue, and the perplexed patient will repeat this futile process endlessly. Ask the patient to pop his tongue firmly two or three times, and then prepare to pop again, making sure that the frenum is stretched. The resulting sensations in his tongue and palate should feel exactly the same when he seals the water in place.

A very common problem, of course, is the impulse to merely scoop up the water, as though the tongue were a shovel and the water a solid element. The patient tends to scoop with mouth open or closed, head forward or erect, and tongue starting from any position. This scooping action can become almost compulsive if it is permitted to start. Warn against it in advance and be alert for its inception.

Testing lingual seal

Should the patient successfully negotiate the entire process of trapping a liquid bolus as required, the conscientious therapist is faced with a quandary: how do you, or the patient, actually *know* that the water is there, poised on that straining dorsum, and not long since passed on to some gastric haven? The strongest impulse of the tongue thruster, at the moment his mouth closes to inaugurate this procedure, is to swallow the water instantly with his usual thrust and remove its bothersome presence. This action happens so quickly and is so disguised by other facial contortions that neither patient nor therapist is aware of its occurrence in some cases. Therefore, the true state of affairs should be investigated.

Watching or feeling laryngeal movement is not a dependable gauge of this situation. At times it is possible for the water to escape into the pharynx without perceptible movement, its passage unfelt even by the patient. Conversely it frequently happens that during the patient's effortful preoccupation with trapping the water, he may execute an involuntary /k/ type of swallow that removes nothing from his mouth. In neither case has the true status been revealed by the larynx.

ACTUALITY OF SEAL. When the patient believes that he has securely trapped the water, he is asked to open his mouth, maintaining the palatolingual seal, and to tip his head forward again over an empty cup held ready by the therapist. If the water is still present but has not been sealed in place, its drainage into the cup will assure the patient of his shortcoming. If the patient bends over without mishap, he is asked to release his tongue, permitting the water to drop into the cup and thus advertising his notable victory. If the water has been prematurely swallowed, the tongue is released without noticeable aftermath; a single drop of saliva may plink dejectedly into the cup.

Repeated efforts are usually necessary to conquer this aspect of the problem: the ability to establish and maintain a palatoglossal seal. Some patients exhaust the entire repertoire of errors, whereas most perseverate a single mistake. Whatever the problem, if trouble arises, *slow down*. Stop after every three or four unsuccessful attempts and explain the entire procedure again, allowing the patient to identify the source of his failure. Stop and discuss the weather or current events with the parent—or just stop. It has been thought by some authorities that we learn to ice-skate in the summer and to swim in the winter because of the tendency for the human nervous system to forget inappropriate movements; during the time that we are not engaged in an activity, we tend to forget our mistakes and remember best the things we did correctly. Quote this to the patient, for want of anything better, but get away from the task at frequent intervals and do not permit a faulty movement to become a habitual response.

Watch also for early signs of frustration in the patient; it is quite easy to end this session abruptly in a flood of tears if you pursue this endeavor to the point of "just one more try," or if the parent reacts emotionally to the child's failure. If even such a possibility appears imminent, or if it becomes apparent that you are at the point of stalemate, terminate the session immediately with a gentle comment on the frequency of such occurrences and a statement of your implicit faith in the patient's eventual triumph after a few relaxed attempts at home. Ask the parent to place the water in the child's mouth with a spoon, eliminating the need for a syringe, and request that as the child succeeds, the amount of water be gradually increased to a heaping teaspoonful. Rigidly restrict the amount of time to be devoted to a practice period: at the most, 10 minutes can be spent practicing, and if the patient is still unsuccessful, a wait of several hours will be necessary before the next attempt. It is amazing how many children return home, wait a few hours, and succeed brilliantly on their first try.

STRENGTH OF SEAL. Only occasionally is it necessary to interrupt the session, providing the therapist remains calm and supportive. If your instructions at the outset have been adequate, some patients accomplish a fairly competent seal on their first attempt, although they are allowed to feel that they are quite remarkable. It is routinely achieved in ten or twelve attempts; if not by then, success becomes doubtful.

When the patient attains some proficiency, to the point of trapping a teaspoon of water consistently, you should test the strength of the lingual seal. When he has trapped the water, opened his mouth, and bent over the cup, ask him to maintain this posture while you count aloud slowly to ten. No particular hazard is present if the musculature has been adequately strengthened; otherwise, the water drips off the tongue as the seal fails.

Note one last source of trouble in this regard: because of the continuing tendency to protrude the tongue, some patients will attempt to trap the water with the edges of the tongue thrust against or between the teeth. Air is thus permitted to enter between the teeth, destroying the seal. As the water is trapped, the tongue must be sucked on up and back until the tip is in contact with the "rubber band spot."

ALTERNATE PROPOSALS. Other therapy programs have proposed different methods of establishing an anterior seal. Some of them may be more to the liking of the individual therapist; a few deserve comment.

One is the "rapid" approach: the patient is asked to trap a bolus on his tongue, without bothering with the details of how this action is to be accomplished. An ingenious patient may occasionally figure it out, true enough, but if it is achieved with promptitude, the patient probably had no great abnormality in his original pattern of deglutition. On the other hand, if the patient fails in his original attempt, we have noted that more time is lost in overcoming his errors than would have been required to instruct him properly at the outset.

Another approach is to explore this area briefly without the use of any type of bolus; when the patient appears to have the anterior tongue elevated, he is requested to maintain this posture when he eats. Regardless of the impressions of those involved, this patient probably continues to swallow by displacing the bolus backward as he thrusts in an unchanged pattern. Products of this approach have been examined; when swallowing on command they exhibit a reasonably accurate facsimile, but if given a sip of water and asked to repeat the same pattern, they are undone.

Still another suggestion has been to proceed from the first with a modicum of peanut butter. This approach appears to be self-defeating in several respects. First of all, it seems somewhat cruel to expect the manipulation and eventual deglutition by the neophyte in normal function of a substance so adhesive. Second, it could not possibly fall from the tongue, so that there is no assurance that the anterior seal has been formed; the tongue may have been braced against clenched teeth and the bolus displaced backward

without negative pressure to assist its gluey progress. Finally, it would not be possible to determine the degree of accuracy with which peanut butter is swallowed. Even normal swallowers may modify their pattern, reinforcing a bit, when faced with peanut butter. In none of the above approaches is it possible to actually test the existence or strength of the seal.

We also employ a solid bolus, as shall be seen in a moment, but it is of somewhat different consistency. Sugarless wafers are used, so that a chewing element is incorporated into the situation. These wafers, too, stick to the tongue if they are improperly swallowed, and the number of crumbs remaining on the dorsum is a fair barometer of the vacuuming, hydraulic assist with which negative pressure has contributed to deglutition.

Application of normal function

When the patient has demonstrated his ability to trap a suitable liquid bolus and hold it suspended for a 10-second period, we are at long last in a position to expect completely normal function in a practical situation, rather than as a trick or an esoteric rite.

Up to this point in the session, the patient has either swallowed correctly or has prepared a bolus for normal swallowing, but he has not combined the two actions. As a final preparation, assist the patient through the total pattern: place water under his tongue again, after which he should keep his head erect, trap the water, and then swallow it as outlined on the fourth practice card (Fig. 20-4, *A*). There is seldom any difficulty in taking this step. In fact, the remainder of this session is fairly routine, since the patient is guided progressively in the application of this routine to the ingesting of food and drink.

However, the most frequently recurrent problem for the *therapist,* particularly the novice, probably occurs at just this point. This problem can be traced directly to the therapist's failure to assure, as an actual functioning element of the total pattern, the required repositioning of the posterior segment of the tongue. The therapist has accepted a counterfeit procedure in home practice, has failed to elicit proper carryover into the complete act of deglutition, or has simply not clarified this aspect in the patient's thinking or his own.

It then transpires, when the patient is requested to swallow a bolus, particularly one of solid food, that two patterns alternate with regularity, and both are frustrating: the patient swallows with seeming exactitude, and then mournfully reveals a tongue still loaded to capacity; or, if the bolus vanishes, it is because he thrusts his tongue in a desperate effort to conjure the bolus away, with the margin of his tongue painfully obvious at some point between his teeth. This full cycle can be repeated with little variation, and it is a touching scene as both therapist and patient begin to weep.

DRINKING FROM CUP. Ordinarily, persons who swallow normally seal their lips about the rim of a glass or cup, sucking the liquid directly onto the dorsum, and then forming the anterior seal and swallowing as a single unified procedure; the tongue remains poised within the oral cavity as the liquid is drawn into the mouth. This routine is not always precise because some of the liquid usually spills down into the floor of the mouth, and many individual differences are found. Nevertheless, the two points in which we are interested are essentially unchanged: lips seal the rim, and the tongue remains in the mouth.

Deviant swallowers, on the other hand, have a tendency to approach the rim with protruded tongue, lay the rim on their tongue, form some type of funnel with their lips, and *pour* the liquid into their mouth. There are many individual differences in this pattern also, but the tongue-to-rim contact is almost invariable. When the very young thruster imbibes a glass of milk, the imprint of a large segment of his tongue is often left on the outside of the glass; with age, only the tip of the tongue is in contact, as a rule.

This touching of the tongue to the rim of a glass or cup is another trigger mechanism for deviant swallowing; it must therefore be forestalled. We will require for a time that the patient drink through clenched teeth, physically preventing the undesired contact. In patients with open bite, closing the teeth does not actually restrain the thrust of the tongue, of course, but even these patients receive support from consciously arranging for molar occlusion before approaching the rim with their lips. Certainly a permanent habit of drinking through clenched teeth is not expected; it is abnormal, just as swallowing with open lips is abnormal, but it serves our purpose very well until the time when the tongue remains and functions, efficiently and subconsciously, within the mouth.

We instruct the patient accordingly. Demonstrate the full procedure: close your teeth and have the patient feel your face to note that the /t/ muscle does not move from beginning to end of such a swallow. Ask him to close his teeth and take a sip from a fresh cup of water, allowing only his lips to touch the rim. In case of gross upper protrusion, the tendency is to push the cup into the teeth, sending the rim to meet the tongue, since the tongue is not coming down to meet the rim. Advise parents to be cautious of this error during the coming week. It often helps to ask younger patients to bite their teeth, say "oo," and hold this posture when they approach the cup.

The patient is to take the water into his mouth and seal it in position without relaxing molar occlusion. When it is trapped in place, he should open his lips, retract the posterior tongue, and swallow. Trouble arises only when the teeth are parted during trapping; in this case, the tongue is once again thrust between the teeth and seemingly fixed there, the patient straining to no avail in his effort to seal the water in the palatal vault. Ask him to cease his struggles, occlude his molars, and start again. Continue in this way until he is sipping easily.

DRINKING FROM STRAW. We discussed previously the thruster's proclivity for mashing straws with his tongue. It is usually helpful at this point to assist him in something less troublesome. It will be necessary for him to manipulate the straw with his fingers, something he has previously managed with his tongue. He is asked to occlude his teeth as with the cup, and again touch only his lips to the straw, thus preventing the insertion of an inch or more of the straw into the dorsum of the tongue. Thereafter, the procedure is identical to that with the cup: suck a small amount through clenched teeth, move the straw away *with his fingers,* trap the water, retract the back of the tongue, and swallow.

Many patients believe that they cannot suck with their teeth closed. The negative pressure that draws liquid through a straw is ordinarily produced in part by retracting the tongue, which enlarges the cavity of the mouth without allowing additional air to enter, thereby creating a partial vacuum. The thruster has instead achieved this effect by dropping his mandible, since his tongue has remained in the anterior space. It is a relatively easy matter to teach him the more usual manner.

HOT AND COLD LIQUIDS. Something similar to the tongue-thrust pattern may be observed when the average person is faced with a cup of very hot beverage: the tongue is protruded as if to test the heat of the liquid; the tongue overlies the entire lower arch, with margins in contact with labial and buccal surfaces; and the liquid is taken into the mouth without subjecting the lower teeth to any marked change in temperature. The deviant swallower usually consumes all drinks in no other way. It is thus a common occurrence that nothing hot or cold has ever touched his teeth: the back of his upper incisors and the anterior segment of the entire lower arch have been insulated by his tongue.

Therefore, anything other than tepid liquid may be experienced as painful when drawn through and around these teeth which are unaccustomed to being nude. The immediate reaction is to revert to the thrust, preventing the pain. Although this reaction is certainly understandable, it is just as surely ruinous to therapy and must be overcome in some manner.

There are toothpastes on the market, such as Sensodyne and Thermodent, that are produced specifically to reduce the sensation of heat and cold in the teeth. The use of such a toothpaste may be advised as a temporary measure. It can be bought at any drugstore and is widely recommended by dentists where its use is indicated. It is not a quick anesthetic but requires several days for the active ingredient to penetrate the enamel to the level of the thermal sensors. It also requires several applications daily. It nevertheless provides salvation for many patients.

These patients can also avoid much of the problem by abstaining from extreme temperatures for a brief time. It is the inordinate chill when milk is poured directly from the refrigerator onto the teeth that hurts; if a glass of milk is allowed to stand at room temperature for even a few minutes, it is still cold milk, but the toothache has been removed. This measure also is a temporary imposition. Some relief is quickly found as the teeth become acclimated to wider extremes and steeper gradients of temperature. Moreover, as soon as normal tongue function is habituated, in a matter of only a few weeks, the teeth may safely be parted, when drinking, in a more normal manner, reducing the exposure of the teeth and eliminating the problem entirely. Explain this fact to the patient; the mountain is less steep when the patient can see the top.

SOLID BOLUS. The deviant swallower experiences great difficulty, as a rule, if presented with a solid bolus as an introductory task; his performance is usually uncertain, haphazard, and poorly understood. Having reached this point in the session, however, we can expect some degree of skill and precision in the handling of solids. A pattern has been established; it needs only to be refined somewhat to proceed from water to wafers.

The distraction of chewing is absent with liquids, as is concern about the collection of crumbs. Then, too, liquids receive some benefit from gravity once they are properly aimed, whereas solids require more active attention and detailed coordination. Yet there is rarely a problem with a solid bolus if its use is delayed until this time and a few minor points are clarified.

As indicated above, we prefer sugarless wafers for this purpose; other materials have been tried and may be more agreeable to the individual therapist. Wafers appear to be fairly universally acceptable to patients of all ages and are easily purchased in assorted flavors. When given a choice of vanilla, chocolate, or strawberry, few children react with anything but pleasure; a number have adamantly refused to consume other types of solids. The crumbly texture also presents a genuine challenge to the patient, not only in bolus formation, but in actual deglutition; those crumbs are sometimes hard to find, and do pile up on the tongue when improperly swallowed.

The patient is offered the cooky jar from which to make his selection. A very small bite is attempted first; it usually eventuates in more saliva than cooky, but it builds confidence. A second, larger bite is usually handled much better than the first, and the patient is instructed to collect all the crumbs possible, suck them into a cohesive bolus positioned in the center of the tongue, and seal the bolus in place before swallowing. This concept can be amplified with the remaining wafer; when it is chewed and collected on the dorsum, ask the patient to look in the mirror and protrude his cupped tongue, observing the manner in which the bolus is positioned in the middle portion of the tongue. He should also observe his own behavior as the bolus is positioned and swallowed. The visual image can be a strong reinforcement for the kinesthetic pattern.

ASSIGNMENT

The patient's deglutition, with both liquids and solids, is usually rather crude and awkward at this point. He needs a period of time in which to try out the new process, lay it down for a time, and then return to it repeatedly before he arrives at the highly coordinated, truly effective pattern that we wish to make habitual.

Solids

Asking that one legitimate meal each day be consumed entirely with the new procedure will suffice for solids. Many patients report that the first three days are the most difficult, for during this period each of the separate elements involved tends to slip back toward the original routine, one part will go astray even though everything else is functioning properly. After the first few meals, the entire process seems to jell, to become welded into a unitary pattern, working with greater efficiency while requiring less attention to detail.

It is an act of kindness, therefore, to suggest that the lightest meal of the day be chosen for these first three or four days. It is understood, however, that once a meal is started with the correct swallow, it must be consumed entirely in this way; it is of small benefit, and sometimes harmful, to eat a few bites of each meal correctly and gulp the remainder. Doing so can be particularly damaging later, in the process of habit formation.

It is often advisable at this time to renew the requirement that all food must be chewed with lips closed. The need for this rule is usually made visible by the patient's handling of the cooky.

Liquids

The proper management of liquid is far more difficult than solids in actual daily practice, simply because of the greater speed that is demanded. When tongue thrusters are permitted to go home and utilize continuous drinking with the meager ability they have at this point, the anterior seal is soon destroyed, the tongue thrusts against the teeth rather than trapping the liquid, and the desired pattern is never established.

Therefore, a slower version of drinking, something within the conscious capability of the patient, is essential for a time as a stepping stone to normal drinking. The patient should be asked to drink for the next week by taking small sips; he should trap each sip, open his lips, and swallow in such a way that both he and the observer can be certain of tongue function. A positive image is thus supplied, and it must be thoroughly instilled.

This feature is always disagreeable, but alternatives never seem to succeed. A minimum of three or four glasses daily, water-tumbler size,

are necessary to complete this phase safely. With most children, however, it is unwise to count glasses: they "chug-a-lug" the one at hand, with every intention of sipping the next, and before they know it, the week is gone. It is far safer to assign *all* liquid.

The patient should be reassured, as he was told in the first session, that he is never expected to employ these practice measures in public; only in the privacy of home are we asking for cooperation. He should also be assured that the sipping of liquids will require only one week, if properly and consistently done.

Pharyngeal reinforcement

The routine exercises that are assigned this week are designed to reinforce the pattern of movement in the posterior segment of the tongue. Not infrequently, problems arise in the later weeks that can be traced to a failure of the musculature in the posterior region to make a smooth transition from chewing to swallowing. In fact, the desired downward and backward trajectory may be lost entirely if not given positive encouragement.

When properly done, the desired movement can be fostered by producing vowels, which remove the tongue from the velum, with the previously used sound of /k/. In this case, however, we will ask for a much more forceful production of the /k/ sound, something that the patient can definitely feel and experience as the posterior tongue crashes into the velum.

A single combination of vowel and /k/ sound would serve the purpose if repeated over and over but would be boring. The list shown on the fifth practice card (Fig. 21-1, *A*) requires less than 1 minute to complete, even when properly done, but accomplishes our objective.

The patient will also be asked to start becoming familiar with the appearance and sensation in his own mouth and throat when he yawns. Few children have a valid image of this function, and they give a distorted performance if asked to yawn voluntarily. The yawn will be modified to achieve voluntary velar control on the next step, and this control, in turn, is used to activate and strengthen velopharyngeal participation in deglutition thereafter.

Rest posture

By this time, the ability to close the lips firmly without undue strain may logically be expected. Accordingly, the therapist will now supply a "lip

5

R. H. BARRETT

SPEECH PATHOLOGIST

TELEPHONE 793-1101

———————

Eat ONE MEAL each day with the new swallow.

Drink ALL liquids (at home) sip by sip.

The new swallow, for both eating and drinking, must have:

1. Teeth tightly CLOSED.
2. Lips wide OPEN.
3. NO tongue showing.

———— ◄●► ————

Twice daily practice the following, making the K sounds very HARD:

Ka, Ke, Ki, Ko, Ku. Ache, Eek, Ike, Oak. Cake, Keg, Kick, Coke, Cook.

With elastic in place, close lips over plastic SCREEN for one hour each day.

Each time you YAWN, notice how it feels, what it does. At least once each day, WATCH yourself yawn in a mirror.

From here on, WORK less — THINK more.

	ONE MEAL	K's	REST POSITION	YAWN
1st DAY				
2nd DAY				
3rd DAY				
4th DAY				
5th DAY				
6th DAY				
7th DAY				

A

B

Fig. 21-1. A, Practice card, step 5. **B,** Chart on reverse side.

zipper'' designed to nurture this component of the resting posture. The method currently suggested entails the use of a modified oral screen; this can be combined with continued use of an elastic, stimulating tongue elevation as well as lip closure.

In its formal version, the oral shield is also used in a dental procedure. The usual oral shield, or vestibular screen, is carefully built of acrylic from a model of the patient's teeth, as shown in Fig. 21-2. This type of shield is beyond the needs or competence of the clinician. However, a light, flexible creation based on the same idea may serve admirably for present purposes.

Two basic sizes are made, as in Fig. 21-3, and stored individually in coin envelopes; one of them can then be cut to fit the patient's requirements. The screen is made of low-density polyethylene plastic 0.030 inch in thickness, the same as that used for lids on many coffee cans and soft margarine cups. This product is difficult to acquire in localities that do not have a well-stocked plastics distributing company. However, many glass and mirror companies are in contact with such distributors and may be willing to put in a special order for you. A minimum quantity is often a 4 by 8 foot sheet, costs very little, and is sufficient to fill your needs for several hundred years. Share it with a friend.

The notches in the center must be sufficiently deep to avoid contact with the upper and lower labial frena, since the frena may be quite sen-

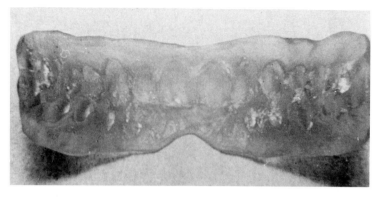

Fig. 21-2. Vestibular screen made of acrylic.

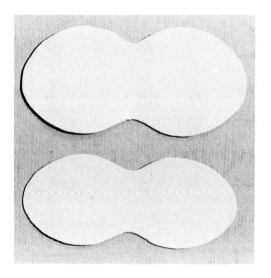

Fig. 21-3. Child and adult oral screens of polyethylene.

sitive to pressure. Nevertheless, the overall size of the screen should be adequate to fill the vertical dimensions of the vestibule just short of discomfort.

When it is properly fitted, the patient can occlude both teeth and lips, although lip action is stimulated by the need to maintain the screen in place. It is now impossible to breathe through the mouth, for the inner surface of the lips seal against the plastic, and any attempt at oral breathing strengthens the seal. Therefore *oral screens should never be used in the presence of nasal blockage*. Should temporary blockage occur, the patient has only to touch the screen with his tongue in order to dislodge it. Some shields have been produced with breathing holes cut along the midline; this arrangement defeats

the very purpose for which we are striving. The air holes convert instantly to whistles.

It has often been found valuable, after the patient is accustomed to maintaining the screen for an hour or more during the day, to require that he keep it in place during sleep. Many patients who habitually mouth-breathe at night are later found to be sleeping with their mouth closed.

In certain orthodontic relapse cases that are caught early, or in some Type I cases in which only incisors are disturbed, it has seemed advisable to suggest that the dentist construct a formal acrylic shield, thus effecting tooth movement at the same time that lips are being closed. The dental version is invariably more effective.

Lip exercises

It is strongly felt that the patient should not be asked to engage in unnecessary exercises or peripheral activities, which frequently scatter the attention and weaken the end product. When lip exercises have been necessary, the status of lip function should be reevaluated at this time, with observation of both strength and posture. If exercises were assigned as the first step of therapy, they have by now been practiced to the point of exhausting their usefulness.

All such procedures should now be terminated, in any event. Any remaining need may be noted, but correction should be postponed until the final session, when attention will be directed even more forcefully toward maintaining closed lips in repose. For the moment, all efforts should focus on deglutition.

THERAPY MATERIALS

Some half-dozen items have been employed in this session, a few of which might be profitably described further. A certain type of material is not a determining factor in the program, and the therapist should feel free to use whatever is preferred. Therapy hardly hinges on the color of the facial tissue presented; perhaps some of the detail below is picayune, but the motivating influence so derived has often been welcome.

Thus, cups are much more intriguing if they are brightly colored. Pallid white cups, or those with a pale-blue border, are certainly less expensive. They also smack of the doctor's office and may evoke unpleasant emotion that is detrimental even though not conscious or apparent. Colored cups, to the contrary, are more likely to be associated with picnics, soft drinks, and pleasure; the small extra cost is well spent.

So, too, with the straws. The candy-striped variety does well, and the type that also has a flexible section that allows bending is even better.

Even the type of cooky jar may deserve a moment's thought. Whereas we may wish to titillate the younger child, we hardly dare present a container bearing bunny rabbits or a cuddly kitten to the teenager. A jar of solid color, or one decorated with bright stylized flowers, accomplishes our purpose and renders insult to no one. It should also be small enough for easy handling.

The cookies themselves were discussed above, and the syringe was discussed in Chapter 20. No specific mention was made of the tissue; with this item, quantity is more important than style.

Chapter 22

STEP 6:
THE CONSCIOUS HABIT

The task at this stage is to inaugurate a specific program by which the new capability for normal deglutition can be made habitual—to supply the patient with definite tools whereby he can remove from this function the necessity for conscious thought. We should expect this session to be brief, pleasant, and relatively easy; many patients find it the most enjoyable step in the program. However, it does not always work out that way. Some patients experience a marked letdown after the fifth step: they achieved a certain goal in learning the complete pattern, they are now sure that they *can* swallow correctly, and they feel no great compulsion to be concerned thereafter. Some of those who are outstandingly excellent on the fifth step return as miserable failures for this session: When they find themselves able to swallow as desired with some ease and smoothness, overconfidence is an understandable reaction, leading to a secondary startle reaction when they encounter another cooky at today's session and find themselves ambushed by their own carelessness.

When things have gone as expected, the entire focus at this session will be to implement correct deglutition as an invariable response during waking hours.

EVALUATION OF PREVIOUS WEEK

One of the dividends of using wafers is now redeemable: one has only to "count crumbs" to garner a fairly accurate assessment of the previous week.

The patient is asked to chew and swallow an average-sized bite. His performance as he does so gives some indication of what he is *able* to do; when he protrudes his tongue after the swallow,

the therapist can readily form a judgment of how faithfully the assignment has actually been carried out. We expect that the patient will chew with closed lips, secure the bolus, occlude his molars, open his lips, and swallow with no trace of lingual protrusion. He should then be able to reveal a tongue untainted by the presence of a single crumb. Anything else should be investigated.

A few crumbs along the lateral borders of the tongue may be acceptable, providing the balance of the dorsum is swept clean; the crumbs indicate some remaining difficulty in bolus formation. Even on the center portion of the tongue, one or two crumbs may be reasonably expected, depending on the general performance. Anything more implies a problem.

If all is well except that the posterior portion of the tongue has functioned improperly, one of two patterns is usually seen: either the swallow is executed with apparent precision, after which the lips close and a *second* swallow actually voids the mouth; or the tongue reveals a concentration of crumbs banked across the posterior segment. Back to the /k/ exercise!

If the tip of the tongue has been retroflexed or otherwise positioned too far back in an effort to avoid protrusion, the concentration of crumbs usually covers the blade. A second swallow to complete the evacuation of the mouth frequently follows.

If there is a generalized scattering of crumbs over the entire dorsal surface, one of two additional situations may be inferred: the sucking element has not been incorporated into actual function and deglutition is still being attempted with sheer lingual force; or the patient has not practiced at home or has done so indifferently. Tea leaves may be adequate for predicting the future, but reading crumbs is much more reliable for divulging the immediate past and present!

Most of the mistakes that are made at this point are evident in only a few scattered patients; with rare individuals there is a specific disability causing some single facet to be particularly difficult. However, the majority of problems result from failure to practice correctly, rather than from any lack of ability. After all, the patient was able to function adequately last week, or you would not have given the previous assignment.

A second cooky is occasionally required before an accurate appraisal is possible; the uncertain patient may be *too* careful, under the clinician's searching eye, and distort his usual procedure completely by attempting to employ added security measures. Care should also be taken to avoid the use of cookies that are enhanced in their lustrous chocolate appearance by the generous addition of a coloring agent; the food color stains the tongue, and what at first appears to be a disastrous performance of deglutition may in fact be only the result of a merchandising gimmick.

The obvious mechanics of deglutition, which the observer has been asked to supervise, should naturally be evaluated. If the teeth are allowed to part, mechanical advantage is lost to the tongue, and we could only expect to find some residuum after swallowing. If lips close during the swallow, nothing of value has been accomplished. If the tongue is still visible between the teeth, ground has been lost during the week. Should any of these failures be apparent, it is a safe assumption that neither patient nor observer has functioned properly.

Failure to swallow a solid bolus with reasonable proficiency requires, of course, that further improvement be completed before the present step is attempted: an erroneous pattern must not become habitual. It is thus more frequently necessary to repeat an assignment at this point than at almost any other session. The patient's best effort must be required; otherwise, the inevitable deterioration that occurs after the intense period of therapy may cause collapse of the entire project within a few months.

The patient's management of liquids should also be inspected. It usually reflects a duplication of the pattern with solids; the patient who has been conscientious throughout one meal daily has also sipped an adequate volume of liquid, as a rule, whereas any error or carelessness can be detected in both situations. The only area of trouble peculiar to drinking is the result of continued reaction to cold liquids, which is usually manifested when the patient handles the solid bolus adequately but approaches the cup of water with tongue still protruding, or at least with teeth apart. The tongue never quite gets into position for the resulting swallow. Interrogation usually reveals that the suggested toothpaste has not been obtained or was not adequately used, or that the child has insisted on liquids far too cold to be tolerable or necessary. This situation must be resolved, of course, before correct rapid drinking can be anticipated.

The patient should also demonstrate the manner in which he has practiced the exercise combining /k/ sounds with vowels. If insufficient force has been applied to the /k/ element, this exercise may be reassigned as a portion of the present session.

The single item most frequently overlooked in the patient's home practice is yawning. A multitude of excuses are given. It is essential nevertheless, and some provision must be made for acquiring voluntary velar control. If it seems feasible to the therapist, this practice also may be carried forward with the sixth step providing it is the only flaw present. This session is completed as planned, including instruction in obtaining control of the velum; practice in this entire area is to be intensified, with the goal of gaining mastery of the velum by the following visit, on schedule. Should it become apparent within a few days that this deadline cannot be met, the patient should call and extend the time before his next appointment.

In those cases in which yawning has been observed but other factors make it necessary to repeat the fifth step, some advantage may be gained by proceeding with the instructions for controlling the velum; should this ability prove difficult to acquire, a week of grace has been provided.

In certain instances it may appear that every aspect of the previous assignment is *possible* of execution by the patient, but with no leeway: there is no indication of ease or security in the new pattern, even though it is technically correct. This degree of proficiency is not adequate to the task we now face. A few additional days of practice before moving on are strongly indicated; the alternative frequently proves to be the repetition of both the fifth and sixth steps, with an understandable loss of enthusiasm.

RAPID DRINKING

The first innovation of this session is the transforming of discrete sips into a pattern of consecutive swallows in drinking. When the previous assignment has been adequately followed, there is no great problem, for the only added ingredient is speed. With the teeth closed and the lips occupied with sealing about the rim of the cup, the tongue is less enticed into error and is thus enabled to function with some rapidity in a fairly normal manner. The most difficult aspect of this achievement usually lies in keeping the lips *closed:* after weeks of practice with parted lips, and particularly as a result of the preceding week, many patients find that keeping their lips sealed to the cup is a near impossibility on the first few attempts. However, this problem is quickly conquered.

It is helpful to demonstrate what is expected before asking the patient to do so. With molars in occlusion, simply drink from the cup. It is safer to ask that the patient position the tip of his tongue in advance on the "rubber band spot," in order to further discourage its efforts to establish contact with the rim of the cup. He can then suck the water through his teeth and around the sides of his tongue, trap it, and swallow. If he attempts to maintain his tongue in some unspecified location within his mouth while sucking in the water, this indefinite posture often becomes a definite thrust after a few swallows. Again, this requirement will be relaxed at the conclusion of therapy to eliminate closed teeth and prepositioned tongue; for the coming two weeks or so, they provide his greatest security.

Ask the patient to perform this action, taking only small sips for now, and then allow him a few moments to digest mentally what he has just experienced. Utilize this time to explain to the observer that we expect drinking to be accomplished with a total absence of facial movement. If the tongue succeeds in reestablishing contact with the cup, a generalized puckering movement is usually seen throughout the chin and lower lip; it can easily be demonstrated if the therapist will place his tongue in similar position and drink. If the patient's teeth remain closed, but his tongue slips down onto the lingual surfaces, a crinkle is usually detected at the corners of the mouth just at the instant that the larynx lifts in the pharyngeal stage of deglutition. This fleeting crease most often extends at a downward oblique angle from the corners of the mouth but may take the form of vertical parentheses a short distance away on the cheeks, or dimples slightly above the angle of the mouth, etc., depending on the specific muscle arrangement in the individual face. It is nonetheless obvious to the informed viewer and usually ceases immediately when the patient is asked to elevate the tip of his tongue slightly. Although this crease may eventually prove to be less diagnostic than it appears, it serves as a useful guide.

INITIATING THE HABIT

Once the patient is capable of an adequate performance in rapid drinking, we should be ready to take direct steps toward habitual use of the new pattern of deglutition. Since there would be little point in expecting subconscious change until the correct pattern is the accustomed response on a conscious level, the latter will be our goal this week.

We may anticipate that, by the following appointment, the patient will be employing the desired pattern on an automatic basis if awake or oriented to his environment. In order to achieve this state of deglutition, the patient is now required to voluntarily eliminate the tongue thrust and replace it with the desired procedure during every instance of swallowing. In actuality, we can hope for very few in comparison to the total number of swallows that occur; nevertheless, the patient's goal should be *every possible conscious swallow*. We will worry about the other swallows next week.

THE REMINDER. To increase the patient's awareness of deglutition, to achieve a sharper focus on this activity, and to increase the number of swallows that can be brought to consciousness, every patient is required to construct a "reminder sign," a free-standing card of some type designed and executed by the patient, which is then placed behind his plate at every meal to assist his memory. Other reminders may be stuck to the refrigerator door, dangled near the kitchen sink, or placed on the television, but they are optional. The one on the table is an absolute requisite and must be turned in to the therapist at the conclusion of therapy, suitably spattered with food and finger marks.

The ingenuity of children in creating these reminders is astounding to behold. A few examples are shown to the patient during this session, so that he knows in general what is expected; some very ordinary and unimaginative specimens should be included among the more original, so that the patient does not feel overpowered by previous geniuses.

The primary requirements are only two: that the patient make the reminder *himself,* and that the resulting creation be able to stand alone. This latter consideration makes it much less likely that the reminder will be lost, hidden under dishes, or otherwise overlooked. As for investing his own efforts, it increases motivation, lends added importance to therapy in the patient's mind, and gives needed impetus to the program, an effective shot in the arm, by creating greater personal involvement of the patient.

The materials employed in constructing re-

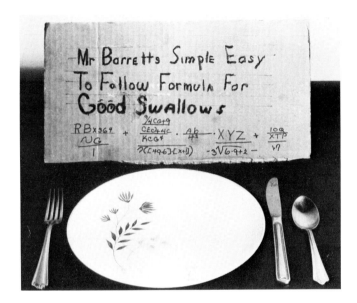

Fig. 22-1

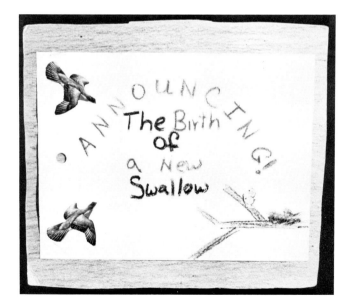

Fig. 22-2

minders cover quite a range in themselves (Figs. 22-1 to 22-7): tablet backs, the cardboard that some laundries place in shirts, shoe boxes, used greeting cards folded in reverse—an endless profusion. They are made to stand upright through a variety of methods almost as great. They are given easels, the ends are bent backward, or a card is folded over with the crease across the top, in addition to the esoteric numbers made of wood, wire, toothpicks, clothespins, etc.

The legends they bear are still more varied, from the single, glaring command, "SWALLOW" (spelled with unexpected originality at times), to anatomical representations of the function itself. Jingles are common, of course, from the little girl's effort

> *I hope I can think*
> *And swallow right*
> *Or Mom will yell*
> *Both day and night.*

to her adult counterpart's rhyme

> *Straight teeth can give more lasting joy*
> *Than a fine fur coat of mink,*
> *And since they're costing just as much,*
> *Before you swallow,* THINK!

Patients who must eat in school or college dining halls have a problem trying to avoid attention. The sign is either of such low profile as to be hardly visible to the patient, much less surrounding students, or sufficiently large to provide a screen behind which to dodge when swallowing with lips apart. One university student who sought concealment kept a file folder opened and upright behind her plate to foster the deception that she was studying; the inside of the folder contained the following classic:

> *Some teeth and a tongue*
> *Two lips and some gums*
> *And exercises that they must follow.*
> *The palatal slurp*
> *The uvular burp*
> *And that's how we learn to swallow.*
>
> *My mouth stuffed with cotton*
> *Lips stretched by a button*
> *A rubber band poised on the tongue.*
> *Slurp, swallow, and sigh,*
> *Gag, upchuck, and die—*
> *The rubber band's stuck in my lung.*
>
> *My fingers were ready*
> *My tongue very steady*
> *To give the /k/ sound a good blast.*
> *But the /k/ wasn't silent:*
> *The reaction was violent*
> *And that's why my hand's in a cast.*
>
> *My heart filled with fear*
> *The time had drawn near*
> *For the public my swallow was ready.*
> *The effort was strong*
> *But something went wrong*
> *And my uvula got wrapped in spaghetti.*

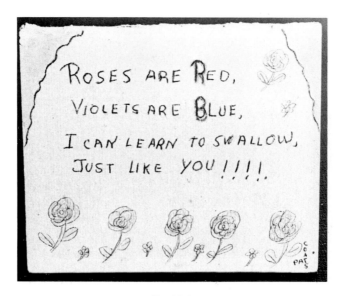

Fig. 22-3

The proximity of San Juan Capistrano Mission to Tucson has inspired a number of reminders. One photograph taken through the arches of the building and showing a sky filled with swallows was placed above the stern admonition: "These swallows can come back, *but mine better not.*" Another depicted a surprisingly accurate pharyngeal section, complete with velum, uvula, and rather hypertrophied tonsils, one of which observed, "This must be Capistrano—here comes another swallow."

Some reminders are in other languages, either native or acquired, whereas some are concerned with a specific aspect of therapy. Tongues are made of numerous materials, given distinctive personalities, and even thrust and retract in some versions. The therapist himself is present in many guises, not all complimentary, although the intentions are good. It is so easy to cut colored letters from magazines to spell out: "Grin and Barrett." One heavily ornamented card, using drawings of the bird in lieu of the word "swal-

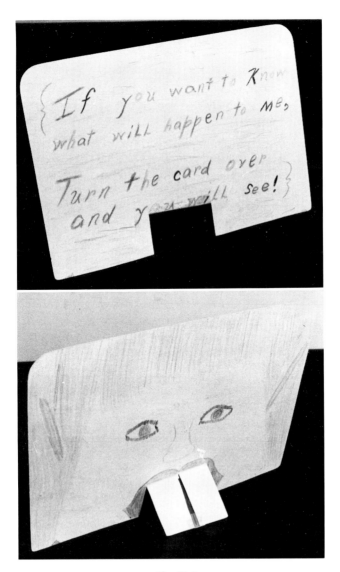

Fig. 22-4

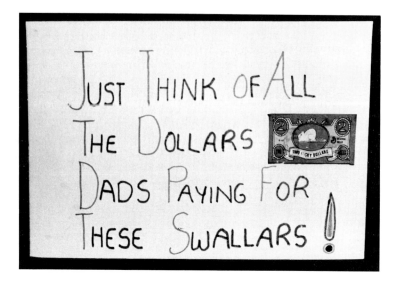

Fig. 22-5

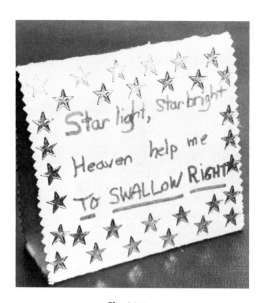

Fig. 22-6

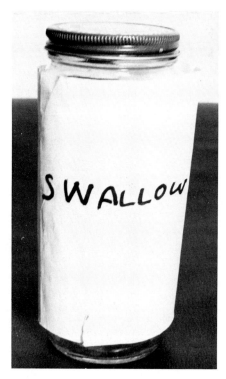

Fig. 22-7

low'' made the following observation:

The Barrett (swallow) has not wings,
The Barrett (swallow) never sings,
But if you learn the Barrett swallow,
Pretty teeth are sure to follow.

The therapist will soon acquire a private collection of reminders but is warned against becoming sentimentally attached to each one; when they begin to overflow one complete closet at home, it is time to arrange for their demise.

VELAR CONTROL

The goal in velar control should be to generate as much velopharyngeal activity as possible. We will accept as a minimum some voluntary ability to contract the levator veli palatini, the tensor veli palatini, and the palatoglossal muscles, resulting in raising and lowering of the velum and constriction of the faucial isthmus. We are not concerned with ability to wiggle the uvula, a common misconception.

This skill is not difficult to acquire, given the right attitude and some specific image of what should be done. If the patient has concentrated on yawning during the previous week, both requirements are present. Relaxation is the key; the patient should allow his jaw to drop, tongue lying flaccid within the lower dental arch, and look in the mirror toward the velum. If the pa-

---

6

R. H. BARRETT
SPEECH PATHOLOGIST
TELEPHONE 793-1101

Please make a "reminder sign" AT ONCE. After you make it, USE it, WATCH it, and THINK about it. This week, you must try to eat EVERY bite with the new swallow.

Remember—KEEP YOUR LOWER LIP AWAY FROM YOUR TEETH for each swallow, and of course NO TV during meals.

Drink ALL LIQUIDS the new fast way, but KEEP TEETH CLOSED TIGHTLY, with tongue held up in front. Your face should not move as you drink.

Once each day, look in mirror and practice moving your SOFT PALATE up and down. Practice MORE than once daily if palate does not move easily. It must go up and down at least six times, without stopping to rest, before you return next time.

The new rest position, with tongue up, lips closed and teeth touching, must support the new swallowing habit. Continue using SCREEN for an hour each day, keeping tongue up without elastic.

Except to talk or eat — KEEP YOUR
MOUTH SHUT!

	SIGN	PALATE	REST POSITION
1st DAY			
2nd DAY			
3rd DAY			
4th DAY			
5th DAY			
6th DAY			
7th DAY			

A

B

Fig. 22-8. A, Assignment card for step 6. **B,** Chart on reverse side.

tient merely recalls the sensations present and the appearance of his throat in yawning, the velum usually lifts a bit. By maintaining relaxation in surrounding muscles that are more responsive to voluntary contraction, the ability to lift the palate can be isolated and brought to consciousness. It is necessary to pause frequently and close the mouth, especially at first, in order to prevent the contraction of unwanted muscles. Tensing the throat, locking the jaw or even forcing it open too far, protruding the tongue, or attempting to lift the soft palate through brute force—all block the desired movement.

Occasionally, patients are helped by having them prepare as above and then emit a short, sharp "ah" or "huh" sound, observing the palatal response. The resulting movement is still not voluntary, of course, but they can achieve a similar velar reaction by merely *starting* to make the sound; working from this point, they gradually learn to move the palate at will. This method is much more difficult for most patients and is completely ineffective with some. Working from the positive mental image of yawning is a much more direct and rapid procedure.

Once voluntary control of the velum is achieved, other pharyngeal movements are accomplished with ease. Since these muscles will require exercise over a period of time, patients are warned that the following step will not even be started until they are able to perform such exercises. As in swallowing with lips retracted, no patient has yet been found who *could not* gain control of velopharyngeal muscles; quite a number *think* that they cannot.

REST POSTURE

The assignment last week marked the most extensive use of mechanical assistance in maintaining the rest posture; we will now begin to transfer responsibility to the patient's own neuromuscular system. The oral screen should be continued for another week, but we expect the tongue to remain elevated without elastic reinforcements, as specified in Fig. 22-8, *A*.

Chapter 23

STEP 7:
THE SUBCONSCIOUS HABIT

The orientation throughout this program is toward the achievement of change through voluntary efforts of the patient. We wish to avoid coercion and mechanical gadgetry, which must eventually terminate, and to secure instead modifications that are more permanent, since they are entangled with the patient's personality. This program is done *by* the patient, not *to* the patient. If volition weakens, some mechanical reinforcement may be supplied; if volition fails, the failure is complete.

Accordingly, at this point, the patient is asked to *voluntarily* assume the responsibility for transferring the correct procedure in swallowing from a conscious level to an *involuntary* response. If he succeeds, the change is relatively quick, permanent, and pleasant. If he does not, it is doubtful, in most cases, that any use of force would yield better results.

The element of speed in making the desired change is an important factor just here—an importance not always comprehended. The method is frequently proposed, and probably more frequently indulged, of bringing the patient to the point of correct conscious deglutition and then assuming that if he continues to practice, it will at some indefinite point in the future, weeks or months hence, become subconscious. This assumption is hardly realistic.

Granted that we have no truly accurate figure for the number of times that deglutition occurs daily in the average patient: we have seen figures ranging from a probably erroneous 590 to a perhaps excessive 2000. In any event, it is a constantly recurring response. How many of these swallows, do you suppose, could be executed *consciously* by the most motivated patient you are likely to see? A few hundred daily? That estimate is probably generous.

At this stage, unless swallowing is performed consciously, it is performed incorrectly. Were it possible to pull each discrete instance, or even a majority of instances, of deglutition up to a conscious level, then practice might truly make perfect. We are faced, instead, by a patient who has a lifelong, subconscious pattern of abnormal function and who continues to reinforce this aberrant pattern many times throughout the day and night compared to each instance of conscious, normal function.

Even the newly acquired conscious pattern is not yet perfected and tends to degenerate quickly—the accustomed method feels comfortable, requires less effort and no thought, and is being maintained through constant repetition: failing some positive combative force, why should we not expect the eventual elimination, rather than the ultimate establishment, of the desired pattern?

EVALUATION OF CONSCIOUS READINESS

Whereas last week we expected considerable agility and smoothness in the patient's performance, this week we expect the pluperfect: normal deglutition should be an accomplished fact, given only awareness.

Solid bolus

Observe the patient's management of one final wafer. The point of progress is usually fairly obvious. The food should be properly chewed and swallowed, with no remaining trace and with the effortless appearance of routine behavior. Crumbs along the lateral margins of the tongue

305

are no longer acceptable. If the patient's mouth has been dry, a scattered crumb or two may be noted without undue alarm, but not many. The patient's general appearance is often more indicative: we seek not only a smooth performance but an obvious effortlessness. When things have not gone well at home, the situation is usually manifested in more than crumbs.

PREVALENT PROBLEMS. The most frequent failure at this stage is closure of the lower lip. Despite everything the therapist said last week, in the face of capital letters on the practice card, notwithstanding five previous weeks of indoctrination, and regardless of the ministrations of the observer, some patients still close their lower lip prematurely. They can produce a crumbless tongue, but when they are required to depress their lower lip, the tongue is either forward of the proper position or there is obvious effort in keeping it back. Again, they have been "rehearsing" their original thrust as they ate.

There are also the micrometer-minded patients. They have tried to gauge how closely they can approach their upper teeth with their lower lip without actually making contact. While they concentrate on keeping their lower lip 1 mm. distant, the swallow goes to pot. We are considered to possess a certain equanimity but find the boundary line of forbearance at about this point.

Next in frequency among the problems we find the patient who flatly has not practiced. He has made no reminder, has dashed off something and left it in his room, has found the conversation at dinner too fascinating to avoid, or has simply decided that therapy is not worth the effort.

Each of these problems arises from the attitude of the patient. Given an honest effort, failure seldom occurs. Excluded, of course, are those rare patients with an individual handicap and the patient who was ill the preceding week; they may require only an additional week in order to gain the required proficiency.

REMEDIATION. For those patients who have closed their lips, indicating a disregard for therapy, or who have not practiced, proving their disregard, some decision is now necessary. Appeals to their better nature are seldom effective, or else they would not be necessary. This situation may be the most difficult one you are required to handle; it does not go away if ignored. It certainly would be illogical to proceed with the present session, depending, as it does, entirely on the volition of the patient.

Some discussion with patient and observer should come first, in an effort to clarify present attitudes. Occasionally, a sore point can be revealed and alleviated, and the previous step repeated profitably. More often, a more drastic change is required. We have come too far in the program to drop the patient from therapy lightly, and yet suspension is usually the most sensible recourse.

Although we view the following procedure with a somewhat jaundiced eye, it has occasionally been found efficacious to twist an arm slightly. The situation is spelled out for the patient, including the fact that this entire program, as well as any dental treatment to follow, is designed to benefit only him. It will not make his parents any prettier or healthier—only poorer—and yet they are willing to offer their time, money, and effort, all they can do, in order to help *him*. It would hardly be fair for him to expect all this beneficence when he does not supply the small amount of effort that is being asked, and still expect his parents to grant all his desires and whims; it simply is not fair, nor is it the way life goes. Therefore, we may take the nonessential that he most enjoys—whatever is nearest and dearest to his heart, be it Little League, television, or association with a certain group or individual—and make his participation dependent on sincere practice. He is not being asked to give up anything; he can see every television program that he ordinarily watches—if he has honestly practiced first. If he has not, the switch is flipped off, or he remains in his room while others watch, but that is *his* choice. He has only to exert this small effort, which is for his own benefit, in order to light up the screen.

This motivation is artificial and may prove to be no motivation whatever, but it is effective in selected cases. One all-star third baseman rode the bench for only one game then developed normal deglutition with amazing skill and rapidity.

Whatever course you choose, do not allow the situation to degenerate into parental nagging. This is worse than futile—it assures present failure and usually foredooms any future improvement. The decision should be clear-cut: either the child is going to do this work himself, or it will not be done.

Liquids

As was the case in the previous step, drinking behavior usually duplicates the pattern with solids. Exceptions occur with sufficient frequency that it is essential to observe the patient as he drinks a cup of water. A few patients actually are more secure in drinking than in managing solids. More often, any difference is to the detriment of the liquids. Excessive speed trips up a few, and carelessness reaps a small harvest. On the whole, errors are uncommon, easily detected, of a minor nature, and can often be accommodated in the present session. For example, if teeth are inconsistently closed, allowing some relapse of the tongue, palpation of the masseter by the fingers for a day or two during drinking often allows everything to fall into place.

Velar control

Proficiency in velar control should be examined, with a muttered prayer that it is adequate. It usually is found to be so, and many patients have already begun to embroider their ability with individual twitches of their own.

When the patient lacks the ready ability to lift and drop the velum, it is probable that he has not practiced, has done so with excessive tension, or has been waylaid in an effort to move only the uvula. The first on the list is the most common: the patient makes an initial attempt at home, sees that the velum does not immediately fly up and down, and proceeds to convince himself and his parents that he is the one exception who *cannot* do this exercise. The problem might easily be handled by telephone, and one session salvaged, providing the patient has called; the defeatist has rarely done so.

This patient should understand that velar control is simply a matter of practice. No one moves the soft palate at will without practice. If he merely sat and stared at his palate in the mirror long enough, wishing it would move, it would probably move eventually; it is quicker if he tries to recapture the sensation of yawning. You may stimulate his velum with a tongue depressor, and in rare instances it has proved necessary to have the parent repeatedly lift the palate in this way, but success is eventually achieved.

The patient who has tried *too* hard, who has strained every fiber above his shoulders, is obvious: the only thing that lifts and falls are his eyebrows. Once you convince him of the value of relaxation, the problem is ordinarily solved. If it appears feasible, you may even complete the present step with a double assignment of velar practice. The misguided soul straining at his uvula may also profit from this approach; once

he broadens his field of action, relief is almost immediate.

RATIONALE OF SUBCONSCIOUS PROCEDURE

Space does not permit, or circumstances require, a dissertation on subconscious brain function at this time. This area is poorly understood at best. Neither will we become embroiled in distinctions between *un*conscious and *sub*conscious function; it is probable that one does not swallow in any event if truly *un*conscious, whereas deglutition continues at a steady pace in sleep and during other *sub*conscious activities.

Magnitude of subconscious need

Swallowing correctly on a conscious level has carved but a small foothold in the total need of the patient. We noted that, even in the waking state, it is impossible to call each swallow to consciousness, or even a majority of them, for the secretion of saliva is a fairly continuous process. Even in sleep the mucosa of the throat must be constantly bathed in saliva; otherwise, evaporation resulting from respiration would render it stiff and nonfunctional. Salivation is stimulated by eating, drinking, and speaking, so that we swallow more frequently during waking hours, but the estimate of one swallow a minute in sleep may not be too far afield. At least it provides a convenient figure for our use at this session. Several studies of swallowing incidence during sleep have been conducted, with such widely differing results as to leave considerable doubt of the true figure or even a fair average.

It must become obvious that we need to supply the patient with some *specific* device by which to modify his subconscious behavior. It has long been felt that teaching a patient to swallow with some semblance of normalcy is no great task; making this ability subconscious has seemed impossible.

Available alternatives

We have tried a considerable number of devices and procedures that might fill the need for subconscious mutation; others have been considered. Little of a helpful, specific nature is available in the literature of speech, dentistry, or psychology. There are some beautiful generalities and a number of wild guesses, but there are no "directions for use" on the package. It may be helpful to evaluate a few of them. Knowledge of what does *not* succeed can also be valuable information: it can save time otherwise squandered in covering ground already proved sterile.

MECHANICAL AIDS. The use of mechanical aids harks back once again to the area of hay rakes, oral screens, and electrical shocking devices. Even at this point in therapy, when conscious learning is not required, the use of such appliances seems undesirable. We have rejected all forms of coercion, preferring to inspire the patient to effect all change on a voluntary basis. When all else fails, there are certain cases in which a physical reminder may prove helpful, but even it would probably not be profitable if the appliance were not *subconsciously* acceptable to the patient; verbal agreement is not always a true reflection of attitude.

Perhaps more importantly, we require some solution that can be routinely applied by clinicians who are not prepared to introduce such devices. A positioner, installed after therapy has been completed, has often proved to be helpful, but installation is primarily a dental procedure.

RECORDING DEVICES. The "sleep teaching" recordings were considered in early cases. They would seem to offer some attractive features; however, investigation revealed that researchers at the Bell telephone laboratories, the Rand Corporation, and elsewhere had made extensive tests of this well-publicized method and found nothing of value. They were evaluating the acquisition of conscious knowledge, of course, but found a steady decline in learning as subjects approached sleep, and *no* learning in the sleeping state. This finding substantiates what harried teachers have known for generations: that original learning occurs only on a conscious level.

Some studies[1,2] have shown, however, that while original learning is not acquired during sleep, responses learned in a waking state can thereafter be evoked even in the deeper levels of sleep. Working from this premise, a device has now been perfected which combines several attractive features.

Termed the *Satellite* of the biofeedback machine described in Chapter 13 (see Appendix 2), some rather complicated electronic circuitry is built around a small cassette recorder. A key, retained by the clinician, unlocks the cover, giving access to a jack for the microphone and the controls which allow for various time delays. A series of messages in the therapist's own voice is recorded; these can be spaced to replay at intervals during the night. When locked and sent home with the patient, the only controls available are those to play, rewind, and stop.

The manufacturer points to many uses in addition to the habituation of deglutition, such as assistance with sucking habits, bruxing, mouth breathing, and the reinforcement of posthypnotic suggestions. It is felt that it might have genuine value as an adjunct to the procedure recommended below.

USE OF HYPNOSIS. Hypnosis, of course, can be an effective tool by which to transport the desired pattern to the subconscious and to secure the support of the subconscious. The details of utilizing hypnosis in deglutition were stated earlier. As noted at that time, however, there are limitations and disadvantages to its routine use.

Some parents would doubtless seize their child and run screaming at the mere mention of the word, despite the fact that the child may spend hours in a hypnotic state, reading, watching television, or merely daydreaming, not aware of the parent's call (hypnotic deafness), not feeling the throb of a lacerated knee (anesthesia), and with time distorted to the point that an hour is telescoped into a few minutes.

Then, too, hypnosis is usually ineffective as a "one-shot" procedure; repeated sessions are required for reinforcement before change is secure in a function as basic as deglutition. More sessions may thus be consumed than in the balance of the program. Some patients are such difficult hypnotic subjects for the average clinician that no amount of reinforcement would suffice.

Primarily, hypnosis for this problem is avoided when possible because it is not completely voluntary. Even though the patient voluntarily seeks hypnosis, and despite the fact that the hypnotist can merely guide and direct, the patient seldom feels an adequate personal responsibility for bringing about change. He often seeks hypnosis as a means by which to *avoid* personal commitment. Hypnosis is incapable of such magic. It can provide wonderful support, but only of conscious desire and voluntary effort. Failing these elements, hypnosis fails.

There should be no hesitancy in suggesting hypnosis when it appears that it might succeed where other measures have already failed. Patients who have proved inaccessible through every other approach have, as reported in Chapter 13, succeeded completely with support from hypnosis.

Twilight zone

A few other techniques, less well defined, have been proposed and have proved to be toys or blind alleys. At some unrecorded moment, the results of these trial-and-error procedures were combined with a few concepts and principles from psychology as well as from clinical hypnosis, were seasoned with common sense and brewed during sleepless nights, and were catalyzed, at last, by pure desperation. No effort will be made to defend the particulars of this specific approach. It has been used effectively by many clinicians for several years.

There is some overlap in terminology, since the framework of this procedure contains elements of autosuggestion, psychosomatic influence, "bio-feedback," and cybernetics, as well as something analogous to the "goal-directed imagining" routinely employed in behavior therapy by some psychologists. In defending this last technique, Spanos and colleagues[3] found that carefully directed patient imagining was an adequate substitute for formal hypnosis. They reported four sets of variables that appear to play a role in mediating the changes in behavior seen in both hypnotic and behavior therapy situations: (1) motivation, (2) attitude and expectancy, (3) specific wording of the suggestions or instructions, and (4) the circumscribed cognitive processes occurring in response to the suggestions or instructions. These four variables do, indeed, appear to be crucial in applying the routine outlined below.

What we are seeking to implement is a type of *self*-hypnosis. This approach places the onus completely on the patient. The manner in which self-hypnosis is employed seeks to take advantage of the transition period between full waking and full sleep, a hazy, twilight interlude during which it appears that subconscious modifications can be wrought, given strong motivation for such change by the subject.

We are utilizing here a natural phenomenon that has been recognized for many centuries but that to this day is not fully understood. It is the process by which the mathematician, for example, unable to retrieve an equation from his brain, puts it aside until bedtime, asks his subconscious, in effect, to produce the desired data, and then awakens in the morning and writes down matter-of-factly what he was unable to sort out the previous day. Leonardo da Vinci wrote in his diary about his own discovery of this ability, although he confessed his lack of understanding concerning how his mind was able to accomplish such feats.

Forgotten names of former acquaintances may be similarly retrieved, providing such recall would not cause emotional discomfort; we do apparently have a built-in safety valve that suppresses many painful memories.

Despite the fact that we still have not found the clock in our brain, it is the proper use of this "twilight time" that permits us, on any given morning when we are sufficiently motivated, to awaken at a specific time much earlier than our routine, often missing our goal by only minutes; if we would really prefer to sleep, the alarm clock may scream in vain.

Even "maternal instinct" becomes entwined with this phenomenon. The mother may sleep undisturbed through the nocturnal stumblings of her spouse, even his snoring, and yet be alert at the mere whimper of her infant. It has been noted that when the father assumes this responsibility because of an ailing wife, the mother now sleeps through some rather assertive infant howls, and it is the father who awakens in an instant.

These manifestations could only result from some change in orientation as sleep is approached, activating some type of sensor or alarm system, or making conscious demands on the subconscious. "Sleeping on it" to resolve a problem appears to be a worldwide practice. Concentrating on a feared area of weakness as the student falls asleep may prove to be his salvation the following morning during an examination. It is believed that some portions of this manuscript would never have found exit from Barrett's skull had it not been for the judicious application of this phenomenon.

PATIENT ORIENTATION

The patient is first made aware of the comparatively few times that he is able to swallow consciously, so that he can appreciate the enormity of the task before us. He should also understand that swallows occurring during sleep will be the most difficult to change, since they require a very large measure of both understanding and desire—that is, he must understand what, why, and how he is bringing about change, and he must want, very sincerely, to change. No one else can want for him.

He is given some concept of the conscious and subconscious facets of his brain; "waking mind" and "sleeping mind" serve as adequate synonyms with younger patients. He should learn three contrasting characteristics of these two aspects of his mind and understand them well enough to explain them to someone else before bedtime this first night. Specifically, concerning the conscious mind, these characteristics are (1) it must obey, (2) it learns from outside the skin, and (3) it forgets.

These characteristics should be made real to the patient and related to his own daily experience so that he understands them as fact, not meaningless phrases. It is not hard to realize that his conscious mind must think of whatever he directs it to focus on; failure to obey may indicate psychosis. The second point is made clearer if you ask him to remember times when he has been reading with his eyes while his conscious mind was busy thinking of something else. He read down the page but had no idea of what he had just read. He may be asked to look at a window and after a few moments look away; then he is asked if the window was open or closed. He probably was conscious of what was outside but not of the status of the window itself. Alternatively, he may be asked to observe a holder of paper cups on the wall, and then asked for the color of the top cup when he looks away. In either case his eye sees the requested detail, but he does not actually learn it until he looks again with his conscious mind. The third point, forgetting, is relatively easy to clarify: he does forget a few things.

He can see that the conscious portion of his brain now knows how to swallow correctly. He has ordered it to learn, and it has obeyed. He has learned this habit pattern from an agency outside his skin, the clinician. Hopefully, he has not yet forgotten. After he falls asleep, however, his conscious mind—the only part that knows the new swallow—also goes to sleep. His subconscious takes command in sleep, and this part of his brain has not learned to swallow correctly and moreover does not even care whether or not it learns. We do have a subconscious resistance to change, which probably is a strong stabilizing influence in our daily life; still, the road is tilted uphill when we insist that the subconscious acquire the new pattern. Our problem is further compounded by the fact that the three specified characteristics of the conscious mind are found to be just the opposite of subconscious function.

The subconscious is not easily made to obey. It tends to concoct dreams of its own choosing, only occasionally honoring a request. Furthermore, when awakened in the midst of a pleasant dream, it refuses to complete that dream when sleep returns. Thus, we cannot simply order it to swallow correctly.

Although the subconscious is able to learn with fantastic ease, it is not capable of taking in original material from outside. Instead, it tends to learn only from the material supplied by the conscious mind. Were it actually possible to learn from a tape recording during sleep, we would long since have stopped building schools and started educating our children at night. With the subconscious thus limited, the patient should realize that unless he continues to swallow correctly at every opportunity during the day, thereby setting the conscious pattern, there is little hope of change on a subconscious level.

The patient must also realize that his subconscious *never* forgets. Every detail of his life will be stored in his subconscious more securely than when placed in the memory bank of a computer. He may have conversed with a great-grandmother or other person approaching senility and noticed that whereas recent events may be lost to consciousness, old memories from childhood are poured out from subconscious storage in accurate detail. The patient may then appreciate that since the subconscious never forgets anything, it will never forget how to swallow the wrong way.

The implication is that there are two impossible tasks before us, and if the conscious pattern is not maintained, there will be three impossible jobs. True enough, we can never force the subconscious to forget the old swallow; we might, however, persuade it to store the old tongue thrust back among all the other memories long lost to consciousness. Yet to do so, it would be necessary to command the subconscious to rearrange some mental furniture, an assignment that we have just described as very difficult.

The patient is then made aware of the "twilight" preceding sleep, a time when both parts of the brain are working as equals. The subconscious is striving to take control, but the conscious mind yet retains the ability to pass along some direction. Some of the potential uses of this time are shown. For example, although youngsters may require physical contact to awaken on school mornings, they often are up much earlier on Saturday in order to watch televised cartoons, and without being called. Our proposal to "sleep on it" finds an echo in almost every language; the Spanish say "I'll consult my pillow," the Portugese feel that "your pillow is your best adviser," whereas the French realize that *"la nuit porte conseil"*—"the night brings advice."

We will ask the patient to utilize this time. Starting tonight, and for eight *consecutive* nights, he should begin to think about correct swallowing when he goes to bed. As soon as his head touches the pillow, he should swallow a few times consciously to set the pattern afresh. Any swallows thereafter should also be good ones, since the last waking swallow should be correct. He should then start talking to his subconscious silently, since it can hear his thoughts. There is a value, however, in almost giving the subconscious an identity, in mentally ordering it about as he would if it were a real person. Tell it that he wants this project completed, that he wants his teeth straight, that he wants to swallow correctly. Continued repetition induces sleep.

Again remind the patient that success will depend on his *understanding* and *desire*. He should discuss the entire routine at bedtime tonight and be able to recount all salient details. Primarily, he must *want* to change his habit, since it is not possible to mislead his own subconscious: it lives right there, inside, and needs only to glance across to see if he means what he says.

The saddest situation arises when the patient forgets for a single night to carry out this routine. The failure wipes away all efforts up to that point, he must start anew for another eight-night period. Forgetting a second time often brings total defeat, since it becomes more difficult to convince the subconscious of his genuine desire.

Attempted modifications

Numerous variations of the present technique have been tried in this program. Rather than making the patient fully responsible for "talking to his sleeping mind," parents were required to "talk" their child to sleep, reassuring him of their love and approval and of his capability for success, talking quietly, calmly, and positively, and avoiding any negative implications. Such a procedure is something employed by pediatricians in problems of enuresis, thumb sucking, etc. It was found that many parents were not successful in this endeavor, others resented the necessity of it, and some patients found their own concentration disturbed by the parent's voice.

As the burden was shifted to the patient, it became obvious that overly brief instruction,

simply asking the child to go through the motions, was not sufficient. As instructions were amplified to include more detail and stronger motivational elements, results improved perceptibly. Thereafter, efforts were made to eliminate portions of the explanation given to the patient, since this session routinely requires at least 45 minutes to complete. Results again dropped disastrously; it appears that this procedure is operative only when it is done from a state of knowledge—when the patient understands the ramifications inherent in the task.

Notwithstanding some of the preceding statements, it has proved quite effective as a reinforcement technique to have a parent talk to the child *after* he is sleep. Once the child has fallen asleep carrying out the above instructions, it can be productive to have a parent partially arouse the child and feed in a similar message, calmly and quietly repeating it several times.

One group of fifty mothers, now anonymous martyrs, volunteered to stare down at the faces of their children at intervals throughout the night, for a series of nights, observing behavior and bringing in reports. They must have felt some animosity toward the clinician, and their heavy-lidded study could hardly be considered scientific data, but their sacrifice deserves some recognition. Many of the assumptions implicit in the present procedure are based on their inferences. A large number of additional parental reports, less painfully attained, have served as confirmation.

Requirements and provisions

One such assumption resulting from parental observation serves as justification for the requirement of eight consecutive nights of concentration on this project. The actual period required for completion naturally varies from one patient to another; it is believed that eight nights provide a reasonably safe standard. An impressive number of parents have reported definite changes in swallowing behavior after the seventh or eighth night. A fresh approach to entering sleep will begin the next week, on the final step, thus providing some "cushion" regarding the time factor and making additional nights available, if necessary, without openly calling this fact to the patient's attention. For the sake of specificity, and to maintain adherence to the program until it is safely completed, a perhaps excessive emphasis is given to the practice period of eight nights.

A supportive basis for this emphasis may be found in the phenomenon of cyclic behavior. Many body functions are influenced by the passage of specific periods of time, recurring consistently at the same phase of the cycle. Cycles of twenty-four hours, seven days, and twenty-eight days have thus been identified as actuating governors of body reactions, along with longer and shorter sequences. Possibly we are involved here with such a seven-day cycle, although this idea is obviously speculation.

It should be noted that there is usually only one true, complete transition from wake to sleep: the first time the patient falls asleep in the evening. Although the patient may thereafter rouse, speak, go to the bathroom, or find another blanket, there is little of consciousness in these activities; in fact, they frequently are not even remembered the following morning. This phenomenon has at least two points of significance for us.

First, an effort was made to reduce the number of nights required to complete this procedure by having someone awaken the patient periodically throughout the night; the patient was asked to sit erect in bed, say something, feel awake, and then go back to sleep, concentrating once more on deglutition. No abridgment could be noted. Resentment, rather than the patient, was more often aroused.

Second, it should be apparent that when a patient watches television in the evening and falls asleep while so engaged, that night is lost to our purpose. Even though he then walks to his room, dons pajamas, and goes to bed, seemingly awake, he has missed his single opportunity for that night.

Care should be taken that the patient truly be allowed to fall asleep undisturbed in his accustomed bed. Radios are turned off with the light. Talkative siblings are sometimes asked to sleep in another room for eight nights or more. Slumber parties and ''sleeping over'' are, of course, out of the question.

Any tendency toward insomnia, even mild, should be discovered; it is essential that the patient fall asleep within 10 or 15 minutes after going to bed. Although this project need not be given the absolute final thought before full sleep, it must be *one* of the last. In such cases, the patient's physician might be consulted regarding sedation throughout this period. Phenobarbital or certain tranquilizers suffice in some cases, but one of the newer sedatives with a bit more power may be required. Most physicians feel no hes-itancy, considering the brief time involved, and are happy to telephone the prescription to the drugstore once the situation is explained. With children who have not consumed aspirin to the point of immunity, one or two tablets as they are preparing for bed may suffice.

For the chronically forgetful patient, of any age, it is ordinarily helpful to suggest an additional reminder device. If the child says prayers at bedtime, an association of ideas can often be established so that he begins to think of swallowing immediately after prayers. For older patients, some incongruous object may be placed on the pillow when the bed is made up in the morning and left there throughout the day. If it is necessary for the patient, on retiring, to remove an eggbeater, a turtle shell, or a soup ladle from the pillow, it will be difficult to ignore its implication. In the rooms of some boys, it is difficult to find an object that would be sufficiently out of keeping. The boy who originally made this suggestion, as a means of ''pounding it into his head,'' employed a hammer on his pillow. Another alternative is a patient-produced sign, made with luminous paint and hung in commanding alignment with eyes approaching sleep.

For those who read after going to bed, further precaution must be taken. They are *never*, of course, to fall asleep while reading. Even so, there is a proclivity to drift off thinking of the incidents just read about rather than deglutition. In order to avoid this pitfall, they are asked to find a scrap of material, 3 or 4 inches square, of an unusual texture: either coarse and rough, or quite smooth and silky. It is then placed over the light switch and taped in place at the top; it hangs like a curtain over the wall switch or is draped like a skirt around the lamp. Later, when drowsy fingers encounter the material, rather than the accustomed switch, attention is safely returned to the essential project.

It has been noticed, incidentally, that when this project is properly carried out, there are occasional mornings toward the end of the week when the patient is not positive of his performance the previous night; after his assignment becomes routine, he may question whether he was actually thinking of deglutition during his hazy journey into sleep. No such uncertainty is found if he has truly forgotten, unless he has a very poor attitude. In the case of the motivated patient who forgets, his eyes are hardly open in the morning before the horrible realization hits. When the failure is genuine, he has no doubt.

In the verbalization of this session, you will

observe that every possible point is tied into the experiental background of the patient, or he is given a concurrent opportunity to experience your explanation, to test what you are saying and relate it to reality as he knows it. The resulting sense of comprehension and security leads him into the project with a heightened confidence in his imminent success. Such an attitude is a strong ally.

Some clinicians, using a technique that is similar but that may differ in some essential respects, report small success, whereas others encounter no such difficulty. Some facet of the interpersonal relationship may be more vital than apparent. Perhaps the degree of confidence displayed by the therapist, and his overt faith in the patient, has a bearing; certainly, the strength of the patient's motivation is the single most forceful factor. However, the conclusion is still drawn that success is dependent on the occurrence of this sincere desire in a patient who is able to understand and accept what he is being asked to perform.

WAKING BUT SUBCONSCIOUS SWALLOWS

It is probable that the procedure outlined above, combined with a thoroughgoing awareness of waking deglutition, would complete the task. Yet, a marked increase in the stability of the new habit is noted when the patient is supplied with a means to influence the many swallows that occur subconsciously even during wakefulness. We can implement this rather directly.

The patient is asked to occupy his conscious attention with something from which he is not easily distracted. With children, television is often an admirable situation, whereas adults may become more engrossed in reading. While so engaged, the patient is to sip a few ounces of liquid in the manner required on the fifth step of therapy. He may eat a light snack, if he prefers, but not in lieu of one meal; we desire as many conscious swallows as possible this week, and thus every meal is important.

Whereas these swallows are executed quite consciously at the beginning of the week, they gradually become so routine and automatic that little attention is wasted on them. They then become part of the pattern that is made subconscious.

It is not difficult to understand the rationale of this assignment. Human beings would not have time to lead life as we know it if they were required to make every movement on a conscious level. Certainly we would never learn to drive a car or achieve connected speech if each muscular adjustment demanded conscious thought. Instead, we perfect highly coordinated skills slowly, painstakingly, on a conscious level but find this process overly taxing once proficiency is gained. Later, when consciousness is occupied with other thoughts, any concurrent demand for this intricate skill brings a gradual transfer of the necessary control to a subconscious level, leaving the conscious mind unencumbered by the details of such control and thus free to engage in more desirable pursuits. Few of these skills are as basic to existence as deglutition, but the same rules govern here as with any other function.

This procedure involving swallowing while conscious attention is elsewhere is certainly not very difficult, nor is it overly dramatic. Therefore, it is easily forgotten in the hubbub at home. It is valuable, nevertheless, and the patient would be cautioned about overlooking this aspect. It would have little effect if done occasionally; to exert an influence, it must be done daily (Fig. 23-1).

ASSIGNMENT

The crux of this step lies in the "twilight time," which is presented most effectively when the patient is fresh and waiting to discover what the session holds. It is thus made the initial order of business at this session. Modification of the waking but subconscious pattern is quickly explained, and better comprehended, once the nighttime procedure is understood.

The minimum requirement for velar exercise is the minute or so each day needed to lift the palate twenty times. The number may be increased as needed, and additional velar or velopharyngeal exercises may be assigned for patients with special need. The latter are seldom necessary.

Some rejuvenation of attitude during eating and drinking may be required and can often be incorporated with the discussion of subconscious function, but it should be reemphasized when the assignment is made. The patient can make subconscious only the pattern that he is maintaining *consciously*.

The oral resting position now becomes increasingly essential, while time grows short in which to solidify the gains that have been made in lip closure and tongue elevation. Accordingly, we will ask that normal posture be sustained for one

R. H. BARRETT
SPEECH PATHOLOGIST
TELEPHONE 793-1101

———————

Your new swallow will NOT become a real habit until these are completed:

1. Keep your LIPS APART for one more week each time you swallow solid food, EXCEPT when you are away from home.

2. Exercise your SOFT PALATE once each day. Make it go up and down at least twenty times.

3. The FIRST TIME each day that you watch TV, or read, drink a few ounces of liquid, SIP BY SIP.

4. Talk to yourself just BEFORE SLEEP for at least eight nights.

5. Hold TONGUE UP, with lips closed, for ONE HOUR each day. Use screen or elastic only if necessary.

These things will only help if they are ALL done, and done EVERY DAY. Call me if you miss any one of them even ONE DAY!

Losers make promises
　　　　　Winners make commitments

A

	LIP DOWN	PALATE	SIP	SLEEP	REST POSITION
1st DAY					
2nd DAY					
3rd DAY					
4th DAY					
5th DAY					
6th DAY					
7th DAY					

B

Fig. 23-1. A, Assignment card, step 7. **B,** Chart on reverse side.

full hour each day on a formal basis, and we anticipate that artificial aids will no longer be necessary. We will also expect to find the mouth closed occasionally at odd moments throughout the day. Optimism counts.

REFERENCES

1. Foulkes, D.: The psychology of sleep, New York, 1966, Charles Scribner's Sons.
2. Granda, A. M., and Hammack, J. T.: Operant behavior during sleep, Science **133**:1485-1486, 1961.
3. Spanos, N. P., De Moor, W., and Barber, T. X.: Hypnosis and behavior therapy: common denominators, Am. J. Clin. Hypnosis **16**:45-64, 1973.

Chapter 24

STEP 8:
FINAL CONCERNS

Today is the bittersweet day of parting, for active therapy should be completed with this session. The patient turns in his reminder sign as a final report, and prepares to depart. Despite the relief from pressure, or perhaps because of it, girls bestow unsolicited kisses on the clinician and weep occasionally, and even boys are not averse to an arm around their shoulders as they leave the therapy room today. However, the clinician should not view this parting as final. You have not lost a patient but have gained another name on your recheck roster, a name that may seem far too permanent before it is eventually filed away.

When this scene is replaced by one in which the patient comes to the session with impatience and sighs openly as if to say, "Thank heaven, that's done!" we may justifiably wonder where we went astray.

Either way, it is a memorable occasion for the patient, and we are not being unscruplous if we capitalize on the situation to the extent of augmenting motivation for carry-over of the newly perfected skills. We have given the patient nothing of value unless the new abilities are permanent. The danger of relapse begins to loom immediately, since there is the ever-present possibility that the patient will drop his new habit on the doorstep as he leaves the office today. We do not wish to end therapy with that degree of finality.

EVALUATION OF TOTAL PATTERN

There is little to be gained in asking the patient to swallow consciously at this session; conscious swallows were evaluated last week. Instead of feeding him, the clinician should observe the pa-

tient closely throughout this entire session, assessing the demonstrated swallowing behavior. Many swallows will be obviously executed on a conscious level, and certainly there is some stimulation supplied by mere presence in the therapy room, but once the patient's attention is distracted by some of the explanations required during the session, many swallows may be observed that are largely subconscious. They form our basis for judgment.

TWILIGHT TIME. An effort is made to conduct this session precisely one week after the seventh step, on the afternoon preceding the eighth night of effort on the subconscious aspect. The final, eighth night still remains to be completed, therefore, as you observe the patient today. Nevertheless, given the impetus of the therapy situation, you should be quite disturbed if a single instance of abnormal swallowing is observed. Usually, the face that you studied during the initial interview only weeks ago, contorting in deglutition, is today passive and unaffected by repeated swallows even when lips are closed, as they usually are once the discussion begins.

It should be established at the outset that there has been no lapse in the nightly routine of the previous week. This fact has supposedly been reported by telephone; nevertheless, an occasional patient will bounce into the therapy room as though everything were complete, and then innocently announce that he went out the previous evening, forgot all about swallowing, and thus assassinated the entire week. It is unclear why these people bother to come in, knowing full well they will only be sent home to repeat the previous week's project; perhaps they feel a certain expiation in verbalizing their guilt.

The clinician has little choice under the foregoing circumstances. The patient is marched directly out of the therapy room with instructions to return if and when seven nights or more have been conscientiously completed. When the establishment of normal subconscious function occupies the preeminent position required for this program to be effective, foregetting a night, without great provocation, casts a heavy pall over the prognosis for future excellence.

Somewhat more frequently a patient will telephone to report in wailing tones the uninvited guest, the sudden illness, or the late, late show, which proved to be his undoing. The patient is simply instructed to begin anew his quest for eight consecutive nights, and the appointment is rescheduled accordingly.

In rare instances it will be apparent to the therapist, as the session progresses, that no detectable inroads have been made on subconscious behavior; questioning will reveal either a deliberate fib about consecutive nights, a gross misunderstanding of the process involved, or an attitude sadly decayed. These situations must be met individually.

OTHER ASPECTS. You will be required to accept the consensus of patient and observer as to whether something has been sipped each day during some other conscious activity. When this assignment has been done only haphazardly, it must indicate a rather poor attitude and create some doubt that anything has been accomplished; after some discussion, the previous step should be reassigned if it seems that any improvement might be gained.

It is not unusual for the patient to be forgetful once or twice during the week; therefore, the sipping assignment is printed on the practice card for the eighth session and may be continued as a part of today's session for an additional week, with dire prophecies for the future if it is not completed. For the patient who has done the sipping routinely, you may cross this section from the practice card or, if further reinforcement seems to be of value, simply let the assignment stand.

You should also ascertain that velar exercise has been carried out. Knowing that you will inquire is usually sufficient motivation to discharge such a simple requirement. If it has not been done, you are helpless at this point. Any further work would have little value for the subconscious pattern that is already set, or that will be, after today. You may point this fact out to the patient, with a prediction of future trouble; however, both of you may "luck out" if there has been even moderate effort.

Reminder signs, incidentally, are accepted with sincere thanks and scrutinized with great care. Regardless of their composition, they are placed on display in an honored location for the balance of the session; they usually represent real effort and are never to be tossed aside. Spaghetti sauce, bacon grease, and other evidence of actual use earn special commendation; after two weeks a pure and spotless sign indicates an excessively tidy eater or a reminder that was never used.

TESTS FOR SUBCONSCIOUS FUNCTION

The bridge between the preceding step and the present session is the "test" of the subconscious response. In actuality, the best tests are those which the therapist conducts personally, through observation, at this session and during rechecks later. The ultimate test is found in the reaction of the dentition. However, something more specific and immediate is essential from the patient's point of view.

USE OF ELASTIC AT NIGHT. After eight nights of concentration as he enters sleep, the patient will be asked to continue his now-familiar conversation with his subconscious but also command it to maintain an elastic on the tip of his tongue throughout the entire night, and to do so nightly for one week. The elastic may be one of those used for the initial exercise, one of them cut in half, or a standard rubber band cut into ¼-inch pieces. We consider this project victoriously accomplished if even once during the entire week the patient finds himself in oral possession of the elastic on the following morning. However, he is to continue this project for the full week, regardless of successes along the way.

We do not accept as adequate an elastic found under the tongue or at any vestibular site outside the teeth; however, any place on the dorsum of the tongue is satisfactory. It is possible to keep the elastic in place all night and then run the tongue around the teeth before being fully aware while awakening, thus sliding the elastic distally without losing it.

This multipurpose assignment is expected to have three different benefits: (1) primarily, it assists in establishing an unconscious rest posture that includes an elevated tongue; (2) it provides a seven-day extension of the "twilight zone," since it would be difficult, even without specific instruction, to attempt this procedure and not think about it nightly with some degree of desire as the patient falls asleep; and (3) it probably does yield some indication of the manner in which subconscious deglutition is performed.

If the swallowing pattern were sufficiently abnormal, it is quite possible that the tip of the tongue might be protruded as the patient fell asleep, carrying the elastic beyond the incisors, or the tongue might be left on the floor of the mouth and make no contact with the palate throughout the night, thus retaining the elastic on the tongue. However, we are asking that the elastic be placed on the tongue tip, then put in position against the original "rubber band spot," and held in the top of the mouth. If the tongue then thrusts in swallowing, the effect is to slide the elastic posteriorly with each swallow, resulting in eventual ingestion of the elastic. Under these conditions, producing a piece of rubber band off the top of the tongue the next morning would indicate fairly normal function. With very few exceptions, patients who have performed adequately in therapy are able to succeed in this endeavor; those who have worked halfheartedly never achieve it.

Of course, there are many reasons why the elastic might be lost *out* of the mouth during sleep. Talking in sleep, snoring, coughing, sneezing, etc. invariably dislodge the elastic outward. Smacking or licking the lips, bruxism, or even sudden inspiration of breath can cause the elastic to be swallowed, even with normal function. Therefore this test is never to be viewed as a *negative* test: inability to succeed certainly does not necessarily indicate abnormal deglutition.

We prefer to supply the patient with a brightly colored rubber band, choosing one that contrasts with the color of the bedroom floor. The patient can then cut it into pieces that are more readily found when lost out of the mouth, although they also reappear routinely in the patient's hair or stuck to the wall behind the bed.

A supply should be kept in a saucedish or cup beside the bed. Should the patient wake during the night and find the elastic gone, a replacement should be made immediately, since we value this influence during every moment of the night. Even if he is able to maintain the elastic for only half the night, we would deem the subconscious function to be secure.

Fear has been voiced in some quarters that a snip of elastic might be aspirated in the course of this assignment. We perceive no such threat. We have asked this performance of thousands of patients; in not a single instance has anything harmful occurred. We have trained hundreds of other clinicians, who in turn have made the identical assignment to other thousands of patients. Their experience has duplicated ours.

On any given night, many thousands of children go to sleep with chewing gum in their mouth. They may swallow it or be required to cut it from their hair the next morning, but they do not inhale it. To the consternation of dentists, children may not brush their teeth before bed and as a result go to sleep with particles of hamburger—larger than our bit of elastic—embedded in the dental embrasures. Although these particles may be dislodged during the night, we know of no documented case of nocturnal aspiration. In several situations such as oral surgery, measles, or tonsillar pustules, bits of tissue are sloughed off during sleep without threat of injury.

Certainly we are aware that children do aspirate foreign objects on occasion. To our knowledge, such incidents have occurred only during a waking state, when the child was struck on the back, laughed suddenly, or was subjected to other stimuli not usually present in sleep. If oral function were such as to make such occurrences commonplace or even probable in sleep, the average person's lungs would be a treasury of bric-a-brac. Instead, each pattern of function and every homeostatic instinct join in protection of the airway. Realistically, our patients would be more likely to fall in the therapy room and break an arm than to introduce elastics into their bronchioles.

EYEDROPPER TEST. As previously stated, almost all patients who truly establish normal deglutition on a subconscious level manage to retain the elastic at least once. Regardless of their nocturnal oral habits, at least one night out of any given seven, the tendency is to simply sleep. However, given enough bad luck or bad habits, the normal swallower may still fail the elastic test.

Without exception, patients are requested to telephone the results of their efforts. It is the cause of great rejoicing, and an opportunity to reinforce the entire program, when the patient's breathless call announces triumph. When, instead, his parent's mournful tones report failure, a substitute test should be available as confirmation. The parent could, of course, merely spend an hour or more standing at the bedside, hoping to evaluate swallowing behavior; this tribulation can be avoided.

Medicine droppers are frequently at hand in the home; if not, they can be purchased quite inexpensively at any drugstore. The parent should be armed with a clean dropper and await a time when the patient is sleeping, preferably face up; when the parent is required to pry him away from the wall, the patient may not remain completely asleep. When an opportunity arises, the parent can fill the dropper with warm water, near body temperature so as not to arouse the child, and simply place a few drops in the patient's mouth, observing the reaction.

Should the patient's mouth be open, the resulting swallow is easily classified. The tongue slams into the teeth in a most convincing manner if the thrust is still present. When normal function has been gained, the patient usually closes his teeth, but not necessarily his lips, swallows with his tongue retracted, and then drops his mandible once more.

Should the patient's mouth be closed, a good indication in itself, the pattern may still be determined. However, in this case it is advisable for the parent to warm the fingers of the free hand and place them gently on the patient's larynx. Two or three drops of water are placed on his lips; the usual reaction is to lick the water into the mouth and swallow. Should deglutition remain abnormal, there is ordinarily an exaggerated contraction of facial muscles in an unmistakable pattern. If the swallow is normal, little or nothing moves in the face, the only indication that swallowing has occurred being throat movement; when the sheet is pulled up to the chin, or a shadow covers the throat, the parent would seldom realize what had transpired without feeling with the fingers. At one period, when parents were being invited to stand and observe their child's behavior during sleep, Barrett learned to appreciate the beautiful significance of the exasperated call from the parent: "My kid doesn't swallow at night!"

This test could be administered with a spoon and a glass of warm water. However, these items tend to clatter, arousing some sleepers; the spoon is handled with less than precision and agility, often resulting in the splashing of a spoonful of water into the patient's face; etc. It is not that difficult to secure a dropper.

TYING LOOSE ENDS

The bulk of this brief session is consumed in presenting the foregoing concepts. With these disposed of, we bring the session to a rapid close. Ascertain that velar exercise has been performed, and then clarify the remaining items to be assigned.

GARGLING. At one time, gargling was initiated early in therapy, purely for activation of velopharyngeal muscles. Its influence in this connection came to appear quite negligible. However, it had been our policy to require, at the conclusion of active therapy, that the patient select some frequently seen object at home, a certain lamp perhaps; each time he passed this object he was to point at it and say, "Swallow!" The result was expected to be a situation in which the patient would be unable to avoid thinking about deglutition daily for a period of time until the newly acquired pattern could become established more firmly, to "grow roots in his brain."

This proved to be a difficult and objectionable task in many cases, and so the responsibility for supplying this effect was simply transferred to gargling. The latter is made a concomitant of toothbrushing, thus increasing the probability that it will be executed, until the initial recheck. Any benefits of the act itself are probably still derived, but it is presented to the patient in such a way that it would be very unlikely that he could gargle and avoid some momentary thought, conscious or otherwise, concerning deglutition. This situation is somewhat analogous to commanding a listener, "For the next 2 minutes, don't think of the word hippopotamus!"

LIP CLOSURE. The day has finally arrived when deglutition may safely be completed with closed lips. The ability to do so has been rehearsed, hundreds of times daily, during unconscious swallows and meals eaten in public. Nevertheless, sudden and complete change to closed lips is an invitation to tragedy. Even when patients were required to keep their lower lip retracted for an additional period after therapy, and then terminated this aspect on a given day, there was a tendency toward some regression. It has been found much safer to arrange for a transition week, a more gradual removal of this crutch.

Therefore the patient will be requested to continue for one week, at only one meal each day, to swallow solids with the lower lip removed from the teeth. This measure appears to be sufficient to eliminate all trouble in this regard.

REST POSTURE. The clinician will now hope to deliver his last discourse on the subject of rest posture, even while knowing in his heart that the end may not be yet. We now expect the mouth to be closed invariably, with the tongue a safe distance from the teeth.

Any final admonition that you can supply will probably not be wasted. Since this matter is of such critical importance, a backup system or two should also be available. When previous assignments have not been rigorously carried out, or appear to have been inadequate, one or more of the following procedures may be called on for support.

An excellent method, when it can be employed, is the association of this venture with reading. The patient is asked to sit down daily with a book or magazine and to arrange the orofacial structures in the specified manner. He is then to read and to establish a habit of checking his resting position *each time he turns a page*.

8

R. H. BARRETT
SPEECH PATHOLOGIST
TELEPHONE 793-1101

———————

1. GARGLE every time you brush your teeth until you return for your first checkup.

2. Keep your LIPS APART for one meal each day. After this week, lips should always be closed in swallowing.

3. Continue to SIP LIQUID, during some other activity. Do this every day for one week, then discontinue.

4. Try to hold elastic on tip of tongue ALL NIGHT for 7 nights.

5. From here on, lips should NEVER be open at rest. Continue quiet time for one hour each day this week, but check yourself throughout the day.

6. Return for a checkup at .... on ....

CONGRATULATIONS! You've finished the hard job. The new habit will stay if you WANT it—and if you keep your tongue UP!

Fig. 24-1. Assignment card, step 8. No chart is given with this step.

He is to do this checking for 30 minutes on each of the first six or seven days, after which it must be continued daily, for an uninterrupted hour, during another week or two or until it appears that the neuromuscular reeducation has occurred. Some conditioning usually occurs also; a point is reached when, regardless of his surroundings, the patient turns a page in a book or magazine and his tongue lifts and his mouth closes.

Television may be put to use with many patients. Obviously, mere willpower in keeping structures in alignment would be of small benefit: the average thruster has already become conditioned to oral collapse as the television program begins. Partly as an antidote for this specific tendency, the patient may profit from reversal of the routine. When television is to be the setting, ask the patient to equip himself with a hand mirror of some type. The mirror is to be held before him with his own hands at all times; the schedule remains unchanged from that specified for reading. Although the ceaseless necessity to hold the mirror calls his attention repeatedly to the basic task at hand, he is to actually look in the mirror and observe his face no less frequently than the beginning and end of each commercial.

Note that assistance by the observer is usually required, regardless of the patient's age or the technique being employed, at least for the first few days. Reminding is permitted when oral droop is seen. Even the most optimistic could hardly expect that the patient would not lapse back quickly to his habitual posture until self-criticism develops some strength through repetition.

Even homework may be forced to give assistance, particularly if it involves arithmetic or other study in which a problem is taken from a book and worked out on a separate sheet of paper, and then another problem extracted. The book is opened to the assigned page and covered with a sheet of paper. Each time the sheet of paper is lifted to secure the next problem, the patient checks his rest posture. Variations of this theme can be devised with a bit of ingenuity. For later reinforcement, a sheet of paper may be cut into strips 1 inch wide and somewhat shorter than the height of a book; a large red X is placed at each end of the strips, on both sides. The strips are taken to school, each book in the child's desk is opened to the coming assignment, and a strip is placed like a concealed bookmark.

Thereafter, each time a red X appears as a book is opened, the patient checks his orofacial posture and moves the strip to the next assignment.

With younger children, we may capitalize on coloring. A new and special coloring book and crayons are purchased, and each time a different crayon is selected for use, the child checks rest posture. Puzzles may similarly serve if conscious attention is jogged as each new piece is picked up. If a trip is planned, the child may check with the passing of each red truck or at each traffic sign, side road, etc. Whatever the exigency of the situation, some specific countermeasure should be supplied for as long as the need persists.

CONCLUSION

This is truly "Until I see you," not "Goodbye." Although active therapy is herewith concluded, the long recheck period now begins. We will hope to see the patient on several future occasions before final dismissal. Although many patients pass every future evaluation with ease, at least half of them require some additional reinforcement, most often for the rest posture. Thus, if the patient whom you now face does not return for rechecks, the chances are very good that you have wasted all your efforts—a possibility that is not pleasant to contemplate.

It seems most effective to simply maintain your attitude that *of course* he will return and that everything will be satisfactory. Not to leave anything more to chance than necessary, however, a definite date is agreed on for the first recheck. Therapy should blend into the recheck period with a jolt as unnoticeable as possible (Fig. 24-1).

It is usually not difficult to find expression at this time for some well-deserved congratulations for both patient and observer; parents deserve a public citation; the child may at least gain the status symbol of "braces." Whether or not an appliance is forthcoming, they have mastered a very difficult problem, much more intricate and demanding than many routine speech defects, and have done so quickly and, in most cases, enjoyably. It is always a valuable and major achievement to conquer any aspect of self, and it is the therapist's truest reward to be permitted a part in that victory. Even the occasional obnoxious youngster, whose seven or eight weeks have seemed as years, deserves warm words today: the therapist has been given the opportunity to conquer almost as much of himself as the patient has. Too bad the good kids seem to finish so quickly!

Chapter 25

RECHECK PERIOD

A turn of the page and here we are, three weeks later; that is characteristic of swallowing therapy. Times flies for patients, also. Several months pass, they intend to run by for a recheck one day next week, someone suddenly notices that months have gone by and that they are no longer swallowing correctly, and then—frantic calls, chagrin, resentment, and other overreactions.

The clinician should do everything possible to prevent such lapses; although he cannot take full responsibility, he should feel at least some obligation. One telephone call or a postcard is often sufficient. There will remain a few who seem impervious to such appeals and are therefore hopeless.

It almost never transpires that patients fail their appointment for the first recheck; those who do usually prove to be, as might be expected, the ones who can least afford a delay. Indifference and procrastination have quickly unhinged the new pattern of deglutition, it was unpleasant to face this fact, and thus they have speedily exhumed the practice cards and sought a futile refuge in once-miraculous exercises: "See, Mom, I can still do it."

The therapist will have two primary concerns throughout the recheck period, twin plagues that this period is expected to subdue. In order of importance, they are orofacial rest posture and subconscious function in deglutition. Since both are easily misrepresented and thus prone to false evaluation, it is necessary that guile and deception become likewise the forte of the therapist. It would be simple indeed if we were compelled to evaluate only conscious posture and function; they are apparent at a glance. At this point, of course, patients know how to swallow correctly:

you have taught them well, and for months thereafter they will be models of perfection—on a conscious level. This accomplishment has little meaning for the future, however. We must look below the surface behavior presented by the patient and seek weaknesses in the subconscious pattern, sources of possible later failure, even elements that are satisfactory now but might be menaced or reversed by prospective dental treatment, etc. There is a great need, still unmet, for brief, definitive tests that truly reflect the desired answers.

Much will depend on the practiced eye of the therapist. Many valid indicators are fleeting, difficult to define, and often far too subjective for research purposes. A movement that is consistent or inconsistent with the desired pattern, the oral position from which the tongue initiates speech, the flicker of tension in muscles still unaccustomed to a closed-mouth posture—these things do not lend themselves to overt verification. For the novice clinician, everyone seems to swallow correctly because he *wishes* them to do so and therefore sees no evil; as he becomes more objective, his success ratio drops a bit.

With this in mind, some of the specific techniques that we employ in an effort to elicit telltale behavior will be presented. You may well prefer a different approach if you have a more diagnostic procedure.

As specified in Chapter 15, the duration of the recheck period depends in great part on the performance of the patient. As a minimum routine, the patient should be followed for nine months. If no flaw is detected in that time, any later regression would be unlikely. When the patient appears to be doing well on the initial evaluation, three weeks after the final therapy session, he is released for a two-month period; the follow-up procedures employed at that time are somewhat more extensive and usually require a bit more time. Should these tests also be accomplished satisfactorily, a three-month period is planned, followed by a second three-month hiatus. If the patient appears secure at that time, he is dismissed from the program.

About half our patients proceed on such a course; the other half require some further reinforcement along the way, usually of a minor nature if it is supplied promptly and carried out conscientiously. However, since the novelty of any exercise is quickly gone, taking motivation with it, a small arsenal of devices and procedures is required, and these are applied in turn as the need becomes apparent. The time between rechecks varies accordingly. The patient may be required to return for a later recheck in only three weeks or six weeks, depending on the circumstances and the assigned tasks.

EARLY TESTS OF COMPLETION

In addition to the array of corrective exercises, it is advisable to be prepared with an assortment of testing routines, formal windows through which to glimpse the interior. It is seldom possible to use any test a second time, for even the most slow-witted patient will make adjustments on subsequent visits, thus jeopardizing the validity of your observations.

These initial procedures may safely be brief and simple, for the patient has had but a short time in which to develop a camouflage for any possible frailty. More intensive measures should be preserved for later use, when sophistication is greater on both sides of the therapy table.

Evaluation of rest posture

If you have a receptionist, train her powers of observation; the patient does not expect evaluation from this source. Another possibility is the installation of a one-way mirror in the waiting room. When the patient is kept waiting for a few minutes, prior to seeing the therapist, he follows a fairly predictable route: he enters with closed mouth, sits down and executes a series of perfect swallows, to assure himself that he has not lost it on the way, and then gradually relaxes into whatever comprises his habitual posture and performance. Having reached this point, a few veiled glances may prove fairly diagnostic. The receptionist may attach a slip of paper to the history card, bearing such impressions as she has gleaned in this way, so that the patient is occasionally condemned or vindicated before he enters the formal situation.

Customarily, the therapist may compile similar data by greeting the patient and then visiting for a moment or two with the observer while unobtrusively studying the patient. Some idea of the current rest position must be gained immediately. Converse with the patient briefly about subjects unrelated to deglutition and observe his oral behavior. Be alert for any unconscious swallows that are thus occasioned and for any tendency to complete a sentence, and then leave the mouth ajar for a time. At times, it is quickly apparent that normal posture is not yet habitual merely from the obvious effort required to maintain position: the lips are so rigidly fixed that the face appears ready to break. As a final resort, inquire of the parent or other observer what has been noticed at home; there is usually sufficient interest so that some opinion of present status has been formed. This person is therefore the best available authority on the subject, provided he or she is candid.

Evaluation of deglutition

To provide a quick appraisal of subconscious deglutition, two simple techniques are usually employed—in addition to eagle-eyed scrutiny throughout. Provide a cup of water and instruct the patient to take a small sip but *not* to swallow it; he is to take the sip, just a few drops, and hold it in his mouth, but not swallow. Having come prepared to swallow, he will be a bit disconcerted. When he has taken the water, study his face for a moment, and then gently depress his lower lip with your thumb. If the water is in the floor of his mouth, there will be a strong resistance in the lip as you attempt to press it down, or you will receive a handful of water. Either way, you can have some assurance that normal swallowing is not yet subconscious. Those patients who have established the desired pattern seem instinctively to trap the water as it enters the mouth, in the absence of any implication that they are to do so. Although there are a few in whom this behavior is not a true indicator, it is fairly consistent. Regardless of the patient's reaction, ask him to swallow the water.

Next, suggest that he pick up the cup and drink about half of the water. Observe any lingering impulse to approach the rim with his tongue. The manner in which the water is imbibed is invariably correct: he is swallowing consciously and thus takes care to assure that it is correct. However, we do not empty our mouth completely with each swallow during drinking. At the conclusion of such a series, as the cup is being lowered from the mouth, a clearing swallow is required to complete the process. This final, clearing swallow is usually unconscious. The patient who has failed to complete his assignments in therapy drinks beautifully, but then, as the cup comes down, his tongue drops in unison, for he is through showing off, and the final swallow is obviously defective. Occasionally the patient is so aware of his situation that even the clearing swallow is conscious, but such a swallow is usually so obviously and dramatically performed that you would not misjudge its character. If you are unsure, ask him to complete the cup, providing you with a second opportunity to judge.

Remediation

It is a rare patient who is not swallowing subconsciously in the desired fashion at this point, most such patients having been screened out on the eighth step of therapy. The few who eluded you are asked to make another half-hour appointment as quickly as possible. The basis for their failure is assessed at that time, and corrective measures are instituted if it appears that they would truly be effective. Repetition of the seventh step is usually indicated. However, if repetition is required, the assignment was obviously performed improperly the first time: unless there is a change in attitude, there is small gain in going through the same motions again. The prospect for these people is usually quite pessimistic.

Should everything appear reasonably satisfactory, but you retain some undefined reservations, ask the patient to return again in one month, rather than allowing the full two months.

Much more commonly, deglutition will appear to be proceeding adequately for the time being, but the requisite rest position is still not established. For such patients there is hope, providing they are rescued quickly and wish to be saved. No magic gadget will force the behavior we seek. The patient may sit for a resentful hour, holding an elastic on his tongue and alternately eyeing the television and the clock, so that on the final stroke of the penalty period he may flop open his mouth for the balance of the day. It would be wrong to offer hope to such a patient unless he has a change in attitude. We can provide crutches to assist him and spell out positive and negative consequences to inform him, but it is not possible to influence his habitual posture without his firm and resolute determination.

With this in mind, you should select the procedure that seems most appropriate for the individual need of this patient and assign its use for a period of at least three weeks. The patient should return after the assignment is completed so that you can evaluate its efficacy. Knowing that he must return and face you in a few weeks does much to implement the assignment. It is also motivating for him to learn that you have no intention of stopping the procession of assignments until he has truly established a normal rest posture.

At this stage, it is necessary to determine what specific weakness needs support. Is it only that the tongue is low, that the lips are frequently separated, that the entire mandible is sagging, or is it a combination of these weaknesses? The assigned procedure should be selective in purpose.

ELASTICS. The mouth may be closed with some regularity while the tongue continues to repose flat on the floor. Although far from uniform, this tongue position tends to be accompanied by an increased freeway space, which is betrayed by a dejected droop at the corners of the mouth. It may also be detected when the tongue habitually appears between or below the teeth during a smile, or when the tongue appears never to be poised within the mouth but instead begins and ends every speech effort from the depths.

Should it appear that further elevation of the tongue is the basic need, we may return to the crossbite elastics with which we originally began this project. When the need is extreme, or when a single elastic has failed to achieve results during the recheck period, we may even ask that two elastics be held in the position assigned on the third step of therapy. Thus the tip is secured in place but the tongue is prevented from merely hanging suspended from the tip. Whether one or two elastics are used, a minimum requirement of an hour daily is set.

With the elastic in place, there is a sound basis for keeping the mouth closed also; it is not comfortable to sit with tongue up and mandible down, the muscles in active opposition. Nevertheless, it may seem advisable in some cases to combine the use of an elastic with one of the "mouth closers" enumerated below. Such a paired project—holding an elastic while using some other device to strengthen lip closure—may accomplish more than assigning a succession of individual techniques.

STOMAHESIVE. An alternative for the elastic that combines well with lip-closing procedures is the use of Stomahesive; this product, made by Squibb, is a double-sided adhesive sheet designed to adhere to the skin. It is composed of gelatin, pectin, celluose fiber, and other harmless ingredients, and is perfectly safe if eaten. It is sold by the orthopedic shop, the medical supply, and some drug stores.

Narrow strips, approximately one quarter of an inch wide or slightly less, may be cut from the sheet and sent home. Small squares are then snipped from the end of the strip; the "rubberband spot" should be wiped dry with a tissue, the square of material placed on a dampened finger, and pressed lightly against the spot. The resulting bulge is intended to attract the tongue tip, and will endure for some time. It dissolves eventually and the residue drops free.

Management at home is simplified if the method of cutting the squares is demonstrated. The original sheets are covered on one side by a heavy paper, on the other with very thin polyethylene. The paper backing is readily removed, once the sheet is cut into strips, but the plastic is quite difficult to peel off. It has seemed easier to pull away the paper a short distance, press a thumb nail down at the desired quarter-inch from the end of the strip, then scrape the square from the polyethylene; it will no longer be square, but it is free of the backing and is usable.

DISCS. When elapsed time since therapy has not been great, it is not unusual to find the following rest posture: the teeth are closed or nearly so, the tongue is apparently in a reasonable position, but the lips are slightly parted. This posture is merely the portent of worse things to come if we fail to take action. An effective countermeasure is the use of the small plastic discs, shown in Fig. 25-1. This once-plentiful item is no longer produced by the original manfacturer, but is occasionally imported from Hong Kong, Japan, or England; toy stores yield up the resulting treasure.

These discs are slightly larger than a quarter and are notched around the edge so that they may be fitted together. Coin envelopes containing five of them in assorted colors may be pre-packaged, with a separate set kept at hand for demonstration purposes.

The patient is instructed to begin with only two discs fitted together. He is to place the edge of one disc parallel to his lips and *against the labial surface* of his upper incisors. He should then close his lips and thus maintain the discs in position; if his lips part, the discs fall, and he has some idea that his mouth is open. Every two days, he adds one disc to those being held until he is maintaining the entire five in a horizontal manner. They may be placed together in any design he chooses, so long as it does not incorporate a chin rest. All five weigh less than 1 ounce, but leverage is supplied as more discs are added. Few patients object to using these discs, and excellent results have thus been achieved.

It is often wise to suggest that the envelope of discs be stored on top of the television set. Some parents have simply made the discs a condition for television: no discs, no television. However, there is nothing to prevent homework, reading, or similar pursuits from including a few discs. Be particularly careful to caution against holding the discs in the teeth, or between the upper incisors and lower lip.

Many variations of this procedure are found.

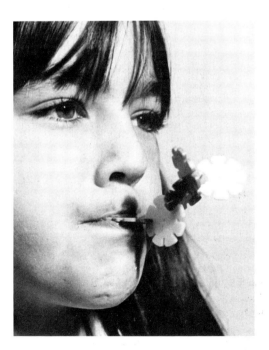

Fig. 25-1. Interlocking discs that help strengthen lip closure.

The patient may be asked to hold a quarter in a similar manner, which works well with some persons. However, the quarter may be too heavy initially or too germ-laden, or it may be spent, causing confusion. The patient may hold a business card or slip of paper between his lips, but this approach is too easy and seldom achieves the desired effect.

As with all such supplemental procedures, if they require attention at all, they should be done for at least an hour daily. Doing more never hurts.

ORTHODONTIC APPLIANCES. The patient who is failing to keep his tongue aloft may also be wearing an upper retainer of some type. This acrylic sheath covering the entire surface of palate and gingiva may totally confound proper tongue placement, since all that the patient feels with his tongue is a slick surface of unidentifiable location, whereas the palate senses only a generalized pressure regardless of where the tongue presses. Yet the retainer may be used to our great advantage with orthodontic cooperation. With patients who have recently completed myofunctional therapy and who are now scheduled for a retainer as part of their orthodontic program, it is logical to ask the dentist for an artificial ruga on the retainer. The incisal papilla is usually imprinted in the plastic, and its posterior end is not difficult to find when viewed from the lingual surface. At just this point we would like a definite landmark of some type. It may take the form of a bit of arch wire bent into a square "U," with the arms embedded into the acrylic; a dental drill may be used to dig a groove of no great length or depth, running laterally across the surface; or an extra drop of acrylic, ⅛ inch or only slightly more in diameter, may be added to the finished appliance. The patient is then expected to keep his tongue in contact with this focal point during every possible moment.

Headgear appliances may also be friend or foe. Of whatever type, they tend to destroy lip closure when first installed. The kind that employs cranial anchorage is often the most harmful, since the extraoral attachment may serve as an effective retractor for the upper lip; we can only hope that the patient wearing this appliance has superb singleness of purpose in keeping his mouth closed.

The neck-strap type offers greater promise. A metal face-bow runs distally around the cheeks to the cervical strap. In front, the face-bow is welded to the intraoral arch wire. When first in-

stalled, this weld usually remains slightly anterior to the lips. As the molars are driven back, however, the weld comes within the grasp of the lips. It would then be reasonable to ask that the lips remain in contact with the weld at all times. As a stimulating nudge, we might request that a single thickness of adhesive tape be wrapped around the weld for a few hours each day, thus altering the texture felt by the lips and attracting greater attention.

Positioners may also be enlisted in our cause. They certainly prevent mouth breathing. As with monoblocs, they may also strengthen a thrusting pattern of movement in the tongue should the tongue retain a low resting posture. However, the upper lingual edge of a positioner provides a convenient shelf for the tongue tip, and when the positioner is so used, the situation is almost

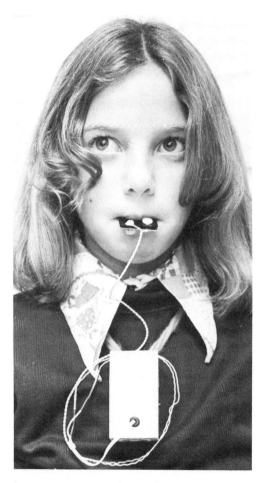

Fig. 25-2. Watching television while "Lip-Ex" signals any weakening of lip closure.

ideal. Any patient receiving a positioner should be urged to exploit its potential.

LIP-EX. An item of recent birth is the "Lip-Ex" pictured in Fig. 25-2 (see Appendix 2). It was designed for our purposes. It consists of a small plastic case containing a transistor-type battery and a buzzer. It is equipped with a clip that may be slipped on the belt, shirt pocket, or collar, or a ribbon may be inserted through the clip and tied around the neck. A detachable mouthpiece is connected via electric cord when in use. The mouthpiece, lightly spring-loaded, is held between the lips and with even moderate pressure all is still. However, should the lips begin to sag, the spring closes a circuit and the buzzer sounds. The buzzer unit can be reused with the installation of a new battery; since each patient is provided with his own mouthpiece, sterilization is not necessary.

ANTISNORE MASK. One final device is occasionally employed, usually as a last-ditch measure. This product is sold to prevent snoring and is stocked by certain prescription pharmacies. It consists of a cupped webbing that fits under and around the chin and is held in place by an ad-

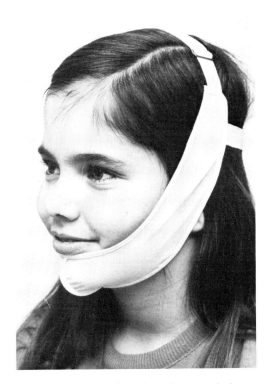

Fig. 25-3. Antisnore mask used to enforce mouth closure. (Courtesy Winco Affiliates, Inc.)

justable elastic band over the top of the head and a second strip of elastic around the occiput (Fig. 25-3). It is designed for adult heads, so that tucks must be taken in the elastic for use with younger children. Certain types of cosmetic chin straps, used to prevent double chins, are more adjustable but are also more expensive.

Our mild aversion to this device stems from its implication of force; it has the flavor of taping lips closed. It is possible to open the mouth while wearing the antisnore mask, but it is necessary to stretch a double thickness of elastic to do so, thus requiring some effort. The mouth certainly does not remain closed as a result of muscle tonus. Nevertheless, the device has proved efficacious in a few resistive cases, perhaps as a bargaining point in securing a more voluntary effort. It does, indeed, provide a central image of a rest posture that includes a closed mouth. On the whole, it is suggested for use at night, its intended milieu, to supplement volitional procedures during the day. Its use should be terminated as soon as possible to avoid building a dependence on its antigravity crutch effect; otherwise, when the mask is removed, the mandible may drop below its original posture.

CELLOPHANE TAPE. A disparaging attitude was reflected above toward the practice of taping lips, a proposal that continues to resurface. The futility of this procedure is seen in the fact that the patient is relieved of all responsibility for maintaining lip closure, whereas such tonicity as may be present is debilitated as the patient relaxes against the adhesive restraint.

However, a version requiring active volition has been successfully applied in a few scattered cases. A single strip of cellophane tape is placed diagonally over closed lips. This tape does not provide sufficient grasp to hold the lips closed forcibly—if there is any sagging of the mandible, the tape pops free. It does, however, supply a stimulus to which some patients make a favorable response. The slight tug experienced when the lips begin to part brings resurgent effort, and the general level of tonus is thereby enhanced.

The special variety of tape made for use on the hair may be the most effective, since it is designed to adhere to the skin. However, some boys reject its "feminine" coloration.

LATER TESTS OF RETENTION

We are now some months removed from therapy, our exact position depending in part on the competence displayed by the patient at the initial recheck. In any event, a careful appraisal of the subconscious pattern of deglutition should be made within three or four months after therapy.

When everything has appeared to be ideal on the first two rechecks, evaluation may be deferred somewhat. If interim measures have been required, it should be made earlier; even so, the patient should be allowed some time to settle into a routine, so that the results of this examination may be assumed to be his usual response.

Rest position

The rest posture, of course, continues to be the first point of inspection on each succeeding recheck. There would be little use in applying the longer, more detailed tests of deglutition until normal rest position *has been attained;* otherwise, subconscious swallowing behavior would be subject to sudden relapse at any time, even if it remained normal today. The greater the delay in establishing normal repose, the greater the odds against retaining a normal swallow.

Therefore, when it develops that you were blinded by the halo of the patient who seemed perfect on the first recheck, and he now evinces a continued lack of muscle tonus, select a supplemental procedure from the previous section and postpone a detailed evaluation of the swallow for an additional three or four weeks.

It has been found that for some patients, even those who were apparently beginning to slip a bit in their pattern of deglutition, thorough completion of the rest position was the only requirement to bring them back to total normal performance. As a corollary, faulty rest posture is the first suspect should any later deterioration be found in deglutition.

Speech evaluation

Another evil influence to which the clinician should be hypersensitive at this time lies in the patient's speech pattern. This is the time for speech correction should it be necessary. Thus, speech must be evaluated as carefully as deglutition within three or four months after therapy.

The interaction of these two functions—speech and deglutition—places a limit on the time that may safely be allowed for spontaneous speech correction. Unless there is marked and immediate improvement in the speech pattern, the persistent interdental or low-tongue production of sounds that normally lift the tongue can have a damaging effect on the patient's tenuous hold on the recently acquired potential for normal deglutition.

If an articulatory defect of a pertinent type continues in evidence, immediate correction should be arranged. The situation at this point provides an existing relationship between speech clinician and patient, a terminology familiar and meaningful for the patient, and a ready muscular ability for normal speech. Given such advantages, it should not be surprising to find that speech correction is routinely completed in a very brief time. A bit of ear training and discrimination, some instruction in phonetic placement, and an opportunity to rehearse in the presence of a congenial critic may be the sole remaining needs. Carry-over can be accommodated during future follow-up procedures, with some continued parental assistance, so that the time and expense demanded are cut below anything the average speech pathologist has previously known. Again, it is primarily a matter of timing.

General observation

As always, once you begin to evaluate deglutition, general observation of the patient may provide the most reliable indicator of present status. After several months out of the therapy routine, normal swallowing, if not the accustomed procedure, becomes rather conspicuously studied. Certainly the patient will have been refreshing his skills for the preceding day or two, in preparation for today's visit, but a period of conversation on his exploits of last weekend, where he went or is going on vacation, or what he wants for his birthday may reveal some inconsistencies in deglutition. Your objective will consist of being acutely aware of oral behavior without appearing to be and providing as much distraction as possible without allowing yourself to become distracted.

Only through practice and personal experience does the clinician become adept at this method of observation and at translating the behavior so observed. Listing minutiae herein would prove futile indeed: they might well be inappropriate for the first dozen patients you see. You will probably misjudge a few early patients. Your errors will be glaringly evident later, and from them you will gain precision.

It is good practice to delay the announcement of your decision, whatever it may be, until you have discussed the situation as candidly as possible with the patient. Inquire as to his honest opinion of his present swallowing habits, and correlate it with the opinion of the parent or observer. Naturally, the swallows of which the patient is aware are hardly subconscious, but valuable impressions may be expressed, and they can often be turned into stepping-stones for further work that may be required.

As cherished as such observation may be, its validity is not beyond question, and thus we must usually look further for a positive answer.

"Squirt" test

The "squirt" test is the most definitive test we know by which to judge subconscious function at some interval after therapy. As such, it is hoarded against the day when it will have greatest significance. If there are any indications of present weak spots, its use may be delayed until more obvious defects, detected through general observation, have been eliminated.

When overt scrutiny reflects nothing amiss, the patient is asked to drink a cup of water. Note again any persistent tendency to approach the rim with the tongue, as well as the manner in which the final clearing swallow is executed. Should these maneuvers also appear satisfactory, explain to the patient in some detail the balance of the test. This procedure was mentioned in Chapter 9 but was not fully elaborated at that time.

You are going to fill with water the syringe with which he is now familiar. The syringe will then be aimed at his mouth. You will then announce a number, large but less than 100, and as soon as you specify the number, the patient is to begin counting aloud, as rapidly as possible, *backward,* in countdown fashion. While he is thus engaged you will now and again, when it seems logical, shoot a bit of water into his mouth. It is best to demonstrate how this will be done before you fill the syringe: a mighty leap of surprise often accompanies the initial burst from the syringe, and the patient's head jerks up and backward, resulting in a stream of water jetting under his chin and down his neck. You can get these initial head jerks out of the way aridly with an empty syringe.

Later, as soon as you shoot water into the patient's mouth, he is instructed to swallow it; failure to do so results in the dribbling of water out of his mouth, but you will hold a tissue or two under his chin at all times to absorb such errors

and to assure proper elevation of the chin so that you may observe his oral behavior accurately. The instant the water enters his mouth he is to swallow it—but he must not stop counting. He should swallow the water and *immediately* say the next smaller number.

The last is the critical factor. We learn to count *up* and are thus usually able to think of other details, continuing without interruption to count in ascending order. However, it requires the entire conscious attention of the average person to count in reverse from a large number. Therefore, if the patient succeeds in following directions, the swallowing that you observe will quite dependably reflect his subconscious pattern. Should the patient switch his attention to deglutition, in order to assure the desired pattern, he is almost never able to produce the next sequential number: he quickly says the next number *higher* than the previous one, takes a number at random out of midair, or simply sits with mouth agape and stares into space until he is able to reorient his thoughts. The degree of conscious attention to swallowing is usually obvious.

You will place your shots most accurately as the patient enunciates the numbers 9, 8, 5, and 1. Beware, until you gain some skill, of the number 3: when the advancing tongue meets the charge of water, it is the clinician, rather than the patient, who is drenched. Nevertheless, it is well to place an occasional round just before or after a number 3, in order to see whether the interdental numeral will have any influence on deglutition.

Most patients enjoy this test uproariously; such hilarity may well be encouraged, for it further distracts attention from swallowing. However, observe closely and accurately the early results. Only an instant is available in which to judge; adaptation sets in rather quickly, and with a bit of practice the intelligent patient can soon flick his attention back and forth with some degree of deception.

In actuality, the most diagnostic swallows are not those which occur when the water is injected. These swallows are hurried, often inefficient, and thus allow part of the water to remain in the mouth. Periodically, while the patient is concentrating intently in an effort to dredge up a number, an incidental clearing swallow, totally and clearly subconscious, will unfold in full glory. It points true north.

This test is continued until you feel that you

have seen two or three legitimate examples of the subconscious pattern. Almost never is it necessary to descend into the twenties. Should a child be too young to count backward, a rare situation unless you are starting patients in therapy too young, an attempt should be made to teach this ability. If you are unsuccessful, there is reason to believe that counting *upward* would require some attention, and thus an ascending order may be permitted. Regardless of how it is done or what the results, no patient ever again enters your office without rehearsing reverse counting beforehand. It is a valid test—but only once.

One or two bits of significant behavior should be recognized if presented during this procedure. As a rule, swallowing behavior will conform either to normal behavior or to the original anomaly. However, the clinician should be ever alert for gross lateral movement of the sides of the tongue; it is readily reflected by this test. If the patient originally displayed a lateral thrust, such action can only mean relapse. If the original thrust was an anterior type, any lateral movement now observed, causing the margins of the tongue to pass between the occlusal surfaces, indicates an incomplete mastery of the velo-pharyngeal mechanism and an immediate need for repetition of the exercises designed for correction.

Should there be single edentulous spaces in the molar region when this test is administered, it is no cause for alarm if the lateral margins of the tongue appear to be pressing lightly into such spaces. Remember that the teeth normally box in the tongue during deglutition, and some contact is to be expected. Nevertheless, when multiple extractions have recently occurred, resulting in great gaping holes in both arches, serious question is raised concerning the validity of the test; the lateral excursion of the tongue may or may not be confined when the spaces close.

Another member of the sabotage squad exposed by this test is found in the gathering stage. Although no thrust may be evident during the swallow proper, obvious malfunction may be seen in preparation to swallow. Appropriate saliva-gathering procedures should be instituted at once. More extensive measures may be required by some patients, but all that is needed by most is a return to a quiet hour or more each day with an elastic on the tongue tip. When the elastic remains in place, it tends to enforce the suck-ing of saliva onto the tongue rather than scooping it or otherwise mismanaging it.

The clinician should also be prepared for a pattern of tongue movement in which deglutition appears basically correct, but with some lag in the elevation of the lateral margins of the tongue: the tip darts into position, followed by a slack, ponderous lift of the sides. This pattern is quite indicative of a tongue still resting on the floor of the mouth, although deglutition has not yet relapsed. The latter contingency will soon occur, failing immediate corrective measures, and further attention to the rest posture, primarily by means of the use of two elastics on the tongue, is strongly indicated.

Final examinations

When all has appeared normal on the "squirt" test discussed above, the patient is released for another two or three months and evaluated at least once more before final dismissal. When minor adjustments have been required along the way, it may then approach one year since the patient was first seen.

As time increases, so does the effort required to swallow in a manner that is not habitual. General observation of the patient's behavior thus also becomes increasingly trustworthy as a diagnostic guide. Younger children have started to forget specifics of the therapy program or have distorted memories, and even adults find gaps in conscious recall. It is now less difficult to trick the patient into betraying his subconscious pattern of deglutition.

Conversation is again a valuable gambit. Normal rest posture should be maintained with ease and comfort; speech should reflect no related articulation problem and no hypernasality. It is often possible to touch the patient's neck by way of distraction while an unobtrusive thumb lies gently on his jaw; a flicker of masseter movement should herald every swallow.

Trapping a bolus is quite awkward and inconvenient unless it is constantly practiced. This ability is then lost rather quickly by unconsciously reverting to abnormal swallowing. At this stage it is possible to take advantage of this area where the relapsing patient might be vulnerable. After you have explained briefly, but have not demonstrated, what you wish the patient to do, he should be asked to drink a cup of water and, when you signal, quickly lower the cup and swallow with lips apart. No special hazard is encountered if it is the patient's usual practice to swallow correctly; otherwise, there is an inclination for a mouthful of water to cascade out of the patient's mouth as the lips part. He should know better!

There is one absolute test of swallowing excellence: spontaneous movement of the teeth toward normal position. Open bites, in whatever location, should be closing at this time. Lower incisors should be uprighting, and protrusion of the uppers should be reduced; even in the absence of an orthodontic appliance, some change for the better should be noted.

If the patient is nearing the conclusion of orthodontic treatment, it is occasionally possible for the dentist to leave the bands in place but remove the arch wire for a week. There is always some tendency for the teeth to return to their original posture, which is the reason that retainers are routinely necessary. However, the patient who has done an adequate job in swallowing therapy and has established a normal rest position shows little ill effect when pressure is removed from his teeth for a week. Abnormal pressures in deglutition can cause noticeable damage to occlusion, even in one week. By the same process, the orthodontist should suspect a continued abnormal tongue pressure when he finds it more difficult than expected to close the bite.

In a few cases, and with orthodontic approval, patients who have been in retention for some time have been asked *not* to wear their retainer for a week; although no apparent damage was found when normal swallowing was subconscious, one older relapsed patient was unable to force his retainer into place at the end of the week.

This chapter would be shorter if there were only a few simple tests that were quicker, more efficient, and more valid. As indicated earlier, even a portable cinefluorographic unit would not provide the ultimate: these films can be misleading. Until something better is provided, train your eye, sharpen your wit, and trust your hunches—and beware of the operator who is *never* wrong in his judgment.

RELAPSES *DO* OCCUR

The one phenomenon concerning tongue thrust that has been universally noted by those who have worked with the problem and carried out adequate follow-up procedures is the propensity of these patients to relapse into their original pattern. The incidence of "relapsed" patients is augmented by quite a number who never learned to swallow correctly in the first place, despite impressions to the contrary. It is well that this predisposition to relapse is so well recognized; it spurs the clinician to greater care during therapy and makes it possible to complete many cases after formal therapy has ended that were only partially accomplished on the first attempt.

In an effort to improve our results, we should give some attention to the specific reasons for relapse. Thereafter, we will be better prepared to deal with the situation.

Causes of relapse

It is a simple matter to find *excuses* for failure. One or two factors that are not even excuses should be trimmed away as a preliminary measure. Parents of relapsed patients have been heard to remark later that their child attempted therapy but "just wasn't able to do it." This is nonsense. Although the child may be too unstable or immature to make any sort of progress, physical *inability,* short of gross pathology, has not in a single instance been found to be a deterrent. The same holds true for *type of swallow:* although much has been written about the impossibility of correcting certain types, no single pattern has been found to be more susceptible to failure or relapse than the others. We must look elsewhere for expiation.

Even an acceptable *excuse* will not increase the percentage of success. The list of problem cases could be wiped out of existence with only one or two good alibis: "poor cooperation" and "failed to return for rechecks" would suffice. We must delve at least one layer below such labels if we wish to advance our knowledge.

Before excavation begins, we may pause to examine one of the generalities above: failure of recheck appointments. It must be obvious that there is nothing inherently therapeutic about mere evaluation of the patient's status. For the 50% who require no further attention after active therapy, it would appear that the rechecks are a waste of time. In addition to their ostensible purpose, that of allowing the clinician to probe for incomplete facets and bring them to perfection, there is a beneficial concept implicit in the situation itself—that is, the day of reckoning, the necessity to demonstrate ability before an authority figure, the difference in the student's study habits when he knows that an examination lies in the future. This inability to drop the subject—the preclusion of the idea that he has mastered his defect by making seven or eight visits to the clinician's office—provides the final trimester of the gestation period and prevents the stillborn product that has typified some of the efforts in this field.

Failure to return for rechecks may in turn have many causes, such as overconfidence, guilt feelings (when the assignment has not been completed), emotional fatigue, resentment of several factors, or sheer forgetfulness. When it occurs, true enough, neglect of follow-up may be assumed to indicate eventual relapse.

There are a number of more specific sources of relapse or of failure to achieve normal deglutition in the first place, which for our purposes are identical situations. Five of these sources deserve attention; they are presented in what appears to be their order of frequency.

PATIENT ATTITUDE. Although a discussion of patient attitude may not seem to be narrowing down to specifics, this factor still remains the single most common obstacle to success. The pivot on which this program turns is the attitude of the patient—his willingness to accept voluntary responsibility for correction, with assistance. Many are unwilling to accept this responsibility, or they lend only lip service, so that there are the inevitable few who never complete the series of sessions proper. Of those who finish, there are just as inexorably the additional number who do so with nothing to spare, who think that all those exercises were unnecessary, who went through the motions under protest, or whose histrionic abilities far surpassed their deglutitory zeal. These types gradually settle to the bottom and are then easily identified. Performance of the acquired pattern cannot be expected by these people.

REST POSITION. The reader may well be growing weary of the term "rest position"; patients become tired of hearing about it also when they have not completely established it as a stable, automatic constituent.

Failure in this regard is not always voluntary or the result of neglect. Recurrence of hay fever during the recheck period, for example, can nullify all efforts. The patient should be cognizant of this possibility and adhere scrupulously to his medication regimen if one has been prescribed. Even a prolonged head cold, inauspiciously timed, can provide an escape corridor for the nebulous new habit. Nevertheless, we refer again to the study conducted by Toronto[1] and discussed in Chapters 6 and 9. This study was a longterm follow-up of patients who had received the program herein presented. His subjects included a routine 42% who had originally reported an allergic condition. Whereas he found 28% who displayed at least some partial relapse, only 2% of the total sample were allergy patients who had regressed. Yet the most salient basis for relapse that Toronto reported was continued mouth breathing (open-mouth rest posture). The indication is that the failures were not those contending with nasal obstruction but instead were patients who simply did not bother to establish a normal resting posture.

Certain severe malocclusions pose an additional barrier; when upper incisors in extreme labioversion remain untreated, making bilabial closure a strenuously effortful undertaking, we could hardly expect total compliance with our requirements. Some of these things we must live with; we can never afford the superficial or spasmodic pursuit of normal rest posture.

INCOMPLETE PRACTICE. Although the clinician should certainly be able to judge with some accuracy the results of each exercise during therapy, he cannot actually count the number of repetitions that the patient has performed. The therapist will occasionally be misled by the patient's report or a seeming facility that is not based on thorough practice. Furthermore, the needs of an individual patient for a certain type of exercise may have been greater than anticipated; the assignment, rather than the patient's efforts, may have been insufficient.

During the recheck period, you may thus find that a certain aspect of the normal swallow is beginning to slip. This problem occurs most frequently with posterior tongue function; you may then discover that the patient did not do as many /k/ swallows as he said, did not really exercise his velum, or, worst tragedy of all, did not actually complete the procedures designed to attain subconscious function. It then becomes necessary to repeat the therapy program from the point of failure, or somewhat *ante mortem*.

DENTAL TREATMENT. Several aspects of the hazard of dental treatment should be faced. We noted before that injudiciously timed oral surgery, involving multiple extractions, can so disorient the patient that he reverts entirely to his original abnormal pattern of deglutition. The same effect may be seen when orthodontic appliances are installed during therapy or during the week or two after therapy.

Nevertheless, for many patients some orthodontic treatment should either precede, or follow as quickly as is safely possible, the attainment of normal deglutition. Tongue thrust encapsulates itself. Possibly no other habit builds its own image to such an extent as does abnormal deglutition. This anomaly, this entity, is carved into the orofacial structure as a brick molds its surrounding mortar. Nothing else fits the resulting space quite as well as the original creative force, so that sheer comfort may entice relapse. Only in a reasonably normal environment can the tongue be expected to persevere in normal function.

SPEECH DEFECT. The influence of speech has been adequately treated in previous sections. By way of summary, however, we may note that it is an infrequent, if inexorable, cause of relapse. Many patients have no speech involvement originally, some who do have a defect spontaneously correct after deglutition therapy, and most of the others have had correction during the recheck period. There is left a very small percentage who persist in an articulation defect and thus revert to abnormal swallowing.

Remediation of relapse

Gaining a clear understanding of the actual cause for later failure almost obviates the need for further discussion here. The nature of the problem dictates its own remedy. Only a few words of advice, perhaps superfluous, will be appended. The procedures suggested apply both to those patients who are found in various stages of decay during the later portion of the recheck period, and to those who suddenly appear after a prolonged absence, having failed to follow the recheck route.

The clinician should naturally perform a careful evaluation, not only to determine the nature and extent of the relapse, pinpointing the patient's position in relation to the base line of skills required in normal deglutition, but also to establish with some accuracy the cause of failure, thus providing a solid basis on which to proceed. It rarely develops that the patient has entirely lost the physical ability to swallow correctly, built during the first four steps of therapy. Positioning the posterior tongue is now often impossible, and certain other elements may also be noticeably weak; however, it is usually feasible to plan one intensive week of muscle exercises that will review each facet of the first four steps, with special emphasis on weak areas. Thereafter, it is possible in many cases to complete the work of the fifth step in only a few days, rather than a full week, after which the balance of the program is simply repeated on its original schedule, including the rechecks.

When relapse is found to be the result of original failure to complete certain assignments or caused by omission or oversight in dental treatment, such a program may be instituted forthwith, provided the dental considerations can now be coordinated with it. On the other hand, if relapse is occasioned by an articulation problem, it would make little sense to consider deglutition until the speech defect is effectively eliminated. This holds true, even more definitely, when an abnormal rest posture is the subverting influence; a thoroughgoing program designed to establish normal posture is assigned—and completed—before any attention is turned to swallowing.

It should only be expected that the patient's attitude would be the most common source of trouble. It therefore demands the most detailed examination. Occasionally there has been a genuine change of heart, a greater maturity has been attained, or dental deterioration or orthodontic relapse has brought a new realization. Welcome home! These people usually make wonderful patients during their reenlistment period.

Unfortunately, attitudes are not always so easily changed. Certainly the demands of therapy do not change. Should the attitude remain the same, the results will remain unaltered, and it is futile to continue in this circular fashion. This aspect should be discussed frankly with the patient and the pertinent facts brought to his attention. You are not justified in retreating the patient who cannot come to therapy with sincerity and enthusiasm, especially in view of his retread status.

In every case where a change in attitude is professed, certain guidelines should be clearly understood before therapy is resumed. The first assignment that is not thoroughly carried out by the patient is the last one. It cannot be otherwise, under the circumstances, if you are to retain any hope for success.

REFERENCE

1. Toronto, A. S.: Permanent changes in swallowing habit as a result of tongue thrust therapy prescribed by R. H. Barrett, Thesis, University of Utah, 1970.

Chapter 26

ALTERNATIVE PROCEDURES OF HANSON

My training from Richard Barrett began 15 years ago. Since that time each of us has continually modified his treatment for tongue thrust. The detailed description of Barrett's therapy found in the preceding chapters bears little resemblance to that I learned years ago. Every nine or ten months I revise my basic set of lessons and print up enough to last for that period of time. As the months go by, the lesson sheets I hand out to my patients become more and more filled with handwritten revisions and new assignments. I try to incorporate procedures and assignments that I hear about from my colleagues, and that I read about in the literature, retaining those which seem effective for me and rejecting others after a trial period.

Barrett's therapy approach and mine are essentially similar. We start with a series of pre-planned lessons and assignments and modify them according to the needs of the patient. Each lesson builds on the skills taught in the preceding lesson(s). We emphasize tongue and lip resting postures throughout training. All associated oral habits are eliminated along with the tongue thrust. Very specific assignments are made to assure subconscious habituation of all swallows and pre-swallow muscle activities. The patient is seen until all orthodontic treatment is completed. The parent is an important participant in therapy.

Salient features of my treatment are (1) the hierarchy of areas of emphasis; (2) the utilization of basic "organismic" principles; (3) frequent reliance upon behavior modification procedures, including the use of isometric exercises and attention to the development of perceptual skills; (4) incorporation of neuromuscular facilitation

exercises; and (5) my approach to the correction of dentalized speech sounds. Each of these features will be described briefly. Then the lesson sheets I am currently using will be presented and specific assignments explained.

THE HIERARCHY OF AREAS OF EMPHASIS

The usual components of a tongue thrusting problem will be listed in *descending* order.

1. *Resting postures of the tongue and lips.* These constitute the beginning position for all muscle movements related to tongue thrust. The law of physiologic economy applies here: If the tongue rests against the anterior teeth habitually, and returns to that position after any movements, such as those occurring in chewing, swallowing, or speech, it will probably move away from that anterior position as little as possible during the activity. Thus, resting postures become the key to the frequency and extent of linguodental contacts during the day and night. Orthodontists and researchers agree almost unanimously on the greater importance of light, constant forces, such as are found in resting postures, over the stronger, less frequent lingual pressures against the teeth during swallowing. For these reasons lingual and labial resting positions receive primary emphasis in my program.

2. *Saliva moving.* Most programs give inadequate attention to the *preparatory* phase of saliva handling. Saliva normally collects forward in the mouth, under the tongue. It must be moved posteriorly without a tongue thrust. If the saliva swallow is corrected, but saliva moving continues to be effected by a linguodental seal, the tongue thrust is likely to return during swallowing of saliva as the weeks and months go by.

3. *Saliva swallowing.* Saliva handling is given precedence over food because of the frequency of saliva swallows and because of the strong relationship between saliva handling and resting postures of the lips and tongue.

4. *Food chewing.* Chewing pressures may occur from five to twenty times per mouthful of food. Proper chewing involves very little contact between the tongue and the anterior teeth. The patient is taught to allow the lips to move the food posteriorly, and the tongue to move it laterally.

5. *Food swallowing.* The *efficiency* of the food swallow is stressed. If food remains in the mouth after an initial swallow, an additional swallow is required, which is nearly always preceded by a "clean-up" action of the tongue against the front teeth. The tongue thrust swallow may have accomplished the same task with only one swallow, and again the law of physiologic economy will promote a return to the more efficient type of swallow. The preparatory phase of swallowing, after chewing is completed, is carefully explained to the patient.

6. *Speech.* Speech pathologists usually notice dentalized /s/ and /z/ sounds, because the anteriorization changes the acoustical characteristics of these sibilants. Dentalization of other linguoalveolar sounds, such as the /t/, /d/, /n/, and /l/, however, may escape detection. These latter sounds involve much greater pressure against the front teeth than do the /s/ and /z/, and should be corrected by a speech pathologist. If the oral myologist does not have the necessary training to be able to work on speech, he or she should make a referral. My approach is to work on dentalization as a distinctive feature, rather than to correct the problem one sound at a time.

7. *Liquids.* Liquid swallows occur relatively infrequently, and require very little pressure. Since they are often a part of the total problem, nevertheless, they should be corrected. Therapy includes instruction in continuous drinking, sip-at-a-time drinking, and drinking from a fountain and through a straw.

ORGANISMIC PRINCIPLES

These principles, originally applied to the treatment of stuttering by Kopp, have provided a philosophical basis for my treatment of tongue thrusters.

1. Old neuromuscular patterns are never erased. Although therapy replaces unwanted psychomotor patterns with new ones, the former are always subject to recall under certain physiological and/or emotional conditions. The parent, the patient, and the clinician should always be alert for any signs of relapse.

2. Attention to each of the component parts is necessary when a habit is an integration of several related habits. This is the case in oral myofunctional disorders. Therapy must encompass the total problem and all its aspects.

3. Habits gain strength as time passes. One implication of this principle has to do with the difficulty of eradicating the thrusting habit, which in most cases has been present from birth. Another implication deals with the establishment of correct habits, which should be accomplished as soon as the patient is mature enough to carry out necessary assignments and to benefit from the treatment.

BEHAVIOR MODIFICATION

Operant conditioning principles have helped to systematize my therapy. The three traditional steps are discussed in the following paragraphs.

Establish base line

Most clinicians do this during the diagnostic sessions, but many fail to utilize the information they glean in planning therapy. This step consists of determining precisely what the patient is doing correctly and what behaviors need to be changed. The initial telephone call made by the parent or patient to the therapist begins the process of establishing the base line. The caller briefly describes the behavior of the patient, names the referral source, and usually gives an indication of attitude toward therapy. The second step is the initial consultation, where the complete case history is obtained and the behavioral patterns are observed and recorded. Direct questions concerning motivation and attitude are often productive in establishing base line. The clinician looks for total behavioral patterns. If tongue thrust is present, what form does it take? Does the thrusting occur during the swallowing of saliva, liquids, and solid foods? The strengths of involved muscles and the appropriateness of the timing and nature of their movements *during function* are assessed. A patient may not habitually occlude the molars during swallowing, but the masseter and temporalis muscles may be normal in strength. If so, the patient would be assigned exercises to increase *awareness* of the contraction of those muscles, and to systematically establish the *habit* of their contraction during swallowing, rather than to strengthen them. Does the tongue rest habitually against the upper or lower anterior teeth, or between the maxillary and mandibular teeth? Is there a frontal lisp? Are the linguoalveolar sounds produced with contact between the tongue and anterior teeth? Is there linguolabial contact in the rest position or during swallow? Are swallowing patterns consistent? Is there a difference between the swallow done on command and the one done subconsciously? Is there anything about the dentition or about the bone or soft tissue structure that might promote the perpetuation of a thrusting pattern? How stimulable is the patient when he is given a brief explanation of how to swallow correctly? Might the base line be altered if remediable conditions, such as large tonsils or adenoids or a deviated septum, were treated medically or surgically? Is there an overjet to such a degree that habitual juxtaposition of the lower lip would be extremely difficult? If so, some preliminary orthodontic work would help to provide a base line responsive to treatment.

The third part of the process of establishing the base line is in the form of an assignment given to the patient and to the parents or spouse of the patient. The patient and one other person are asked to be very observant during the next week or two of various aspects of the habit needing correction. If the problem is digit sucking, both are asked to try to determine exactly under what conditions the finger or thumb is placed in the mouth, the manner in which it is positioned, the length of time it is left in place, and whether there is any relationship between the occurrence of the sucking and fatigue, emotional state, time of day, hunger, or happenings during the day. In the case of tongue thrusting, it is important to know when the mouth is most likely to be held in an open position; where the tongue usually rests when the mouth is open; the relative involvement of tongue and lips during the chewing process; the positions of the tongue and lips during sleep; and any other abnormal behavior involving any of the oral musculature. A questionnaire given to the patient lists these points, and the patient is asked to complete it before returning for the next visit. The completion of these three steps in the establishment of base line assures the therapist that he sees the total pattern and

enables him to prescribe and individualize a plan of therapy for the patient. It eliminates unnecessary and ineffectual use of stock exercises and assignments and greatly improves the quality of therapy. A tongue thrust is a complex pattern that may take various forms and may be accompanied by any of several related habit patterns.

Modify behavior

The phase of therapy in which behavior is modified can be completed for most patients with the use of social praise as the only reinforcer. For younger children, and for the older children who have been difficult to motivate, token or primary reinforcers are used. Whenever possible, the child is made responsible for his own practice and for keeping current the practice charts he brings to therapy with him. If for some reason the parent is unable to observe a given practice session and wants to know whether the practice has actually been done, she need only look at the practice chart. For the patient, the knowledge that someone trusts him to keep up his practice chart and praises him for having done so at the next therapy session provides effective motivation. In therapy for thumb suckers, the children telephone the clinician daily, or at least periodically, to report their progress on assignments. The verbal approval given on the telephone seems to be enough to motivate them to persist in their efforts.

Throughout this phase of therapy, certain subgoals are set that are related to the achievement of skills involved in the swallowing process. These are presented to the child in list form at the beginning of therapy. With the younger child, the parent and child ar asked to decide on a small reward for the completion of each of the subgoals. When the child demonstrates the ability to swallow food, liquid, and saliva correctly and to maintain correct lip and tongue postures for certain periods of time or during certain activities, he has reached a major goal, and it is recommended that a greater reward be given at that time. The following are a few achievements that might be included on the list:

1. Location of correct spot on roof of mouth for placement of tongue
2. Tight seal between blade of tongue and roof of mouth
3. Sufficient strength in contraction of masseter muscle

4. Ability to chew while keeping lips closed and tongue away from anterior teeth
5. Movement of saliva posteriorly in mouth without pushing tongue against teeth
6. Formation of proper bolus of food
7. Drinking of liquids without unnecessary movement of facial muscles

Another behavioral modification is that of "time-out," which is a punishment device. The therapist might punish any unwanted behavior in therapy by simply turning away from the child for a certain number of seconds or minutes, and then facing him again; by leaving the room; by turning out the light; or by simply giving a signal to indicate to the child he is to stop talking for a prescribed period of time. My program uses this principle, in a modified form, in an effort to secure consistent practicing on the part of the patient. The child who is correcting a tongue-thrust pattern is required to practice assignments three times every day, every day of the week, but if he misses more than one practice a week, he is to call and inform the clinician. Without criticizing him in any way, I advise him that I will not see him for the scheduled appointment; he is to practice the same assignment for another week and then come for another session.

It is important during this stage of therapy for the clinician to define very specifically the role of the parent in providing reinforcement or punishment. Probably most important is the insistence to the parent that all types of punishment, other than that prescribed by the therapist, be avoided. It is also important to avoid using facial expressions that convey disgust or anger to the child if he misses practices or performs an exercise in an imperfect manner. It is usually more effective when the parent avoids punishing the child and instead gives much praise and encouragement.

ISOMETRIC EXERCISES. Muscle strengthening is accomplished by having the patient contract a muscle or muscle group for ten seconds, relax, and repeat the procedure a specified number of times.

PERCEPTUAL SKILLS. The patient must first become aware of and later accustomed to new resting positions and movements of the tongue and lips. Several exercises require that positions be maintained for a number of seconds or that movements be performed very slowly in order to give the patient time to heighten stimulus awareness.

Extend stimulus control

The "carry-over" part of therapy consists of extending the stimulus control. The child has learned proper posturing and is able to swallow all media correctly. He now must apply what he has learned to all swallows that occur day and night, and to the lip and tongue postures throughout the day. Of course, the careful structuring and carrying out of the preceding phase of therapy is an important step in facilitating the success of the extension process. At this time, whatever type of reinforcement has been used during therapy has to be gradually modified to conform with the very sporadic and infrequent reinforcement he will receive in everyday life. He will need to receive feedback from many sources. Parents, siblings, friends, and teachers should be called on to help, unless the child objects to assistance from any of these people. The feedback is less objectionable if it is given in the form of a simple signal, such as touching the forefinger to the thumb, or touching the cheek or chin to let the child know that his mouth is resting in an open position or that his tongue is resting against his teeth. The three hundredth time the child receives this signal is less painful to him than the three hundredth time he is *told* to close his mouth. The child is provided with "Remember" buttons, rings, or signs to place in conspicuous places in various rooms in the house. He is assigned to make his own signs. He takes bookmarks to school to put in all his school books so that every time he opens one of them he is reminded that his tongue should be positioned correctly or that his lips should be closed or that he should not be biting on his lower lip. He is given a list of reminders from which he can choose one or two. Some children stick with a given reminder for several months; others need to change reminders every week or two. The following list provides examples:

REMINDERS

1. Every time you *see*:
   a. A clock or watch (you will think, "It's time to . . .") (one technique that seems to work for many children is to have them wear their watch upside down)
   b. A certain color or type of car
   c. A pleasant smile
   d. A reminder sign you have made
   e. A certain color
   f. One polished fingernail

g. A sticker, picture, or initials such as TOS (tongue on spot) on your hand

h. A person with crooked teeth

2. Every time you *hear:*
   a. A bell of any kind (school, phone, doorbell)
   b. A clock ticking
   c. A horn honk

3. Every time you *feel:*
   a. A rock or weight of any kind in your pocket
   b. A bracelet on your wrist
   c. A ring on your finger (adjustable rings are good because they can be moved from finger to finger each day)
   d. A sugarless mint on your tongue

4. Every time you:
   a. Go through any doorway
   b. Turn the light on or off
   c. Turn the radio, TV, or record player on or off
   d. Practice the piano or other musical instrument
   e. Walk up or down stairs
   f. Smile
   g. Sit down or stand up

PLUS-MINUS CHARTS. Another useful technique is a "plus-minus" system for working on tongue and lip postures. During the fourth or fifth session, the patient and parent are instructed in using the plus-minus system. When the child (on his honor for the first 15, 20, or 30 minutes he is at home after school, after the evening meal, or at any specified time during the day) has kept his tongue and lips in the proper position for that period of time, he so informs the parent by saying simply, "I have earned a plus." He then places a plus on the chart on the wall. Or when either parent sees that the child's lips have been closed for that period of time he tells the child, "You get a plus," and the child puts the plus on the chart. At any time the parent sees the child with the lips in an open position at rest for 10 seconds or more, or with the tongue forward at rest, he informs the child, "You get a minus," and the child places a minus on the chart. No marks are made on the chart without the parent so advising the child or vice-versa. At the end of each day, the pluses and minuses are tallied. If there are more pluses than minuses, the child receives a plus for the day. At the end of the week, if there are more plus days than minus days, a predetermined reward is given to the child. If there are more minus than plus days appropriate punishments (tasks, restriction on hours, or limitation of activities) are meted out. During the second week the earning of awards is made more difficult by requiring the patient to earn at least twice as many pluses as minuses to

receive a plus for the day. During the third week a plus for the day requires at least three times as many pluses as minuses, and the fourth week the ratio becomes four to one. The next step is usually to set a goal for a maximum number of minuses that are allowed each day, and pluses are no longer counted. If necessary, the number of minuses allowed can be progressively decreased each week.

It is recommended to the parent that if the child, following this progressive schedule, achieves weekly rewards four weeks in a row, he be given a relatively greater reward at that time.

"COUNTERS." When the patient has learned to gather and swallow saliva proficiently and effortlessly (usually after six or seven sessions), he is given a little pocket "adder" such as shoppers use to determine how many dollars' worth of groceries are in the cart, or a wristwatch counter such as golfers use to tally their strokes. He is to count a certain number of correct saliva "gatherings" and swallows each morning, afternoon, and evening. Even teenagers seem to enjoy keeping track of their swallows in this way. The first counting assignment will usually total 100 to 300 swallows a day. When the patient returns with his report on number of swallows counted, he is asked how many he thinks he should count for the next week or two. Nearly always he chooses to count more than he did the week before. His decision is influenced a little by the signs we have posted in the office, showing photographs of our current counting champions. Compared to their records of number of proper saliva swallows in a week or month, his own performance pales. After a few weeks of allowing him to set his own goals, the clinician and patient together decide to taper off the counting, both with respect to number of swallows counted per day and number of days per week the counting is done.

PERCENTAGE CHARTS. The most meaningless question a clinician asks of a patient in advanced stages of therapy is: "How are you doing with your swallowing?" It is inevitably answered: "I don't know. When I think about it I'm doing all right." Then, of course, the clinician asks, "How often do you think about it?" And so it goes. To avoid this unprofitable exchange, the patient keeps weekly percentage charts on which are listed seven or eight swallow-related habits he should be strengthening, including the following:

1. Tongue-resting postures

2. Lip-resting postures
3. Saliva gathering
4. Saliva swallowing
5. Chewing
6. Food swallows
7. Liquid swallows

The chart contains several columns, each for the goals for a week; each week new goals are set. The chart is placed in a conspicuous place in the home so that the patient and members of his family might be kept aware of the various aspects of the behavior to which they should be attentive. By now, therapy sessions are infrequent, and the patient brings the chart to each recheck visit. In this way more meaningful comments and assignments can be made by the therapist.

MAINTENANCE PROGRAM. The activities and assignments listed above can all be part of a rather permanent set of assignments given to the patient. Until all orthodontic work has been completed and the retainer has been shed for good, it is advisable to have the former tongue thruster carry out some brief daily-to-weekly assignments. The patient helps to make decisions regarding frequency and nature of these assignments, because in order to be effective they have to be activities he can live with, usually for a period of several months. He is to phone the clinician periodically or drop a card in the mail reporting his compliance with these assignments. When he comes in for rechecks at critical points during orthodontic treatment, the clinician reviews his progress on the maintenance program. Parents are encouraged to continue to provide social reinforcers for proper oral behavior. The orthodontist observes the patient and provides reinforcement when warranted.

I have found the application of these operant conditioning principles to be highly effective in assisting in the establishment of permanently correct habits. The patients enjoy knowing exactly what to do and how often, and they appreciate the concrete evidence of their changing behavior that they see as therapy progresses.

NEUROMUSCULAR FACILITATION

A modification of the Falk approach, based on Rood's procedures, forms a part of the early stages of therapy. The dorsum and sides of the tongue are tapped and stroked, respectively, a given number of times each practice, for three or more practice periods each day. The hard palate is stroked with ice or frozen fruit a number of times each practice. These exercises, performed by the patient prior to each meal, reportedly result in the development of proper tonicity in the muscles of the tongue and encourage a reflexive, protective lifting of the dorsum of the tongue against the palate. It is too early for me to be able to determine whether they are as efficacious for my patients as Falk found them to be in his practice. A tentative impression is that they are especially beneficial for those patients whose tongue movements during initial testing are obviously lacking in fine control.

CORRECTION OF DENTALIZED SPEECH SOUNDS

I postpone work on these sounds until the seventh or eighth week of therapy. By this time, proper lingual resting postures are fairly strongly habituated, and it is relatively easy to teach the feature of linguoalveolar contact. Even though there is a central aperture for the air to escape on the /s/ and /z/ sounds, the general similarity in tongue position among the six linguoalveolar sounds makes a distinctive feature approach viable. I have the patient imagine that the tip of the tongue is connected to the upper alveolar ridge by a tiny tubular (spiral) spring, which draws the tongue tip back to its proper "home" position as often as possible during speech or reading. Normally only four to six sessions are required to establish correct patterns in everyday speech following this procedure.

LESSONS

INITIAL VISIT. Base line data are taken. Malocclusions are described and measured. Proper resting postures for tongue and lips are explained. The level of motivation is ascertained as much as possible, and explanations and encouragement are given as deemed advisable. Reminder signals and signs are presented to the patient, and he/she is assigned to keep a log on progress with resting postures. Any medical or dental work which seems advisable before the initiation of therapy is recommended. If nose breathing is difficult, a referral is made to an ear-nose-throat specialist.

LESSON NUMBER 1. Progress records kept by the patient are examined. The lesson given the patient is reproduced below. For each exercise and assignment in this lesson, as well as for all the lessons which follow, the purpose will be explained, and some instructions to the clinician given.

LESSON 1 Date _____

Watch the mirror closely for all exercises!

PRACTICE THE FOLLOWING EXERCISES THREE TIMES EACH DAY, SEVEN DAYS EACH WEEK!

1. Tongue tapping. Let your tongue rest on the floor of your mouth. Tap the upper front part of your tongue rapidly for 30 seconds.
2. Tongue stroking. Stroke one side of your tongue gently, from back to front, 15 times. Then do the same to the other side of your tongue.
3. Icing. Ice the middle of the front half of the roof of your mouth, from back to front, for 20 seconds.
4. Plus-Minus chart. To help make a strong habit of keeping your tongue in the right place and resting your lips together you will use a plus-minus system for the next few weeks. Whenever you have kept your tongue and lips in their proper positions for about 15 minutes, mark a +, either on your note pad or on a chart on a wall. Any time you or your observer (parent, spouse, friend) catches you with your lips apart at rest, or with your tongue forward, record a −. Observers are to signal you, rather than tell you, when they see your lips apart.

At the end of each day, count the pluses and minuses. If there are more pluses than minuses, you have had a + day. If there are more minuses than pluses, you have had a − day. If you have more + days than − days during the week, you have a + week. This may earn you a small reward, according to the agreement between you and your parents.

For Lesson 2, you must earn twice as many pluses as minuses to earn a + day. For Lesson 3, you need three times as many pluses as minuses, and for Lesson 4, four times as many. Four + weeks in a row may earn you a special award, if your parents agree to it.

	Day						
	1	2	3	4	5	6	7
1. Tongue tapping							
2. Tongue stroking							
3. Icing							
Number of +'s							
Number of −'s							
+ or − day?							

Exercises one through three are my modifications of the Falk adaptations of the Rood procedures for neuromuscular facilitation. These will be carried out just before each meal, for six weeks or more.

Exercise one: *Tongue tapping.* I use a "steak marker," a stick rounded at one end and pointed at the other, for this and the other two Falk exercises. The rounded end is used for the tapping of the anterior half of the dorsum of the tongue. The stick is held at an approximate 45-degree angle as the clinician taps, in turn, all the areas of this part of the tongue. The patient is instructed to simply relax the tongue. This is continued either by the parent or by the patient for 30 seconds each practice.

Purpose: This action promotes a flattening of the tongue and a concavity of its dorsal surface. The tongue normally also withdraws posteriorly, away from the lingual surface of the anterior teeth.

Exercise two: *Tongue stroking.* Again using the rounded edge of the stick, the anterior half of the sides of the tongue are stroked, from back to front, slowly. Falk uses a brush for this purpose. Each side is stroked 15 times.

Purpose: This exercise narrows the tongue.

Exercise three: *Icing.* The pointed end of a steak marker is inserted into a grape, pitted cherry, or rounded partition of an ice cube tray and frozen. Beginning at the junction of the hard and soft palates, the patient slowly strokes the median line of the hard palate from back to front, stopping when reaching "the spot" (the incisal papilla). This is repeated for 20 seconds.

Purpose: The icing of the palate results in a protective "snuggling" of the tongue against the roof of the mouth, with the tongue tip placed in the proper place.

Plus-minus chart. I like to give the patient a choice between the assignment as explained above, and the use of a pocket adder for counting pluses and minuses. If he/she chooses the latter, instead of having to hold correct tongue and lip resting postures for 15 minutes in order to push the "plus" button, credit is given for a plus whenever the patient finds the tongue and lips in correct positions. A *limit* of one plus per 15 minute period is allowed.

LESSON 2   Date _____

Watch mirror closely!

1, 2, and 3. Repeat tapping, stroking, and icing exercises.

4. Tongue popping. Place the tip of your tongue on the spot. Suck your tongue up against the roof of your mouth. Keep the frenum stretched as you slowly count to ten. Then pull your tongue down rapidly, causing a popping sound. Ten times each practice.

5. Biting exercise (masseter muscle). Place your fingers on each side of your face, just in front of your ears. Bite and feel the muscles tighten. Hold for ten seconds, then relax. Try to keep the tip of your tongue on the spot, and the whole top part of your tongue against the roof of your mouth. When a parent is present, he can place a hand on one of your cheeks while you touch your other cheek.

6. Plus-minus work. In order to get a + for the day, you must earn at least twice as many +'s as −'s.

Even though the Falk exercises are simple, they are also simple to do incorrectly. The execution of each of them is carefully observed.

Exercise four: *Tongue popping.* This is a classic exercise in oral myofunctional therapy, modified only to make it isometric.

Purposes: To strengthen the muscles which assist in making a linguopalatal seal, and to introduce the patient to the *feeling* of proper tongue placement for swallowing.

Exercise five: *Biting.* Muscle contraction on both sides must be about equal. If not, I examine molar occlusion to see whether symmetry is feasible. The patient is instructed to bite hard enough so that after ten performances of the exercise, the jaw muscles are very tired, but is cautioned against continuing any degree of tightening that produces pain.

Purposes: Strengthening and perception.

Continue the plus-minus work as described.

LESSON 3   Date _____

Watch mirror closely!

1, 2, and 3. Repeat tapping, stroking, and icing exercises.

4. Open and close. Suck your tongue up into the roof of your mouth, as if you were going to pop your tongue. Open your mouth as wide as possible and hold your tongue sucked up for five seconds. Then bite slowly down on your back teeth, keeping your tongue sucked up, and again hold to a count of five. Relax, then begin again. Ten times each practice.

5. Beginning swallow. Place a small plastic straw just behind your upper cuspids. Lift your tongue up against the roof of your mouth, then bite down. The tongue should be held against the roof of your mouth, but should *not* touch the straw. Squirt water into your mouth. Keep your lips spread wide. Slurp back *hard* and swallow. Do not let either the tip or the under part of your tongue come forward and touch the straw while you *slurp* or while you *swallow*. Do this five times. Then remove the straw, and watch the mirror closely as you do it five more times. Then put the straw back in between your teeth and do it five times more. (A total of 15 times each practice.)

6. Plus-minus work. In order to get a + for the day, you must earn three times as many +'s as −'s.

The Falk exercises are numbers 1, 2, and 3.

Exercise four: *Open and close.* This is similar to the tongue-popping exercise, but requires greater control over the muscles which suck the tongue against the hard palate. Until the patient is corrected, a common error is to protrude the mandible as the jaws are approximated during the exercise.

Purpose: To continue the strengthening of the tongue-lifting muscles.

Exercise five: *Beginning swallow.* For some patients, the straw is more of a hindrance than a help, and is excluded from the exercise. I like to include it whenever possible, because of the focus it gives to kinesthetic and tactile sensations. The slurping is simply to facilitate movement of the liquid to the back of the mouth for swallowing. Keeping the tongue from "sagging" during slurping, though, is an important part of the exercise.

Purpose: To give the patient an initial experience with swallowing without *any* tongue thrust. A direct application of the "tongue pop" and "open and close" exercises.

The plus-minus task continues to increase in difficulty.

LESSON 4 Date _____

Watch mirror closely!

1, 2, and 3. Continue tapping, stroking, and icing exercises.
4. Trapping. (1) Stick your tongue way out. (2) Raise the tip of your tongue. (3) Keeping the tip up, raise the sides of the tongue. The tongue should be shaped like a bowl, or a spoon. (4) Squirt water into the "spoon" the tongue has made. Don't let any spill over the tip *or sides* of your tongue. (5) Keeping the sides and tip up, slowly draw your tongue back into your mouth. As you do this, slowly bite down on your back teeth. (6) Lift the whole tongue up to the roof of your mouth, keeping it spoon-shaped. The sides and tip should make a seal all the way around your upper gums. (7) Spread your lips wide, squeeze the middle of your tongue up, and swallow. Watch the mirror closely to see that neither your tongue nor the water comes forward. Ten times each practice.

5. Back-tongue lifting. Keep your head tipped back during this entire exercise. (1) Lift the back of your tongue, as if you were going to say the /k/ sound. (Keep the tip of the tongue on the floor of your mouth.) (2) Squirt water into the throat. (3) Drop the back of your tongue, to let the water drain back. Don't swallow yet. (4) Lift the back of the tongue again. (5) Hold the back of the tongue up for five seconds. (6) Swallow, keeping the back of the tongue up and the tip down. Keep your mouth open wide during the whole exercise. Ten times each practice.

6. Plus-minus work. At least four pluses for every minus.

(Appropriate charts are provided.)

Exercise four: *Trapping.* The explanation of this exercise given above is explicit and needs little elaboration. Many patients are unable to achieve the concavity of the tongue required to begin the exercise until a slight amount of water is squirted onto the dorsum of the tongue. Partly because it is a natural reflex and partly because of the tapping and stroking work the patient has been doing for several weeks, the tongue nearly always responds by elevating its tip and sides to contain the water. The patient observes the cuspid and premolar area closely to notice any lateral tongue protrusion.

Purpose: To achieve a tight, effective linguo-alveolar seal, essential for the normal swallowing of food and saliva.

Exercise five: *Back-tongue lifting.* The most effective way to begin this exercise is to have the patient watch the mirror as he/she produces a few /k/ sounds. Then demonstrate how to stop the production of the sound without moving the back of the tongue, and have the patient try to do the same. Some patients need to hold the anterior part of the tongue down with a tongue depressor as they elevate the posterior portion.

Purpose: To strengthen the muscles which raise the back part of the tongue straight up, and to enhance kinesthetic awareness of this elevation. The tongue tip is kept on the floor of the mouth in order to make the back-tongue lifting muscles exert more effort.

LESSON 5   Date _____

Watch mirror closely!

1, 2, and 3. Continue tapping, stroking, and icing exercises.

4. Back-middle-tip. Keep your head tipped back as you do this exercise. (1) Squirt water to the back of your mouth. (2) Keeping the tip of your tongue on the floor of your mouth, raise the back of the tongue, as if you were going to say a /k/ sound. (3) Without dropping the back of the tongue, *squeeze* the rest of the tongue up; the middle part, the tip. (4) Bite your back teeth together, keep your lips wide apart, and swallow. Do not let the tongue show against the teeth. Swallow with your *throat*. Fifteen times each practice.

5. Trapping with tongue depressor. Trap water as in Lesson 4, Exercise 4. With your teeth still closed, suck your tongue up so the frenum stretches. Then open wide enough to place the tongue depressor edgewise between the upper and lower back teeth. Swallow without letting the tongue come forward or stick out the sides. Ten times each practice.

6. Continue with the plus-minus work only if you did not make the goal of at least four plusses for every minus last week. Choose at least one reminder that can be used outside, and at least one for inside, to help you remember to think about your tongue and lip resting positions.

Visual reminders: Wear watch upside down. Smiles. Your own reminder signs. One polished fingernail. Bracelet. Ring. A certain color. Elastic on pen or pencil. Stickers.

Auditory reminders: Bells. Buzzers. Phone ringing. Horn honking. Your name. Yelling.

"Feeling" reminders: A rock in your pocket. Penny in your shoe. Sugarless mint on your tongue. Upside-down ring.

"Doing" reminders: Go through a doorway. Turn light on or off. Practice an instrument. Go up or down stairs. Sit down or stand up.

Inside reminder: _____ Outside reminder: ___

(Appropriate charts are provided.)

Exercises one, two, and three: *The Falk exercises.*

Exercise four: *Back-middle-tip.* This is the successor to the "back-tongue lifting" exercise. The clinician demonstrates the rolling, lifting motion of the tongue. This is, of course, the reverse of the normal tongue lifting pattern for swallowing, because the patient is required to lift first the back, then the middle, then the tip of the tongue.

Purposes: To continue the work on elevating the back of the tongue. To exercise the muscles raising the middle of the tongue. To continue work on swallowing without any tongue thrust.

Exercise five: *Trapping with a tongue depres-*

sor. A junior-sized tongue depressor is used with younger patients. If a patient is unable to swallow without tongue thrusting or dropping the tongue with the tongue depressor edgewise, it is turned nearly flat. The patient gradually turns it edgewise as the week progressess. This exercise is rarely done well until after a few days of practice.

Purpose: To further strengthen the tongue-lifting muscles and to focus the attention to the back part of the mouth. The patient is asked to "swallow with the throat muscles."

Reminders replace the plus-minus charts if the patient has achieved the goal of four plusses for every minus, or if the plus-minus work is losing its effectiveness.

LESSON 6   Date _____

Watch mirror closely!

1, 2, and 3. Continue doing tapping, stroking, and icing exercises.

4. Squeaky sucking. (1) Put your tongue on the spot. (2) Place a straw between your teeth as in Lesson 3, Exercise 5. (3) Bite down. (4) With the lips spread wide, squirt water into the corner of your mouth. (5) Close your lips gently and suck back, making a squeaking (not a slurping) sound. (6) Spread your lips wide again and swallow. Make sure the tongue tip remains on the spot. Use the muscles in the back of the tongue and throat to suck and swallow. Try not to let the muscles around your lips and in your chin move while you suck and swallow. Fifteen times each practice.

5. Whistle. The purpose of this exercise is to give you more practice in keeping the sides of the tongue against the upper gums, instead of against your side teeth. Say "SSSSSSSSSS." As you hold the "SSSSSSSSS," curl the tip of your tongue slowly back and draw its sides up tighter against your gums. As you do this, the "SSSSSSSS" should begin to sound sharper, and may turn into a whistle. When you have it as sharp as you can get it, keep your tongue in that position for at least *two minutes,* paying attention to the *feeling* of having the sides of the tongue against the *gums.* Every few seconds, test the position by trying to whistle.

6. Beginning food swallows. Take a small bite of a soft food and hold it in the middle of the top of the tongue. Bite down, spread your lips wide, and swallow. See if you are able to swallow all the food on your tongue. WATCH THE MIRROR CLOSELY! Ten times each practice.

7. Continue to use the reminders you chose, if they are working. If not, choose two others. Write the reminders below:

Inside: _____ Outside: _____

(Charts are provided.)

Normally this will be the last week for the patient to do the tapping, stroking, and icing exercises. By now the patient is habitually resting the lips and tongue in correct positions and is able to swallow normally with little effort.

Exercise four: *Squeaky sucking.* The use of the straw is very helpful for many patients, but counterproductive for others. I usually try for the straw first, unless there is a very broad, severe open bite or the cuspids or bicuspids are missing. At times I have the patient do the exercise five times with the straw, five times without, and five times with, again. No slurping is accepted, for this indicates that the lips are slightly apart.

Purpose: This is the first of a series of exercises aimed at habituating proper saliva handling. The water is squirted under the tongue in the area where saliva collects. The purpose of the squeaking is to assure the clinician and the patient that the proper kind of sucking action is being accomplished. With some patients it is helpful to have them palpate the supralaryngeal musculature just lateral to the thyroid cartilage to feel the muscle activity during sucking.

Exercise five: *Whistle.* Some patients can learn the whistle more easily *without* working from an /s/, and others who cannot learn to whistle at all achieve the purpose of the exercise by simply sustaining the /s/. The important thing to stress is that this is a "feeling" exercise, to focus the patient's attention on contact between the sides of the tongue and the lateral maxillary alveolar processes.

Exercise six: *Beginning food swallows.* The clinician takes a small amount of pudding or jello on the end of a tongue depressor and places it in the middle of the dorsum of the patient's tongue. The patient bites down and squeezes the tongue against the palate. Watch for lateral thrusting. If saliva comes forward during the swallow, it is often because the sides of the tongue did not maintain contact with the upper alveolar ridge during swallow.

Purpose: This is an extremely simple assignment for the patient, but it introduces him/her to the swallowing of foods without the sometimes confusing chewing and gathering tasks being required.

LESSON 7   Date _____

Watch mirror closely!

1. Quiet sucking without the straw. This exercise helps you to learn how to move saliva back to get it ready for swallowing. (1) Put your tongue on the spot. (2) Squirt water under the tongue. (3) Bite down. (4) Close your lips gently. (5) Suck back, without making a noise. (6) Spread lips and swallow. Try to keep the lip and chin muscles quiet as you do the exercise. Fifteen times each practice.
2. Beginning chewing and swallowing. Either at a snack or at a meal, eat a food that requires chewing (apple, celery, carrot, cracker, cookie, etc.). As you bring the food toward your mouth, don't let your tongue reach out for it. (1) Take a reasonable-size bite. (2) Chew with your lips closed, moving the food back into your mouth as you chew. (3) Do not touch your front teeth with your tongue as you chew. (4) Collect the food on the middle part of your tongue as soon as the food sticks together. (Check in the mirror to see that the food "bolus" is not too close to the tip of the tongue.) (5) Lift your tongue tip to the spot and bite down on your back teeth. (6) Spread your lips wide. (7) Squeeze your tongue against the roof of your mouth and swallow. Ten bites each practice. Try to practice with a variety of foods as the week goes by.
3. Continuous drinking. When your hand first touches the glass, do three things: (1) put your tongue tip on the spot; (2) bite down on your back teeth; (3) be sure your head is not tipped forward. Stay like that all through your drink. At the end of your drink your head may tip back a little. *Drink three average-sized glasses of liquids each day.* Let your lips rest naturally around the edge of the glass. Tip the glass as you drink. Keep your lip and chin muscles quiet as you drink. Be careful of the last swallow. Don't lick your lips when you're through.
4. Upper lip stretcher. Holding your lower lip quiet and your mouth quite wide open, stretch your upper lip down over upper teeth. Hold for ten seconds. Fifteen times each practice. (Do this one only if we worked on it at our lesson.)

KEEP YOUR TONGUE ON THE SPOT AND YOUR LIPS CLOSED AT REST!

(Appropriate charts are provided.)

Exercise one: *Quiet sucking without the straw.* A few patients who have difficulty managing the squeak required in the predecessor to this exercise in Lesson 6 are able to suck back without a squeak effortlessly. Most, though, find the week of work with the squeaky sucking helpful. If they can perform the squeaky sucking easily when they come for the seventh lesson, you are assured that they will be able to suck properly for this exercise. When the lips are spread after the sucking, and before the swallowing, be sure all the water is gone from the lower vestibule. If not, the patient has not achieved the purpose of the exercise.

Purpose: To train the patient to move saliva posteriorly without any visible effort, and without any forward motion of the tongue.

Exercise two: *Beginning chewing and swallowing.* At no time during eating does the tongue need to push against the lingual surfaces of the anterior teeth. It is important to begin correctly, as the food approaches the mouth, and end correctly, without a "clean-up" motion of the tongue against the incisors, or lip-sucking, after swallowing. I assign only ten swallows each practice because I want them done very carefully. When the bolus is formed and placed properly on the tongue, the correct swallow is easy, for the patient has had a week of practice with soft food.

Exercise three: *Continuous drinking.* The same emphasis to the *total* drinking act is given as was given in beginning chewing and swallowing. I admit to the patient that what I am teaching is not a *normal* drinking pattern, but one that is a little safer than normal. Normally, the teeth are not occluded, the head is not perfectly straight, nor is the tongue tip held on the spot during drinking. The tongue thruster usually exaggerates the postures and movements of the normal swallower, tipping the head too far forward, keeping the mouth wider open, and allowing the tongue to remain forward during drinking. To assist in retention of proper habits, I require him/her to go a bit beyond normal. I expect that in most patients eventually the teeth are again held slightly apart during drinking, but the tongue usually remains on the spot. Patients whose teeth are strongly affected by liquids of even moderate coldness are allowed to drink with the teeth unoccluded.

Exercise four: *Upper lip stretcher.* Lip exercises are discussed by Barrett in Chapter 17. This particular exercise is my mainstay. I feel that most lips are strong enough to create adequate pressure on the teeth, providing they can meet without undue strain or discomfort. Again I turn it into an isometric exercise.

LESSON 8   Date_____

Watch mirror closely!

1. Saliva moving and swallowing. Use a sugarless mint to stimulate the flow of saliva. Place the mint in the side of the mouth between the cheek and gums. Keep your tongue tip on the spot. Whenever you have enough saliva to swallow, bite your back teeth together, suck back with your lips closed and relaxed, and swallow. Do not chew the mint. Keep repeating this action until the mint is gone. Even after the mint is gone, let the taste that remains remind you to keep moving and swallowing your saliva right. Use the mirror occasionally to make sure your lips are *lightly* closed and no muscles of the face are used in swallowing. One mint each practice, three times a day.

2. Sip-at-a-time drinking. (1) Tongue on the spot. (2) Teeth together. (3) Take a *small* sip of water. (4) Close your lips and suck the water back. (5) Bite down, spread your lips wide and swallow. Fifteen times each practice.

3. If you began lip-stretching exercise last week, continue it.

4. Speech work: _____
   _____

5. Chewing and swallowing practice. Eat at least five *different* foods right each day, at meals, snacks, or both. Be sure to watch the mirror from bite to swallow. Spread your lips wide as you swallow. List the foods you practiced with on the Food Chart below.

Day	Foods				
1					
2					
3					
4					
5					
6					
7					

(Other charts provided.)

Exercise one: *Saliva moving and swallowing.* The patient is now weaned from the squirt bottle and practices with saliva instead of water. This is an assignment which is enjoyed by patients of all ages, and I find it to be very effective in habituating correct saliva moving and swallowing. If the patient and parents wish, more than three mints per day may be used.

Exercise two: *Sip-at-a-time drinking.* Often, the clinician explains, we do not drink continuously. When we drink something unusually hot, cold, or tasty, we take a sip, move the liquid back, then swallow. To make sure this is done properly, we include this instruction. This exercise is exactly the same as the quiet sucking the patient has been practicing for a week, except that instead of the liquid being squirted into the mouth, it is sipped. This is easy for most patients to learn.

Exercise three: *Lip stretching.* Work usually continues for at least a month.

Exercise four: *Speech work* is begun at about this point. I have not included instructions on the assignment sheet because they vary so much according to the individual's incorrect patterns. The use of the imaginary coil spring has been explained earlier. I begin, with patients who can read, with reading practice, rather than with words out of context. The patient is asked to slow down enough to give him/herself time to let the spring idea work. I watch the patient at an angle to see if the tongue really returns to the "spot" at every opportunity. Three practice sessions a day are assigned, for two or three minutes each time. The patient is to try to talk in that same way for a specified period of time after each practice.

Exercise five: *Chewing and swallowing practice.* Many of the older patients have found this to be so easy that they ask if they can eat everything right this week instead of only certain foods. Even the adults must spend some time each day watching the mirror closely, however, no matter how easy they say it is for them to eat correctly.

LESSON 9   Date _____

Watch mirror closely!

1. Eat and drink everything right. Keep the mirror on the table during all meals. If you have company, or eat away from home, swallow correctly, but keep the lips closed and don't use a mirror.

Write "+" if you ate and drank everything right: "part" for part right; and "−" when you did not eat anything right during the meal.

Day	Breakfast	Lunch	Dinner
1			
2			
3			
4			
5			
6			
7			

3. TV or reading. Drink about 8 ounces of liquids, a sip at a time, while reading or watching TV. Keep your attention on the TV or the book. Make the 8 ounces last the 30 minutes.

Write number of minutes per day:
1 _____ 2 _____ 3 _____
4 _____ 5 _____ 6 _____
          7 _____

2. Counting saliva swallows. Using your "counter," count at least 100 good saliva swallows each morning, 100 each afternoon, and 100 each evening (total of 300 a day). Write the number in the chart.

Day	Morning	Afternoon	Evening
1			
2			
3			
4			
5			
6			
7			

4. Continue lip-stretching if you have been assigned.
5. Speech work:_____
   _____
6. Think "swallow right" over and over as you go to sleep each night. Be sure your tongue stays on the spot and your lips remain closed until you fall asleep.
7. Posture reminders. If the ones you have been using are still helping you, continue to use them. If not, choose two new ones.
   Inside: _____ Outside: _____

Exercise one: Everything the patient eats and drinks should be handled correctly.

At this point the patient should be able to swallow liquids, solids, and saliva effortlessly, and we begin to emphasize habit-strengthening, by means of the following three exercises.

Exercise two: *Counting saliva swallows.* Most patients enjoy this assignment, because it gives them visible evidence that they are swallowing correctly a number of times per day. Those who find it inconvenient to have a pocket counter handy are not required to use it, but the responsibility for *knowing* that a significant percentage of saliva swallows daily are being carried out

correctly is given to them. Most children can obtain permission from their teachers at school to use the counter. If it is embarrassing for them to do so, again, the requirement is modified. Some will keep a record on a piece of paper, and others prefer to double up on the assignment before and after school.

Exercise three: *TV or reading.* This assignment is explained by Barrett in Chapter 23. I have not altered it.

Exercise four: The assignment to think about swallowing right while going to sleep is also explained by Barrett in Chapter 23. I use it exactly as he describes.

LESSON 10   Date_____

1. Swallow all food and liquids correctly, watching the mirror and spreading your lips for food swallows when at home.
2. Continue the TV or reading assignment, as in Lesson 9.
3. Count at least _____ saliva swallows every day. Be sure to move the saliva correctly. Write the number in the following chart.
4. If you think it would be helpful, ask a friend to signal you when your lips are resting apart.
5. Place one of the tiny elastics I've given you (don't use any others) on your tongue tip when you go to bed at night. Try to keep your tongue on the spot and your lips closed all night. Repeat to yourself, over and over, as you go to sleep, "I will swallow right all night." In the morning, either check yourself, or have someone check you, to see whether the tongue is on the spot, the elastic is still on the tongue tip, and the lips are closed when you awaken. Keep track of the number of successes.
6. Fill out the chart below each night, using either percent signs or the following abbreviations: A= all the time; NA= nearly always; ½; S= some (less than ½); and VL= very little.
7. Speech or lip exercises:_____
_____

Date														
Saliva swallows														

Dates														
1. Mouth closed at rest														
2. Tongue on spot at rest														
3. Proper chewing														
4. Food swallows														
5. Drinking														
6. Saliva gathering														
7. Saliva swallowing														

The three assignments just referred to are continued, with whatever alterations might be needed or helpful for motivation. Instead of simply thinking about swallowing right while going to sleep, the patient attempts to keep a tiny, thin-walled orthodontic elastic on the tip of his tongue during sleep. My requirement is only that the patient try this for about four weeks, and keep a record of his success with it. Patients who have any objection to doing this are not required to use the elastic.

Those who do not seem to have success with the elastic assignment are later given one or both of the following alternate assignments:

1. The parent talks to the patient as he/she sleeps, repeating whatever suggestions may be applicable several times without totally awakening the patient.

2. The patient records on a cassette a message repeatedly at ten-second intervals, which he/she plays while going to sleep.

Progress chart. During this lesson I talk to the patient about systematically transferring the responsibility for making assignments to him. I explain that I can't continue to give assignments so the patient must learn to become his own clinician. The first step in this process is for the patient to become very much *aware* of his swallowing and associated behaviors. To help him to do this, the chart in Lesson 10 has been provided. The chart can help the patient in three ways:

1. Knowing the chart must be filled out each night gives the patient a reason to be aware during the day of seven items it contains. If the goal of increased awareness is to be reached, he must pay some attention to all seven activities each day.

2. Each night as he marks the chart, there will be certain items that receive lower marks than others. These items, along with items which the patient is uncertain what score to give, are the ones which should receive special attention the next day. In this way, no activity will be neglected two days in a row.

3. Percentages or letter-scores should improve as the days go by. The improvement shown on the chart serves as a good motivator for the patient.

Saliva swallow counting. In keeping with the principle discussed relative to the above chart, the patient is asked how may saliva swallows he would like to self-assign for the next couple of weeks. (I begin seeing the patient at this point at gradually longer intervals of time.)

Speech and/or lip exercises are continued if appropriate.

Visits from this point are called "rechecks," and are very much individualized. I have prepared handouts for the first three rechecks, but they are as often unused as used.

RECHECK VISITS

First recheck   Date: _____

1. Swallow all food correctly. Watch the mirror for all chewing and swallowing at home. Spread your lips wide during the first three swallows at each breakfast and dinner. For all other food swallows keep the lips very lightly closed.
2. Count at least _____ saliva swallows each day.
3. Continue to use Daily Progress Chart. Try to reach each five-day goal, then never drop below it.
4. Continue "I will swallow right all night" with elastic. If you have not had success with the elastic, have your parent talk to you about swallowing right after you're asleep, as I have explained.
5. Speech or other assignments: _____
_____

(Two charts are provided. The first is similar to the seven-item chart in Lesson 10, but with every fifth column marked "goal." The second is for recording number of saliva swallows counted.)

At every recheck I observe swallows of food, liquid, and saliva. With each recheck it becomes more and more essential to refer back to the diagnostic sheet so you will know what habits the patient may be returning to.

Patients who have done extremely well on the daily progress chart from the last lesson are ordinarily not required to continue the "goal" chart. Other patients, with the help of the clinician, set five-day goals representing small, attainable daily increments. I expect 100% on all functions related to eating and drinking, and from 95% to 98% on saliva and resting habits.

Second recheck   Date: _____

For the next month you are to choose two assignments, activities, or exercises from any of Lesson 6 through 10 to be done each day of the week. Vary the activities so that all four areas (food, liquid, saliva, and resting postures) will get attention.

For example: On Mondays you might do quiet sucking with a straw, plus watching the mirror as you eat dinner. On Tuesday, use a sugarless mint, plus watch the mirror every time you drink at home. On Wednesday, do the night swallow assignment, plus count saliva swallows. And so on.

Fill in the "Weekly Maintenance Chart" tonight, listing the exercise for each of two assignments for each day of the week. KEEP THE CHART WHERE YOU CAN'T HELP BUT SEE IT OFTEN!

The patient is assigned to choose two assignments for each day of the week. A chart is provided, in which the patient lists assignments for entire week. Assignments which seem particularly beneficial to the patient may be repeated during the week. Since the next appointment is probably a month away, he has the option to change assignments during the month as needs change. This provides a relatively palatable way of maintaining awareness, and continues to give the patient more responsibility for making self-assignments.

At about this point in therapy, I test the patient's progress with some kind of squirt test. The patient either counts backwards from 100 to about 60 and swallows whenever the clinician squirts water into his/her mouth, or attempts to handle the "squirts" as they occur more and more rapidly. Patients whose saliva-handling habits are not correct automatically have difficulty with either of these tasks.

It is also here that I routinely measure anterior malocclusions to see whether there has been any change since the initial visit.

Third recheck   Date: _____

For the next six weeks you will continue to keep a maintenance chart, but instead of doing two things every day, you will do only one (unless I've indicated otherwise).

(A chart similar to the one in the second recheck is provided, but with only a single line for each day of the week.)

The patient who has done reasonably well

with the two-item maintenance chart from the last recheck visit is assigned to make a new chart, this one having only one assignment for each day. To repeat an important point, assignments given at rechecks vary considerably. If everything is going well, the patient will not be seen for six weeks. He is free to modify assignments during that time, just so proper records are kept.

Subsequent visits

Patients who are not going to have orthodontic work done are seen at gradually increasing intervals. Typical intervals after the third recheck for such patients would be six weeks, two months, three months, six months, six months, one year, and one year. Orthodontic patients would be seen at similar intervals, *or* at any time significant changes occurred, such as bands applied or removed, a positioner or retainer inserted or removed, etc. Patients are always seen before the retainer is discontinued. Measurements are again taken as a reference for subsequent movement of teeth.

CONCLUSION

By the time this revised edition is published, the therapy described in the present chapter will have been altered in several ways. The *principles* underlying the lessons and assignments, though, will probably still be being followed.

Every exercise and assignment will have a definite, important purpose. Behavioral changes will be achieved in systematic steps. Organismic principles will be applied. Therapy will be individualized, based on carefully obtained baseline measures and observations. Personalized motivational techniques will continue to be the most essential ingredients for success in treatment. Any new approaches gleaned from colleagues or from the literature which seem promising will be incorporated in my therapy, and, admittedly, evaluated fairly subjectively before being rejected or accepted as a part of routine treatment.

Appendix 1

FORMS USED IN THERAPY

CASE HISTORY FORM

Form A-1 is a form used by Hanson. It can be mimeographed on standard 8½ by 11 inch paper, using both sides of the sheet. It provides specific space for each important bit of datum, preventing oversights and giving a clear visual picture of the case on the face of the form. The reverse side is a record of therapy from the first consultation through the recheck period.

Form A-2 is used by Barrett. It is printed on 5 by 8 inch cards, one side only. It provides basically the same material, except that only pertinent details are noted under "Other conditions," "Remarks," etc. The back of the card offers space to record additional therapy sessions and progress through the recheck period.

LETTER TO PARENTS

Form A-3 is mimeographed on a letterhead and given to parents at the time of their initial interview. It has been found to prevent many later problems when actually read by both parents. Merely explaining this material, rather than sending it home in print, has not been found as effective and requires more time. Many other details were once included, making for a letter of such overpowering length that it was seldom read.

Some of the material deleted from the letter was later incorporated in a pamphlet, *So You Have a Tongue Thrust!* which Barrett prints and distributes in bulk to referral sources to simplify and speed up the referral process itself. The dentist need only hand the pamphlet to a patient rather than take the time to explain and to answer the inevitable queries about tongue thrust.

REPORT FORMS

As soon as the patient has actually appeared for the first appointment, it is helpful to send a card such as Form A-4 so that the referral source may know that referral is complete. When two or three sessions have been completed, and the clinician has some basis for evaluating the situation, a report such as Form A-5 should be completed. Two of them can be mimeographed on a single 8½ by 11 inch sheet and the halves cut apart.

As soon as possible after the first recheck, a report such as Form A-6 should be sent. They also fit two to a page, but their import is more readily recognized if printed on colored paper as discussed in Chapter 12.

REST POSTURE CHART

When additional procedures are found to be necessary during the recheck period, it is advisable to supply the patient with a chart such as that shown in Form A-7. A minimum period of three or four weeks will usually be assigned, during which the patient will not see the clinician. Consistency of performance is increased when a daily record of completion is required. Of course, the chart should be returned on the subsequent visit.

SUCKING HABIT CALENDAR

The use of Form A-8 on p. 365 is described in Chapter 16. It is printed on a full 8½ by 11 inch sheet, to facilitate the insertion of numbers with blunt crayons and to provide enough weeks so that success might be expected before the spaces are exhausted.

Name _____ Birthdate _____ Today's date _____

Address _____ Phone _____ Father _____

Mother _____ Occupation _____

Referred by _____ Siblings _____

Previous therapy _____ Digit sucking _____

Other habits _____ Allergies _____

Mouth breathing _____ Tonsils _____

Tongue: Large _____ Poor movement _____ Short frenum _____ Normal _____

Mentalis: Contracted _____ Normal _____ Large chin button _____

Upper lip: Short _____ Flaccid _____ Normal _____

Lower lip: Tight _____ Flaccid _____ Normal _____

Hard palate: High _____ Narrow _____ Low and flat _____ Normal _____

Soft palate: Short _____ Poor movement _____ Normal _____

Occlusion: Class _____ Overjet _____ Measured at _____

      Overbite _____ Measured at _____ Diastemata _____ Measured at

      _____ Missing teeth _____

      Tongue posture _____

Speech _____ Eating habits _____

	Lip activity	Mentalis	Masseter	Thrust
Solids:	_____	_____	_____	_____
Liquids:	_____	_____	_____	_____
Saliva:	_____	_____	_____	_____
Diagnosis:	_____	_____	_____	_____

Diagnosis: _____

_____

Comments: _____

_____

Recommendations: _____

_____

Continued.

Form A-1

Consultation: Explanation given? _____

                Motivation Talk _____ Materials _____

Therapy sessions:

First _____

Second _____

Third _____

Fourth _____

Fifth _____

Sixth _____

Seventh _____

Eighth _____

Ninth _____

Rechecks:

First _____

Second _____

Third _____

Fourth _____

Fifth _____

Others _____

Reports sent:

Diagnostic _____ Progress _____

_____ _____ Final report _____

Fee _____ Payments _____

Date	Paid	Balance	Date	Paid	Balance
_____	_____	_____	_____	_____	_____
_____	_____	_____	_____	_____	_____
_____	_____	_____	_____	_____	_____

Form A-1, cont'd

Name _____ Age _____ Date _____

Address _____ Phone _____

Referred by _____ Parent _____

Occupation _____ Marital status _____

Siblings _____

_____

Tonsils and adenoids _____ Allergies _____

Emotional status _____ Sucking habit _____

Other conditions _____

Infant feeding _____ Walked _____ First words _____

Orthodontics _____

Swallowing type _____ Occlusion _____

Gag reflex _____ Speech _____

TMJ pain _____ Crepitus _____ Headache _____

Remarks _____

_____

1st _____ 2nd _____

3rd _____ 4th _____

5th _____ 6th _____

7th _____ 8th _____

Form A-2

DEAR PARENT:

Experience shows that if you are aware of the few brief bits of information below, correction may be more certain and easy.

SUPERVISION: Patients of any age are NEVER seen unless accompanied by an observer, for a majority of the necessary exercises cannot be adequately performed without supervision. Oh, the joys of parenthood!

APPOINTMENTS: Missing an appointment or two leads to much additional practice, results in loss of interest and often actual resentment on the part of a child, and in every case places a serious doubt on the eventual outcome. For your sake, as well as mine, please avoid cancellations. A charge will be made for appointments broken without 24-hour notice. It looks so foolish for a grown man to twiddle his thumbs!

FEES: Sessions will vary from 30 to 90 minutes, depending on the tasks to be completed each week. A charge of $ is made for each session, regardless of length, since each is one step in the total therapy program. If extra sessions are required, they are charged at the same rate. Should we finish in the usual eight weeks, the total cost would be $, but THIS IS NOT A FLAT FEE. Should it be necessary to eliminate a sucking habit before therapy starts, an additional charge of $ is made. It is customary to pay for each session as it is received, but in any event your account is to be paid in full by the final therapy session. We all have our problems.

RECHECKS: The above fee includes the cost of such rechecks as may be necessary. THESE CHECKUPS ARE VERY IMPORTANT. If you return for rechecks at the appointed times, and additional work proves necessary, such work will be done without charge for a maximum of three sessions; this promise CANNOT be kept if you delay more than one week in returning as scheduled. This topic is seldom a source of humor around here!

FUTURE PATIENTS: Of course we love little brothers and sisters! It's just that we think they should not be in the therapy room until they are old enough to profit thereby. This project requires rather intense concentration during the short time you are here each week, and the little ones do distract! Baby-sitters usually charge less than we do, and experience shows that sessions often must be repeated if little sister falls in the waste can or turns out to be a faster talker than the therapist. Besides, she is invariably cuter.

Please feel free to ask questions at any time about any aspect of the program; we may not know the answer, but we'll think of something. And thanks for taking the trouble to read this.

Form A-3

ALLOW ME TO THANK YOU FOR HAVING REFERRED

_____

TO ME FOR PROFESSIONAL SERVICES.

R. H. BARRETT
1645 NORTH ALVERNON - - TUCSON, ARIZONA 85712
TELEPHONE 793-1101

Form A-4

**NAME OF
CLINICIAN**

TO _____ DATE _____

_____ has now received _____ therapy

sessions for tongue thrust and has completed work on _____ step of eight-step

program. Cooperation has been _____ and prognosis is

_____.

Thank you very much,

Form A-5

**NAME OF
CLINICIAN**

TO _____ DATE _____

_____ has now been seen for _____ ses-

sions, has completed the therapy program, and was rechecked three weeks after com-

pletion. _____ has accordingly been released from active therapy but will

be kept under observation for a time. The next recheck is scheduled for _____.

Thank you very much,

Form A-6

First week						
Second week						
Third week						
Fourth week						

Form A-7

Name

Month

Sunday	Monday	Tuesday	Wednesday	Thursday	Friday	Saturday

Form A-8

Appendix 2

MATERIALS AND SOURCES OF SUPPLY

A comparatively small amount of material is required to begin tongue-thrust correction. However, much time and travel may be spent in seeking out some of the items that are not standard equipment in either dentistry or speech pathology.

The following list is offered merely as a possibility. Some of the materials may be more readily available from a different source in a particular area, or a substitute product may be preferred. It may seem superfluous to mention some items, but at least with these materials at hand, you may confidently throw wide the door to all comers.

Instead of listing each item alphabetically, it seems more functional to group those which are available from a single source. The remaining items will be alphabetized thereafter.

From the dental supply company
Cotton rolls: sizes No. 2 (small) and No. 3 (large), both in 1½-inch length, usually packaged 2000 per carton.
Elastics: ⁵/₁₆ or ¼ inch, thick wall, packaged in various amounts.
From the medical or surgical supply
Applicator sticks: standard 6-inch length. Inexpensive, several uses.
Eye-flushing bottle (syringe): Zeigler, preferably with full curve of syringe tip; with tip offset only slightly, syringe drips and is messy.
An alternative is to acquire a number of polyethylene squeeze bottles 4 to 8 ounces in capacity. These are available with hose, cap, and nozzle molded in a single piece. They are less convenient in daily use, probably have a less professional appearance and are more difficult to sterilize unless each patient is given his personal bottle. They are sold by scientific supply companies.
Finger cots: tissue, may be offered in small, medium, large; packaged one gross per box.
Glass storage jars: 7-inch height (2) for tongue depressors and applicator sticks; 3-inch height (2) for finger cots and manometer mouthpieces. May be more convenient in 3-inch diameter rather than 4-inch or 5-inch diameter, although one of the latter of 4-inch height is convenient for storing elastics.
Tongue depressors: standard 6-inch length.
Oral manometer components (Chapter 17): connectors (2) made for ¼-inch rubber tubing; glass tubing: ¼-inch outside dimension, 3- or 4-foot length; plastic or rubber stoppers (2): No. 10, 2-hole size.
From a plastics distributing company (if available)
Polyethylene sheets: 0.030-inch thickness, low density, for making oral screen.
Polyethylene tubing: ¼-inch inside diameter, to connect bottles of oral manometer and for mouthpieces.
Rigid-wall tubing: ¼-inch outside diameter, substitute for glass tubing in manometer.
From a scientific supply company
Acquisition of many items (squeeze bottles, glass and plastic tubing, rubber stoppers, etc.) may be expedited if you have access to a scientific apparatus and equipment concern. Almost any university or high school chemistry teacher is a source of information as to which companies operate in your locality. Larger companies, such as VWR Scientific, have outlets nationwide and even internationally. Some of them are willing to sell the relatively small amounts needed by the myotherapist.

From the supermarket
Cooky jar
Paper cups and wall dispenser
Straws, preferably striped and flexible
Sugarless wafers, package of assorted flavors
Tissue, facial type
Miscellaneous
Anti-snore mask: Many prescription pharmacies have them in stock, or write to manufacturer: Winco Affiliates, Inc., 310-328 Dean St., Brooklyn, N. Y. 11217.
Bio-My Products, P. O. Box 154, Fallbrook, Calif.

92028, for Bio-My Master and Satellite, Lip-Ex, etc.

Bottles for oral manometer: Approximately 1-pint capacity, 1¾-inch mouth. May be found in variety store or in housewares section of other stores. Empty pill bottles from drugstore, as described in Chapter 17, may be substituted.

Coin envelopes: From stationery or office supply store. A small size, 2¼ by 3½ inches, is adequate for elastics, lip discs, etc. A large size, 2½ by 4¼ inches, is more appropriate for oral screen and other uses. Packaged 500 per box, may be purchased in smaller quantities.

Flat wooden stirrers: Any type will serve. Available at restaurant supply or ice cream manufacturer. Some appear to be reject Popsicle sticks. Packaged 1000 per box; send home plenty.

Lip discs: From the toy store. Available only occasionally; if you find them, buy plenty.

Penlight: From drugstore or other store. Two-cell type with size AA batteries and positive "on-off" switch is preferred.

Plaster models: Myotherapists may request the orthodontist to run an extra set of models of unusual patients. A number of companies supply sets displaying a variety of malocclusions—some, unknowingly, the result of tongue thrust—as well as normal deciduous and permanent dentition. One such company is Columbia Dentoforms, 49 E. 21st St., New York, N. Y. 10010. This company can also supply greatly enlarged models that hold the attention of children and make explanations easier.

Plastic tubing: In areas where no plastics distributor is accessible, the ¼-inch polyethylene tubing can usually be found at a hardware store. Other possibilities are companies that service refrigeration units, and some foreign car dealers.

Stomahesive: Best bet is orthopedic shop, but may also be found at medical supply or drug store.

Wax bottles: Used in program for sucking habits. Ideally, obtained from wholesale candy distributor. Otherwise, try the candy counter in variety stores or other candy displays. In some localities it may be necessary to ask a retail store to place them on special order.

AUTHOR INDEX

A

Akamine, J. S., 143
Andersen, W. S., 116, 128, 133
Angle, E. H., 28-29, 106
Ardran, G. M., 105, 128, 135
Aungst, L. F., 124
Azrin, N. H., 218

B

Ballard, C. F., 104-105
Barber, T. K., 156
Baril, C., 128
Barrett, R. H., 155, 176, 201
Begg, P. R., 140
Bell, D., 128, 134
Berry, M. F., 14
Bloomer, H. H., 16
Bonus, H. W., 156
Bosma, J. F., 124-127
Brader, A. C., 146
Brauer, J. S., 172
Brodie, A. G., 108

C

Carr, D. T., 119
Case, J. L., 154-155
Christofferson, S., 158
Cleall, J. F., 139, 199
Cohen, M. S., 116, 118, 120, 128-130, 133, 148-149
Collins, T. A., 199
Costen, J. B., 95
Croce, G., 148
Crowder, H. M., 202

D

Davidian, C., 214
Deasy, M. J., 140
Dreyer, C. J., 140

E

Eisenson, J., 14
Eversaul, G. A., 209

F

Falk, M. L., 208-209
Findlay, I. A., 128
Fisher, N. D., 215

Fletcher, S. G., 128, 133, 135
Fuhrer, A. V., 214

G

Gellin, M. E., 214
Gianelli, A. A., 139, 140, 147
Gingold, N. L., 215
Goda, S., 204
Goldman, H. N., 139, 140, 147
Goodhart, G. J., 209
Graber, T. M., 26-28, 151, 200
Gwynne-Evans, E., 103

H

Hale, A., 128, 134
Hanna, J. C., 116
Hanson, M. L., 116, 118-120, 128-130, 133, 148-149
Hanson, T. E., 119
Harvold, E. P., 148
Hedges, R. B., 135
Herman, E., 98
Hoffman, J. A., 8, 154
Hoffman, R. L., 8, 154
Holik, F., 120
Holt, T. V., 172
Hooker, D., 124

K

Kaye, S. R., 199
Kemp, S. H., 105, 135
Kent, J. N., 201
Kesling, P. C., 140
Kilpatrick, S. J., 128
Klein, E. T., 109, 212
Kopp, G. A., 131
Kydd, W. L., 138, 142

L

Lambert, C. G., 202
Lear, C. S. C., 141, 142-145, 146
Leech, H. L., 105, 120
Lind, J., 105
Linder-Aronson, S., 215
Lischer, B. E., 22, 106
Littman, J. Y, 199

M

McDonald, E. T., 124
McGlone, R. E., 145
McWilliams, R. R., 201
Milne, I. M., 139
Moorrees, C. F. A., 142-145
Moss, J. P., 138
Moyers, R. E., 22, 110, 128, 135, 175

N

Najera, A., 115-116, 118
Nanda, R. S., 215
Neff, C. W., 138
Negri, P. L., 148
Neumann, B., 200
Nunn, R. G., 218

O

Overstake, C. P., 155-156

P

Palmer, G. L, 202
Palmer, J. M., 123
Pang, A., 98
Parker, J. H., 98
Paul, J. L., 215
Penzer, V., 139
Picard, C. J., 114
Pierce, R. B., 205
Posen, A. L., 140, 214
Proffit, W. R., 138, 141, 142, 146, 147

R

Rathbone, J. S., 15
Reding, G. R., 216
Reitan, K., 139, 147
Ricketts, R. M., 111, 215
Riedel, R. A., 139
Ringel, R. L., 123, 124
Rix, R. E., 103, 137
Robson, J. E., 156-158
Rogers, A. P., 107, 254
Rubright, W. C., 216

S

Sakuda, M., 154
Salzmann, J. A., 22
Scott, J. H., 135
Secter, L. L., 202
Shelton, R., 149

Shepard, R. S., 210
Silcox, B. L., 124
Smernoff, G. N., 146
Snow, K., 15
Sood, S., 215
Stansell, B., 155
Strang, R. H. W., 108, 119
Straub, W. J., 109, 114, 175
Strayer, E. R., 98
Subtelny, J. D., 138, 150, 154
Swinehart, D. R., 140

T

Thompson, W. M., 119
Toda, J. M., 142
Toronto, A., 98, 158
Toth, S., 208
Truesdell, B., 107
Truesdell, F. B., 107
Tulley, W. J., 75, 105, 133, 135

V

Van Riper, C., 12
Verma, S., 215
Vogel, R. I., 140
von Dedenroth, T. E., 155

W

Walker, R. V., 199
Wallen, T. R., 143
Warren, D. W., 215
Warren, E., 214
Warvi, V., 205
Watson, R. M., 120, 215
Wechsler, D., 218
Weinberg, B., 133, 135
Weinstein, A., 141
Wells, M., 208
Werlich, E. P., 128, 133, 137
Whitman, C. L., 109
Wiesner, G. R., 98
Wilskie, G. H., 142

Z

Zickefoose, W. E., 208
Zimmerman, S. O., 216

SUBJECT INDEX

A

Abnormal swallowing, 172-175
Abrasion, 32
Acrylic, 38
Activator, 38-39
Adenoid facies, 104
Adenoids, 240-241
  as cause of tongue thrust, 119
Age in treatment, 222
Aids, mechanical, 308
Ala, 81
Allergies, 119-120, 241
  respiratory, 98
Alveolar process, 18, 32, 58
Alveolus, 32
American Dental Association, 29
Anatomy, 52-80
  dental, 18
Anchorage, 50
Andresen appliance, 38-39, 200
Anesthetic throat, 120-121
Angle classification system, 28-29
Ankyloglossia, 32
Anodontia, 32
Anterior open bite, 15
Anterior seal, 286-288
Antisnore mask, 327, 366
Anti-tongue thrust appliance, disadvantages of, 200-201
Apical base, 32
  foramen, 18, 33
Aponeurosis, 81
  palatine, 78
Appliance therapy, 198-200
Appliances, orthodontic, 37-44, 326-327
  fixed, 42-44
  reminder, 199
  removable, 38-42
Applicator sticks, 366
Arch, palatal, examination of, 191-192
Arch wire, 42
Arthritis, of temporomandibular joint, 94
Articular meniscus, 54
Articulation of teeth, 33
Articulatory disorders, functional, 13
Atmospheric force, 90
Atrophy, 81

Attitudes, maternal, 233
Attrition, 33
Axioversion, 22

B

Back-tongue lifting exercise, 344
Balloons, in therapy, 250
Band, orthodontic, 42
Banding, of teeth, 47-48
Basal ganglia, 63
Base line, establishment of, 207, 335-336
Begg light wire technique, 43
Behavior modification, 335-339
  therapy, 205-208
Bicuspid, 33
Bilabial gymnastics, 255
Bilabial opposition, 252
Bimler appliance, 39
Biofeedback, 209-210
Bio-My-Master, 248
Bionator, 200
Bite, occlusion, 27
Bite plane, 40
Bite plate, 40, 107
Biting exercise, 342
Black light technique, 187-188
Blade, positioning tongue, 270-271
Bodily movement of teeth, 49
Bonding
  direct, 48
  indirect, 48
Bones, 54-59
  cranial, 55-57
  hyoid, 59
  maxillary, 58
  nasal, 57-58
  palatine, 58
Bottle feeding, 114-116
Brackets, 42
Brain, 60
  injury, 121
  stem, 64-65
Breast feeding, 114-116
Bribery, 230-231
Bruxism, 8, 33, 216-217
  treatment of, 216-217

Buccal, 33
   surface, 20
Buccinator, 81
   muscle, 72
Button exercise, 251

C

Cage, 198-199
Calendar for sucking habits, 358, 365
Canine, tooth, 33
Caninus, 72
Cartilage, 81
   types of, 54
Case history form, 358-361
Cassette program, 208
Caudad, 53
Cellophane tape, 327
Cementum, 18, 33
Central incisor, 33
Central nervous system, 59-64
Centric occlusion, 26
Cephalad, 53
Cephalometrics, 44
Cerebellum, 63-65, 81
Cerebral cortex, 62-63
Cerebrum, 60-62, 82
Cervical strap, 41
Cervical vertebrae, 59
Charts
   percentage, 338-339
   plus-minus, 337
   rest posture, 358, 364
Cheek sucking, 7
Chewing, 170-171, 335
Chewing exercise, 348
Chin pullup exercise, 252
Cilia, 82
Cinefluorograph, 105
Cingulum, 33
Class I occlusion, 28
Class II occlusion, 28
Class III occlusion, 29
   speech, 16
Classical conditioning, 206
Classification, angle system of, 28-29
Classification of tongue thrust, 175-183
Clicking of temporomandibular joint, 94
Clinician, obligations of, 226-227
Closure
   lip, 267-268
   tooth, 267
Conditioning
   classical, 206
   operant, 206
Condyle, 33, 82
Condyloid process, 58
Connective tissue, 53
Consonants
   dentalization of, 7, 335
   dentalized correction of, 339
   order of learning of, 10-11
Contraction, types of muscle, 70
Contralateral, 82
Controversies in tongue thrust, overview of, 4-5
Convolutions, cerebral, 61
Coronoid, 58

Corpus callosum, 60-61
Cortex, cerebral, 62-63
Cotton rolls, 255-256
   description of, 366
Counters, pocket, 338
Cranial bones, 55-57
Cranial nerves, 66
Crepitus, 33, 94
Cribriform, 82
Crossbite, 15, 27
Crown of tooth, 32
Crozat appliance, 40-42
Curtain, 199
Cusp, 21, 34
Cuspid, 34
Cytology, 53

D

Deciduous tooth, 34
Decussate, 82
Decussation, pyramidal, 65
Deglutition, 82; *see also* Swallowing
Delayed speech, 14
Dental
   anatomy, 18
   assistants as oral myotherapists, 6
   development, 22-25
   hygienists as oral myotherapists, 6
   treatment as cause of relapse, 332-333
Dentalization
   of consonants, 7, 335
   of linguoalveolar sounds, 14
Dentistry
   fundamentals of, 18-32
   general, and myofunctional disorders, 162
   preventive, 5
Dentists
   and oral myofunctional disorders, 5
   responsibility of, in treatment, 225
Dentition
   and speech, relationships between, 15-16
   mixed, 25
Dento-alveolar joint, 19
Development
   dental, 22-25
   of normal patterns, deterrents to, 127-128
   of speech, 9-11
Developmental changes
   in infancy and early childhood, 126-127
   in later childhood, 128-130
Developmental theory of tongue thrust, 124-126
Deviant deglutition, 137
Deviate swallow, 137
Deviated septum, 212
Diagnosis, 187-195
Diagnostic
   procedures, 189-195
   questions, 187-189
Diastema, 34
Diet, soft, as cause of tongue thrust, 121-122
Digastric muscle, 81
Direct bonding, 48
Discs, plastic, 325-326
Dislocation of temporomandibular joint, 93-94
Disorders
   of articulation, 13

Disorders—cont'd
  of speech, 11-14
Distal, 34, 82
  surface, 20
Distocclusion, 28
Distoversion, 22
Dorsal, 53, 82
Drinking
  continuous, 298, 349
  from cup, 290
  rapid, 298
  from straw, 290
Dysarthria, 12

E

Eccentric occlusion, 26
Ectopic eruption, 34
Edentulous, 34
Edgewise wire, 43
Elastics, 324-325
  use at night, 317-318
Electroencephalography, 105
Embrasure, 34
Embryology, 82
Emotional problems, in children with sucking habits,
  230
Emotional status of patient, 241
Enamel, 34
Endodontics, 34
Epiphysis, 82
Equilibration, 165
  of teeth, 31
Eruption
  forces of, 88
  teeth, sequence of, 24-25
Ethmoid bone, 57
Etiologies
  of malocclusion, 27-28
  of tongue thrust, 114-131
Evaluation of speech, 328
Examination
  final, 330-331
  oral peripheral, 246-247
Exercises for repositioning lips, 239-258
Existence of tongue thrust, 133-135
Expansion devices, 45
Extension of stimulus control, 337
External pterygoid muscle, 74-75
Extractions, 45
Extraoral appliance, 40-41
Extrapyramidal system, 65
Extrusion, 34
Eyedropper test, 318-319
Eye-flushing bottle, 366

F

Facet, 34
Facial movement, extraneous, 261
Facial network of muscles, forces of, 88-89
Facies, adenoid, 104
Facilitation, neuromuscular, 339
Falk program, 208-209
Fasciculus, 82
Fauces, 82
  pillars of, 78
Faucial isthmus, 78

Fence, 199
Final examination, 330-331
Finger sucking, 7
Fissure, 82
  cerebral, 61
  of Rolando, 61
  of Sylvius, 61
Food swallowing, 335
Foramen, 82
  apical, 18
Forced air exercise, 254
Forces
  atmospheric, 90
  intermittent vs. constant, 146-148
  of occlusion, 86-87
  optimal for moving teeth, 50
  on teeth, 86-90
Forms used in therapy, 358-365
Fossa of tooth, 34
Fossae of teeth, 21, 34
Fragmentation, 223
Frankel appliance, 39
Frenectomy, lingual, 247
Frenum, 34
  labial, 30
  lingual, 247
Frontal bone, 55-56
Fusiform, 82

G

Gag reflex, 192-193, 246
Ganglion, 69
Gap-filling tendency, 118-119
Gargling, 319
Genetic influence on swallowing, 117-118
Genioglossus muscle, 76, 163
Geniohyoid muscle, 81
Gimmicks, 231-232
Gingiva, 19, 34
Gingivitis, mouth breathing and, 167
Glossal, 82
Glossary
  of anatomical terms, 81-85
  of dental terms, 32-36
Glottis, 82
Gnathodynamic system, 162
Gnathology, 35
Grinding of teeth, 8
Grooves of teeth, 21
Group therapy, 242-243

H

Habits
  sleeping, 123
  sucking, 228-238
Handicapped patients, 222-223
Hawley retainer, 40
Hay rake, 198
Headgear, 326
Hearing loss, 14
Histology, 53
Homeostasis, 83
Hyaline cartilage, 54
Hyoglossus muscle, 77
Hyoid bone, 59
Hypernasality, 14

Hyperplasia, 35
Hypertrophy, 35
Hypnosis, 201-202, 308
Hyponasality, 14
Hypothalamus, 63

I

Icing, 340
Incidence of speech defects, 12-13
Incidence of tongue thrust, 134-135
Incisal edge, 20
Incisal papilla, 35
Incisor, central, 33
Inclined planes of teeth, 21
Infantile swallow, 137
Infraversion, 22
Infundibulum, 83
Initial interview, 224
Instruments, musical, effects of playing, 98-100
Integument, 83
Interceptive orthodontics, 30-31
Internal pterygoid muscle, 74
Intrinsic, 83
Ipsilateral, 83
Isometric exercises, 337
Isthmus, faucial, 78

J

Joint, temporomandibular, 25-26; *see* Temporoman-
    dibular joint
    analysis of, 45
Jug, plastic, 251

K

"K" exercise, 279-282, 344
Kinesiology, 209
Kinesthetic pattern recognition, 124

L

Labial frenum, 30
Labioglossal seal, 261
Labioversion, 22
Lalling, 13
Lateral lisp, 13-14
Lessons, used by Hanson, 330-357
Leukoplakia, 35
Levator veli palatini, 79
Lingual
    frenectomy, 247
    frenum, 247
    seal, testing, 288-289
    surface, 20, 35
Linguoversion, 22
Lip
    biting, 7, 217
    closure, 267-268
    discs, 367
    exercises, 239-258, 348
        for repositioning, 253-256
    habits, 217-218
    licking, 7, 217
"Lip-Ex," 326-327
Lipstick exercise, 254-255
Liquids, drinking hot and cold, 290-291
Liquid swallows, 194-195

Lisp
    lateral, 13-14
    occluded, 14
    types of, 13-14
Luxation, 35

M

Macroglossia, 120, 162
Maintenance program, 339
Malocclusion, 35
    etiology of, 27-28
    and oral habits, 214-215
    relationship to tongue thrust, 137-138
    and speech defects, 12
Mandible, 58-59, 83
    prognathic, 163
Manometer, oral, 249
Masseter
    exercise for, 342
    muscle, 271
Mastication, 170-171
    and abnormal swallowing, 173
    muscles of, 73-75
Materials, 366-367
    therapy, 294-295
Maturation, effects on tongue thrust, 150
Maxilla, 83
Maxillary bones, 58
Maxillary protrusion, 15
Mechanical aids, 308
Mechanical stimulators, 253
Medulla, 83
Medulla oblongata, 64
Membrane
    periodontal, 18-19
    synovial, 54
Meniscus, 83
Mentalis muscle, 73
Mesial, 35
    drift, 50
        forces of, 89-90
    surface, 20
Mesiocclusion, 29
Mesioversion, 22
Microglossia, 120
Midbrain, 64
Mint, sugarless, 350-351
Mixed dentition, 25
    open spaces during, 118-119
Models of teeth, 37
Modifying behavior, 207-208
Molar occlusion, 262, 271-272
Morphology, 83
Mothers, blasé, 260
Mouth breathing, 8, 97-98, 193, 215-216
    as a cause of tongue thrust, 120
    treatment of, 216
Movement of teeth, 49-50
Mucous membrane
    of nasal cavity, 97
    oral, 19
Muscles, 69-81
    attachment of, 70
    classification of, 70
    of expression, 70-73
    of mastication, 73-75

Muscles—cont'd
  of the neck, 79-81
  nerve supply, 70
  of the soft palate, 77-79
  of the tongue, 75-79
    extrinsic, 75-77
    intrinsic, 75-76
  types of contraction of, 70
Musical instruments, effects of playing, 98-100
Mylohyoid muscle, 81
Myo-, 83
Myofascial pain-dysfunction syndrome, 95
Myology, 69-81
Myotherapy, 152

N

Nail biting, 218
Names for tongue thrust, 137
Nares, 83
Nasal airway, 96-98
  function of, 97-98
Nasal cavity, 96
  mucous membrane of, 97
Nasal polyps, 212
Neck muscles, 79-81
Nerves
  cranial, 66-68
  spinal, 66
Neurology, 59-69
Neuromuscular facilitation, 208-209, 339
Neuromuscular system, 26
Neuron, 83
Neutrocclusion, 28
Nitinol, 48
Normal swallowing, 4
  description of, 169-172

O

Occiput, 83
Occlusal surface, 20
Occlusion, 35
  centric, 26
  eccentric, 26
  forces of, 86-87
  habitual, 26
  molar, 262, 271-272
  normal, 26
  retruded, 27
Oligodontia, 35
"Open and close" exercise, 343
Open bite, 27
  anterior, 15
  posterior, 15
Open spaces during mixed dentition, 118-119
Operant conditioning, 206
Oral habits, 212-219
  etiologies of, 212-213
  influence on speech, 213-214
  list of, 212
  and malocclusions, 214-215
  review of, 7-8
Oral manometer, 249
  components of, 366
Oral myologists, 6-7
Oral peripheral examination, 246-247
Oral screen, 200; *see also* Oral shield

Oral sensitivity, tests of, 123-124
Oral sensory deficiency, 123
Oral shield, 38
  construction of, 293-294
Oral stereognosis, 123-124
Oral surgery, 162-164, 201
Oral trauma, 123
Orbicularis oris, 71
Organismic principles, 334-335
Oropharynx, 83
Orthodontic appliances, 37-44, 326-327
  fixed, 42-44
  removable, 38-42
Orthodontics
  interceptive, 30-31
  and oral myology, 168
  preventive, 29-30
  treatment, 7
    as cause of tongue thrust, 122-123
Ossify, 83
Ostectomy, 32
Osteology, 54-59, 83
Overbite, 27
Overjet, 27

P

Palatal arch, examination of, 191-192
Palate, muscles of, 77-79
Palatine
  aponeurosis, 78
  bones, 58
  processes, 58
Palatoglossus muscle, 79
Palatopharyngeus muscle, 79
Papilla, incisal, 35
Paraffin, 235-236
Paranasal sinuses, 96-97
Parasympathetic division, 69
Parents, letter to, 358, 362
Patients, handicapped, 222-223
Payne technique, 187-188
Pedodontics, and oral myology, 164-165
Periodontal membrane, 18-19
Periodontics, 35
  and oral myology, 165-166
Periodontium, 35
Perioral, 84
Periosteum, 35, 55, 84
Peripheral examination, 246-247
Peripheral nervous system, 65-69
Perverted swallow, 137
Philosophy of treatment, 220-227
Phonetic placement, approach to treatment, 204
Physical therapists as oral myotherapists, 6
Pictograph program, 205
Pillars of the fauces, 78
Pits of teeth, 21
Planes, anatomical, 53
Platysma, 73
Plus-minus charts, 338
Polyethylene sheets, 366
Polyethylene tubing, 366
Polyps, nasal, 212
Pons, 64
Positioner, 39-40, 326-327

Posterior open bite, 15
Posture, normal achievement of, 274-275
Practice requirements, 259
Pressure
  as a cause of malocclusion, 140-148
  orofacial muscle
    in normal swallowers, 141-146
    in tongue thrusters, 141-146
  required to move teeth, 140-141
Preventive
  dentistry, 5
  orthodontics, 29-30
Procedures
  alternative, of Hanson, 334-357
  in diagnosis, 189-195
Processes, palatine, 58
Prognathic mandible, 163
Prognosis, 8, 195-197
Progress chart, 355
Prosthodontics, 36
  and oral myology, 167-168
Proximal, 52, 84
  surface, 20
Psychological arrest, 122
Psychophysiological approach, 220-221
Pterygoid, 84
  muscles, 74-75
  plate, 57
Pullup exercise, 260
Pulp, 18, 36
Punishment, 206
  in treatment for sucking habits, 231
Pyramidal
  decussation, 65
  system, 65

Q

Quadratus labii muscle
  inferior, 73
  superior, 72

R

Rake, 198
Ramus, 84
Rechecks, 322-333, 356-357
Recording devices, 308
Referrals, from dentists, 225
Reinforcement, 206-207
  primary and secondary, 206-207
  schedules, 207
Relapse, 331-333
  causes of, 331-333
  orthodontic, 51
  remediation of, 324-327, 333
Reminders, 337-338
  appliances, 199-200
  mechanical, 151-152
  sign, 298-299
Report forms, 358
Reports, progress, 227
Resection, 32
Resistance, in muscle strengthening, 251
Resorption, 36
Respiratory allergy, 98
Resting position, 272-276, 328, 334
  as cause of relapse, 332

Resting position—cont'd
  characteristics of, 272-274
Resting postures, 278, 292-294, 319, 320
  lingual, 189
Restraints, mechanical, 151-152
Retainer, 51
  Hawley, 40
Retention period, 50-51
Reverse swallow, 137
Risorius muscle, 73
Rolando, fissure of, 61
Round wire, 43
Rubber bands, 261
Rugae, 36
  examination of, 190-191
Rules of therapy, 244-245

S

Sagittal, 84
Saliva, exercise for moving, 350-351
Saliva swallowing, 194-195, 335
  counting of, 352-353
Salt water, hot
  for exercise using, 260
  for lip conditioning, 254
Screen, oral, 200
Seal
  anterior, 286-288
  labioglossal, 261
  lingual, testing of, 288-289
Self-hypnosis, 309
Sensitivity, oral, test of, 123
Sensory deficiency, oral, 123
Separation of teeth, 47
Septum, 84
  deviated, 212
Serial extraction of teeth, 30-32
Shield, oral, 38
Sinuses, paranasal, 96-97
Skeleton, facial, 57-59
Skull, bones of, 55-59
Sleeping habits, 123
Soft palate, muscles of, 77-79
Solid bolus, swallow of, 305-306
Solids, assignments for eating, 292
Somatic nervous system, 65-66
Sounds, dentalized,
  correction of, 339
  linguoalveolar, 14
  order of learning of, 10-11
Space maintainer, 40
Speech
  acquisition of, 9-10
  and Class III occlusion, 16
  delayed, 14
  and dentition, relationships between, 15-16
  development of, 9-11
  disorders of, 11-14
  evaluation, 328
  and oral habits, 213-214
Speech defects
  causes of, 11-12
  incidence of, 12-13
  malocclusion, 12
Speech pathologists as myotherapists, 5-6
Speech sounds, order of learning of, 10-11

Speech therapy, 335
Sphenoid bone, 57
Spinal cord, 65
Squamous, 56-57
"Squeaky sucking" exercise, 346-347
Squirt test, 329-330
Stabilizing plate, 40
Stereognosis, oral, 123-124
Sternum, 84
Stimulators, mechanical, 253
Stimulus control, extending, 208, 337
Stomahesive, 325, 367
Stomatognathic, 36
Straub program of therapy, 202-203
Study models of teeth, 37
Styloglossus muscle, 77
Stylohyoid muscle, 81
Styloid process, 57
Subconscious function, tests for, 317-319
Subconscious procedures, rationale of, 307-309
Subluxation, 36
Sucking habits, 228-238
    tongue, 238
    treatment for, 232-238
Sulci
    cerebral, 61
    of teeth, 21
Sulcus, 84
Supernumerary, 36
Supraversion, 22
Surgery, 201
    oral, 162-164
Swallow, coordinating the total, 285-295
Swallowing
    abnormal, 172-175
        the oral stage of, 173-174
    beginning instructions for, 343
    esophageal stage of, 172
    genetic influence on, 117-118
    normal, 4
        description of, 169-172
    oral stage of, 171-172
    pharyngeal stage of, 172
    as reflex, 169-170
Swallows
    examination of food, 193-194
    examination of liquid, 194
    teeth apart, 103
    waking, 313
Sylvius, fissure of, 61
Sympathetic division, 69
Symphysis, 84
Syndesmology, 53
Synergy, 84
Synovia, 84
Synovial membrane, 54
Syringe, eye-flushing, 366

T

T exercise, 278
Tape, cellophane, 327
Teeth
    deciduous
        arrangement of, 22
        development of, 22-23
        equilibration of, 31

Teeth—cont'd
    eruption sequence of, 24-25
    examination of, 190
    grinding of, 8
    permanent
        arrangement of, 23
        development of, 22-23
    relationship of, to arch, 21-22
    serial extraction of, 30-32
    supporting structures of, 18-19
    surfaces of, 19-21
Temporal bone, 56-67
Temporalis muscle, 74
Temporomandibular joint, 25-26, 90-95, 247
    analysis of, 45
    construction of, 90-92
    degenerative conditions of, 94-95
    disorders of, 93-96
    movement of, 92
Tensor veli palatini, 79
Tests
    at completion of therapy, 323-331
    of oral sensation, relevance of, 124
Thalamus, 63
Therapists, obligations of, 226-227
Therapy; see also Treatment
    group, 242-243
    localization, 209
    outline of, 223-224
    room for, 245-246
    rules of, 244-245
    successfulness of, 154-158
    tests for completion of, 323-331
    timing of, 152-154, 225-226, 242
Thumbsucking, 7
    as a cause of tongue thrust, 118
Timing of therapy, 225-226, 242
Tipping movement of teeth, 49
Tissues, types of, 53-54
Tongue
    forces of, against teeth, 87-88
    lifting exercise, 269-270
    muscles of, 75-79
    popping, 342
    popping exercise, 277-278
    protrusion of, during nonswallowing activities, 194
    resting postures of, 189
    restricted, 246-247
Tongue sucking, 7, 238
Tongue thrust
    advisability of treatment of, 149-150
    as cause of malocclusion, 138-148
    classification of, 175-183
    effects of maturation on, 150
    existence of, 133-135
    history of, 102-112
    implications of, 243
    incidence of, 134-135
    names for, 137
    normalcy of, 135-137
    relationship to dental malocclusion, 137-138
    types of, 176-183
Tongue-tip, position of, 262
Tonsils, 240-241
    as cause of tongue thrust, 119

Tooth; *see also* Teeth
  closure, 267
  movement, 49-50
Torque, forces of, 26, 89
Torsioversion, 22
Transducers, as artifacts, 146
Transversion, 22
Trauma, oral, 123
Treatment; *see also* Therapy
  approaches to, 198-211
  dental, as cause of relapse, 332-333
  orthodontic, 7
    as cause of tongue thrust, 122-123
  patient age in, 222
  philosophy of, 220-227
Triangularis muscle, 73
Trismus, 36
Trituration, 170-171
Trumpet, effects of playing, 99
Tuberosity, 84
Tubing, polyethylene, 366
Tug-of-war exercise, 260
Turbinate, 84
Twilight time, 313, 316-317
Two-elastic exercise, 278
Two-point discrimination, 124

U

Universal appliance, 43
Universal numbering system for teeth, 23, 24

V

Velar control, 303-304, 307
Velopharyngeal muscle, 79
Velum, 84
  muscles of, 77-79
Ventral, 53
Vertebrae, cervical, 59
Vestibular surface, 20
Vestibule, 85
Visceral nervous system, 66-69
Visceral swallow, 137
Vomer bone, 57-58

W

Waking swallows, 313
Wax, 235-236
Whistle exercise, 346
Wind instruments, effects of playing, 98-100
Wires, types of orthodontic, 42-44

Y

Yawning, 297

Z

Zickefoose program, 208
Zygomaticus, 72